More essential reso

for hand and upper extremity rehabilitation...

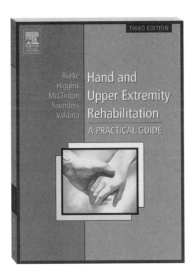

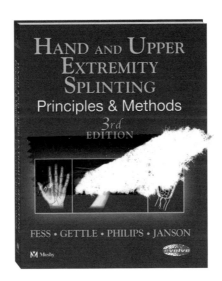

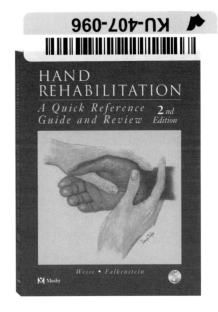

Hand and Upper Extremity Rehabilitation: A Practical Guide, 3rd Edition

By Susan L. Burke, OTR/L, CHT, MBA; James P. Higgins, MD; Michael A. McClinton, MD; Rebecca J. Saunders, PT, CHT; and Lauren Valdata, PT, CHT

This practical resource blends the technical and clinical skills and knowledge of hand surgery and hand therapy for the treatment of common medical conditions affecting th upper extremity. Written in an outline form it covers non-surgical and surgical procedu for these conditions, along with their purpose and rationale. This edition addresses not only the hand, but also features expanded coverage of the wrist, elbow, and shoulder. Both conservative and postoperative rehabilitation are reviewed, and potential postoperative complications are addressed.

2006 • 784 pp., 400 illus.
ISBN: 0-443-06663-9
ISBN-13: 978-0-443-06663-4

Hand and Upper Extremity Splinting: Principles & Methods, 3rd Edition

By Elaine Ewing Fess, MS, OTR, FAOTA, CHT; Karen Gettle, MBA, OTR, CHT; Cynthia

CHECK CD-ROM IN BACK POCKET

splints provides a photographic key to all splints mentioned in the book.

2005 • 752 pp., 1,002 illus.
ISBN: 0-8016-7522-7
ISBN-13: 978-0-8016-7522-5

ALISTAIR MacKENZIE LIBRARY

Hand Rehabilitation: A Quick Reference Guide and Review, 2nd Edition

By Susan Weiss, OTR/L, CHT; and Nancy Falkenstein, OTR/L, CHT

This one-of-a-kind reference provides a comprehensive overview of hand rehabilitation. Featuring a unique, question-and-detailed-answer format, **Hand Rehabilitation** guides you from basic information about hand anatomy through complex topics including the most advanced treatment techniques. Each chapter is formatted as a series of multiple-choice questions, complete with detailed answers and references to other hand therapy resources. Also included are "clinical" gems in each chapter, providing helpful hints and important facts to remember.

2005 • 528 pp., 400 illus.
ISBN: 0-323-02610-9
ISBN-13: 978-0-323-02610-9

Ordering is easy!

ONLINE: www.elsevierhealth.com • PHONE: toll-free 1-800-545-2522

HP-06109

Fundamentals of Hand Therapy

Clinical Reasoning and Treatment Guidelines
for Common Diagnoses of the Upper Extremity

CHECK CD-ROM
IN BACK POCKET

Fundamentals of Hand Therapy

Clinical Reasoning and Treatment Guidelines for Common Diagnoses of the Upper Extremity

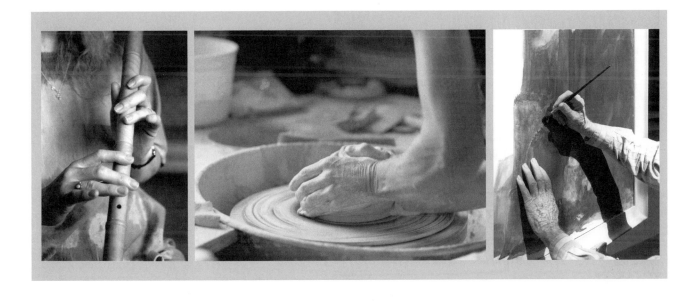

Edited by

Cynthia Cooper, MFA, MA, OTR/L, CHT

Director of Hand Therapy in Arizona
NovaCare Rehabilitation
Phoenix, Arizona

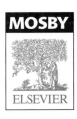

11830 Westline Industrial Drive
St. Louis, Missouri 63146

FUNDAMENTALS OF HAND THERAPY: CLINICAL REASONING   ISBN-13: 978-0-323-03386-2
AND TREATMENT GUIDELINES FOR COMMON DIAGNOSES OF   ISBN-10: 0-323-03866-5
THE UPPER EXTREMITY
Copyright © 2007 by Mosby, Inc., an affiliate of Elsevier Inc.

Notice

Cover and part opener art copyright John Evarts

ISBN-13: 978-0-323-03386-2
ISBN-10: 0-323-03386-5

Acquisitions Editor: Kathy Falk
Developmental Editor: Megan Fennell
Publishing Services Manager: Julie Eddy
Project Manager: Richard Barber
Designer: Kim Denando

Working together to grow
libraries in developing countries

www.elsevier.com | www.bookaid.org | www.sabre.org

ELSEVIER   BOOK AID International   Sabre Foundation

Printed in the United States

Last digit is the print number: 9   8   7   6   5   4   3   2   1

Contributors

Michelle Abrams, MS, OTR/L
Center Manager
NovaCare Rehabilitation
Phoenix, Arizona

Sandra Artzberger, MS, OTR, CHT, CLT
Lecturer, Consultant
Hand Therapy Lecturing and Consulting
Hartford, Wisconsin
Co-Director, Professional Education and Lymphedema
  Services
Department of Outpatient Occupational Therapy
Cedar Haven Rehabilitation Services of Cedar Community
West Bend, Wisconsin

Romina P. Astifidis, MS, PT, CHT
Clinic Manger and Physical Therapist
Curtis National Hand Center at Lutherville
Regional Rehabilitation at National Rehabilitation Hospital
Baltimore, Maryland

Lynn Bassini, MA, OTR, CHT
Owner
Empire State Occupational Therapy
Lynn Bassini Certified Hand Therapy
Brooklyn, New York

Margaret Newsham Beckley, PhD, OTR/L, BCN, BCG
Assistant Professor
Occupational Therapy Division
School of Allied Medical Professions
The Ohio State University
Columbus, Ohio

Jeanine Biese, MEd, OTR, CHT
Assistant Professor
Department of Occupational Therapy
Grand Valley State University
Grand Rapids, Michigan
Hand Therapist
Rehabilitation Professionals
Grand Rapids, Michigan

Mark W. Butler, MPT, OCS, Cert., MDT
Adjunct Associate Professor
School of Related Health Professions
University of Medicine and Dentistry of New Jersey
Stratford, New Jersey
Center Manager
NovaCare
Medford, New Jersey

Lisa Deshaies, OTR/L, CHT
Adjunct Clinical Faculty
Department of Occupational Science and Occupational
  Therapy
University of Southern California
Los Angeles, California
Clinical Specialist
Department of Occupational Therapy
Rancho Los Amigos National Rehabilitation Center
Downey, California

Lori Falkel, PT, DPT, MOMT, CHT
Outpatient Physical Therapy
Mayo Clinic Hospital
Phoenix, Arizona

Sharon Flinn, PhD, OTR/L, CHT, CVE
Assistant Professor
Division of Occupational Therapy
The Ohio State University
Columbus, Ohio
CEO, President
Functional Visions Inc
Columbus, Ohio

Barbara Haines, BS, OTR, CHT
Clinic Coordinator
Hand Clinic
Froedtert and Medical College of Wisconsin
Milwaukee, Wisconsin

Rebecca von der Heyde, MS, OTR/L, CHT
Assistant Professor
Department of Occupational Therapy
Maryville University
St. Louis, Missouri
Occupational Therapist, Certified Hand Therapist
Miliken Hand Rehabilitation Center
The Rehabilitation Institute of St. Louis
St. Louis, Missouri

Linda J. Klein, OTR, CHT
Clinical Specialist
Hand Surgery, Ltd
Milwaukee, Wisconsin

Paige E. Kurtz, MS, OTR/L, CHT
Senior Hand Therapist
HealthSouth Sports Medicine and Rehabilitation Center
Melbourne, Florida

Cornelia von Lersner Benson, OTR, CHT
Area Hand Therapy Director
Hand Therapy and Occupational Therapy
NovaCare Rehabilitation
Cherry Hill, New Jersey

Hope A. Martin, PhD, OTR, CHT
Occupational Therapist
Department of Physical Medicine and Rehabilitation
University Medical Center Health System
Lubbock, Texas

Joel F. Moorhead, MD, PhD
Assistant Professor
Rollins School of Public Health
Emory University
Atlanta, Georgia

Anne M.B. Moscony, MA, OTR/L, CHT
Adjunct Faculty
Occupational Therapy Program
Philadelphia University
Philadelphia, Pennsylvania
Occupational Therapist, Certified Hand Therapist
Crozer Keystone Healthcare
Springfield Hospital Division, The Philadelphia Hand Center
Media, Pennsylvania

Mukund Patel, MD, FACS
Associate Clinical Professor of Surgery
Department of Orthopedic Surgery
Downstate Medical Center
State University of New York
Brooklyn, New York
Attending Hand Surgeon
Department of Orthopedic Surgery
Victory Memorial Hospital, Maimonides Medical Center
Brooklyn, New York
Staten Island University Hospital, St. Vincents Medical
    Center
Staten Island, New York

Teri Britt Pipe, PhD, RN
Director of Nursing Research, Associate Professor of Nursing
Mayo Clinic College of Medicine
Mayo Clinic in Arizona
Phoenix, Arizona

Michael J. Staino, OTR, CHT
Occupational Therapist, Certified Hand Therapist
Occupational and Hand Therapy, New Jersey Shore Region
NovaCare Rehabilitation, Inc
Manahawkin, New Jersey

To my husband,
John L. Evarts,
who helped me learn to take chances.
This project would not have happened
without your full emotional support and technical help.
You are a magnificent man
and the love of my life.

Foreword

Hand therapy has grown exponentially over the past nearly 30 years. We, as occupational and physical therapists with a specialty in hand therapy, will always use, as a reference, Mackin et al's, *Rehabilitation of the Hand* (also published by Elsevier); but this new text is an exciting new entry into the field. One might say that at this time, we already have several good and relevant texts in hand therapy to provide the basic knowledge for occupational and physical therapists who have an interest in becoming hand therapists. The plan for this book is simple, and the format of this book is also unique, just as Cynthia Cooper is unique. It provides us with the basics along with some advanced knowledge and tips to help even the experienced therapist in the clinic.

The distinction to this new text: *Fundamentals of Hand Therapy: Clinical Reasoning and Treatment Guidelines for Common Diagnoses of the Upper Extremity*, is clearly delineated within the title itself. The text provides the basic fundamentals of hand therapy with the important aspect of clinical reasoning associated with each chapter. As students of occupational and physical therapy, we learn early on that we cannot do our job without good clinical reasoning, and although it is difficult to teach, it is always a topic of concern with our development as young therapists. I am delighted this piece is an integral part of this text. Cynthia Cooper starts off the reader with the basic fundamentals of hand therapy concepts that are defined and described to provide us with the information we need to critically think through how to approach a patient with a particular presentation of signs and symptoms associated with a particular diagnosis.

After we review Part One: Fundamentals, an important section but not always as clearly presented is offered in Part Two: Professionalism. I was particularly pleased to see the clear delineation of therapy assistants in hand therapy. It is an area that does not always receive adequate importance in the usual literature and provides attention to concerns of assistants as valued members of the team.

Part Three: Treatment Guidelines for Common Diagnoses of the Upper Extremity, provides us with useful information in a unique arrangement that impressed me with its completeness. Each chapter is arranged so that it identifies and defines the problem for discussion, provides overview of relevant anatomy, discusses diagnosis and pathology, possible operative treatment, precautions, and ideas for what to ask the doctor, what to say to clients about their injury or diagnosis, tips, discussion of complications, possible exercises, and splint needs. Each chapter includes "pearls" that the individual authors have learned and are passing on to the reader to make a particular aspect of the problem easier to deal with, treat, or other relevant information. Finally, where there is evidence to substantiate, this information has been provided in each chapter's review of literature.

The writing is clear; the arrangement of chapters provides added clarity to basic topic discussion and yet provides "pearls" helpful to the new as well as more experienced therapist. We all have a need for learning and relearning over time, and this new text will be a welcome addition to any hand therapist/clinic library.

Writing an introduction to a book on hand therapy can be a daunting task! However, when Cynthia Cooper was in the early stages of developing and planning her new book, I was, without hesitation, pleased and honored to accept her request to write this introduction. Cynthia has accomplished much in hand therapy on diverse topics in which it is evident she keeps the mind and body and its importance to function as key in her work. I am pleased to see that this text continues to follow that line of thinking throughout.

Respectfully,
Donna Breger Stanton, MA, OTR/L, CHT, FAOTA
Past-President, ASHT (2005)
Assistant Professor,
Samuel Merritt College,
Oakland, California

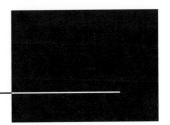

Preface

Changes in health care delivery can restrict clients' access to specialists. Even if their health plans support specialty care, they may live in remote locations where there are no specialists. Therapists who are not familiar with the body of knowledge in hand therapy may inadvertently do more harm than good. Therapists who are unaware of tissue tolerances or who do not know about tissue timelines following injury or surgery can unintentionally injure clients.

The purpose of this book is to educate non-specialist therapists, hand therapists in training, and occupational and physical therapy students about the fundamentals of hand therapy using didactic materials and case examples. It teaches the reader how to apply sound clinical reasoning to determine the needs of their clients with upper extremity problems. In addition, it provides clear treatment guidelines for common upper extremity diagnoses with content that is valuable even for experienced hand therapists.

Good clinical reasoning skills are required in order for therapists to move beyond therapy protocols, to think critically about their clients' needs, and to provide safe and creative treatment. Clinical reasoning allows therapists to treat their clients as unique people with individual needs while applying appropriate and safe treatment.

The scope of the book is broad, with content that includes those diagnoses most typically referred to hand therapy. The book is organized into three parts. Part One lays the foundation and identifies the fundamentals of hand therapy treatment. Part Two covers issues of professionalism. Part Three presents chapters on common upper extremity diagnoses. Pictures of common hand therapy exercises, plus supplemental photographs for some of the chapters are included on the CD. Although the topic of splinting is addressed throughout the book, the reader is referred to those books that are devoted entirely to splinting.

The chapters in Part Three provide diagnosis-specific information. Although the reader should spend time with the entire book, the chapters in Part Three are useful as an easily accessed resource for common diagnoses of the hand and upper extremity. The diagnoses chapters use a similar organizational format that serves as a unifying framework:

- Anatomy
- Diagnosis/pathology
- Timelines and healing
- Nonoperative treatment
- Operative treatment
- Questions to ask the doctor
- What to say to clients
- Evaluation tips
- Diagnosis-specific information that affects clinical reasoning
- Tips from the field
- Precautions and concerns
- Therapy assistants' roles
- Case examples

In addition, clinical pearls and precautions are highlighted throughout each chapter.

This book is unique in that it explicitly aims to teach clinical reasoning in hand therapy. The special features in Part Three—questions to ask the doctor, what to say to clients, tips from the field, precautions and concerns—can be used as mental prompts by therapists when treating their clients. Doing this will help them find their own clinical voices and will strengthen their clinical reasoning skills.

The case examples, many of which are not simple, serve two purposes. First they demonstrate the use of clinical reasoning in treating the client. Second, they highlight the humanistic side of each client encounter. In reality, even a seemingly straightforward clinical case has its special challenges and intriguing moments. The cases were selected to remind the reader of the human side and humane concerns in caring for a hand therapy client.

I am hopeful that this book will spark therapists' passion for hand therapy and will teach them gentle ways of touching their clients' hands and lives.

Acknowledgments

I would like to acknowledge my mother, Delma P. Cooper, and my sisters, Jan Carroll and Linda McGarry, for their interest in and enthusiasm for my work. I am extremely grateful to my editor, Kathy Falk, of Elsevier, for her vision, expertise, and unflagging support. I would also like to thank Rich Barber, project manager, for everything he taught me on the project and his attention to detail, and Megan Fennell, developmental editor, for all her help along the way. Thanks as well to Mark W. Butler and Anne M. B. Moscony for accepting additional editorial and writing assignments; to Michelle Abrams for reviewing certain chapters; to Sandra Artzberger for being my friend and role model; and to Marcia McMurtrey for helping me recognize and create opportunities. Lastly, I wish to acknowledge the memories of my father, Herschel A. Cooper, and my friend, Gerald W. Sharrott, both of whom would be very pleased for me to have this especially wonderful opportunity.

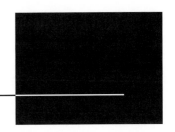

Contents

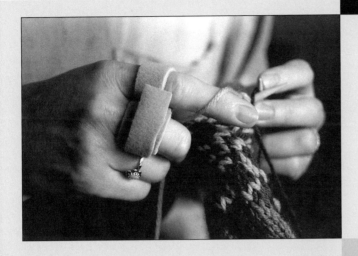

Fundamentals

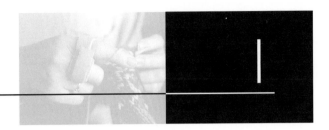

Fundamentals of Clinical Reasoning: Hand Therapy Concepts and Treatment Techniques

CYNTHIA COOPER

"The more you know about something in detail, the less you know about it in general."

From *The Child in Time* by Ian McEwan, Anchor Books, 1987.

KEY TERMS

Antideformity (intrinsic-plus) position

Blocking exercises

Chip bag

Composite motions

Differential flexor tendon gliding exercise

Dynamic splints

Dyscoordinate co-contraction

Edema

Elastic mobilization splints

Extensor habitus

Extrinsic extensor tightness

Extrinsic muscles

Fibroplasia phase

Hard end-feel

Inflammation phase

Interosseous muscle tightness

Intrinsic muscles

Joint contracture

Joint tightness

Lag

Maturation (remodeling) phase

Mobilization splints

Multiarticulate

Musculotendinous tightness

Outrigger

Phagocytosis

Place and hold exercises

Quadriga effect

Serial static splints

Soft end-feel

Static progressive splints

Static splints

Hands are visible, expressive, and vulnerable. When clients use their hands to get dressed, eat, touch, gesture, or communicate, they are performing exquisite and complex movements. Limitations of motion or even a small scar can affect a person's life in profound ways.[1] When we touch our clients' hands, we touch their lives. Although it is very important to be knowledgeable about the details of hand anatomy and to be structure specific in our treatment, it is equally important not to lose sight of the whole person whose extremity we are treating. We must continuously encourage clients to tell us about themselves and their needs so that their therapy can be relevant and successful. While getting to know the person we are treating, we can explain how our interventions and the client's home programs will be helpful. As a rule, I find that if I listen well, clients frequently tell me in lay terms or even show me exactly what motion or function is missing. The challenge is to identify and treat clients' specific tissues effectively while not losing sight of them as people.

HAND THERAPY CONCEPTS

The anatomy of the hand is complex. Many structures are **multiarticulate** (i.e., they cross multiple joints), and little room is available for scar tissue or edema to develop without affecting function. Injury in one area of the hand can result in stiffness in other, uninjured parts. A good demonstration of this is the **quadriga effect,** which illustrates the interconnectedness of the digits. If you passively hold your ring finger extended with your other hand and then try to make a fist, you will notice how limited the whole hand can feel when just one finger is held stiff. In this example, the flexor digitorum profundus (FDP) tendons to multiple digits have a shared muscle belly. Restricting movement at one finger restricts the other fingers when they try to flex. This example reminds us that clients can be limited in motion in areas not originally injured. Therefore the therapist needs to evaluate beyond the isolated area of injury when treating clients with hand problems.

To be competent in hand therapy, therapists must be able to do more than just note decreased range of motion (ROM). They must be able to figure out what structures are restricted and how these restrictions affect function (e.g., The client has decreased digital flexion due to FDP adherence, preventing him from holding the steering wheel); they then must be able to target treatment to those particular tissues. These three elements are part of all the decisions we make as hand therapists. As treatment continues, re-evaluation reveals new findings with different tissues to target, and appropriate modifications and upgrades are made. This chapter addresses treatment concepts and techniques of hand therapy and concludes with some provocative thoughts to stimulate clinical reasoning.

Timelines and Healing

Tissues heal in predictable phases. However, the length of these phases varies depending on client variables, such as age and health. The three phases of healing are inflammation, fibroplasia, and maturation (also called *remodeling*). In the **inflammation phase,** vasoconstriction occurs, followed by vasodilation, with migration of white blood cells to promote **phagocytosis** in preparation for further healing. In this stage, which lasts a few days, immobilization often is advised, depending on the specifics of the diagnosis.[2] If wound contamination or delayed healing is a factor, this phase can last longer.[3]

The **fibroplasia phase** begins about 4 days after injury and lasts 2 to 6 weeks. In this phase, fibroblasts begin the formation of scar tissue. The fibroblasts lay down new collagen, on which capillary buds grow, leading to a gradual increase in the tissue's tensile strength. In this stage, active range of motion (AROM) and splints typically are used to promote balance in the hand and to protect the healing structures.[4]

The timeline for the **maturation (remodeling) phase** varies; this phase may even last years. In the maturation phase, the tissue's architecture changes, reflecting improved organization of the collagen fibers and a further increase in tensile strength. The tissue is more *responsive* (i.e., reorganizes better) if appropriate therapy is started sooner rather than later. In this stage, gentle resistive exercises may be appropriate, and the client should be monitored for any inflammatory responses (also known as a *flare response*). Dynamic or static splinting may also be helpful.[5,6]

Positioning to Counteract Deforming Forces

Predictable deforming forces act on an injured upper extremity (UE). **Edema** (swelling) routinely occurs after injury, creating tension on the tissues. The resulting predictable deformity posture is one of wrist flexion, metacarpophalangeal (MP) hyperextension, proximal interphalangeal (PIP) and distal interphalangeal (DIP)

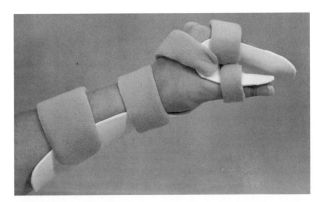

FIGURE I-I Antideformity (intrinsic-plus) splint position. (From Coppard BM, Lohman H, editors: *Introduction to splinting: a clinical-reasoning and problem-solving approach,* ed 2, St Louis, 2001, Mosby.)

flexion, and thumb adduction.[7] This deformity position occurs as a result of tension on the extrinsic muscles caused by dorsal edema.

Use of the **antideformity (intrinsic-plus) position** is recommended after injury unless it is contraindicated by the diagnosis (e.g., it is not used after flexor tendon repair). The antideformity position consists of the wrist in neutral position or extension, the MPs in flexion, the IPs in extension (*IPs* refers to the PIP and DIP joints collectively), and the thumb in abduction with opposition (Fig. 1-1). The antideformity position maintains length in the collateral ligaments, which are vulnerable to shortening, and counteracts deforming forces.

Joint and Musculotendinous Tightness

Joint tightness is confirmed if the passive range of motion (PROM) of a joint does not change despite repositioning of proximal or distal joints. **Musculotendinous tightness** is confirmed if the PROM of a joint changes with repositioning of adjacent joints that are crossed by that particular muscle-tendon (musculotendinous) unit.[8]

Joint tightness and musculotendinous tightness can be treated with serial casting, dynamic splinting, static progressive splinting, or serial static splinting (see section on splinting later in this chapter). With joint tightness, splinting can focus on the stiff joint, and less consideration is needed for the position of proximal joints. With musculotendinous tightness, because the tightness occurs in a structure that crosses multiple joints, the splint must carefully control the position of proximal (and possibly distal) joints to remodel tightness effectively along that musculotendinous unit.

The client in Fig. 1-2, *A,* had an infected PIP joint in the index finger. He was treated with hospitalization, intravenous administration of antibiotics, and joint

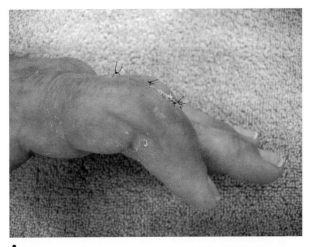

A

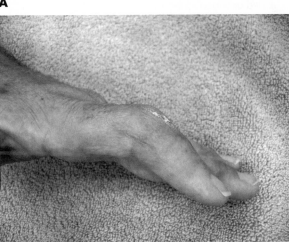

B

FIGURE I-2 **A,** Unsplinted, infected index finger after surgery. **B,** Improvement in edema and improved extension ROM after 2 weeks.

debridement. He arrived for therapy 2 weeks later than his physician had ordered; he had no splint, significant edema, and a severe flexion contracture of the PIP joint. Because the stiffness was localized to the PIP joint, he needed only a digit-based extension splint for that joint. Fig. 1-2, *B,* shows his progress after 2 weeks of edema control and serial static digit-based splinting.

Musculotendinous tightness can be a cause of joint tightness. Clients with tightness of the extrinsic flexors (i.e., lacking passive composite digital extension with the wrist extended) are at risk of developing IP flexion contractures. Instruct these clients to passively place the MP in flexion and then to gently, passively extend the IPs to maintain PIP and DIP joint motion. In these cases, although you should consider night splinting in composite extension to lengthen the extrinsic flexors, the better course may be to splint in a modified intrinsic-plus posi-

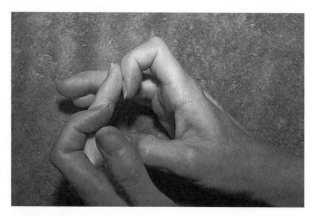

FIGURE I-3 Interosseous muscle tightness. PIP and DIP flexion is passively limited when the MP joint is passively extended or hyperextended.

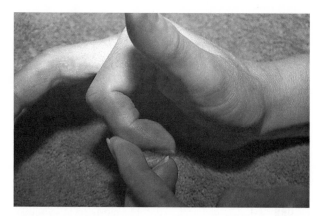

FIGURE I-4   Extrinsic extensor tightness. PIP and DIP flexion is passively limited when the MP joint is passively flexed.

tion with the MPs flexed as needed to support the IPs in full extension. This helps prevent IP flexion contractures.

Intrinsic or Extrinsic Extensor Muscle Tightness

Intrinsic muscles are the small muscles in the hand. **Extrinsic muscles** are longer musculotendinous units that originate proximal to the hand. Intrinsic tightness and extrinsic extensor tightness are tested by putting these muscles on stretch. This is accomplished by comparing the PROM of digital PIP and DIP flexion when the MP joint is passively extended and then passively flexed. With **interosseous muscle tightness,** passive PIP and DIP flexion is limited when the MP joint is passively extended or hyperextended (Fig. 1-3). With **extrinsic extensor tightness,** PIP and DIP flexion is limited when the MP joint is passively flexed (Fig. 1-4).[8]

To treat intrinsic tightness, perform PIP and DIP flexion with MP hyperextension. Functional splints (see splinting section) are very helpful for isolating specific exercise to restore length to the intrinsics while performing daily activities. To treat extrinsic extensor tightness, promote **composite motions** (i.e., combined flexion motions of the wrist, MPs and IPs) with splinting, gentle stretch, and exercise. Instruct the client that performing these exercises with the wrist in a variety of positions is helpful.

Extrinsic Extensor or Flexor Tightness
Extrinsic tightness can involve the flexors or the extensors. To test for tightness, put the structure on stretch by positioning the proximal joint crossed by that structure. With extrinsic extensor tightness, passive composite digital flexion is more limited with the wrist flexed than

with the wrist extended. With extrinsic flexor tightness, passive composite digital extension is more limited with the wrist extended than with the wrist flexed.[8]

Lag or Contracture

CLINICAL *Pearl*

When PROM is greater than AROM at a joint, the active limitation is called a lag.

A client with a PIP extensor lag is unable to actively extend the PIP joint as far as is possible passively (which may not necessarily be full extension). Lags may be caused by adhesions, disruption of the musculotendinous unit, or weakness.

CLINICAL *Pearl*

When passive limitation of joint motion exists, that limitation is called a joint contracture.

Joint contractures can be caused by collateral ligament tightness, adhesions, or a mechanical block. A *joint flexion contracture* is characterized by a stiff joint in a flexed position that lacks active and passive extension. A person with a joint flexion contracture whose passive extension improves may progress from having a flexion contracture to having an extensor lag. In your treatment communications and documentation, it is important to identify such changes, to use these terms correctly, and

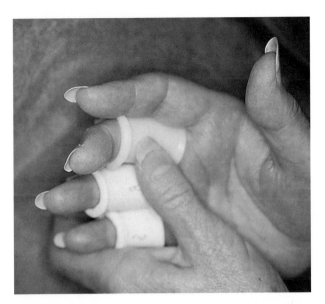

FIGURE 1-5   DIP blocking exercises with the MP in various positions.

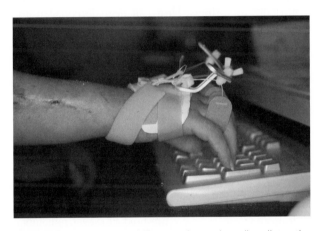

FIGURE 1-6   A dynamic MP extension assist splint allows the client to perform keyboard activities at the computer.

to be joint specific and motion specific. For example, you should note, "The client has full PIP passive extension but demonstrates a 30-degree PIP extensor lag."

When a lag is present (PROM exceeds AROM), treatment should focus on promoting active movement. Blocking exercises (Fig. 1-5), differential tendon gliding exercises (see Fig. 1-18), place and hold exercises (see Fig. 1-19), and dynamic or static functional splints can be helpful (Fig. 1-6). If a contracture is present, promote both PROM and AROM with the same exercises and with corrective splinting, which may be the dynamic, static progressive, serial static, or casting type.

Joint End-Feel

A joint with a **soft end-feel** has a spongy quality at the end-range. This is a favorable quality that indicates a potential for remodeling. Splinting for soft end-feel may be the static type or the low-load, long duration type (see splinting section).

A joint with a **hard end-feel** has an unyielding quality at end-range. This is a stiffer joint, and correcting it may require serial casting or static progressive splinting with longer periods of splint wear.[9]

Documenting the end-feel and explaining the implications of your findings to the client are very important.

Preventing Pain

Precaution. *Pain with therapy is a signal that injury is occurring. Irreversible damage can result when clients or their families or, worse, therapists injure tissue by using painful force and PROM. Avoid pain in your hand therapy treatment. Being overzealous and ignoring objective signs of tissue intolerance is inexcusable.*

Teaching clients and their families that painful therapy is counterproductive can be a challenge. Often clients come to therapy with a "no pain, no gain" mentality. To make matters worse, this philosophy frequently is reinforced by their physicians and friends. Therapists have a duty to explain to their clients that imposing, prolonging, or aggravating pain slows the healing process, fosters more scarring and stiffness, and delays or eliminates opportunities to upgrade therapy.

CLINICAL *Pearl*

Never tell your clients, "Exercise to pain tolerance" or "Go to pain." Instead, say, "Avoid pain when you exercise. It's okay to feel a stretch that isn't painful, but it's not okay to feel pain when you exercise."

Taking Care with PROM

PROM of the hand should be performed gently and with care.

Precaution. *PROM can injure swollen and inflamed joints and tissues.*

Colditz[8] cautions that the only joints for which manual PROM is safe are joints with a soft end-feel. Nevertheless, clients may request more aggressive therapy. They may even be passively stressing their swollen, stiff hands at home. It is very important that the therapist inquire about this and put a stop to it. Explain to your client how injurious and counterproductive it is, emphasizing that delicate hand tissues are all too easily injured (see Chapter 18).

Precaution. *PROM can trigger inflammatory responses, causing additional scar production, pain, and stiffness. PROM used inappropriately or painfully can incite complex regional pain syndrome (CRPS or RSD).*

What to Say to Clients if the Doctor Orders "Aggressive Therapy"

When a physician orders aggressive therapy for a client, I tell the client, "Your doctor wants you to make excellent progress. But the reality is that tissues in the hand are delicate and can easily be injured by too much force or pressure. We will assertively correct the restricted or injured tissues, and you will make the best progress by providing controlled stress to the proper structures. Painful, injurious treatment or exercise will only delay or even derail your progress. What we will do aggressively is to upgrade your program and encourage maximum results."

Hopefully, physicians soon will realize the wisdom of replacing the term *aggressive* with *progressive*. Until that happens, explain to your clients that pain-free, controlled stretching and remodeling have proved to be the best course of treatment for the fragile hand tissues.

Quality of Movement and Dyscoordinate Co-contraction

Dyscoordinate co-contraction is a poor quality of movement that can result from co-contraction of antagonist muscles. Clients may demonstrate dyscoordinate co-contraction when they use excessive effort with exercise or when they fear pain with exercise or PROM, or it may be habitual. The resulting motion looks unpleasant and awkward. For example, you may feel the extensors contract as the client tries to activate the flexors. It is important not to ignore dyscoordinate co-contraction. Instead, teach the client pain-free, smooth movements that feel pleasant to perform. Replace isolated exercises with purposeful or functional activities and try proximal oscillations (small, gentle, rhythmic motions) to facilitate a more effective quality of movement. Biofeedback or electrical stimulation may also be helpful. Imagery offers additional possibilities (e.g., have your client pretend to move the extremity through gelatin or water).[10] Do not bark at the client to "Relax!" Instead, be gentle with your voice and your verbal cues.

Adjunct Treatments

Superficial heating agents can have beneficial effects on analgesic, vascular, metabolic, and connective tissue responses. Analgesic effects are seen in diminished pain and elevated pain tolerance. Vascular effects are evidenced by reduced muscle spasms and improved pain relief. Metabolic effects are related to an increased flow of blood and oxygen to the tissues, with improved provision of nutrients and removal of byproducts associated with inflammation. Connective tissue effects are seen as reduced stiffness with improved extensibility of tissues.[11]

Many clients feel that heat helps prepare the tissue for exercise and activity. The safest way to warm the tissues of hand therapy clients is aerobic exercise, unless this is contraindicated for medical reasons. Tai chi, for example, provides multijoint ROM, relaxation, and cardiac effects.

Application of external heat (e.g., hot packs) is a popular method in many clinics. Although the use of heat is fine if it is not contraindicated, be mindful that heat increases edema, which acts like glue, and this may contribute to stiffness. Heat can degrade collagen and may contribute to microscopic tears in soft tissue.[12] For these reasons, be very gentle and cautious if you perform PROM after heat application. Monitor the situation to make sure that the overall benefits of heat outweigh any possible negative responses. Measuring edema is a good way to objectify these responses.

Cold therapy (also called *cryotherapy*) traditionally has been used to relieve pain and to reduce inflammation and edema after injury (and sometimes after overly aggressive therapy). Cryotherapy typically is used after acute injury to reduce bleeding by means of vasoconstriction. Cold therapy reduces postinjury edema and inflammation and raises the pain threshold. However, remember: *cold therapy can be harmful to tissues; be cautious with this modality.*

Precaution. *Do not use cryotherapy on clients with nerve injury or repair, sensory impairment, peripheral vascular disease, Raynaud's phenomenon, lupus, leukemia, multiple myeloma, neuropathy, other rheumatic disease, or cold intolerance.*

Other modalities used in hand therapy include therapeutic ultrasound, electrical stimulation, and iontophoresis (provision of an agent such as an anti-inflammatory medication into tissue through use of low-voltage direct current). Therapists should study these topics further. However, they also must abide by their practice acts and the regulations of their state licensing agencies regarding the use of modalities. Never use a modality for which you cannot demonstrate proper education and training.

Scar Management

Scars can take many months to heal fully. Treat scar sensitivity with desensitization. If the sensitivity causes functional limitations, provide protection, such as padding or silicone gel. Scars are mature when they are pale, supple, flatter, and no longer sensitive. Scar maturation can be facilitated by light compression (e.g., with Coban, Tubigrip [an elastic support sleeve], or edema gloves).

Precaution. *Always check to make sure the compression on the scar is not excessive (i.e., the wrap, sleeve, or glove are not too tight).*

Inserts made of padded materials or silicone gel pads also help facilitate scar maturation.[13] This padding is thought to promote neutral warmth of the area and may decrease oxygen to the collagen, thus promoting collagen maturation. Evans[14] advocates scar management using micropore paper tape applied longitudinally along the incision line once epithelialization has occurred.

Instruct your clients to avoid sun exposure while the scar is still immature (i.e., pink or red, thick, itchy, or sensitive). Sunlight can burn the fragile scar and darken its color, affecting the cosmetic result when the scar is mature. Frequent use of sunscreen is highly recommended (see Chapter 19).

Although scar massage is often performed, it is important to monitor the client's tissue response.

Precaution. *If scar massage is too aggressive, it may cause inflammation and contribute to more extensive development or thickening of scar tissue.*

Do not encourage aggressive massage; instead, teach the client to perform gentler massage that does not cause a flare of tissues. Further research on this topic is needed.

TREATMENT TECHNIQUES

Splinting

Splinting is a mainstay of therapy for UE problems. Splints can provide immobilization or selective mobilization. They can be used with exercise or to promote function. The topic of splinting exceeds the scope of this book. I strongly advise readers to study more comprehensive resources on this subject.[15,16] In addition to learning about splint fabrication, readers should learn about strap placement for mechanical advantage and comfort.

Static splints are used to immobilize tissues, to prevent deformity, to prevent contracture of soft tissue, and to provide substitution for lost motor function. **Serial static splints** position the tissue for lengthening and are remolded at intervals. Static splints contribute to disuse, stiffness, and atrophy, therefore they should not be used

more than necessary. **Static progressive splints** (also called *inelastic mobilization splints*) apply mobilizing force using nonmoving parts such as monofilament, Velcro, or screws. **Dynamic splints** (also called **mobilization splints** or **elastic mobilization splints**) use moving parts such as rubber bands or spring wires to apply a gentle force. These splints are used to correct deformity, to substitute for absent or impaired motor function, to provide controlled movement, and to promote wound healing or help with alignment of fractures.[17,18]

Forearm-based splints should cover approximately two thirds of the forearm. Have the client bend the arm at the elbow and note the place where the forearm meets the biceps muscle. The proximal edge of the splint should be $1/4$-inch distal to this so that the splint is not pushed distally when the client flexes the elbow. Flaring the proximal edges of the splint is also important to ensure that the splint stays in place on the arm.[19] Clearing the distal palmar crease is extremely important. If the splint crosses this crease, MP flexion will be impeded. When you construct a dorsal forearm-based splint or a forearm-based ulnar gutter, pad the area of the ulnar head, because this bony prominence can become a pressure area. Always incorporate the padding into the molding of the splint; do not place it inside afterward as an addition.

With mobilization splints, the best approach is to provide a splint your client can tolerate for long periods.

CLINICAL *Pearl*

Applying low tension that is tolerable and constant over prolonged periods is much better than applying strong forces over shorter periods.

The amount of safe force for the hand is 100 to 300 g.[9] Clients often ask that more force be used in their splint. These clients need repeated education that low load over a long duration is the safest and most effective way to remodel tissues and make clinical progress.

Precaution. *Painful splinting can be harmful.*

Skin blanching is a sign of high tension or incorrect splint mechanics.[3] The line of pull on the part being mobilized in a static progressive or dynamic splint must be a 90-degree angle from the **outrigger** (the structure from which the forces are directed). An outrigger can be high profile or low profile (Fig. 1-7). High-profile outriggers have certain mechanical and adjustment advantages but are bulkier and less attractive.[20]

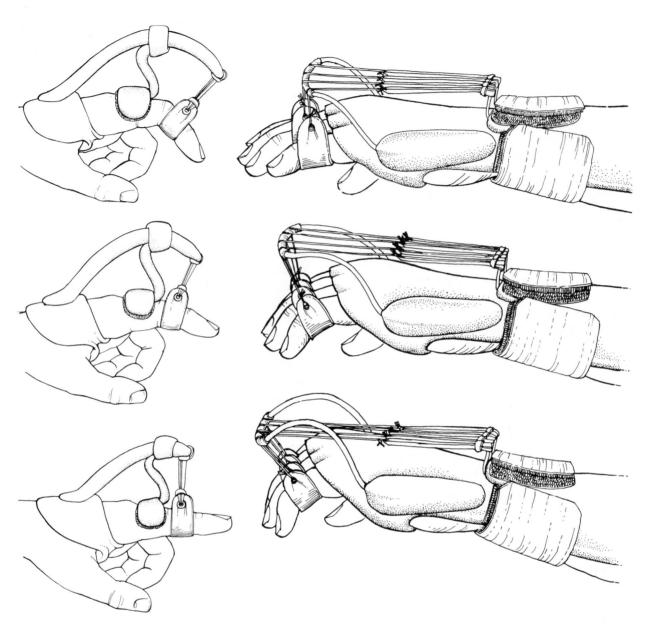

FIGURE 1-7 Examples of the 90-degree angle of pull with high-profile and low-profile outriggers. (From Fess EE: Principles and methods of splinting for mobilization of joints. In Mackin EJ, Callahan AD, Skirven TM et al, editors: *Rehabilitation of the hand and upper extremity,* ed 5, St Louis, 2002, Mosby.)

Splints Used with Exercise

A dorsal dropout splint can be used to correct digital flexion or extrinsic extensor tightness. Mold the splint in a position of comfortable stretch. Use strapping as needed to keep it in place. The client should try to gently flex the digits away from the splint as able (Fig. 1-8). Having an object to reach for, such as a dowel in the palm, can be helpful.

Splinting can be used to achieve various differential MP positions. The differential MP splint in Fig. 1-9 posi-

tions the long finger MP in greater flexion than the index and ring fingers. In this splint, active MP flexion of the index and ring fingers facilitates long finger flexion. Fig. 1-10 shows the opposite differential MP splint, with the long finger MP more extended than the adjacent fingers. A differential MP splint with the small finger MP more flexed than the ring finger might be useful for a small finger metacarpal fracture with limited MP flexion. Active PIP flexion and extension within this type of splint at various MP positions also promotes PIP joint

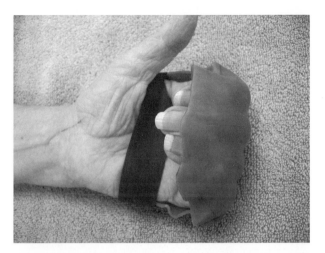

FIGURE 1-8 Client performing active digital flexion in a dorsal dropout splint.

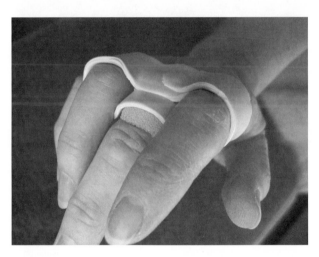

FIGURE 1-9 Differential MP positioning splint with long finger MP more flexed than adjacent fingers.

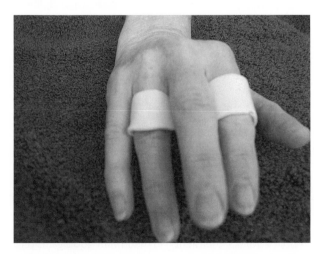

FIGURE 1-10 Differential MP positioning splint with long finger MP more extended than adjacent fingers.

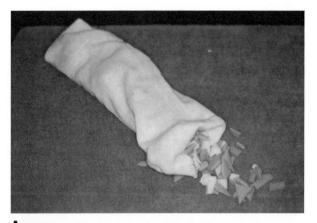

A

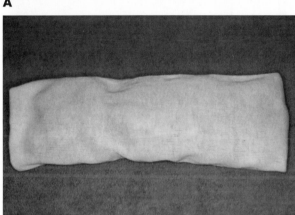

B

FIGURE 1-11 A, Chip bag contents consisting of small pieces of foam placed in a cotton stockinette. **B,** Ends of chip bag can be folded over and taped closed.

ROM and tendon gliding. This splint can be used during a progressive gripping activity (e.g., gripping a handful of dried beans, squeezing some out of the hand, then gripping further).

A scrap of thermoplastic material can be used to create a cylinder to fit the client's available limited fist position. Sustained gripping of or holding onto this cylinder and "pumping" to flex and extend the digits around the cylinder may enhance composite digital flexion.

Chip Bags

Chip bags can be incorporated into splinting regimens to maximize lymphatic flow and minimize the stiffness and adherence that otherwise would worsen as a result of the edema. A **chip bag** is a cotton stockinette bag filled with small foam pieces of various densities (Fig. 1-11). The foam can be cut from a variety of sources, including foam exercise blocks, padding, and soft Velcro materials. Chip bags traditionally have been used in the treatment of lymphedema; they are positioned over indurated areas

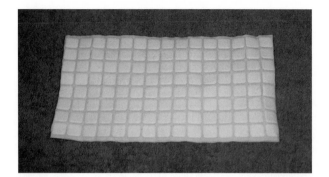

FIGURE 1-12   Gore Procel cast liner.

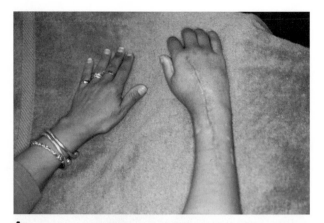

A

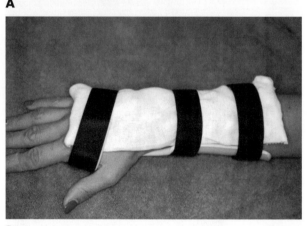

B

FIGURE 1-13   A, Dorsal scars and edema. **B,** Style of chip bag incorporated into the client's volar wrist splint.

of edema within external compressive garments or multilayered stretch bandages. Chip bags provide light traction on the skin, facilitate lymphatic stimulation, and promote neutral warmth. All these effects help reduce edema. The increased body heat under the chip bag and the light pressure exerted by the bag help soften thickened or fibrotic tissue.

In some cases chip bags can be used alone, without an accompanying splint. In such cases they can be held in place with stockinette or a soft Velcro strap that is not applied tightly. Sometimes a less technical approach, such as using chip bags with splints, is a very effective option. Chip bags also can be positioned inside or in conjunction with splints to maximize edema control and reduce scar adherence. Clients find chip bags very comfortable. Some refer to the chip bag as their "pillow," which probably conveys the comfort they experience with it. If the therapist wants less bulk or wants the effect of a chip bag with an existing splint that cannot accommodate the bulk, a product such as the Gore Procel cast liner (Fig. 1-12) can be used instead.

CASE *Studies*

CASE STUDY 1-1

A client was in an altercation with a family member, and her hand was closed in a door during the argument. She was seen for malunion of a right distal radius fracture with right ulnar joint dislocation and extensor pollicis longus (EPL) rupture. She underwent open carpal tunnel release, corrective osteotomy of the distal radius fracture with internal fixation and bone grafting, and intercalary tendon grafting of the EPL tendon using the extensor indicis proprius (EIP). When the client was seen in occupational therapy, her hand was extremely swollen and stiff, and she had severe extrinsic extensor tightness that limited full fisting. She developed complex regional pain

syndrome and was treated successfully for this with a combination of stellate ganglion blocks and hand therapy. Note the dorsal scars and edema (Fig. 1-13, *A*). The style of chip bag incorporated into her volar wrist splint is shown in Fig. 1-13, *B*. This woman was a highly motivated client. At the time her therapy was discontinued, she had regained very good hand function.

CASE STUDY 1-2

A client who underwent surgery for release of a Dupuytren's contracture developed a flare reaction. Note the incisional scar and fullness of the ulnar hand (Fig. 1-14, *A*), as well as the limitation in composite digital flexion (Fig. 1-14, *B*). This client used a chip bag inside an exercise splint designed to block the MPs and promote PIP and DIP flexion exercise; the goals were to resolve intrinsic muscle tightness and promote composite digital flexion. Within 2 weeks, the client had made very good gains (Fig. 1-14, *C*).

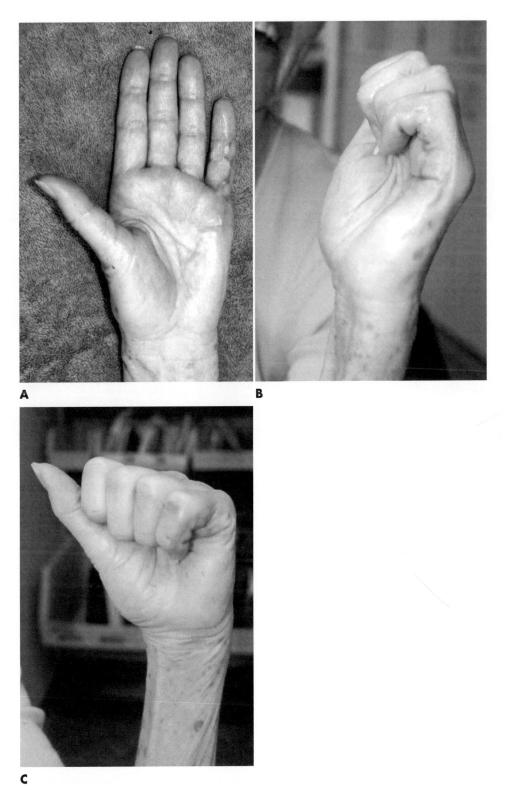

FIGURE 1-14   A, Flared incisional scar that developed after Dupuytren's release surgery. **B,** Limited active composite flexion. **C,** Full active composite flexion 2 weeks later.

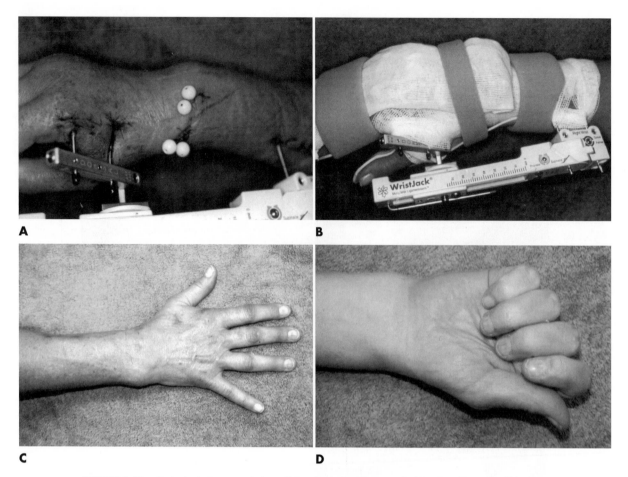

FIGURE 1-15   A, Indentations made by a tight elastic bandage applied by the client. **B,** Chip bags incorporated into dressings and splints with external fixator and pins. **C** and **D,** Resolution of edema and active digital extension and flexion at discharge.

CASE STUDY 1-3

A woman who fell while hiking sustained a displaced distal radius fracture that required external fixation and per-cutaneous pin fixation. More than a week passed after her fall before she went to her physician. The woman explained this by noting that she has attention deficit disorder. She came to therapy 1 day after applying an elastic bandage tightly and irregularly around her external fixator. Note the indentations left on her skin by the wrap (Fig. 1-15, *A*). Chip bags were incorporated into the dressings and splints used in this case (Fig. 1-15, *B*), and the client progressed very well in therapy. She had good composite digital extension and flexion at the time of discharge (Fig. 1-15, *C* and *D*).

Soft Four-Finger Buddy Strap

A soft four-finger buddy strap can be made from Softstrap Velcro loop to provide transverse support that promotes more efficient primary function of the extrinsic flexors and extensors (see Fig. 1-21 on CD). This strap facilitates AROM for composite flexion and extension and for iso-

lated extensor digitorum communis (EDC) and FDP tendon glide. It also stimulates lymphatic flow over the volar proximal phalanges, similar to chip bags. The soft four-finger buddy strap can relieve pain and promote AROM when hand stiffness is present. It also is helpful for symptom management in clients with lateral epicondylitis (tennis elbow) who have EDC involvement and pain on fisting.[21]

EXERCISES FOR UPPER EXTREMITY THERAPY

Precaution. *Shoulder stiffness can develop insidiously and can be very limiting.*

Check the client's posture and proximal motion initially and then at intervals. Incorporate proximal AROM into all home exercise programs, even if this is only a preventive measure (see Chapter 10).

Shorter, milder sessions of exercise performed more frequently are better than longer, intensive sessions done less often. Some clients do well at first, performing 5 repetitions 5 times a day and gradually building to 10 repetitions hourly during the day. Explain that exercises work well if the process is brief and frequent.

When working on isolated wrist extension, be sure to isolate the extensor carpi radialis brevis (ECRB) and teach clients how to extend the wrist with a soft fist that includes MP flexion. Have them hold an object so that the MPs are flexed. It is critical to retrain the ECRB to perform wrist extension. Without this isolation of motion, the client may learn to extend the wrist with EDC substitution instead of using the ECRB.

CLINICAL *Pearl*

Once established, the habit of extending the wrist with EDC substitution can be very hard to break.

To work on wrist active/active assistive range of motion (A/AAROM), put a towel on the table and then place a coffee can (no bigger than the 3 lb size) on its side on the towel. Teach the client to place the involved hand on the can and to use the other hand to hold the involved hand flat on the can. The client then rolls the can using A/AAROM forward and backward. Clients like the feeling of this exercise, which also promotes proximal ROM and stimulates lymphatic flow.

In contrast to this, if extrinsic flexor tightness is a problem, the client would perform exercises involving wrist extension with simultaneous digital extension. Otherwise, exercises for wrist extension should be done primarily with a fist that includes MP flexion.

Always look at the client's wrist position when exercising the digits. Do not exercise or coax the digits into flexion with the wrist flexed unless you are deliberately trying to stretch the extrinsic extensors. It is biomechanically easier to achieve digital flexion with the wrist in extension, to achieve PIP joint flexion with the MP extended, and to achieve PIP joint extension with the MP flexed. If the client cannot sustain a position of wrist neutral or extension, use a splint or have the client self-support the wrist using the other hand when digital exercises are performed.

Instruct clients always to keep the upper arm locked at the side of the body when performing forearm rotation exercises.

CLINICAL *Pearl*

Do not perform forearm rotation exercises with the elbow on a table or even on a pillow; this prevents isolated forearm rotation and allows for substitution with humeral motions.

Teach the client that one way to do this is to keep a towel roll pressed to the side of the body with the arm used to perform forearm rotation exercises, because this requires that the elbow be kept close to the body.

In some cases, AROM through functional activity and exercise may be all that is needed to enable the client to recover full UE flexibility and function. When more isolated and structure-specific exercises are needed, the exercises discussed in the following sections may be helpful.

Blocking Exercises

Blocking exercises are exercises in which proximal support is provided to promote isolated motion at a particular site. They are helpful for clients with limitation of either AROM or PROM or both. Blocking exercises exert more force than nonblocking exercises.

CLINICAL *Pearl*

With blocking exercises, instruct the client to hold the position at comfortable end-range for 3 to 5 seconds; this allows remodeling of the tissues.

Blocking exercises can be accomplished in a variety of ways. You can use either commercially available devices or individual devices made from scraps of splinting materials. Digital gutters or cylinders that cross the IPs help isolate MP flexion and extension. If the cylinder is shortened to free the DIP, then DIP blocking exercises can be performed. These exercises can be done with the MP in extension or in varying degrees of flexion. Often a client exerts too strong a contraction, and the PIP tries to flex within the blocking splint. Explain to the client that isolating motion to only the DIP requires a soft quality of contraction so that the effort is not overridden by other structures. The biomechanical challenge to the FDP is greater when DIP flexion is performed with MP flexion than with MP extension. This positional progression can be used to upgrade the exercises.

CLINICAL *Pearl*

When a digital block is used to promote MP flexion of the small finger, it is very helpful to stabilize the small finger metacarpal.

The ring and small finger metacarpals are more mobile at their carpometacarpal (CMC) joints than are the index and long finger metacarpals. If the metacarpal

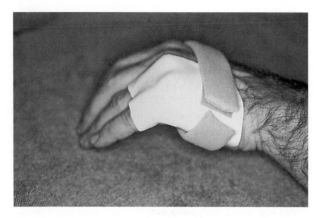

FIGURE 1-16 Blocking splint with the MP flexed helps isolate PIP extension and promotes extrinsic extensor stretch.

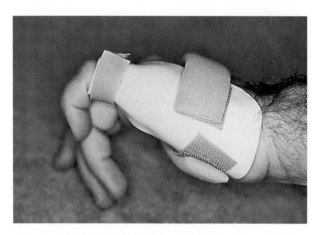

FIGURE 1-17 Blocking splint with the MP extended helps isolate active PIP flexion and FDP excursion and also helps resolve intrinsic tightness.

is supported by your hand or the client's other hand, more effective isolated motion can occur at the MP joint. This isolation and proximal support can be very helpful for clients trying to recover MP flexion after a small finger metacarpal fracture.

A blocking splint with the MPs flexed helps isolate active PIP extension (Fig. 1-16). Extending the PIP is easier biomechanically when the MP is flexed, because this position promotes central slip function. This same blocking splint also promotes composite flexion exercise and can be helpful for normalizing extrinsic extensor tightness. Conversely, a blocking splint with the MPs extended (Fig. 1-17) helps to isolate active IP flexion and FDP excursion and to resolve intrinsic tightness. These types of splints can be used with function, or they may be used only for exercise.

A DIP cap or flexion block diverts FDP excursion to the PIP and thus promotes isolated exercise of the FDS muscle with MP and PIP flexion and DIP extension. This

blocking device may also help the client exercise the flexor digitorum superficialis (FDS) fist position more easily (see following section).

Differential Flexor Tendon Gliding Exercises

Differential flexor tendon gliding exercises are a mainstay of most home programs because they are easy to perform and they promote motion very effectively (Fig. 1-18).[22] They are a standard exercise for conservative management of carpal tunnel syndrome and are also used after carpal tunnel release. These exercises are an important option for all clients with hand or wrist stiffness. Rolling a thick highlighting pen up and down in the palm is an effective way to perform FDP gliding.

Place and Hold Exercises

Place and hold exercises can be helpful when PROM is greater than AROM (Fig. 1-19). Gently perform AAROM to position the finger (e.g., in composite flexion). Then ask the client to sustain that position comfortably while releasing the assisting hand. The assisting hand may be yours or the client's other hand. Watch for co-contraction or force that is too strenuous as the client tries to sustain the exercise position. A combination of blocking exercises and place and hold exercises can be very productive. Also, you can try doing place and hold exercises with a blocking splint in place.

When the client releases the sustained contraction, pain sometimes may be felt in the area of a stiff joint. For instance, if the client performs place and hold exercises for composite fisting and then has PIP joint discomfort when releasing the fist, have the client relax the muscle contraction but stay in the same fisted position. While the client stays in that position, gradually provide assistance to gently begin extending the digit or digits (minimal joint distraction mobilization also can be helpful if not contraindicated). Next, ask the client to slowly actively extend the digits the rest of the way. This technique can be helpful for eliminating pain associated with end-ranges and AAROM.

Resistive Exercises

After clients have been medically cleared for them, resistive exercises are used for strengthening and to improve excursion of adherent tissue. Sometimes clients want to use a greater load than is safe for them. Teach clients that, for isolating wrist curls, they should not use as heavy a weight as they would for biceps curls.

Precaution. *Think carefully and critically about the status of your client's wrist if the person is recovering from a fracture, has had tendonitis, or is at risk for degenerative joint changes. Be very careful with wrist radial and ulnar deviation strengthening exercises, because these may provoke tendonitis.*

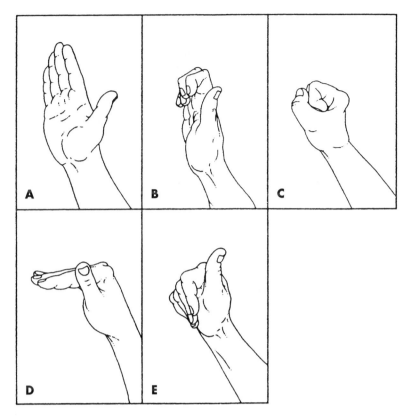

FIGURE 1-18   Differential tendon gliding exercises. **A,** Straight digits. **B,** Hook fist. **C,** Composite fist. **D,** Tabletop. **E,** Straight (FDS) fist. (From Rozmaryn LM, Dovelle S, Rothman ER et al: Nerve and tendon gliding exercises and the conservative management of carpal tunnel syndrome, *Journal of Hand Therapy* 11:171-179, 1998.)

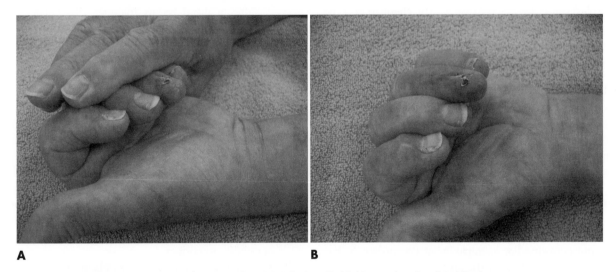

FIGURE 1-19   **A,** Place exercises for digital flexion. **B,** Hold exercises for digital flexion.

Generally speaking, the safest course in performing resistive exercises is to use more repetitions with a lower load. This approach promotes endurance. (A more detailed discussion of resistive exercise is presented in Chapter 4.)

Resistive exercise can take many forms, including progressive resistive exercises (PREs) and exercises performed with graded grippers, rubber bands, squeeze balls, graded clothespins, and putty. For example, marbles or other objects can be embedded in putty, requiring pinch and dexterity to remove them.

Functional Activity

It is essential that the client incorporate the gains made from exercising into functional UE use at home and at work. Practicing or simulating relevant activities in the clinic can reinforce this. Examples of such activities may include tying shoes, folding clothes, manipulating coins, writing with an adapted pen, using the involved hand for handshakes, hammering, using screwdrivers, or lifting. Putty can be used to simulate activities such as turning keys. Adding visualization to the simulation enhances the treatment. The scope of practice for either occupational therapy or physical therapy dictates some of these choices.

Ball rolling can be used for wrist AROM, composite stretching, weight bearing, and closed chain exercise. The ball can be dribbled or thrown for strengthening or sports simulation. Balloons can also be thrown or batted with the hand.

Dried beans can be used for grip and release, for progressive gripping, and for fishing other objects (e.g., marbles) out of the beans. Instruct the client to grip the beans and then to release them with full digital extension. Wrist motions can be varied, and tenodesis can be incorporated. You also can have the client use opposition of the thumb to each finger to pick up one bean and then release it with full digital extension.

Pegs of varying sizes promote tendon gliding, sensory stimulation, and joint ROM. Fine motor activities (e.g., threading beads, in-hand manipulation of marbles, stacking blocks) can be modified with blocking splints to promote isolated ROM or tendon glide.

TIPS FROM THE FIELD

- Look at all your clients and their hands with interest and curiosity. For example, what do you see in Fig. 1-20? See the CD for the answer.
- Be tender when you touch your clients. If your hands are cold, try to warm them up a bit before you touch the person.
- Remember that you do not have to evaluate and treat everything on the first visit.

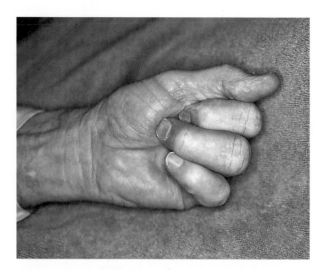

FIGURE 1-20 What do you see wrong with this client's hand?

- Never yell at or order a client to "Relax." Instead, encourage relaxation with a calm, slow voice.
- Working on one area of stiffness sometimes can also resolve stiffness in another area.
  - *Example:* A client who sustained a distal radius fracture had limited AROM and PROM in wrist flexion and extension and decreased ECRB excursion (i.e., passive wrist extension exceeded active wrist extension). Stretching led to improved wrist flexion. It also helped reduce ECRB adherence, which resulted in improved wrist extension.
  - *Example:* A client had extrinsic flexor tightness after a distal radius fracture with edema and decreased wrist and hand AROM. As her extrinsic flexor tightness resolved (she recovered full passive composite extension), the active digital flexion also resolved because she had better mechanical function of the lengthened digital flexors.
- Keep the timeline open for more progress by not performing painful therapy and by avoiding a flare reaction.
- As a hand therapist, you won't be able to resolve every problem in every case. If prolonged, established stiffness is present, if the client has highly fibrotic tissue responses, or if client follow-through has been poor, residual limitations may exist that are beyond our ability to correct.
  - Document explicitly if poor client follow-through is a factor. For example, a client was carrying a glass table, which broke; the client received a laceration to his right-dominant forearm. Several flexor tendons and the median and ulnar nerves also were lacerated. The client missed many

therapy visits and did not perform his Duran home program (see Chapter 16). The client returned to therapy with very poor passive digital flexion, severe edema, and skin maceration. In this case, documentation would include the following: "The patient had been instructed to perform hourly protected passive digital flexion within his splint, but he reports that he did not do so. He states he understands the need to exercise as instructed. He also states he understands that if he does not gain passive digital flexion soon, he may lose the opportunity to make maximum clinical gains." If appropriate, the progress note to this client's physician should report that the patient now agrees to increase the frequency of home exercise program (HEP) exercises, as he was previously instructed to do.

- If a client is not following through as instructed, it is important to investigate why this is happening and to work with the client to correct the situation. Clients can have a number of reasons for failing to follow their regimen. They may be uninformed about the importance of the HEP; they may think they can catch up and make progress later; they may have a secondary agenda, such as avoiding a return to work; they may be depressed; or they may need help to assimilate the HEP into their daily routine successfully. (See Chapter 7 for more information on functional somatic syndromes and challenging behaviors.)
- Help clients learn to be patient. Encourage them to continue with their home program and to celebrate small improvements. Assist them in finding meaningful ways to use their time (e.g., find new interests and hobbies) if participation in an enjoyable activity has been temporarily disrupted.
- Replenish your own reserves so that you have the resources needed for complicated clinical situations (see Chapter 8). Give yourself a few moments to take some deep breaths and focus on the client as a person. Try to sense what it must be like for the client to have this injury. Carefully check for **extensor habitus,** which is habitual posturing in digital extension. The index finger is particularly prone to this response. Extensor habitus can occur after an injury as simple as a paper cut. It is important to identify this phenomenon and to correct it as soon as possible so that it does not become permanent and so that joint stiffness does not occur. Buddy straps and splinting may be helpful.
- Take one day at a time with the therapy. Do not presume that you will pick up where your last session left off. Look at your clients with fresh eyes at each visit. Ask them what is better, what they are noticing about their hands, what they are able to do functionally now, and what they are still unable to accomplish functionally.

THINKING OUTSIDE THE (TREATMENT) BOX

When to Mix and Match

Mix and match your treatment repertoire. After reading the rest of this book, try to think outside the treatment box. Be creative and have some fun. For example, why not perform early protective motions (e.g., place and hold tenodesis motions described in Chapter 22) with most of your patients?

When Less is More

Teaching your client the benefits of a "less is more" approach to UE exercises is very important. For example, a 12-year-old girl underwent flexor tendon grafting. In therapy, when trying to isolate FDP motion at the DIP with the PIP blocked, she was co-contracting and eliciting PIP flexion instead. The therapist taught her to contract more softly so as to isolate the FDP more effectively. The therapist used some helpful verbal cues, such as "Don't try so hard," "Stop trying altogether," and "Stop thinking." The therapist gave these cues in a soft, gentle voice and made sure to compliment the girl and smile when her isolated motion was of better quality. This activity was followed by place and hold exercises, which progressed successfully. Even though this client was very young, she learned the quality of isolated motion well, recognizing that "less is more." She also could see the improvement in her capabilities.

When to Stop Exercising for a Few Days

Another important lesson to teach clients is when to stop exercising for a short time. For example, a 53-year-old, right-dominant woman sustained a distal radius fracture when she fell while shopping. She developed significant, diffuse edema and stiffness of the shoulder, elbow, forearm, and hand. This client demonstrated objective signs of a flare response after efforts were made to upgrade her exercises gradually. She was at risk for IP flexion contractures of all digits. Her sisters came to visit her, and they all went to a spa for 4 days. During this time, the client stopped performing her assigned UE exercises while she pampered herself at the spa. When she came back to therapy, she had diminished flare responses, decreased edema, and improved ROM throughout the upper extremity. It helped her immensely to stop trying so hard. She was then able to resume "trying," but with a better sense of her tissue tolerances.

When to Accept a Stiff Hand and Get On with Life

Unfortunately, hand therapists cannot fix everything. In some cases, the client's injuries may be too severe to permit a full recovery. In other cases, a family crisis may prevent therapy from continuing in a timely manner. Under circumstances such as these, the client's best course of action is to accept the residual stiffness or limitations and to resume otherwise normal living. In such cases, therapists can perform the important role of identifying and teaching compensatory techniques to maximize the client's function.[23] Also, sometimes the therapist has the responsibility to identify a clinical plateau and to help clients realize that they may have achieved all that is possible at that time.

SUMMARY

This chapter has identified fundamental hand therapy concepts that foster clinical reasoning. It also has highlighted treatment techniques and provided guidelines to promote interventions that are safe and appropriate. Most treatment techniques are not diagnosis specific, but rather can be applied to a variety of diagnoses. As a hand therapist, the challenge you face is to be tissue specific, to be aware of clinical precautions, and to adapt the appropriate treatment from your toolbox of techniques to a given diagnosis. As you continue with this book, I encourage you to ask yourself what interventions would be most appropriate and why. I also recommend that you return to this chapter and reread it after you have read the rest of the book. Rereading this chapter at that time will help you appreciate what you have learned; that, hopefully, will be how to apply clinical reasoning in selecting safe treatment choices for clients with many different diagnoses.

Acknowledgments

I wish to thank Sandra M. Artzberger, MS, OTR, CHT, CLT, for reviewing this chapter and for providing me the impetus to explore chip bags in conjunction with upper extremity splinting; Patricia Zarbock Fantauzzo, COTA/L, for her creative ideas for using chip bags on clients with upper extremity problems; and Joel Moorhead, MD, MPH, John L. Evarts, BS, Lisa Deshaies OTR, CHT, and Sharon Flinn, PhD, OTR/L, CHT, CVE, for reading and critiquing this chapter.

References

1. Tubiana R, Thomine J-M, Mackin EJ: *Examination of the hand and wrist*, ed 2, London, 1996, Martin Dunitz.

2. Smith KL, Price JL: Care of the hand wound. In Mackin EJ, Callahan AD, Skirven TM et al, editors: *Rehabilitation of the hand and upper extremity*, ed 5, St Louis, 2002, Mosby.

3. Strickland JW: Biologic basis for hand and upper extremity splinting. In Fess EE, Gettle KS, Philips CA et al, editors: *Hand and upper extremity splinting*, ed 3, St Louis, 2005, Elsevier.

4. Fess EE, McCollum M: The influence of splinting on healing tissues, *J Hand Ther* 11:157-161, 1998.

5. Bryan BK, Kohnke EN: Therapy after skeletal fixation in the hand and wrist, *Hand Clin* 13:761-776, 1997.

6. Fess EE: Hand rehabilitation. In Hopkins HL, Smith HD, editors: *Willard and Spackman's occupational therapy*, ed 8, Philadelphia, 1999, JB Lippincott.

7. Stewart KM: Therapist's management of the complex injury. In Hunter JM, Mackin EJ, Callahan AD, editors: *Rehabilitation of the hand: surgery and therapy*, ed 4, St Louis, 1995, Mosby.

8. Colditz JC: Therapist's management of the stiff hand. In Mackin EJ, Callinan N, Skirven TM et al, editors: *Rehabilitation of the hand and upper extremity*, ed 5, St Louis, 2002, Mosby.

9. Brand PW: The forces of dynamic splinting: ten questions before applying a dynamic splint to the hand. In Mackin EJ, Callahan AD, Skirven TM et al, editors: *Rehabilitation of the hand and upper extremity*, ed 5, St Louis, 2002, Mosby.

10. Cooper C, Liskin J, Moorhead JF: Dyscoordinate contraction: impaired quality of movement in patients with hand disorders, *OT Practice* 4:40-45, 1999.

11. Bracciano AG, Earley D: Physical agent modalities. In Trombly CA, Radomski MV, editors: *Occupational therapy for physical dysfunction*, ed 5, Philadelphia, 2002, Lippincott Williams & Wilkins.

12. Miles CA, Burjanadze TV, Bailey AJ: The kinetics of the thermal denaturation of collagen in unrestrained rat tail tendon determined by differential scanning calorimetry, *J Mol Biol* 245:437-446, 1995.

13. Baum TM, Busuito MJ: Use of a glycerin-based gel sheeting in scar management, *Adv Wound Care* 11:40-43, 1998.

14. Evans RB: Instructional course given at the annual meeting of the American Society of Hand Therapists and the American Society for Surgery of the Hand, San Antonio, September 21-24, 2005.

15. Fess EE, Gettle KS, Philips CA, Janson JR: *Hand and upper extremity splinting: principles and methods*, ed 3, St Louis, 2005, Elsevier.

16. Coppard BM, Lohman H, editors: *Introduction to splinting: a clinical-reasoning and problem-solving approach*, ed 2, St Louis, 2001, Mosby.

17. Coppard BM, Lynn P: Introduction to splinting. In Coppard BM, Lohman H, editors: *Introduction to splinting: a clinical-reasoning and problem-solving approach*, ed 2, St Louis, 2001, Mosby.

18. Deshaies LD: Upper extremity orthoses. In Trombly CA, Radomski MV, editors: *Occupational therapy for physical dysfunction*, ed 5, Philadelphia, 2002, Lippincott Williams & Wilkins.

19. Belkin J, Yasuda L: Orthotics. In Pedretti LW, Early MB, editors: *Occupational therapy: practice skills for physical dysfunction*, ed 5, St Louis, 2001, Mosby.

20. Fess EE: Principles and methods of splinting for mobilization of joints. In Mackin EJ, Callahan AD, Skirven TM et al, editors: *Rehabilitation of the hand and upper extremity*, ed 5, St Louis, 2002, Mosby.

21. Cooper C, Meland NB: Clinical implications of transverse forces on extrinsic flexors and extensors in the hand. Unpublished paper presented at the annual meeting of the American Society of Hand Therapists, Seattle, Oct. 5-8, 2000.

22. Rozmaryn LM, Dovelle S, Rothman ER et al: Nerve and tendon gliding exercises and the conservative management of carpal tunnel syndrome, *J Hand Ther* 11:171-179, 1998.

23. Merritt WH: Written on behalf of the stiff finger, *J Hand Ther* 11:74-79, 1998.

2

Upper Extremity Anatomy

SHARON FLINN AND MARGARET NEWSHAM BECKLEY

An understanding of normal anatomy is essential to the treatment of common upper extremity (UE) disorders. Without the ability to recognize the effects of impairment on the functional demands of our clients, we cannot fully assist them in their recovery efforts. Occupational and physical therapists learn the basic anatomy and neurophysiology of the upper extremity. However, courses in gross anatomy and neurophysiology frequently entail rote memorization of terminology, origins, insertions, nerves, and actions.[1] Hand therapy practitioners need to take the next step in organizing this introductory knowledge of the human body. A presentation of UE anatomy in nontraditional views can assist you in making meaningful connections in the ways the upper limbs operate as a kinematic chain; it also can help you to realize the delicate balance between form and function and to meet the educational needs of your clients.

To further enhance your clinical reasoning skills, this chapter presents a series of scenarios, along with questions and illustrations. These will facilitate your overall reasoning processes with regard to the upper extremity. This line of discovery can help you to appreciate the complexity of the upper extremity and to reflect on the dynamic relationship of various anatomic systems. An anatomic review of the upper extremity begins with the proximal structures and concludes with a review of the distal anatomy. More detailed discussions of specific anatomic features, such as joint function, the lymphatic system, dermatome levels, sensory distributions, and pulley mechanisms for flexor tendons, are provided in other chapters of this book.

SCENARIO 1

How Does Proper Cervical Alignment Facilitate Normal Functioning of Blood Vessels and Nerve Roots?

Proper cervical alignment is necessary for sound neurologic and vascular function in the shoulder, arm, and hand. Symptoms of cervical misalignment may appear distal to the primary injury site and manifest as sensory, motor, or autonomic dysfunction. A thorough understanding of the workings of the cervical spine is necessary to identify the source of injury in some clients with symptoms along the upper extremity. Educating the client in appropriate cervical posture patterns is part of an effective intervention and improves UE rehabilitation outcomes.

The relationships of bones, ligaments, disks, vasculature, and nerves provide the cervical spine with valuable mobility that other segments of the spinal column do not have. The cervical spine supports motions of the head, which consist of rotation from side to side, flexion and extension, lateral flexion to each side, and all the motions in between. The locations of the spinal components are designed to provide increased mobility at the cervical level; however, their anatomic relationships also make them vulnerable to injury.[2] Disorders arising from misalignment of the cervical spine can result in conditions that impair UE function (Table 2-1).

Proper cervical alignment of vertebrae, muscles, and soft tissue provides for normal conduction and excursion of nervous tissue in nerves C1-C8. Proper alignment of these structures also provides for normal blood flow in

TABLE 2-1

Common Cervical Injuries and Disorders and Resulting Impairment

ANATOMIC STRUCTURE	INJURY OR DISORDER	SYMPTOMS
Vertebrae	Subluxation, instability, fracture; abnormal bone development; arthritis; displacement; degenerative changes; stenosis; bony spurs	Disruption of sensory, motor, or vascular function throughout the upper extremity (UE)
Muscle	Weakness; tightness; imbalance; hypertonicity or hypotonicity; spasm; overstretching; sprain or strain	Compression of nervous tissue characteristically results in numbness, pain, paralysis, and loss of function; vascular compression characteristically results in moderate pain and swelling[3]
Soft tissue	Disk protrusion, lax ligament; ligament avulsion; degeneration or thickening of dura; adhesions	
Vasculature	Compression; constriction; mechanical irritation; congestion; reflex response; hemorrhage; stretching	Sympathetic symptoms associated with circulation can manifest in UE; decreased blood flow to UE tissues; temperature changes; pain; edema; decreased healing time
Nerve root and nerves	Decreased movement and elasticity; compression; strain, irritation, axonotmesis, severance	Pain at point of entrapment or along distal distribution in UE; decrease in or loss of sensation, motor control, or strength in UE; decreased UE deep tendon reflexes; decreased UE muscle tone; trophic changes in UE; sensation of deep pain; pain that radiates over shoulders and arms

the vertebral artery and the vertebral and deep cervical veins, ensuring adequate blood flow and drainage for the cervical structures related to UE function. The anterior rami of nerves C5-T1 form the brachial plexus, which innervates the entire UE (Fig. 2-1).[4]

CLINICAL *Pearl*

It is important that therapists look at UE problems as system problems, not conditions isolated to the region of the UE displaying symptoms.

SCENARIO 2

What Movements of the Upper Body Create Additional Tension on the Blood Vessels and Peripheral Nerves?

Movements of the upper body can create additional tension on the neurovascular bundle in the upper quadrant of the body, causing sensory, motor, or vascular symptoms. When these movements are repeated over time, the temporary symptoms caused by compression of

the neurovascular bundle can become frequent or constant and somewhat unrelenting. Fig. 2-2 shows common claviculocostal sites of increased neurovascular pressure with upper body movement. The symptoms that occur at these sites often are referred to as *thoracic outlet syndrome*.

Therapists must always keep in mind that increased neurovascular tension, over time, can lead to compression. Tension occurs with normal upper body movement. If the movement becomes repetitive over time, long-term compression occurs. The effects of upper body movement on neurovascular structures are presented in Table 2-2. Many other upper body and UE sites are prone to neurovascular compression arising from poor posture, injury, and/or muscle imbalance caused by weakness or malnutrition.

SCENARIO 3

What is the Relationship between the Rotator Cuff Muscles and an Intact and Mobile Glenohumeral Joint?

The glenohumeral joint depends on the rotator cuff muscles, rather than bones or ligaments, for its support.[2] The rotator cuff muscles include the subscapularis,

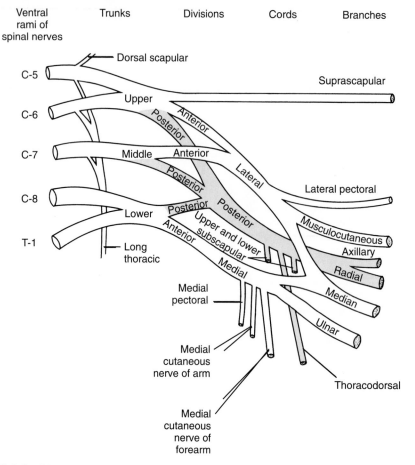

| Ventral rami of spinal nerves | Trunks | Divisions | Cords | Branches |

FIGURE 2-1   Diagram of the brachial plexus. The small nerve to the subclavius from the upper trunk is omitted. (From Jenkins DB: *Hollinshead's functional anatomy of the limb and back,* ed 8, Philadelphia, 2002, WB Saunders.)

TABLE 2-2

Neurovascular Symptoms Associated with Upper Body Movement

BODY PART	MOTION	RESULT	SYMPTOMS
Shoulder	Depression	*Peripheral nerve:* Stretching of upper and middle trunks of brachial plexus over scalene muscle; pulling of lower trunks into angle formed by first rib and scalene tendon *Blood vessel:* No compression of subclavian artery	Numbness and pain, particularly over ulnar distribution; pain worse at night because of positioning; intensity fluctuates throughout the day; arm fatigue, weakness, finger cramps, tingling, numbness, cold hand, areas of hyperesthesia, atrophy, tremor, and/or discoloration of hand
	Retraction	*Peripheral nerve:* No compression *Blood vessel:* Compression of subclavian vein by tendon of subclavian muscle, *not* by clavicle	
	Abduction and retraction	*Peripheral nerve:* Clavicular compression on brachial plexus *Blood vessel:* Clavicular compression of subclavian artery against scalene muscle	
Scapula	Retraction	*Peripheral nerve:* Compression of brachial plexus at point where it passes between clavicle and first rib *Blood vessel:* Compression of subclavian artery at point where it passes between clavicle and first rib	

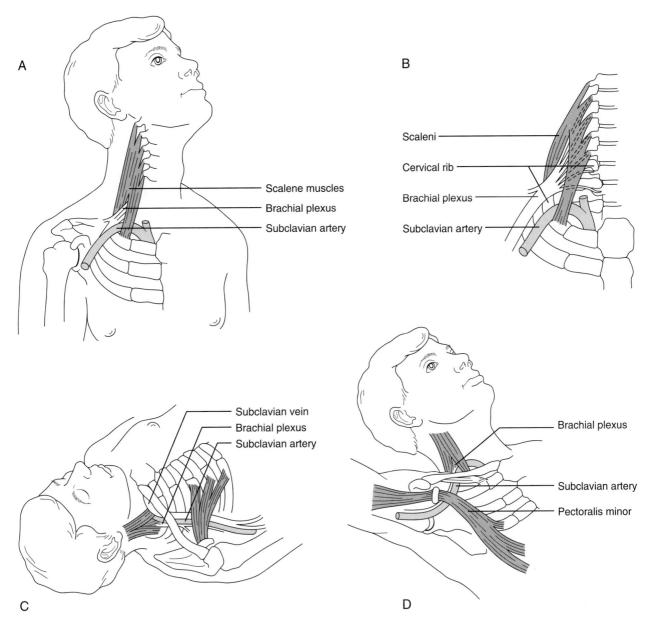

FIGURE 2-2 A, Scalenus anterior syndrome. **B,** Cervical rib syndrome. **C,** Costoclavicular syndrome. **D,** Hyperabduction syndrome. (From Magee D: *Orthopedic physical assessment,* ed 4, Philadelphia, 2002, WB Saunders.)

supraspinatus, infraspinatus, and teres minor muscles. The glenohumeral joint is a ball-and-socket synovial joint that moves in multiple axes. The motion of the glenohumeral joint provided by the rotator cuff muscles is related to the angle of pull of each muscle. Table 2-3 presents the locations and motions of the rotator cuff muscles.[5]

Besides providing the primary motions of the glenohumeral joint, the rotator cuff muscles act as part of force couples. For instance, the deltoid and supraspinatus muscles work as a force couple to produce glenohumeral abduction or flexion. The deltoid and teres minor muscles work as a force couple to produce depression and stabilization of the humeral head. Another force couple, the deltoid muscle and the rotator cuff muscles, produce depression of the humeral head and flexion of the humerus.[6] The therapist also must keep in mind the impact of forces and how the impact may change with different positions or postures. For instance, painting a ceiling requires glenohumeral stabilization and flexion proximally—but how do the forces change when the position is held for an extended period with the cervical spine extended? The therapist must look at the entire system, not just the isolated motion of shoulder flexion, in such cases.

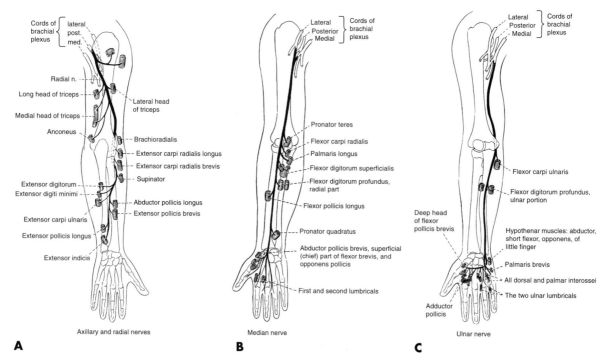

FIGURE 2-3 **A,** Axillary and radial nerves. **B,** Median nerve. **C,** Ulnar nerve. (From Jenkins DB: *Hollinshead's functional anatomy of the limbs and back,* ed 6, Philadelphia 1991, WB Saunders.)

TABLE 2-3

Location and Motion of Rotator Cuff Muscles

MUSCLE	LOCATION	MOTION
Supraspinatus	*Proximal attachment:* Supraspinous fossa of scapula *Distal attachment:* Superior facet of greater tubercle of humerus	Abduction and rotation
Subscapularis	*Proximal attachment:* Subscapular fossa *Distal attachment:* Lesser tubercle of humerus	Medial rotation and adduction
Infraspinatus	*Proximal attachment:* Infraspinous fossa of scapula *Distal attachment:* Middle facet of greater tubercle of humerus	Lateral rotation
Teres minor	*Proximal attachment:* Superior part of lateral border of scapula *Distal attachment:* Inferior facet of greater tubercle of humerus	Lateral rotation

SCENARIO 4

If You were to Perform A Manual Muscle Test by Assessing Nerve Function, Which Muscles would be Evaluated for the Median, the Ulnar, and the Radial Nerve Distributions? Why would it be Useful to Evaluate These Muscles by This Grouping?

Manual muscle tests frequently are performed by evaluating the synergistic action of muscle groups, such as wrist extension or finger flexion. However, manual muscle testing can be a valuable tool for viewing muscle function from other perspectives. A new therapist may identify unrecognized impairments of the upper extremity caused by muscle imbalances arising from a condition such as peripheral neuropathy.

The findings of a manual muscle test are more precise when the test involves muscles innervated by various nerve distributions. Fig. 2-3, A, shows the distribution of the muscles associated with the axial and radial nerves. It is important to note that more than finger, as well as wrist extension, can be involved in impairments in this area, especially with trauma to the nerve proximal to the elbow, such as in the midhumeral or brachial plexus regions. The muscles evaluated should include wrist and finger extensors and the muscles responsible primarily for elbow extension, elbow flexion with the forearm in midposition (i.e., forearm in neutral position), supination, and thumb extension/abduction.

The same approach can be used to identify the muscles innervated by the median nerve (Fig. 2-3, *B*). Note that the pronator teres and several extrinsic muscles (muscles that originate outside the hand and have tendons that cross the wrist) are innervated by the median nerve. In some cases the musculotendinous units can cross the elbow, forearm, wrist, fingers, and thumb. The median nerve also innervates several intrinsic muscles (muscles that originate in the hand). These muscles potentially may provide movement to the thumb, index finger, and middle fingers. Fig. 2-3, *C*, shows the muscles innervated by the ulnar nerve. Motor function is supplied to a wrist flexor, finger flexors to the ring and little fingers, and to many intrinsic muscles of the fingers and thumb. Delineating patterns of weakness based on nerve distribution presents a picture of function very different from that obtained from a generalized manual muscle test.

SCENARIO 5

If You were to Identify the Muscles That Originate on the Lateral and Medial Epicondyles, Which Muscles would They be? Why would it be Useful to Evaluate These Muscles by This Grouping?

Even though all muscles that originate from the lateral epicondyle are innervated by the radial nerve, a different picture of function can be obtained by evaluating each muscle individually. Evaluating each individual muscle in this grouping can be useful because these muscles commonly are overused, and they may require a longer recovery time than muscles surrounded by sheaths that bathe them in cooling lubricants.

When you test the muscles that originate from the lateral epicondyle, keep in mind that full joint motion, muscle and connective tissue pliability, and muscle strength are critical for full function. Muscle insufficiency occurs when the full length of a muscle is compromised; this can result in limited range of motion for many joints and reduced muscle strength.[6] A knowledge of the origin of a muscle and the joints it crosses from origin to insertion is critical to understanding the function of that muscle. For example, to obtain a full passive stretch of the extensor digitorum communis muscle, the elbow must be extended, the forearm must be pronated, the wrist must be flexed, and the fingers must be in a fisted

position. The muscles that originate from the lateral epicondyle, their origin, their action, and the positions in which full musculotendinous flexibility can be achieved are presented in Table 2-4.[7]

The muscles that originate from the medial epicondyle present a different picture of function (Table 2-5).[7] These muscles all are innervated by the median nerve except for the flexor carpi ulnaris muscle, which is supplied by the ulnar nerve. Despite the different nerve innervations, the same principles apply for stretching these muscles as were suggested for the muscles originating from the lateral epicondyle. For example, to obtain a full passive stretch of the flexor digitorum superficialis, the elbow must be extended, the forearm must be supinated, the wrist must be extended, and the fingers must be in a fully extended position.

SCENARIO 6

If You were to Check the Excursion of the Extensor and Flexor Tendons to the Fingers, You would find That the Location and the Type of Supportive Structures Affect Movement in What Ways?

You have learned that a muscle, such as the extensor digitorum communis, can cross the elbow, forearm, wrist, and fingers. In addition to these anatomic descriptions, a classification system has been developed to identify the location of the extensor tendons, as well as other structures that can affect tendon gliding. The seven zones of the extensor tendons to the fingers and thumb are presented in Fig. 2-4. In the most proximal zones (zones VI and VII), which is made up of the dorsum of the hand and wrist, the influence of an extensor tendon crossing multiple joints is important. Within this area, other important contributors to the function of extensor tendon gliding are the six compartments created by the deep layers of the dorsal fascia. Fig. 2-5 shows the tendons in each of the numbered dorsal compartments of the wrist. Testing the independent movement of each extensor tendon by compartment provides a picture of the effectiveness of tendon excursion through the dorsal pulley system and can supplement the findings of a more generic range of motion or manual muscle test.

Similarly, an appreciation of the extensor tendons to the fingers in zones I through V provide a different perspective on the way location can affect function. In Fig. 2-6 the extensor mechanism of a finger proximal interphalangeal (PIP) joint is presented in a dorsal view and in a lateral view with digital metacarpophalangeal (MP) joint flexion and extension. This shows the balance that must be achieved between the intrinsic and extrinsic muscle groups to allow full extension of a digit.

TABLE 2-4

Muscles Originating from the Lateral Epicondyle

MUSCLE	ORIGIN	ACTION	POSITION FOR FULL MUSCULOTENDINOUS FLEXIBILITY
Anconeus	Lateral and posterior surfaces of proximal half of body of humerus, and lateral intermuscular septum	Extends the elbow	Elbow flexion, forearm pronation
Brachioradialis	Proximal two thirds of lateral supracondylar ridge of humerus and lateral intermuscular septum	Flexes the elbow, assists with pronating and supinating the forearm	Elbow extension, forearm pronation or supination
Supinator	Lateral epicondyle of humerus, radial collateral ligament of elbow joint, annular ligament of radius, and supinator crest of ulna	Supinates the forearm	Elbow extension, forearm pronation
Extensor carpi radialis longus	Distal one third of lateral supracondylar ridge of humerus and lateral intermuscular septum	Extends the wrist in a radial direction, assists with elbow flexion	Elbow extension, forearm pronation, wrist flexion in an ulnar direction
Extensor carpi radialis brevis	Lateral epicondyle of humerus, radial collateralligament of elbow, and deep antebrachial fossa	Extends the wrist, assists with wrist radial deviation	Elbow extension, forearm pronation, wrist flexion
Extensor carpi ulnaris	Lateral epicondyle of humerus, aponeurosis from posterior border of ulna, and deep antebrachial fossa	Extends the wrist in an ulnar direction	Elbow extension, forearm pronation, wrist flexion in a radial direction
Extensor digitorum communis	Lateral epicondyle of humerus and deep antebrachial fossa	Extends the metacarpophalangeal (MP) joints of the second through fifth digits; in conjunction with the lumbricals and interossei, extends the proximal interphalangeal (PIP) joints of the second through fifth digits; assists with abduction of the index, ring, and little fingers; and assists with extension of the wrist in a radial direction	Elbow extension; forearm pronation; wrist flexion; and MP, PIP, and distal interphalangeal (DIP) flexion of the fingers
Extensor digitorum minimi	Lateral epicondyles of humerus and deep antebrachial fossa	Extends the MP joint of the fifth digit; in conjunction with the lumbricals and interossei, extends the PIP joints of the fifth digit; assists with abduction of the fifth finger	Elbow extension; forearm pronation; wrist flexion; and MP, PIP, and DIP flexion of the little finger

TABLE 2-5

Muscles Originating from the Medial Epicondyle

MUSCLE	ORIGIN	ACTION	POSITION FOR FULL MUSCULOTENDINOUS FLEXIBILITY
Pronator teres	Medial epicondyle of humerus, common flexor tendon, and deep antebrachial fascia	Pronates the forearm, assists with elbow flexion	Elbow extension, forearm supination
Flexor carpi radialis	Common flexor tendon of medial epicondyle of humerus and deep antebrachial fascia	Flexes the wrist in a radial direction; may assist with pronation of the forearm and elbow flexion	Elbow extension, forearm supination, wrist extension in an ulnar direction
Flexor carpi ulnaris	Common flexor tendon of medial epicondyle of humerus	Flexes the wrist in an ulnar direction; may assist with elbow flexion	Elbow extension, forearm supination, wrist extension in a radial direction
Palmaris longus	Common flexor tendon of medial epicondyle of humerus and deep antebrachial fascia	Tenses the palmar fascia, flexes the wrist, and may assist with elbow flexion	Elbow extension, forearm supination, wrist extension
Flexor digitorum superficialis	Common flexor tendon of medial epicondyle of humerus, ulnar collateral ligament of elbow, and deep antebrachial fascia	Flexes the proximal interphalageal (PIP) joints of the second through fifth digits; assists with metacarpophalangeal (MP) and wrist flexion	Elbow extension; forearm supination; wrist extension; and MP, PIP, and distal interphalangeal (DIP) extension of the fingers

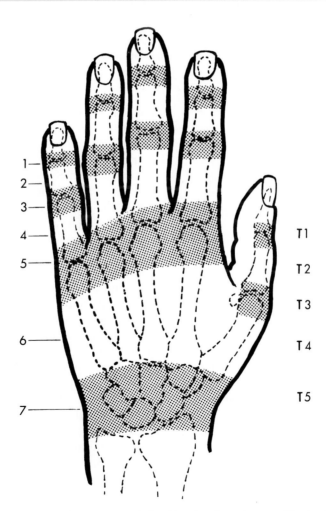

FIGURE 2-4 Extensor tendon zones as defined by the Committee on Tendon Injuries for the International Federation of the Societies for Surgery of the Hand. (From Kleinert HE, Schepel S, Gill T: *Surg Clin North Am* 61:267, 1981.)

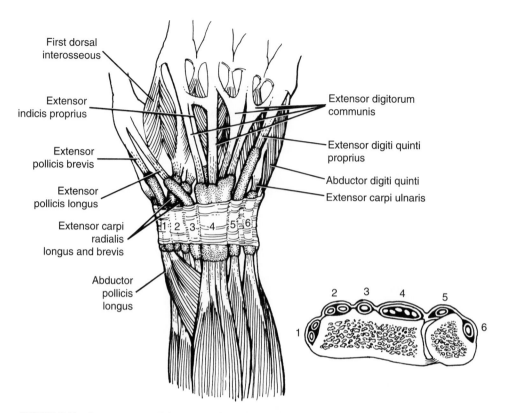

First dorsal
interosseous

Extensor
indicis proprius

Extensor
pollicis brevis

Extensor
pollicis longus

Extensor carpi
radialis
longus and brevis

Abductor
pollicis
longus

Extensor digitorum
communis

Extensor digiti quinti
proprius

Abductor digiti quinti

Extensor carpi ulnaris

FIGURE 2-5 Arrangement of the extensor tendons in the compartments of the wrist. (From Fess EE et al: *Hand and upper extremity splinting: principles and methods,* ed 3, St Louis, 2004, Mosby.)

CLINICAL *Pearl*

To assess the contribution of the extrinsic muscles to PIP extension, stabilize the wrist and MP joints in extension; in this position, the power of the intrinsic muscles is minimized.

When the PIP joint is held in extension and the distal interphalangeal (DIP) joint is actively flexed, a passive stretch to the lateral bands is completed; this ultimately facilitates balanced extension between the PIP and DIP joints. A knowledge of the extensor tendon anatomy, the location of these tendons by zone, and the surrounding structures is an important component of the therapist's skill in assessing conditions of the hand.

The finger flexors have similarities and differences with regard to the extensor tendons. Fig. 2-7 shows the five flexor tendon zones to the fingers and the three flexor tendon zones to the thumb. Flexor tendons located in zone V are located proximal to the carpal canal and are not subject to many of the challenges that affect the excursion of flexor tendons in other zones of the hand. Zone IV includes the structures in the carpal tunnel; Fig. 2-8 provides a cross-sectional view of the carpal tunnel

anatomy. To examine the excursion of the flexor tendons at this level, start your assessment with the superficial tendons and progress to the tendons in the deeper compartments of the carpal tunnel. The flexor digitorum superficialis (FDS) to the middle and ring fingers is the most superficial structure, followed by the FDS to the index and little fingers, and finally the flexor digitorum profundus (FDP) to all the fingers. Two other compartments are contained within the carpal tunnel, the flexor pollicis longus and the median nerve, and the synovium that encases and lubricates the flexor tendons. Overall, isolating the excursion of these tendons by compartments can be useful, because more superficial injuries, such as burns, may have a greater effect on the FDS than would a deeper injury, such as a fracture to the distal one third of the radius.

Other considerations become evident in flexor tendon zones I through III. In zone III, the flexor tendons are not encased in a lubricating sheath, and injuries to the area may involve the lumbrical muscle. In zones I and II, the relationship between the FDP and the FDS changes. Before entering zone II, the FDP lies deep to the FDS. In zone II, the FDP passes through the decussation of the FDS (Fig. 2-9). Therefore isolating a tendon is very important to assess its excursion.

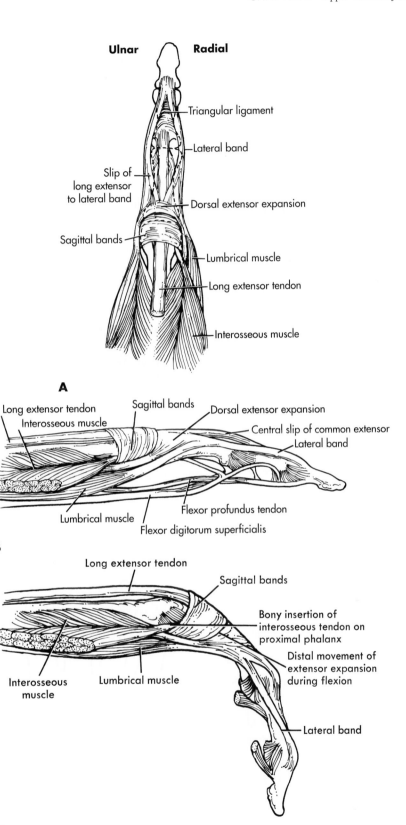

Ulnar   **Radial**

Triangular ligament

Lateral band

Slip of long extensor to lateral band

Dorsal extensor expansion

Sagittal bands

Lumbrical muscle

Long extensor tendon

Interosseous muscle

A

Long extensor tendon
Interosseous muscle

Sagittal bands

Dorsal extensor expansion

Central slip of common extensor

Lateral band

Lumbrical muscle

Flexor profundus tendon

Flexor digitorum superficialis

B

Long extensor tendon

Sagittal bands

Bony insertion of interosseous tendon on proximal phalanx

Distal movement of extensor expansion during flexion

Interosseous muscle

Lumbrical muscle

Lateral band

C

FIGURE 2-6   Extensor mechanism of the digits. The figure shows distal movement of the extensor expansion with metacarpophalangeal joint flexion. (From Fess EE et al: *Hand and upper extremity splinting: principles and methods*, ed 3, St Louis, 2004, Mosby.)

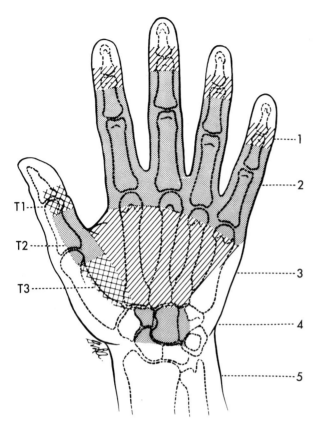

FIGURE 2-7   Flexor tendon zones of the hand. (From Kleinert HE, Schepel S, Gill T: *Surg Clin North Am* 61:267, 1981.)

When you test the FDS, eliminate the effects of the FDP by holding the DIPs of the nontested fingers in extension and allowing each individual finger to actively flex at only the PIP joint.

To test the FDP, support the PIP joint in extension to allow only DIP flexion. In this way, isolated range of motion exercises can be performed to facilitate the independent function of these two important flexor tendons to the hand.

SCENARIO 7

What are the Major Structures that Support the Wrist, Fingers, and Thumb? How Do They Change in Different Positions of Movement and How Do They Contribute to the Strength of the Wrist and Hand?

The collateral ligaments provide joint stability while functional activities occur within multiple planes of movement. Fig. 2-10 shows the ligamentous anatomy of the wrist. The palmar wrist ligaments provide support between the carpal bones. The dorsal wrist ligaments provide support between the carpal bones and the radius.

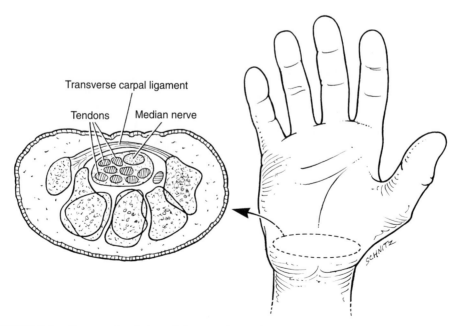

FIGURE 2-8   Cross-sectional view of the carpal tunnel anatomy. (From Fess EE et al: *Hand and upper extremity splinting: principles and methods,* ed 3, St Louis, 2004, Mosby.)

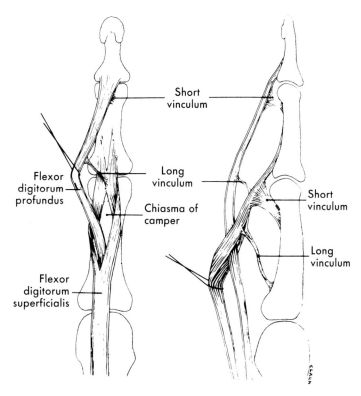

FIGURE 2-9 The flexor digitorum superficially lies volar to the flexor digitorum profundus as the tendons enter the sheath. (From Schneider LH: *Flexor tendon injuries,* Boston, 1985, Little, Brown.)

The palmar radioscaphoid lunate ligament provides support for the radius, the scaphoid, and the lunate. The triangular fibrocartilage complex (TFCC) provides support between the carpal bones, the ulna, and the distal radial-ulnar joint. Each of the supporting structures is important for stabilizing the wrist in extreme ranges of wrist extension, flexion, radial deviation, and ulnar deviation.[8] The stability of the joint affects more than just mobility; without adequate support on the ulnar border of the wrist, the amount of pinch strength can be diminished.

The ligamentous structures in the fingers differ considerably from those of the wrist. Fig. 2-11 presents the supporting structures of the finger MP and PIP joints. The collateral ligament is designed to ensure lateral support. When the MP joint is flexed, the collateral ligament lengthens to accommodate the movement; when the joint is in an extended position, the collateral ligament becomes slack. Essentially the opposite process occurs at the PIP joint. (See Chapters 15 and 23 for splinting implications related to collateral ligament length.)

In addition to the lateral support of a joint, volar reinforcement is provided through strong membranous

connections with the collateral ligament. The palmar plates (also called *volar plates*) are slack in flexion but become taut when the joint is extended, thereby protecting the joint from hyperextension stress or dislocation.

The thumb has ligamentous supports at the interphalangeal (IP) joint, the MP joint, and the carpometacarpal (CMC) joint. The ulnar collateral ligament (UCL) of the MP joint is particularly noteworthy. The location of the UCL suggests the importance of this strong band of tissue in supporting pinch, especially lateral pinch. (See Chapter 15 for treatment implications related to the thumb MP collateral ligaments.)

SUMMARY

It is critical that therapists understand the roles *and* interrelationships of nerves, vascular systems, muscles, tendons, and ligaments in order to appreciate the mechanisms of hand function. Continuing study and application of knowledge are vital if you are to provide the level of rehabilitation expertise needed to help these clients recover from the devastating effects of injury, disease, and aging.

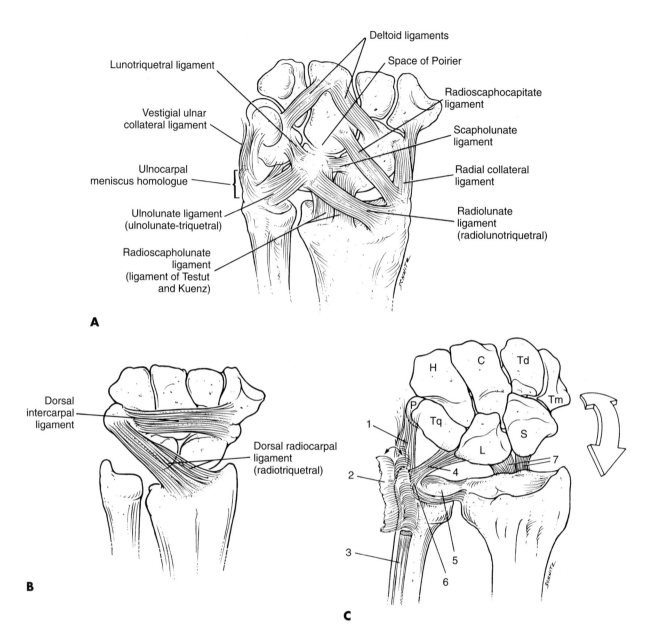

FIGURE 2-10 Ligamentous anatomy of the wrist. **A,** Palmar wrist ligaments. **B,** Dorsal wrist ligaments. **C,** Dorsal view of the flexed wrist, including the triangular fibrocartilage. *1,* Ulnar collateral ligament; *2,* retinacular sheath; *3,* tendon of extensor carpi ulnaris; *4,* ulnolunate ligament; *5,* triangular fibrocartilage; *6,* ulnocarpal meniscus homologue; *7,* palmar radioscaphoid lunate ligament. *P,* Pisiform; *H,* hamate; *C,* capitate; *Td,* trapezoid; *Tm,* trapezium; *Tq,* triquetrum; *L,* lunate; *S,* scaphoid. (From Fess EE et al: *Hand and upper extremity splinting: principles and methods,* ed 3, St Louis, 2004, Mosby.)

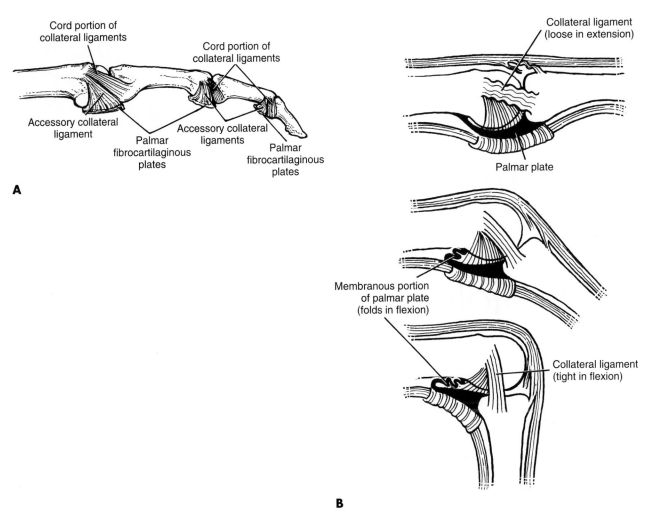

FIGURE 2-11 A, Ligamentous structures of the digital joints. **B,** At the metacarpophalangeal joint level, the collateral ligaments are loose in exertion but tighten in flexion. (**A** from Fess EE et al: *Hand and upper extremity splinting: principles and methods,* ed 3, St Louis, 2004, Mosby; **B** modified from Wynn Perry CB et al: Rehabilitation of the hand. In Fess EE et al: *Hand and upper extremity splinting: principles and methods,* ed 3, St Louis, 2004, Mosby.)

References

1. Miller S, Perrotti W, Silverthorn D et al: From college to clinic: reasoning over memorization is key for understanding anatomy, *Anat Rec* 269:69-80, 2002.
2. Magee D: *Orthopedic physical assessment,* ed 4, Philadelphia, 2002, WB Saunders.
3. Schafer R: Cervical spine trauma, monograph 22, manuscript prepublication copyright 1999.
4. Lundy-Ekman L: *Neuroscience: fundamentals for rehabilitation,* ed 2, New York, 2002, WB Saunders.
5. Jacobs M, Austin N: *Splinting the hand and upper extremity: principles and process,* Baltimore, 2003, Lippincott Williams & Wilkins.
6. Rybski M: *Kinesiology for occupational therapy,* Thorofare, NJ, 2004, Slack.
7. Kendall F, McCreary E: *Muscles: testing and function,* ed 5, Baltimore, 2005, Williams & Wilkins.
8. Fess E, Gettle K, Phillips C et al: *Hand and upper extremity splinting: principles and methods,* ed 3, St Louis, 2005, Mosby.

3

Edema Reduction Techniques: A Biologic Rationale for Selection

SANDRA ARTZBERGER

Editors Notes: Before the importance of Sandra Artzberger's work on the treatment of edema was recognized, the edema techniques that hand therapists were taught were not specific to the lymphatic system and sometimes even damaged this delicate and amazing part of the body. Artzberger has done much to delineate the anatomy and physiology of posttraumatic edema. She has changed our thinking and has overhauled the treatment repertoire, creating an approach that is based on science. Her technique of manual edema mobilization has resulted in much-improved management of edema in clients with upper extremity injuries.

Unlike in the past, the treatment of hand edema no longer needs to be partly a guessing game. Modern treatment selections are more firmly grounded in anatomic and biologic principles and therefore are more successful. To treat edema effectively, the therapist must know the difference between the lymphatic and venous systems, including the role these systems play in edema reduction. It also is essential that the therapist understand the different types of edema. This chapter describes acute, subacute, and chronic edema. It reviews vascular and lymphatic anatomy and biology, and it describes appropriate interventions for edema, including the technique of **manual edema mobilization (MEM).** Special emphasis is placed on the clinical reasoning involved in selecting the appropriate treatment.

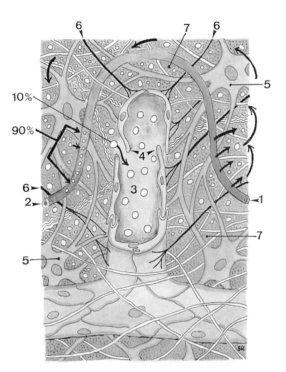

FIGURE 3-1 Incorporation of the lymph capillary into the interstitium. *1,* Arterial section of the blood capillary; *2,* Venous section of the blood capillary; *3,* Lymph capillary; *4,* Open intercellular groove-swinging tip; *5,* Fibrocyte; *6,* Anchor filaments; *7,* Intercellular space. Small arrows indicate the direction of blood flow; large arrows indicate the direction of intercellular fluid flow. (From Foldi M, Foldi E, Kubik S: *Textbook of lymphology for physicians and lymphedema therapists,* Munich, 2003, Urban & Fischer Verlag.)

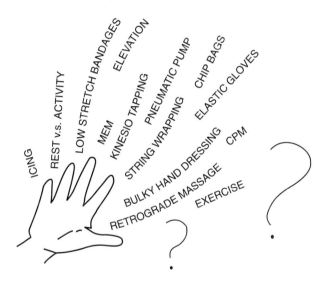

OVERVIEW OF ANATOMIC INTERSTITIAL CAPILLARIES: VENOUS AND LYMPHATIC CAPILLARIES

An overview of the capillary vascular structures and their relationship to each other is a prerequisite for a more detailed discussion of these systems. The vascular structures include the interstitium, the arteriole, and the venule. The **interstitium** is the space between cells. It contains both the smallest arterial vessel, called an **arteriole,** and the smallest venous structure, called a **venule.**[1,2] Both the arteriole and the venule terminate in capillaries, which are joined histologically (Fig. 3-1). The heart is responsible for pumping blood through these structures.

The lymphatic system originates in the interstitium with the smallest of the lymphatic vessels, called the **initial lymphatic** or **lymphatic capillary,** and culminates in the largest lymphatic structure, called the **thoracic duct.**[2] The venous system has a continuous-loop pump system, but the lymphatic system does not (Fig. 3-2).[3] Therefore the lymphatic system must be stimulated to activate a *force pump,* creating a vacuum and drawing the lymph proximally.[3] Initial lymphatics, which are larger than venules, are finger-shaped tubes that are closed on the distal end and lined with overlapping, oak leaf–shaped endothelial cells. Anchor filaments extend from the endothelial cells to the connective tissue. Movement of the connective tissue pulls on the anchor filaments. This, in turn, pulls on the overlapping flaps (junctions) of the endothelial cells, and water and large molecules are admitted into the initial lymphatic. Large molecules also enter the initial lymphatic when a change in the interstitial pressure causes the junctions of the endothelial cells to spread apart. The initial lymphatic connection forms a netlike structure (see Fig. 3-1).[1-3]

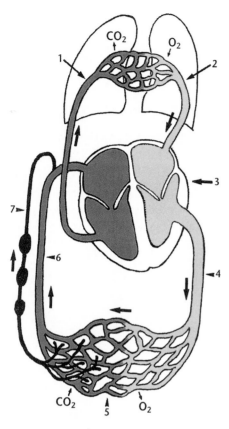

1 Pulmonary artery ⎫
2 Pulmonary veins ⎬ pulmonary circulation
3 Heart
4 Aorta – arterial system ⎫
5 Capillaries   ⎬ systemic circulation
6 Venous system   ⎭
7 Lymph vessels and lymph nodes

FIGURE 3-2 Blood and lymph circulatory systems. (From Foldi M, Foldi E, Kubik S: *Textbook of lymphology for physicians and lymphedema therapists*, Munich, 2003, Urban & Fischer Verlag.)

The balance between fluid moving into and out of the vascular vessels on a cellular level, first described by Ernest Starling in the early 1900s, is called **Starling's equilibrium.**[1,2] This balanced movement of fluid functions as a gradient system from high to low pressure. On the capillary level, **arteriole hydrostatic pressure** (the pressure of the blood fluid exerted on the arteriole vessel wall) is 30 to 40 mm Hg, which is enough pressure to cause filtration of electrolytes, fluid, a few small plasma proteins, and other nutrients into the interstitium.[1,2] The **osmotic pressure** (also called the **oncotic pressure**) in the interstitium is determined by the concentration of proteins in this intercellular space; this pressure is approximately 25 mm Hg.[2] Tissue cells in the interstitium absorb the nutrients, electrolytes, and other substances filtered out of the arteriole. Of the remaining substances, 90% diffuse by osmosis into the venous

system.[1-3] The residual 10% of leftover substances are large molecules, which are absorbed by the lymphatic system.[1-3] These large molecules consist of plasma proteins, minerals, ions, hormone cells, bacteria, fat cells, and fluid.[1-4] Once the cells enter the initial lymphatic, they make up a substance called **lymph** (see Fig. 3-1).[2]

ACUTE EDEMA RELATED TO THE VASCULAR ANATOMY

The venous and lymphatic systems have many pumplike structures that help propel the blood back to the heart. Because of the descending gradient of hydrostatic pressures from the arteriole capillary to the venule capillary, small-molecule substances diffuse easily and are reabsorbed into the venous capillary through its thin wall.[2] Active muscle contraction acts as a pump as it compresses and empties the large deep venous vessels. As this blood is propelled proximally toward the heart, a negative pressure is created, which draws blood from the periphery into the deep veins.

Edema develops when the descending gradient of Starling's forces are disrupted by an interruption and an imbalance. The cascade of events that occurs after tissue laceration is a good example. Initially, an outflow of water and electrolytes **(transudate edema)** into the wound occurs. The mast cells then release histamines, which greatly increase capillary permeability, and plasma proteins, phagocytic cells, and other substances leak into the area. Plasma protein fibrinogen is converted to fibrin, which plugs the endothelial cells lining the lymphatics.[5] This prevents the lymphatics from temporarily removing the large molecules as the various **phagocyte cells** perform their "cleanup" function.[5] Edema results when excess fluid and plasma proteins are trapped in the interstitium. Starling's equilibrium is disrupted, because the trapping of excess proteins in the interstitium increases the osmotic pressure.

The immediate goal of treatment by physicians and therapists is to limit the amount of outflow into the wound bed, thereby preventing excessive swelling, accumulation of blood, and further tissue damage. After 2 to 5 days, the swelling begins to subside as the surrounding intact venous capillaries start to absorb the transudate and the lymphatic vessels absorb the large-molecule plasma proteins not phagocytized by the **macrophages.**

Reduction Techniques for Acute Edema

Bulky Dressing

Several techniques can be used to reduce excessive fluid outflow (edema). For example, a bulky hand dressing applied at the time of surgery gives counterforce to the outflow (filtration) by changing the tissue pressure. It is composed of appropriate wound care dressing, fluffy gauge sponges, and rolled-on gauze. After soft tissue trauma, immobilization for up to a week in a bulky dressing or plaster splint facilitates healing of involved structures by preventing stress on fragile tissue, which could cause microscopic rupture of vessels with resulting edema. The therapist should check the dressing or splint to make sure it is not too tight and should contact the physician immediately if this is a possibility. A bulky dressing that is too tight causes vascular changes, temperature changes, increased edema, or severe, painful compression of the fingers and can lead to tissue breakdown. The capillary refill test can be used to check vascular status (see Chapter 5). The therapist also must teach the client that any vascular changes (i.e., changes in tissue color) or sensory changes must be reported immediately to the physician. Procedures such as tenolysis and flexor tendon repair involve minimal or no immobilization in a bulky dressing. However, even with these diagnoses, limited motion can increase edema, therefore early motion must be balanced with rest to prevent this. In an animal study, high-voltage pulse current (HVPC) used on very acute edema was reported to retard the high capillary permeability outflow.[6] This finding has not yet been replicated in human subjects. (HVPC is discussed later in the chapter.)

Elevation

Elevation of the hand above the heart, if not contraindicated, also reduces outflow because it reduces the arterial hydrostatic pressure.[7] Elevation in the acute stage facilitates lymphatic flow because hydrostatic gradient pressure is increased along the lymphatic trunks.[8] Ideally, the involved extremity is elevated in a plus 45-degree "ski hill" position; this means that pillows are placed such that the elbow is above the shoulder, and the hand is above the elbow and wrist.

Keeping the arm elevated while sleeping can be difficult. Often clients use pillows on either side of them. A belt can be fastened around the pillows to keep them together. Also, the bed can be moved against the wall so that one set of pillows is pushed up against the wall, preventing them from falling. For clients with finger replantation, elevation no higher than the heart is recommended to avoid compromising arterial blood flow.[9]

Precaution. *Extreme elevation of the right arm must be avoided in stroke clients with right-sided heart weakness. Extreme upper extremity elevation may cause fluid to flow too quickly into the right side of the heart, because the right upper quadrant is drained by the right lymphatic duct that empties into the right subclavian vein.*

Cold Packs

Cold packs, if not contraindicated for vascular and tissue ischemia reasons, cause vasoconstriction and thus reduce the outflow of fluid in the acute stage. However, the temperature of the cold pack is a consideration. Research shows that when the temperature is lower than 59° F (15° C), proteins leak into the interstitium from lymphatic structures.[10] Excess proteins in the interstitium cause edema.

Precaution. *To prevent "ice burn" to tissue, always place a dry towel between the skin and the cold pack. Cold packs should not be used on a client with a replanted hand or digit because of the effect of vascular compromise on tissue viability.[11] A nerve repair may be injured by cold postoperatively. Clients should get explicit care instructions from their physicians, including precautions on the use of cold packs.*

Retrograde Massage

Light retrograde massage with elevation facilitates diffusion of small molecules into the venous system. The elevation reduces capillary filtration (outflow) pressure, and the light pressure from the retrograde massage aids in venous absorption of the small molecules.

Precaution. *The pressure is kept light to avoid damaging the single-cell initial lymphatic structures in the dermal layer of the skin.*

Compression

Light compression, such as from an elastic glove, Coban lightly spiral-layered on a digit (see Fig. 3-6, A, on CD), or low-stretch finger bandage wraps (see Fig. 3-6, B, on CD), facilitates small molecule absorption by the venous system and absorption of large and small molecules by the lymphatic system. A loose but compressive glove generally is one in which the glove material can be pulled away from the hand and fingers at least $^1/_8$ inch (see Figure 3-6, C, on CD).

Precaution. *An elastic glove should be fitted to give some compression but should feel loose on the hand and fingers. If the compression is too tight, fluid flow is restricted, which increases edema.*

Kinesio Tape also promotes absorption of the large and small molecules in the interstitium because it increases the space between the skin and connective tissue (see Fig. 3-6, D, on CD).[12] Increasing this space creates a pull on the connective tissue anchor filaments attached to the endothelial cells of the initial lymphatics; this separates the planted endothelial junctions, thereby increasing lymph and fluid flow.

Indications for Manual Edema Mobilization

Many wonder why MEM is not started in the acute stage. In 1989, Hutzschenreuter and Brummer[13] did a research study on this point using sheep. They compared the results in two groups, one in which **manual lymphatic drainage (MLD)** was performed and one in which it was not, over a defined period (i.e., immediate postoperative to 3 weeks postoperative). They found that both groups showed minimal fluid reduction during the first week after surgery. However, after the first week, the MLD group had a significantly greater increase in fluid movement and edema reduction than the control group.[13] These results are not surprising because initially, acute edema is transudate that is changing to **exudate edema** as the plasma proteins invade and are contained. Only the lymphatic vessels can remove excess proteins from the interstitium. MEM and **manual lymphatic treatment (MLT)*** programs are designed to activate lymphatic vessels. A multicenter study compared the results of retrograde massage with those of MEM in clients with subacute edema from a wrist injury 4 weeks after injury.[14] The study found that both groups showed improvement, but the MEM group showed statistically greater improvement in all but one category.

CLINICAL *Pearl*

Remember, edema at 4 weeks is subacute and has a high protein content. To be successful in these cases, reduction treatment must stimulate the lymphatics.

Some physicians prescribe proximal active motion of an extremity or gliding of the involved structures, or both, during the acute stage of wound healing. Proximal trunk and shoulder motion is excellent. It decongests the lymphatic vessels and removes tissue waste products, resulting in better oxygenation to tissue and faster wound healing. However, movement must be balanced with rest of involved structures. This is done by progressively grading the exercise so as not to increase hand inflammation, pain, and swelling. Always respect the fragility of healing tissue and vascular structures. When moving the involved structures, start with limited movement and check for signs of increased pain, swelling, or redness. If edema increases, rest the involved hand for a day (consider applying a static splint). Resume activity, but do less than previously and gradually increase the exercise over the next treatment sessions. I usually begin with the *rule of three or five:* three (or five) repetitions of an exercise three (or five) times a day. If this does not increase swelling, gradually increase repetitions or frequency, or both. Remember, edema and pain limit motion and retard progress.

Manual lymphatic treatment is the generic term used to describe the massage principles common to all schools of lymphatic drainage.[15]

CLINICAL *Pearl*

Reducing edema is almost always the first priority; do this, and the client will gain motion.

In the early poststroke stages, hand and arm edema is a transudate swelling because fluid leaks into the interstitium as a result of lack of muscle pumping activity on the vascular vessels. Elevation, light retrograde massage, and light compression from an elastic glove or elasticized arm stockinette are effective treatments that promote diffusion of leaked electrolytes and water back into the venous system.

Precaution. *When using an elasticized garment, observe two important precautions: (1) make sure it is not too tight (i.e., it does not cause color or temperature changes in the hand or digit) and (2) with elasticized stockinette, make sure it cannot roll down, causing swelling distally.*

A body garment glue can be used to prevent the elastic stockinette from rolling down on itself, which can cause distal swelling. Keep in mind that some body garment glues are latex based, therefore always make sure your client does not have a latex allergy before using such a glue.

Summary of Reduction Treatment for Acute Edema

- Bulky hand dressing (usually applied by the surgeon postoperatively)
- High-voltage pulse current (HVPC) (used only for very acute edema; benefit in humans not yet proven)
- Elevation
  - Lesser degree of elevation is needed for replanted digits and/or hands.
  - Extreme elevation is contraindicated if right-sided heart weakness is present (i.e., poststroke client).
- Cold packs (used in the first 24 to 48 hours only as directed by physician)
  - Cold packs should not be used for replants because cold causes vasoconstriction.
  - Precautions should be clarified with physician if a nerve is involved.
- Light retrograde massage
- Loose elastic glove or elastic stockinette
- Coban (loosely placed on digit in spiral, distal-to-proximal pattern)
- Finger bandage wraps
- Limited active motion of uninvolved areas (excessive trunk/shoulder motion increases edema)
- Balance of activity and rest for all structures to prevent inflammation or increase in edema

SUBACUTE AND CHRONIC EDEMA RELATED TO THE LYMPHATIC ANATOMY

As mentioned earlier, the initial lymphatic capillary (initial lymphatic) is the lymphatic system's smallest structure. The initial lymphatic is not connected to the venous or arterial system. As described previously, the initial lymphatic is composed of finger-shaped tubes that are closed on the distal end and lined with overlapping, oak leaf–shaped endothelial cells; these tubes are connected to each other in a netlike structure in the dermal layer of the skin (see Fig. 3-1).[1-4] The lymphatic system is also a negative-pressure pump system that absorbs large molecules out of the interstitium ending in the venous system at either the right or left subclavian vein.

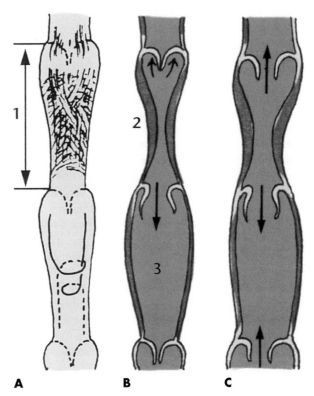

FIGURE 3-3 Structure and function of the valve segments in the collector lymphatics. **A,** Arrangement of the musculature. **B,** Normal function. **C,** Dilated lymph vessel with valvular insufficiency and reflux. (From Foldi M, Foldi E, Kubik S: *Textbook of lymphology for physicians and lymphedema therapists,* Munich, 2003, Urban & Fischer Verlag.)

CLINICAL *Pearl*

The anatomic differences between the lymphatic and venous systems determine the anatomically based treatment of edema.

The lymphatic system does not have a continuous pump system, such as the venous system and the heart (see Fig. 3-2). Also, unlike with venous capillaries in the interstitium, molecules do not diffuse into the lymphatic capillary. Rather, large molecules that cannot permeate the venous system are absorbed into the initial lymphatic when pressure changes in the interstitium cause the junctions of the endothelial cells to spread apart.[2,3] Then the large molecule substances (plasma proteins, fat cells, bacteria, hormones, tissue waste products, ions), and the small water molecules move into the lymphatic capillary.[1,2,8] This arrangement is often called a *force pump.*[8]

As lymph enters the initial lymphatic, it causes pressure changes that open the valve connected to the next lymphatic vessels, the three-celled **collector lymphatics** (Figure 3-3). Clinically, the most important features of the tubelike collector lymphatics are a middle layer of muscle cell and the presence of valves every 6 to 8 mm along the tube.[1,3] The chamber between two valves is called a **lymphangion.**[3] As a bolus of lymph enters a lymphangion, the single layer muscle cell contracts against the expanding lymphangion and pushes the bolus proximally into the next lymphangion (Fig. 3-3). This process continues until the bolus reaches the afferent lymphatic pathways of the lymph node.

The pumping movement of the lymphangions resembles the peristaltic movement of the small intestine. The lymphangions pump at a rate of 10 to 20 times per minute,[3] and exercise can increase this pumping motion

by 10 to 30 times.[1] Recent theories hold that peristalsis also creates a negative pressure that opens the junctions of the endothelial cells, enabling large-molecule substances to move from the interstitium into the initial lymphatic.[3]

CLINICAL *Pearl*

Exercise moves lymph faster through the collector lymphatics and increases the rate of lymphatic uptake from the interstitium.

Eventually the bolus of lymph moves into the afferent lymphatic pathways of the **lymph nodes.** Lymph nodes, which perform several immunologic functions, are composed of a series of complex sinuses and therefore often are considered "dams" or "kinks in the hose" in the movement of lymph. Excessive swelling distal to the lymph nodes does not increase their rate of filtration, but rather causes further congestion distally.[8] Venous vessels do not connect to lymph nodes and therefore do not reflect this slowing of fluid movement. Also, venous vessels do not carry bacteria or tissue waste products and therefore do not pass these substances through the lymph nodes for cleansing. Lymph nodes present significant resistance to the flow of lymph and must be massaged to facilitate a faster flow of the distal congested lymph.[8] The MEM method of massaging healthy and uninfected nodes or uses **MEM pump point stimulation,** which is a method of simultaneously massaging two groups of nodes, bundles of lymphatic vessels, or **watershed areas,** which speeds up the movement of lymph through the nodes.

From the nodes, lymph can enter the venous system directly, through **lymphovenous anastomoses** (areas where the small vessels of the lymphatic and venous systems join), or it can continue on in the lymphatic vessels and empty into either the right lymphatic duct or the largest lymphatic vessel, the thoracic duct. The thoracic duct lies anterior to and parallel with the spinal cord from approximately L2 and empties into the left subclavian vein.[2,3] The right lymphatic duct terminates in the right subclavian vein.

The movement of lymph in the thoracic duct is affected by changes in thoracic pressure. **Diaphragmatic breathing** expands the abdomen, causing changes in thoracic pressure that move the contents of the thoracic duct more proximally.[1,3] This action creates a vacuum, drawing lymph from the more distal vessels toward the thoracic duct.[1,3] Treatments such as MEM, therefore, begin with diaphragmatic breathing and trunk exercise. This is analogous to removing the plug from a drain or a clog from a backed-up sink. The clog must be removed before the water can flow out. In terms of clinical application, the vacuum created by diaphragmatic breathing moves lymph more proximal in the thoracic duct, creating a space into which the more distal peripheral edema can move.

CLINICAL *Pearl*

The key to successful edema reduction is to "remove the plug" by starting proximally at the trunk with diaphragmatic breathing and proximal exercise.

Before they reach the thoracic duct, the deep lymphatic trunks share a common vascular sheath with the venous and arterial structures.[3] Therefore exercise increases the rate of arterial flow and passively stimulates the lymphatic vessels, increasing the rate of lymph flow. Also, at least 200 lymph nodes are located centrally and around deep venous and arterial structures. Exercise of the abdominal muscles increases the pumping of blood, which stimulates the lymph nodes, moving lymph through them more rapidly.

"Exercise is key to lymphatic activation"[16]—this is a frequently quoted statement. Yet therapists know that in most cases, simply exercising the edematous hand or arm in the subacute phase does not significantly or permanently reduce edema. Lymphatic structures can exceed 30 times their normal capacity before edema becomes visible[1]; this means that proximal to the visible edema is the beginning of nonvisible edematous congestion.

Exercise and light massage significantly proximal to the visible edema create a negative pressure, drawing lymph proximally and thus removing the "clog." The results of research by Pecking and colleagues[17] present a strong argument for stimulating lymphatic absorption and conduction significantly proximal to visible edema. In these researchers' study, MLD was performed exclusively to the contralateral, normal upper quadrant on 108 women with lymphedema caused by mastectomy; this resulted in a 12% to 38% lymph uptake in the hand, even without massage of the involved area.[17] The contralateral massage created a negative pressure (vacuum), drawing the lymph from the involved to the uninvolved area, where it could be absorbed into the normal system.

If we synthesize these findings with the theory that changes in thoracic pressure move lymph proximally, and add the knowledge that muscle contraction stimulates lymphatic uptake on many levels, we arrive at a very strong rationale for beginning edema reduction at the trunk even if edema is visible only in the hand. Clinically, this means that therapists should not begin edema reduction treatment where edema is visible; rather, they must begin in a normal, uninvolved area significantly proximal to the visible edema. Appropriate treatments include diaphragmatic breathing, trunk stretching and muscle contraction exercises and activities, and MEM massage that begins in the area of the uninvolved axilla. (MEM is discussed in more detail later in the chapter.)

Reduction Techniques for Subacute and Chronic Edema Based on the Lymphatic Anatomy

To review, the lymphatic system is an independent pump system that works on a negative pressure gradient. When lymph vessels fill (high pressure is created), lymph moves to an area of lower pressure.[8,12]

The two keys to activating the lymphatic system are as follows:

CLINICAL *Pearl*

The sooner lymphatic decongestion occurs, even with non-visible edema, the less the chances of developing tissue and scar thickening, fibrosis, and contractures.

1. Proximal, uninvolved lymphatic structures must be stimulated (massaged), creating a lower negative pressure to draw the most proximal edema out of the involved area.
2. Molecules are absorbed into the lymphatics from the interstitium because only changes in the interstitial fluid pressure (low to high) cause the endothelial cells lining the lymphatics to open.

Key 1 is based on the theory that negative pressure causes a suction effect that moves the more distal lymph proximally in the trunk and extremities.[1,3] Appropriate treatments to achieve this include MEM massage that starts at the uninvolved axilla, diaphragmatic breathing, trunk exercise, trunk exercise combined with breathing, proprioceptive neuromuscular facilitation (PNF) techniques combined with exhaling and inhaling, and easy yoga trunk stretching exercises.

Key 2 facilitates the uptake of lymph from the interstitium by creating changes in the interstitial pressure; by causing stretching of the anchor filaments attached to connective tissue; and by creating negative pressure, which causes the opening of lymphatics through lymphangion pumping. Appropriate treatments to achieve this include MEM, Kinesio Taping, gentle myofascial release (MFR), bombardment of tissue with fluidotherapy particles at a machine temperature *no higher than 98° F (36.7° C)*, continuous passive motion (CPM) machine therapy, and active and passive exercise. The movement and slight compression of a *loose* elastic glove or elastic stockinette causes interstitial pressure changes and lymphatic absorption. It is critical to absorption that the glove fit loosely. Kinesio tape provides light stimulation of tissue because it increases the space between the skin and connective tissue. Courses providing instruction in the use of Kinesio Tape are available.

Massage or compression on tissue must be light to avoid collapsing the single-cell initial lymphatics in the dermal layer. Miller and Seale[18] reported that the initial lymphatics began to collapse at a pressure of 60 mm Hg and that they closed completely at 70 mm Hg. Eliska and Eliskova[19] found that a 3-minute friction massage on edematous tissue at 75 to 100 mm Hg caused temporary damage to the endothelial linings of both the initial lymphatics and the collector lymphatics.

Contrast Baths

Some therapists use contrast baths to reduce edema, although currently no research is available that supports this practice. If contrast baths are to be used, research findings on temperature need to be considered. Kurz[20] states that lymph flows best at temperatures between 71.6° F (22° C) and 105.8° F (41° C).[20] For therapy purposes, the hot temperature should not exceed 98° F (36.7°

C) to avoid increasing capillary permeability (which is enhanced by heat) and thus edema. With regard to the cold temperature, as mentioned earlier, research has shown that the initial lymphatics actually leak protein into the interstitium at temperatures below 59° F (15° C).[10] Therefore, to avoid the leakage of more plasma proteins into the interstitium (potentially increasing edema), the cold temperature should not be lower than 59° F (15° C).

Precaution. *To avoid worsening the edema, set the temperatures for contrast baths between 71.6° F (22° C) and 98.6° F (36.7° C).*

Therapy with contrast baths commonly is performed by having the client immerse the hand in warm water for 3 minutes and then in cold water for 1 minute. This sequence is repeated four times, ending on cold.

High-Voltage Pulse Current

HVPC is also a consideration for subacute and chronic edema. Griffin and colleagues[21] found that HVPC did not reduce pre-existing edema.[21] However, a subsequent study by Stralka and coworkers[22] on employees with cumulative trauma disorders provided new insights and raised more questions.[22] In this study, both the control and experimental groups used a splint that incorporated HVPC. However, the device was energized only in the experimental group. According to the study's findings, the experimental group showed a reduction in edema, whereas the control group did not. Considering that there are various types of edema, this raises the question of whether the members of the experimental group had a combination acute and chronic edema and, if so, which type the HVPC affected, or whether it affected both types.

Pneumatic Pump

If a pneumatic pump is used on subacute or chronic edema, two research-based guidelines must be considered. First, the maximum pressure should not exceed 40 mm Hg to avoid collapsing the initial lymphatics.[8] Even though the initial lymphatics do not begin to collapse until 60 mm Hg, the 40 mm Hg level is recommended to account for any calibration or pump errors. Second, high pressure is not necessary, because the pneumatic pump only softens lymph, it does not cause protein uptake.[23]

Continuous Passive Motion

CPM initially was designed to maintain gliding of tendons and joints after surgery. However, the movement of the CPM machine pulls on connective tissue. This means that the anchor filaments running from the initial lymphatics to connective tissue are stretched, which pulls apart the junctions of the endothelial cells lining the initial lymphatics. In extremely edematous tissue, the motion may or may not stretch the anchor filaments because tissue expansion caused by the edema may already have ripped off the anchor filaments.[8] Giudice[24] used CPM on edematous hands more than 4 weeks after the injurious incident and found that although edema diminished initially, it returned to pretreatment levels once the CPM treatment stopped. I would conclude that because no proximal massage of the lymphatics was performed before the CPM technique was used, the fluid content of the lymph was merely pushed into adjacent areas. The **hydrophilic** plasma proteins (plasma proteins that attract the water molecule) remained congested in the interstitium and reattracted the water molecules, causing edema to return. The CPM treatment might have had a more permanent effect if two full MEM treatment sessions, as well as the MEM pump point technique (discussed later in the chapter), had been done before the CPM was applied. Also, a short MEM home treatment program performed three or four times daily would continue to decongest the edema, aiding the anatomic lymphatic pump. A comparison of the use of CPM with and without MEM on subacute hand edema clients would be a valuable research study.

Summary of Reduction Treatment for Subacute Edema

- Diaphragmatic breathing
- Trunk stretches, trunk exercises, easy (appropriate) yoga trunk stretches
- MEM
- Kinesio Taping
- Gentle myofascial release
- Continuous passive motion machines
- Fluidotherapy machine (set at 98° F [36.7° C] or lower)
- Active and passive exercise (avoid excessive exercise, which can cause reinflammation of tissue)
- Loose elastic glove; loose elastic stockinette; cotton finger wrap bandages; Coban
- Pneumatic pump to soften lymph (set at 40 mm Hg maximum)
- Chip bags (see Fig. 3-7, *A* and *B*, on CD)

CLINICAL *Pearl*

Starting proximal at the trunk is the key to lymphatic decongestion; this is the first technique that must be done so that the other edema reduction techniques are effective.

Reduction Techniques for Chronic Edema

Chronic edema is persistent edema that lasts longer than 3 months and is **indurated** (hard) and difficult to pit.[25] As a result of the long-term entrapment of plasma proteins in the interstitium, the tissue becomes fibrotic. In part, treatment is the same as for subacute edema, but it includes softening of the fibrotic tissue to facilitate uptake by the initial lymphatics. Softening of indurated tissue can be accomplished with low-stretch bandaging, chip bags (convoluted foam pieces covered with stockinette), foam-lined splints, silicone gel sheets, and elastomer pads (see Fig. 3-7 on CD). Neutral warmth builds up under these inserts, causing an enzymatic reaction that softens the indurated tissue. The varying densities of the foam chips in a chip bag can result in tissue pressure differentiation, stimulating protein uptake.

Low-Stretch Bandaging

Low-stretch bandages are cotton, nonelastic bandages that have a 20% stretch because of the weave of the bandage. These bandages are rolled on rather than stretched on. Because of the low stretch factor, Dr. Judith Casley-Smith and Dr. John Casley-Smith[8] call the bandages "high working, low resting bandages." When a muscle contracts, it bulks up under the bandages. Because they stretch only 20%, they provide a light counterforce, which is not enough to collapse the initial lymphatics. When the muscle relaxes, the bandages only collapse 20%, again not enough to collapse the initial lymphatics. Thus variation in tissue pressure facilitates lymphatic uptake and prevents refilling of stretched tissue. Research has shown that use of a combination of low-stretch and foam bandages on the forearm, along with exercise, increases protein uptake.[26]

Low-stretch finger wraps also soften lymph and facilitate lymphatic absorption. (see Fig. 3-6, *B*, on CD) These are often used when a client's hand is so edematous that it does not fit into an elastic glove. Low-stretch finger wraps are not used to squeeze the edema out, because that would collapse the delicate lymphatic structures. The distal-to-proximal spiral pattern in which the wraps are applied, the neutral warmth maintained by the finger bandages, and the effect of finger movement all soften the indurated tissue, improving lymphatic flow and edema reduction.

Chip Bags

Chip bags vary in size, depending on the area they are to cover. They consist of stockinette bags filled with various densities and sizes of foam. The ends of the bag are either taped or sewn closed. Chip bags can be worn under low-stretch bandages, loose elastic gloves, or splints (see Fig. 3-7, *C* and *D*, on CD). Various types of commercially fabricated chip bags made of foam or wheat hulls are also available for purchase.

Coban

Coban is used by many therapists on edematous fingers. When placed on the finger or digit circumferentially, it creates a squeezing effect, pushing fluid distal or proximal, or both. Lightly overlapping spirals of Coban distal to proximal down a digit facilitates the absorption and movement of fluid proximally (see Fig. 3-6, A, on CD). Coban also creates a buildup of neutral warmth. A small stockinette or powder can be put on Coban once it is on the finger so that the wrapped fingers do not stick together.

CLINICAL *Pearl*

For chip bags, Coban, or low-stretch bandaging to be successful, proximal MEM, or at least pump point stimulation (discussed later in the chapter), must be done first to decongest the lymph ("pull the drain plug") and move it proximal.

Summary of Reduction Treatment for Chronic Edema

- All techniques listed for treatment of subacute edema
- Methods to soften indurated tissue (i.e., tissue that is hardening or already hard), including chip bags, convoluted foam in stockinette, elastomer and elastomer-type products, silicone gel sheets, foam-lined splints, low-stretch bandages, cotton finger wraps, and loose elastic stockinette and/or gloves (on CD, see Fig. 3-6, A to C; also Fig. 3-7, A to F).

OTHER TYPES OF EDEMA AND APPROPRIATE TREATMENT

Lymphedema

Lymphedema is a chronic, high-protein edema that results when a permanent mechanical obstruction of the lymphatic system creates a lymphatic overload.[27] Permanent obstruction can be caused by surgical removal of the lymph nodes, irradiation of the nodes or skin, **filariasis** (an infestation of worms that destroys the lymph nodes), or a congenital deficit of the lymph nodes and lymphatic vessels. Clients with lymphedema must be treated with a full MLT program performed by a trained

therapist. Treatment includes multiple rerouting of lymphatic flow patterns around deficit areas. MEM is not appropriate for these clients.

Precaution. *MEM is a treatment for clients with an overloaded but intact lymphatic system.*

Therapists working with hand clients may see a permanent deficit of the lymphatic system, resulting in persistent, sustained swelling. This is seen with circumferential scars, as with a replanted digit. It may also occur with circumferential skin grafting. Primary (congenital) or secondary lymphedema (e.g., from the removal of diseased nodes) causes lymphatic congestion (slow outflow of lymph) in the subcutaneous, epifascial tissue space[28]; which means that only the superficial lymphatic vessels are affected. Therefore a client whose fingers are edematous as a result of this type of lymphedema does not develop joint contractures (Fig. 3-4). If surgical or traumatic invasion into the deeper lymphatic structures around joints has occurred, joint contractures may develop. Soft tissue contractures are caused by laceration of superficial and deep lymphatic capillaries, high capillary permeability that causes leakage of plasma proteins,

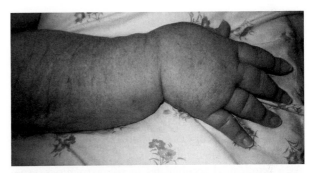

A

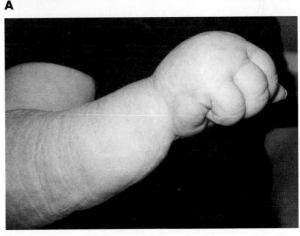

B

FIGURE 3-4 Lymphedema of the hand with no loss of mobility.

and prolonged congestion of plasma proteins around these joint and tendon structures.

Complex or Combined Edema

Complex or combined edema is initially a transudate edema, such as acute flaccid stroke hand edema. With flaccidity, no muscle pump facilitates vascular flow, and water and electrolytes leak into the interstitium, resulting in a transudate edema. The treatment is the same as for acute edema. During this phase, night splinting might be considered to prevent shortening of the extensor tendons. Three months later, the edema may have a viscous feel, but it is relatively fast to rebound and it does not significantly or permanently reduce with elevation and/or the use of an elastic glove. The edema now has an exudate component. At this point, the lymphatic system, which initially was aiding in the removal of the excess fluid (transudate edema), has reached its maximum capacity. The lymphatic system is overloaded and has slowed down, resulting in lymphatic congestion. The congested plasma protein content of the fluid makes the edema feel viscous. The treatment is the same as for subacute and chronic edema. Often a splinting program is needed to prevent or overcome joint contractures.

Precaution. *Overexercising or forcing joints in a flaccid or hemiparetic hand can cause microscopic rupture of tissue, resulting in inflammation and increased hand edema. Therefore a balance must be attained between gentle, progressive motion and rest of structures.*

Cardiac Edema

Cardiac edema occurs with a decline in the heart's ability to pump blood completely through the circulatory system. As a result, fluid accumulates in the extremities, especially around the ankles. Often cardiac edema manifests as bilateral ankle swelling with a slight pinkish tone to the tissue. Hand therapists treating older adults need to look for this type of edema.

Precaution. *MEM and many of the edema reduction techniques are contraindicated for clients with cardiac edema, because movement of more fluid can further overload the already compromised cardiac system.*

Low-Protein Edema

Low-protein edema can manifest as extremity swelling caused by liver disease, malnutrition, or kidney failure (e.g., nephrotic syndrome).[1,4] Edema results because too few plasma proteins are present in the interstitium to bond with the water molecule and bring fluid back into the vascular systems.

Precaution. *Low-protein edema has a systemic cause and must be treated with medication. MEM and many of the edema reduction techniques are contraindicated because they may overload the kidneys or liver. Also, even if these edema control techniques are used, this type of edema will return because of its systemic cause.*

EVALUATION OF EDEMATOUS TISSUE

Edema reduces range of motion (ROM) both actively and passively because it increases the size of the fingers or hand. This, in turn, can reduce functional use and coordination of the hand. Once the edema has been reduced, if decreased ROM persists, the therapist can effectively evaluate and treat joint and/or soft tissue limitations. The sooner the edema is reduced, the less the buildup of plasma proteins in soft tissue, the less the fibrosis of the tissue, and the less the thickening of scar tissue.

Precaution. *Reducing edema does not reverse existing joint contractures.*

By taking circumferential measurements, the therapist can determine where on the hand specifically the edema is prevalent. For consistency, always use the same measuring device; also, take measurements at the same time of day and after the same amount of hand activity.

Edema rebound tests (see Chapter 5) can help determine whether treatment has reduced some of the viscous congested edema. For instance, if the edema rebound time was 65 seconds before treatment and 40 seconds after treatment, this indicates that lymph was moved out. To make this subjective test more consistent, devise a protocol for how much pressure used and for how long it is applied.

Volumeters repeatedly have proved that they provide reliable, valid edema measurements.[29] These measurements indicate whether volume reduction has occurred; they do not specify the location of the reduction.

The criteria for tissue quality assessment, another evaluation method, are as follows:

- *Acute edema:* Tissue pits deeply, rebounds rather quickly, and can be easily moved around.
- *Subacute edema* or *early stage chronic edema:* Tissue pits, is very slow to rebound, and has a viscous quality.
- *Chronic edema:* Tissue pits minimally and has a hard feeling.
- *Severe edema:* Tissue has no elasticity and is shiny, taut, and cannot be lifted.
- **Lymphorrhea:** Weeping of tissue occurs with an extremely congested edematous hand or arm. Lymph, a clear. yellowish fluid, escapes from the interstitium to the outside of the skin. Techni-

cally, weeping tissue is considered an open wound and must be treated as such. MEM techniques can rapidly decongest the lymph and stop the lymphorrhea.

NOTE: Always perform the capillary refill test if the client's hand has a bulky dressing or if the client is wearing finger bandages.

Precaution. *Color, temperature, and sensory changes may be signs of a problem. A purple color often indicates pooling of venous blood, and a whitish color means that arterial blood flow to the tissue is compromised. Immediately notify the physician of these signs.*

CLINICAL *Pearl*

Macrophages are less effective in edematous tissue because it has less oxygen; phagocytic activity therefore is diminished.[8]

The therapist must be able to distinguish between congestion and infection. With an open wound, the classic signs of infection are redness, warmth, pain to the touch, odor, and/or cloudy drainage. With a closed wound, the signs of a subclinical infection are a pinkish red color and slight warmth; also, the wound may be painful to the touch and the tissue may be hard.[30] This is often seen with a very edematous extremity or hand if the first course of antibiotics hasn't fully resolved the infection. Extremely edematous hands often need a second course of antibiotics.

Precaution. *If infection is suspected, MEM should not be started before a full course of antibiotics has been completed and the physician has assessed the status of the infection.*

The signs of congestion frequently are the same as those of a subclinical infection. The client's history can help determine whether the condition is congestion or infection (or both). Often congestion (and, possibly, infection) can be prevented if the therapist begins treatment of an uninfected extremity early, before visible edema is present, with the short version of MEM. Prolonged tissue congestion can lead to infection because congestion reduces oxygen delivery to tissue, diminishing the effectiveness of the phagocytic cells.

Both old and new scars can create a barrier to lymph flow. Check for proximal scars (e.g., on the shoulder, back, or axilla). Soften both old and new scars with gentle myofascial release techniques, silicone gel sheets, and/or Kinesio Taping. Instruct the client in MEM techniques to reroute edema around scars and to soften scars.

Sensory testing is very important for an edematous extremity because edema often reduces sensation. As edema is reduced, the degree of sensation usually improves. Sensory testing therefore becomes an objective test that shows limitations and improvements that can be related to function.

Coordination often is diminished by edema in the hand. A nine-hole peg test can become a repeated, scheduled test for assessing hand function. Reducing hand edema should improve coordination, unless an underlying problem exists.

Pain assessment is very important. As edema declines, pain usually diminishes. Clinically, pain reduction often is noticed before ROM shows improvement. Keep in mind that pain can have many sources. For example, in a client with a Colles fracture, edema reduction can relieve the pain caused by the pressure of edema on the nerve receptors; however, the client still may have chronic pain specifically related to the fracture site. Therefore other, appropriate methods must be used to reduce that pain, which differs from edema-related pain. Even during treatment for a different cause of pain, the client should follow a MEM home program twice daily to eliminate any new, not yet visible congested edema.

MANUAL EDEMA MOBILIZATION

MEM is an edema reduction technique for persistent edema in the hand, arm, or leg in which the lymph system is intact but overloaded. MEM specifically activates the lymphatic system to facilitate absorption of the excess and congested large plasma protein molecules, other large molecules, and small water molecules from the interstitium. This technique reduces both visible and not yet visible edema. It is a modification of MLT techniques used for lymphadenectomy and/or lymph node irradiation, primary (congenital) lymphedema, and lymphedema arising from filariasis. For those types of edemas, MLT very appropriately involves extensive rerouting of lymph flow around missing or permanently damaged nodes and lymphatic vessel areas.

I developed MEM after I became certified in lymphedema treatment and learned about the anatomic functioning of the lymphatic system. My study of anatomy and physiology led me to realize that the traditional treatments for upper extremity edema could be improved if they were based on this knowledge. I realized that the subacute edema I struggled to reduce in my surgical, trauma, and stroke clients with hand edema was a lymphatic overload edema. In these cases, because the lymphatic system, although overloaded, was still intact, extensive rerouting wasn't necessary, just decongestion, starting at the trunk.

MEM is a significant modification of MLT in several ways: (1) it involves only one trunk rerouting technique; (2) it requires exercise after each segment is massaged; (3) it has its own light hand massage patterns; (4) it includes scar rerouting patterns; (5) it relies heavily on client follow through with a self-management program; and (6) it incorporates pump point stimulation, which is unique to MEM.

The full MEM program takes 30 minutes. The short version, consisting of trunk rerouting and pump point stimulation, takes 15 minutes. *MEM can be combined with other edema reduction techniques, but it should be done before those techniques are performed.* The reason for this is simple: MEM decongests the most proximal edema and moves that edema proximally, creating a space into which the more distal edema can move by means of a proximal negative pressure vacuum. The more traditional edema reduction techniques will be more effective after MEM, after there is space cleared to which the edema can be moved proximally.

Principles and Concepts

MEM is grounded in the following principles and concepts[25]:

1. Light massage is provided, ranging from 10 to 20 mm Hg, to prevent collapse of the lymphatic pathways and arterial capillary reflux.
2. When protocol allows, exercises are performed before and after the MEM session; these exercises are done in a specific sequence, starting proximal to the edematous area or in the contralateral quadrant if possible.
3. Massage is performed in segments, proximal to distal, then distal to proximal. Massage ends in a *proximal* direction (i.e., toward the trunk).
4. When possible, the technique includes exercise of the muscles in the segment just massaged.
5. Massage follows the flow of lymphatic pathways.
6. Massage reroutes around scar areas.
7. The method of massage and the types of exercise do not cause further inflammation of the involved tissue.
8. A client home self-massage program is devised that is specific to the pathologic condition of the hand.
9. MEM can be adapted to various diagnoses and stages of high plasma protein edema.
10. Guidelines are included for incorporating traditional edema control, soft tissue mobilization, and strengthening exercises without increasing in edema.
11. Specific precautions are observed.
12. When necessary, low-stretch compression bandaging or other compression techniques are used.
13. Pump point stimulation is used extensively.
14. MEM is beneficial in clients whose lymphatic vessels are intact but overloaded from congestion.

Contraindications

The precautions and contraindications for MEM include those that are common to most massage programs and others that are specific to the movement of a large volume of fluid through the system. Always consult a physician if you are concerned about the client's current or past cardiac and/or pulmonary status. For instance, if an 80 mL volumetric difference exists between the client's two extremities, inform the physician that with MEM, that much fluid may be moved through the heart and lungs. Ask whether this would compromise the client's cardiac status.

Therapists should not use MEM in the following circumstances:

- If infection is present, because the infection may be spread by the technique.
- Over areas of inflammation, because inflammation and pain may be increased; MEM should be performed proximal to the inflammation to reduce the amount of congested fluid.
- If a hematoma or blood clot is present in the area, because the clot may be activated (i.e., it may move).
- If active cancer is present. A controversial theory notes the potential for spreading cancerous cells. MEM should absolutely *never* be done if the cancer is not being medically treated. The therapist should always seek the physician's advice.
- If the client has congestive heart failure, severe cardiac problems, or pulmonary problems, because the cardiac and pulmonary systems may be overloaded.
- In the inflammatory stage of acute wound healing, because theoretically the cellular cleanup process and the invasion of fibroblasts may be disrupted.
- If the client has renal failure or severe kidney disease, because the edema in these cases is a low-protein edema, and the renal system may be overloaded and/or the fluid may be moved to some other undesirable site.
- If the client has primary lymphedema or lymphedema arising from a mastectomy. Successful treatment of this condition requires a knowledge of ways to reroute lymph to other parts of the body, as well as specific techniques beyond the scope of this chapter.

MEM Massage, Drainage, and Term Definitions

U's Hand Movement Pattern

U's are a pattern of hand movement that involves placing a flat but relaxed hand lightly on the skin. The hand gently tractions the skin slightly distal and then circles back up and around, ending in the direction of the lymph flow pattern. The movement is consistently a clockwise or counterclockwise motion in a **U**, or teardrop, configuration. Very light pressure (10 mm Hg or less) is used to move just the skin, thereby stimulating the initial lymphatics. Clinically, this is taught by having the therapist first place the full weight of the hand on the client's arm; then, while the entire palm and the digits remain in contact with the client's skin, the hand is partly lifted so that only half its weight rests on the arm. MEM massage proceeds at this very light pressure, moving in a **U** while tractioning (pulling), not sliding, the skin. This is a "skin" massage—just enough pressure to make the skin move.

Clearing U's Skin Tractioning Pattern

Clearing **U**'s is a pattern of skin tractioning performed in segments. It starts proximally and moves to the designated distal part of the trunk or arm segment (i.e., upper arm, forearm, or hand). A minimum of five **U**'s are done in three sections for each segment. The purpose is to create interstitial pressure changes that cause the initial lymphatics to take up lymph. The direction of "flow" movement follows the lymphatic pathways toward the heart (i.e., flowing proximally, not distally). If not contraindicated by the diagnostic protocol, active muscle contraction is done in each segment after it has been "cleared." This increases the rate of lymphangion contraction, which moves the lymph out of the area more quickly.

Flowing U's Lymph Movement Pattern

Flowing **U**'s is a pattern of sequential **U**'s that starts in the distal part of the segment being treated and moves proximally past the nearest set of lymph nodes. This could be described as "waltzing" up the arm. The process of moving one **U** after another from distal to beyond the node is repeated five times. After the final repetition is completed, the flowing **U** motion is performed all the way to the contralateral upper quadrant. The purpose is to move the softened lymph out of the entire segment and facilitate its eventual return to the venous system and the heart (Fig. 3-5).

Pump Point Stimulation

Pump point stimulation involves simultaneous, synchronous movement of the therapist's two hands in a **U** pattern over areas of **lymphatic bundles** (groups of initial and collector lymphatics), watershed areas, and/or lymph nodes.[25] Because nodes pose resistance to the flow of lymph, pressure from the full weight of the hand is used. Typically the therapist does 20 to 30 **U**'s in one area before proceeding to the next area of pump points. After pump point stimulation is performed in an area, exercise

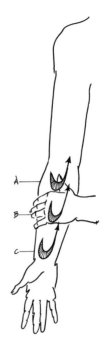

FIGURE 3-5 Forearm: Clear A, B, C. Flow C, B, A. (From Mackin EJ et al, editors: *Rehabilitation of the hand and upper extremity*, ed 5, St Louis, 2002, Mosby.)

is done either in that area or proximal to it. Sometimes an MEM flow massage is done before the next area of pump points is stimulated (see Fig. 3-8, *B*, on CD).

Therapists should not attempt MEM unless they have been trained in the technique. Two- and 3-day courses are available and encouraged for any therapist who would like to use MEM as a course of treatment. The following case study is an example of the short version of MEM, which is presented here to offer the reader a sense of what the MEM program entails (see Fig. 3-8 on CD).

Case *Study*

This case study, presented by Karin Ronhoj, OTR, CLT, an occupational therapist in Denmark, is offered as a clinical reasoning tool to help readers synthesize the material in this chapter. This case represents the first time Karin used MEM. Her problem-solving approach is valuable for readers not already familiar with MEM. The answers to the six questions posed below can be found at the end of the case study.

HISTORY

An 84-year-old woman fractured the first (thumb) metacarpal bone of her left (L) hand when she hit a door with her hand. The client was treated in the emergency department (ED) with casting of the fracture. After 2 days this cast became too tight. She returned to the ED, where a new cast was applied. At neither visit was the client instructed in any edema reduction techniques. During her third visit to the ED, 10 days after injury, the ED physician called in a hand surgeon. The surgeon immediately sent the client to Karin in occupational therapy (OT), knowing that she had expertise in edema reduction techniques (see Fig. 3-9, *A* and *B*, on CD).

1. What edema reduction techniques could the ED physician or nurse have advised the client to perform for this acute stage while wearing the cast?
   a. Elevation of hand above heart
   b. Use of ice/cold pack for 24 hours
   c. Use of hot pack first 24 hours
   d. Continue all activities, use hand as much as possible
   e. Restrict activities for first 24 hours, rest as much as possible with hand elevated above heart, move shoulder and elbow when arm is elevated

CLINICAL EVALUATION FINDINGS

- Social history: widow, lives alone in large house, responsible for all self-care and household chores; client is ambidextrous but prefers using L hand.
- Hematoma covering two thirds of the dorsum of the hand; multiple bruising of volar surface forearm and fingers; fingers pale and also purplish from bruising.
- Hand girth measured along descending angle of MCPs was 6.5 cm larger than same area on unaffected (R) hand. Proximal phalanges of index-small digits averaged 2 cm greater than on the right. Skin was taut, shiny, couldn't be lifted, and felt viscous (spongy) when compressed.
- Sixty-second rebound time on index proximal phalanx, the most edematous digit.
- Average of 10 to 15 degrees of active and passive motion of all finger joints; thumb not measured.
- When client actively made a fist, distance to palmar crease ranged from 10 cm on index finger to 11 cm on small finger.
- Client reported extreme pain when the therapist touched her hand or when she moved it actively or passively.
- Client needed a replacement splint, to be made of thermoplastic material, for L thumb; hand surgeon had ordered the splint.
- Slight swelling of both ankles, but no heat or redness.
2. The type of edema the client had was subacute because
   a. The tissue had a viscous feel.
   b. The tissue was slow to rebound when pitted.
   c. The physician had given it that label.

   d. The patient had pain and decreased active and passive ROM.
3. The therapist must plan an edema reduction program 10 days after the injury. What types of treatment techniques should be considered?
   a. Ice packs
   b. Light retrograde massage
   c. Vigorous active and passive ROM of the entire upper extremity
   d. Intermittent elevation to reduce dependent edema
   e. Kinesio Taping to reduce the hematoma and swelling
   f. MEM
   g. Elevation of the arm/hand as much as possible
   h. Gentle, progressive active ROM of the arm, including the fingers but not the thumb
   i. Light spiral Coban wrapping of the digits
   j. Elastic glove on all fingers and the hand, including the thumb with the splint
4. Why wouldn't you consider fluidotherapy for this client, even at 98.6° F (36.7° C)? Why wouldn't you use contrast baths within the recommended range?

INITIAL TREATMENT

Karin's treatment of this client for the first session consisted of fabrication of a thumb immobilization splint, MEM treatment to the upper trunk (diaphragmatic breathing, MEM exercises before and after treatment, upper trunk massage, active muscle contraction for the shoulders) and an activities of daily living (ADL) evaluation. The client borrowed appropriate assistive devices for temporary one-handed use.

5. Why didn't Karin do MEM for the entire extremity or trunk and all pump points at the first session (MEM short version)?
   a. She ran out of time.
   b. It was contraindicated because of the extent of bruising on the arm and the hematoma on the hand.
   c. A potential cardiac problem was a concern because of bilateral ankle swelling.
   d. She wanted to go slowly with the client so that she could watch for contraindications and observe the rate of edema reduction.

CONTINUING CARE

The client was seen for a second therapy treatment 5 days later. Her entire medical chart was obtained and showed no cardiac problems. The bilateral ankle swelling was from venous insufficiency. The bruising was fading on her arm, the color of the fingers had become more normal (i.e., less congestion), her pain had decreased, and she had some increase in ROM. Karin then did the entire MEM program and put low-stretch bandages on the fingers and forearm (see Fig. 3-9, *C to E,* on CD).

6. Low-stretch bandages were used to:
   a. Squeeze fluid out of the fingers and hand
   b. Prevent refilling of tissue with fluid after MEM massage
   c. Reduce indurated (hard) tissue

SUBSEQUENT CARE

Four days later, the client returned for her third hand therapy treatment. Edema continued to decrease slowly, pain continued to decrease, active and passive ROM of digits continued to improve, the client was successfully following her self-management exercise program, self-massage, and rebandaging wearing 23 of 24 hours daily. Karin noted that the edema was reducing slower than she had thought it would with the MEM method. At this point, she had done MEM massage only up to the wrist because of the contraindication for doing MEM on the area of a hematoma. Karin contacted me, and I advised her to do the Kinesio Taping hematoma/edema reduction method on the dorsum of the hand. She obtained the proper instruction for Kinesio Taping for hematoma/edema reduction. The Kinesio Tape was applied (see Fig. 3-9, *F,* on CD).

At the client's fourth therapy visit, 19 days after the start of treatment, she had reduced hand pain with a resulting increase in ROM, such that a composite fist was only 4 cm from touching the palm. Originally the fingers were 10 to 11 cm from touching the palm. This was 4 days after application of the Kinesio Tape, and the hematoma was almost gone.

RESULT OF CARE

Four weeks after treatment began, the thumb splint was discontinued. The next week Karin discontinued the low-stretch bandages and stopped performing MEM during clinic visits. The client continued her home MEM program for 2 more weeks. The client was discharged 2 months after treatment was initiated with a nonedematous, functional thumb and hand (see Fig. 3-9, *G and H,* on CD).

DISCUSSION

Q: If Karin had known Kinesio Taping methods for hematoma reduction before treating this client, could she have applied the Kinesio Tape at the first treatment session, 10 days after injury?

A: Yes, this would have reduced the hematoma, and the digit edema would have been reduced more quickly.

Q: If Kinesio Taping for hematoma reduction had been applied during the first treatment, could the same MEM trunk program been performed?

A: Yes. However, this was Karin's first experience with using both MEM and Kinesio Tape. It is advisable not to do two new techniques at one time. It is best to observe the reaction and extent of edema reduction before applying the second technique. This gives a frame of reference for future application. In this case, it was especially important to do just one technique at a time and gradually add techniques because of the extent of bruising.

Q: Is there edema normally related to a healing fracture?

A: Yes, it is not uncommon to see moderate swelling during the first 2 weeks of the healing process. Usually the secondary edema in the surrounding tissue can be reduced during this time with MEM.

Q: Could two or three different treatment techniques have been used to reduce edema during those first three treatment sessions?

A: No. Currently, with subacute edema, MEM is the only method that follows lymphatic anatomy for proximal decongestion. This proximal decongestion must be done first so that the peripheral edema has a space into which it can move. Other techniques will be more effective after trunk MEM and a home MEM program have been done for a week. If edema isn't reducing as quickly as you think it should, re-evaluate as Karin did.

CLINICAL PROBLEM SOLVING

What is the effect of the hematoma? Are there scars or old injuries proximal to the edema that are barriers to lymph flow? Does the client have fascial restrictions or ROM restrictions proximally? Is the client following through with an MEM home program and doing a light stroking massage? Add more treatment techniques according to your evaluation findings.

ANSWERS

1. A, B, E
2. A, B
3. D through H
4. Because the client must wear the thumb splint at all times. Also, heat would soften the splint.
5. B, C, D
6. B, C

Acknowledgment

I would like to thank Karin Ronhoj of Denmark for the case study and for her passion for MEM. Her dedication has prompted her to conduct an MEM research study (in progress) and to become an expert in the teaching of MEM. Her efforts doubtless will help to further develop this area of expertise.

References

1. Guyton A, Hall J: *Textbook of medical physiology*, ed 9, Philadelphia, 1996, WB Saunders.
2. Hole JW: *Human anatomy and physiology*, ed 4, Dubuque, IA, 1987, William C Brown.
3. Kubik S: Anatomy of the lymphatic system. In Foldi M, Foldi E, Kubik S, editors: *Textbook of lymphology for physicians and lymphedema therapists*, Munich, 2003, Urban & Fischer Verlag.
4. Chikly B: *Silent waves: the theory and practice of lymph drainage therapy with applications for lymphedema, chronic pain and inflammation*, Scottsdale, AZ, 2001, I.H.H.
5. Bryant WM: Wound healing, *Clinical Symposium* 29:1, 1977.
6. Reed B: Effect of high voltage pulsed electrical stimulation on microvascular permeability to plasma proteins, *Phys Ther* 68:491-496, 1988.
7. Vasudevan S, Melvin J: Upper extremity edema control: rationale of treatment techniques, *Am J Occup Ther* 33:520, 1979.
8. Casley-Smith JR, Casley-Smith JR: *Modern treatment for lymphedema*, ed 5, Adelaide, 1997, The Lymphoedema Association of Australia.
9. Buncke HJ et al: Surgical and rehabilitative aspects of replantation and revascularization of the hand. In Hunter JM, Schneider LH, Mackin EJ, et al, editors: *Rehabilitation of the hand: surgery and therapy*, ed 4, St Louis, 1995, Mosby.
10. Lievens P, Leduc A: Cryotherapy and sports, *Int J Sports Med* 5:37-39 (Supplement), 1984.
11. Villeco JP, Mackin EJ, Hunter JM: Edema: therapist's management. In Mackin EJ et al, editors: *Rehabilitation of the hand and upper extremity*, ed 5, St Louis, 2002, Mosby.
12. Kase K, Wallis J, Kase T: *Clinical therapeutic applications of the Kinesio Taping method*, Tokyo, 2003, Ken Ikai.
13. Hutzschenreuter P, Brummer H: Die manuelle lympdrainage bei der wundheilung mit decollement, *Lymphologica* 97:100, 1989.
14. Rodrick R, Howard S: Sub-acute edema reduction in patients with wrist disorders: a pilot study comparing the effectiveness of traditional retrograde massage versus manual edema mobilization. Paper presented at the meeting of the International Federation of Societies of Hand Therapists, Edinburgh, June 2004.
15. Consensus Document of the International Society of Lymphology Executive Committee: The diagnosis and treatment of peripheral lymphedema, *Lymphology* 28:113, 1995.
16. Ganong WH: *Review of medical physiology*, ed 18, Stanford, CN, 1997, Appleton & Lange.
17. Pecking A et al: Indirect lymphoscintigraphy in patients with limb edema: progress in lymphology, *Proceedings of the Ninth International Congress of Lymphology* pp 201-296, 1985.
18. Miller GE, Seale J: Lymphatic clearance during compressive loading, *Lymphology* 14:161, 1981.
19. Eliska O, Eliskova M: Are peripheral lymphatics damaged by high pressure manual massage? *Lymphology* 28:21, 1995.
20. Kurz I: *Textbook of Dr. Vodder's manual lymph drainage*, ed 4, Heidelberg, 1997, Haug.
21. Griffin JW, Newsome LS, Stralka SW et al: Reduction of chronic posttraumatic hand edema: a comparison of high voltage pulsed current, intermittent pneumatic compression and placebo treatments, *Phys Ther* 70:279, 1990.
22. Stralka S, Jackson J, Lewis A: Treatment of hand and wrist pain, *AAOHN J* 46:5, 1998.
23. Leduc O et al: The physical treatment of upper limb edema, *Cancer* 15(12 suppl Am):2835, 1998.
24. Giudice M: Effects of continuous passive motion and elevation on hand edema, *Am J Occup Ther* 44:10, 1990.
25. Artzberger S: Manual edema mobilization: treatment for edema in the subacute hand. In Mackin EJ et al, editors: *Rehabilitation of the hand and upper extremity*, ed 5, St Louis, 2002, Mosby.
26. Leduc O et al: Bandages: scintigraphic demonstration of its efficacy on colloidal protein reabsorption during muscle activity, *Progress in Lymphology XII* 887:421, 1990.
27. Casley-Smith JR: Modern treatment of lymphedema, *Mod Med Aust* May, 1992.
28. Szuba A, Rockson S: Lymphedema: classifications, diagnosis and therapy, *Vasc Med* 3:145, 1998.
29. Waylett-Rendall J, Seibly D: A study of the accuracy of a commercially available volumeter, *J Hand Ther* 4:10, 1991.
30. Marcks P: Lymphedema pathogenesis, prevention, and treatment, *Cancer Pract* 5:1, 1997.

4

Tissue-Specific Exercises for the Upper Extremity

LORI FALKEL

KEY TERMS

Agonist

Antagonist

Arthrokinematics

Chondroblasts

Chondrocytes

Closed chain

Collagen

Covalent bonds

Cross-bridges

Extracellular matrix

Fibroblasts

Glycosaminoglycans

Golgi tendon organs

Ground substance

Hypermobility

Hypomobility

Imbibition

Instability

Isometric maximum

Kinesthesia

Mechanoreceptors

Metabolites

Muscle fiber length equilibrium

Myofibroblasts

Nociceptive

1 IM

1 RM

Open chain

Osteoblasts

Osteoclasts

Osteocytes

Osteoid matrix

Osteophytes

Phasic muscles

Plyometrics

Procollagen

Proteoglycans

Pseudarthrosis

Reflex disturbance

Resistance maximal

Sliding filament theory

Steady state respiratory rate

Tonic muscles

Tropocollagen

Tissue-specific exercise progressions can be thought of as the science of prescribing an accurate dosage of exercise. Tissue-specific exercise allows us to use our knowledge of exercise physiology to address the specific pathologic tissue conditions. When physicians prescribe medicine, they do not arbitrarily select a medication from the pharmacy and administer it. They prescribe medicine based on the pathologic condition.

With proper knowledge, exercise is the therapist's area of expertise. For optimal outcomes, exercise dosage must not be assigned arbitrarily; it should be dosed accurately according to the physiology of the tissue(s) involved. When designing an exercise program effectively to promote the recovery of the target tissue, one needs to consider multiple variables. Some of these variables are the appropriate resistance; the repetitions and sets that will promote the desired response; the speed, frequency, breaks, and duration of exercise; the appropriate positioning of the limb and/or client; and the precise range of motion. Proper exercise equipment, to provide support, can be critical for restoration of physiologic motion. The types of muscle work (e.g., concentric, eccentric, and isometric) are also important considerations.

The Ola Grimsby Institute developed Scientific Therapeutic Exercise Progressions (STEP), which is a concept of dosing exercises according to the specific pathologic condition and tissue tolerance of each client. STEP is based on principles of medical exercise therapy. It was developed in Norway and has been practiced throughout Europe for many years with excellent results. STEP addresses musculoskeletal dysfunctions with respect to their histologic, biomechanical, and neurophysiologic significance.*

JOINT DYSFUNCTION

Joint dysfunction occurs because of a compromise in connective tissue integrity. This may result from capsular, ligamentous, or cartilaginous causes. In cartilage, symptoms of joint dysfunction present as an inability to withstand compressive forces. If the joint dysfunction is capsular, joint swelling will be present. A ligamentous injury has point tenderness. The end result is altered mobility. Joint dysfunction can be labeled as a **hypomobility,** a **hypermobility,** or an **instability.** A joint is considered to be hypomobile when movement takes place about a physiologic axis but is less than normal. A hypermobile joint has greater than normal motion around a physiologic axis. Joint instability is motion around a nonphysiologic axis.[1] All synovial joints can

be categorized by a joint mobility grading system[2] (Table 4-1).

MUSCULOSKELETAL DYSFUNCTIONS

The two main *causes* of musculoskeletal dysfunctions are acute trauma and cumulative trauma. Acute trauma is associated with an excessive contraction (muscle strain) or an externally applied force. Chronic overload or cumulative trauma is associated with prolonged static work, stress, and often reduced aerobic activity.

CLINICAL *Pearl*

A large percentage of clients who have cumulative trauma injuries are deconditioned because of a fairly sedentary job or lifestyle.

Co-morbidities Associated with Increased Prevalence of Musculoskeletal Dysfunction

The vast majority of clients who present for treatment in a hand clinic do not have only a hand injury. The therapist must be aware of the client's co-morbidities and provide comprehensive treatment that addresses the client as a whole, rather than just an extremity. Some of the more common diseases that are associated with lowered tolerance of the musculoskeletal system are diabetes, hypothyroidism/hyperthyroidism, gastric ulcer, chronic/recurrent infections, colitis, and cardiovascular and respiratory diseases.

Diabetes causes the production and use of insulin in the body to be impaired. This results in an abundance of sugar in the bloodstream. With diabetes the pancreas secretes little or no insulin (type I diabetes), or the body becomes resistant to the action of insulin (type II diabetes). If the disease is not treated, the level of sugar in the bloodstream builds up and leads to diabetic complications.

The thyroid gland affects all aspects of metabolism. The thyroid releases hormones that regulate heart rate, the strength of bones, how quickly calories are burned, and sensitivity to heat/cold. If the thyroid gland is underactive or overactive (hypothyroidism/hyperthyroidism), medical treatment is necessary to avoid complications.[3]

A gastric ulcer is an open sore that develops in the lining of the stomach. The ulcer may result from diet, stress, medication, or bacterial infection.

Infections can occur when the immune system is suppressed or comes in contact with an organism to

---

*The Ola Grimsby Institute offers courses on a range of subjects pertaining to exercise and physical therapy if more information is needed.

TABLE 4-1

Joint Mobility Grading Scale

GRADE	JOINT MOBILITY	TREATMENT
0	Ankylosed	Surgery/no therapy treatment
1	Considerable limitation	Joint mobilization/avoid exercise
2	Slight limitation	Joint mobilization/self-mobilization
3	Normal	No treatment needed
4	Slight increase	Postural correction/taping/self-stabilization
5	Considerable increase	Postural/bracing/self-stabilization
6	Pathologically unstable	Surgery/no therapy treatment

which it does not have resistance. Bones and joints become susceptible to chronic infections that originate elsewhere in the body and are passed to them via the bloodstream.[4]

Colitis is a painful and debilitating chronic inflammation of the digestive tract.[5] Cardiovascular and respiratory disease includes any of a multitude of problems involving the heart, lungs, and blood vessels. Some of these disease processes are preventable and are acquired over a lifetime; others are congenital. Cardiovascular disease is more prevalent than all of the previously mentioned diseases combined.[6,7]

Exercise Considerations

Always use caution and discretion when prescribing the intensity of exercise. A thorough evaluation provides the necessary information regarding cardiovascular compromise or risk factors, pulmonary disease, diabetes mellitus, hypertension, obesity, peripheral vascular disease, arthritis, and renal disease.[6]

Precaution. *An exercise program may not be recommended for uncontrolled diabetes. A rigorous strengthening or aerobic exercise program, in this case, may cause a hyperglycemic effect because cellular absorption of glucose is restricted. Insulin-dependent diabetic clients may need to decrease insulin or increase carbohydrate intake when exercising. They should monitor their glucose more frequently when starting an exercise program. For this client population the exercise should be dosed at a lower level of intensity and duration initially and should progress at a much slower rate.[3]*

OSTEOPOROSIS

An estimated 30 million Americans have osteoporosis. This disease is responsible for 1.5 million individuals sustaining bone fractures per year (200,000 wrist frac-

BOX 4-1

Traits That Have Been Shown to Increase Risk for Fractures

- Slender build
- Fair skin
- Family history of osteoporosis or osteoporotic fracture
- Small muscle mass
- Sedentary lifestyle
- Small peak adult bone mass (approximately age 35)
- Low calcium intake
- Cigarette smoking
- Excessive consumption of protein, sodium, and alcohol
- One or more osteoporotic fracture(s)
- A situation that increases the likelihood of falling (i.e., wet floor, throw rugs, or small pets)

tures, 300,000 hip fractures, 300,000 non-wrist extremity fractures). Osteoporosis costs more than $13.8 billion per year in health care expenses and lost productivity. Bone mass attains a peak in males and females at approximately 30 to 35 years of age, with total bone mass beginning to decline 5 to 10 years later. Boxes 4-1 and 4-2 list traits and age-related changes associated with osteoporosis.[8,9]

Males are less affected by osteoporosis than females. Males usually ingest more calcium and have higher levels of calcitonin. They also produce testosterone into the seventh and eighth decades of life as opposed to the decline in hormone production that females experience with menopause in the fourth or fifth decade. The increased calcium and hormone levels reduce the loss of

Common Age-Related Changes Affecting Bone Loss

- Gradual increase in parathyroid hormone secretion as a result of chronic calcium deficiency
- Decreased intestinal absorption of elemental calcium
- Lower circulating calcitonin
- Decreased sunlight exposure and dietary vitamin D intake
- Decreased ovarian function causing altered estrogen balance

BOX 4-3

Some Considerations for Exercise Selection

- Weight-bearing activities and strength training are ideal for bone stimulation.
- Increased strength improves balance and decreases the risk of falls.
- Walking is ideal because it is weight bearing, dynamic, and repetitive.
- Swimming or cycling use less weight-bearing forces and are less effective than walking.
- Nonimpact loading may cause damage to weakened bone.

BOX 4-4

Contraindicated Exercises for Advanced Osteoporosis

- Vigorous aerobic workout
- Exercises that require twisting or bending
- Abdominal machines
- Biceps-curl machines
- Rowing machines
- Tennis
- Golf
- Bowling

bone mass, which in turn reduces the potential for development of osteoporosis.

Several factors can affect bone resorption levels. A lack of weight bearing and of activity in antigravity muscles changes the resorption rate, as does excessive thyroid and parathyroid hormones. Corticosteroids also have an impact.

Determinants of bone mass and loss are genetic, mechanical, or hormonal. Genetics can cause large-boned individuals to gain a relative immunity to osteoporotic fractures. The mechanics of bone density can aid in the prevention of fractures, but they also can be a possible cause. Increasing loading yields lead to increased bone mass, and decreased loading yields lead to decreased bone mass.

Exercise for Prevention/Treatment of Osteoporosis

Exercise can help prevent or slow down bone loss, improve posture, and increase overall fitness. For clients who are at risk of osteoporosis, a bone density test before beginning an exercise program is recommended. Box 4-3 lists factors to consider when selecting an exercise.[8]

Although walking is the best of all of the options listed in Box 4-3, those clients who are unable to tolerate walking because of co-morbidities or advanced osteoporosis have other options. These options provide benefit by generating muscle tension, which provides needed stress to bone. To prevent injury to those with advanced osteoporosis, clients absolutely should avoid the exercises listed in Box 4-4.

Client Education for Osteoporosis

Education of the client on what impact osteoporosis will have on his or her life and what the client can do to prevent fractures or falls is important. Teach clients about proper body mechanics by demonstrating proper posture. When teaching lifting and carrying techniques, show the client how to hold loads close to the body. Explain that strengthening exercises improve balance and decrease the risk of falling. Address fall prevention. Wearing of proper shoes, removal of throw rugs, sufficient lighting, and use of handrails decrease the risk of a fall or fracture.

Precaution. *Avoid forceful, unguarded motions such as opening a stuck window or bending forward to lift a heavy object. Instead, teach clients how to squat when lifting.*

HISTOLOGY OF COLLAGEN, BONE, AND CARTILAGE
Collagen

Collagen is the fundamental component of the connective tissues of the body, including fascia, fibrous cartilage, tendons, ligaments, bones, joint capsules, blood vessels, adipose tissue, and dermis. Collagen is the most abundant protein in the human body. It accounts for approximately 30% of all protein. Before 1970, researchers believed that all collagen was identical. Now, 19 types of collagen are known that are differentiated by their protein composition. Type I and type II together compose approximately 90% of human connective tissue. Type III collagen is produced first, in the initial reparative phase, before type I collagen. Type III collagen also is found in arteries, the liver, and the spleen.[9]

Type I collagen constitutes about 90% of total body collagen. Type I collagen is found in bone, tendon, fascia, fibrous cartilage, derma, and sclera. This collagen is synthesized by **fibroblasts, osteoblasts,** and **chondroblasts.** Its primary function is to resist tension.

Type II collagen is found in hyaline and elastic cartilage and intervertebral disks. Type II collagen is synthesized by chondroblasts. Its primary function is to resist intermittent pressure.

Fibroblasts produce type I collagen fibers that are found in tendons, ligaments, and joint capsules. **Procollagen,** the precursor of collagen, is produced in the endoplasmic reticulum and is made up of polypeptide chains of lysine, glycine, and proline. **Tropocollagen,** is the basic molecular unit of collagen fibrils and is found in the interstitial spaces; this collagen is the building block of collagen. The bonds of procollagen and tropocollagen are weak and easily deformed or ruptured. One must understand that collagen bonds are remodeled from mobilization or exercise.

Fibroblasts also produce **glycosaminoglycans.** These are **proteoglycans,** the fundamental components of connective tissue, which make up the **extracellular matrix** of tendons, ligaments, and articular cartilage. **Imbibition** is the primary nutritional source for avascular tissues such as tendons, ligaments, cartilage, and vertebral disks. When tension/pressure increase, fluid is forced out of tissue and the volume of the tissue decreases. This causes an increase in the concentration of proteoglycan substances and an increase in osmotic pressure, which in turn produces imbibition. Glycosaminoglycans provide the fibers with nutrition via imbibition and lubrication. They allow space for elastic deformity of the tissue.[9] The half-life of glycosaminoglycans is 1.7 to 7 days. Immobilization for more than 1.7 to 7 days causes a 50% decrease in glycosaminoglycans. Therefore lubrication is decreased and the elastic range of collagen is decreased. A decrease in glycosaminoglycans causes a decrease in nutrition, which damages the tissue.

Bone

Bone is the protective and supportive framework that has rigid and static, elastic and dynamic properties. The properties and geometry of bone can be altered in response to internal and external stress and also in response to mineral demands. Bone has plastic qualities; it absorbs and stores compressional forces and transmits tensile forces. Bone also has elastic qualities. Long bone can deform up to 5%. The ability of bone to deform decreases with age.

Bone is composed of approximately 5% water and approximately 70% minerals (calcium hydroxyapatite, phosphate, magnesium, sodium, potassium, and fluoride carbonate); approximately 20% organic compounds, mostly type I collagen; and approximately 5% noncollagenous proteins. Osteoblasts are the functional building blocks of the **osteoid matrix;** they are located only at the surface of bone tissue. **Osteocytes** are mature osteoblasts. **Osteoclasts** are responsible for bone dissolution and absorption. Bone homeostasis balances synthesis, dissolution, and absorption with the forces that are applied on the skeleton.[9]

Cartilage

Cartilage is a semirigid connective tissue that is less dense and more elastic than bone. The functional unit of cartilage is the chondrocyte. Chondroblasts are immature **chondrocytes,** and they produce the **ground substance** or extracellular matrix of cartilage. This extracellular matrix consists of glycosaminoglycans and type II collagen. Water composes 65% to 80% of articular cartilage. Like fibroblasts, chondroblasts synthesize collagen and glycosaminoglycans when stimulated by mechanical tension. Mature cartilage is avascular and lacks nerve supply. Cartilage gets nutrition through imbibition. The mechanical forces of motion stimulate imbibition and removal of waste products.

The three types of cartilage are the following:

1. Hyaline cartilage, which is the most common and is found on articular surfaces of peripheral joints, sternal ends of the ribs, nasal septum, larynx, and tracheal rings
2. Elastic cartilage, which is found in the epiglottis, laryngeal cartilage, walls of eustachian tubes, external ear, and auditory canal
3. Fibrocartilage, which is found in intervertebral disks, some articular cartilage, the pubic symphysis, dense connective tissue in joint capsules, ligaments, and the union of tendons to bone

The two primary functions of articular cartilage are to promote motion between two opposing bones with minimal friction and wear and to distribute the load applied to the joint surfaces over as great an area as possible.[9]

Optimal Stimulus for Regeneration of Collagen, Bone, and Cartilage

Collagen

The optimal stimulus for fibroblastic function in the regeneration of collagen is modified tension along the line of stress. This modified tension is not to exceed the level of tension that the newly formed polar bonds of tropocollagen can withstand. The tropocollagen is an immature, precursor to the stronger, more resilient collagen. Once a certain level of tension is exceeded, tissue breakdown will occur instead of proliferation.

Precaution. *If tension exceeds this critical level, the signs and symptoms will be pain, inflammatory reaction, muscle guarding, decreased range of motion or loss of flexibility, and secondary scarring.*[9]

Bone

The optimal stimulus for osteoblastic production in the regeneration of bone is modified compression in the line of stress. Wolff's law states that bone will change its internal architecture according to the forces placed upon it.

Precaution. *Abnormal shear force may cause a pseudarthrosis.*

Pseudarthrosis or "false joint" occurs at the site of nonunion. **Osteophytes** are bony outgrowths that develop as the body attempts to provide stability or to repair itself. Shearing force stimulates undifferentiated mesenchymal cells to produce cartilage, and a false joint may be created at the fracture site.[9]

Cartilage

The optimal stimulus in the regeneration of cartilage is intermittent compression/decompression with glide. Joint movement (shear) is necessary to distribute synovial fluid over the cartilaginous surface and provide oxygen and other necessary nutrients. Intermittent compression forces the extracellular fluid within the joint to be compressed into the cartilage matrix. With joint immobilization, an alteration in joint mechanics and a decrease in the normal contact areas of cartilage occur. This eventually leads to joint dysfunction, hypomobility or hypermobility, and muscle guarding.

Precaution. *The body responds to the stresses placed upon it. With abnormal stresses there will be dysfunctional remodeling. This manifests as joint degeneration, osteophytes, bone spurs, or pseudarthrosis.*[9]

Effects of Immobilization versus Early Mobilization

CLINICAL *Pearl*

Early mobilization within a pain-free range of motion promotes faster healing of connective tissue, stronger collagen bonds, reduced scar tissue adhesions, and improved collagen fiber orientation.

After 9 weeks of immobilization, there is 14% loss of total collagen, and by 12 weeks there is a 28% loss. The half-life of glycosaminoglycans is 1.7 to 7 days. The half-life of collagen is 300 to 500 days. For this reason, under normal physiologic conditions, it takes between 1 to 2 years for full healing to occur. Immobilization of cartilage causes a decrease in thickness and number of collagen bundles, a decrease in proteoglycan content, an increase in water content, a decrease in load-bearing capacity, softening of the articular surface, decrease in tensile strength of cartilage, and a decrease in oxygen content. To decrease these adverse effects of immobilization, one should institute an exercise model of high repetitions with low to no resistance. This model increases the oxygen content within the tissues by improving blood flow and imbibition. For maximal benefit, mobilization exercises should be performed several times a day.[10] A home exercise program helps accomplish these goals. Box 4-5 lists the qualities of a good home exercise program.

NEUROPHYSIOLOGY

Muscle Spindles

Muscle spindles are proprioceptors that consist of intrafusal muscle fibers enclosed in a sheath (spindle). They run parallel to the extrafusal muscle fibers and act as receptors that provide information on muscle length and the rate of change in muscle length. The spindles are stretched when the muscle lengthens. This stretch causes the sensory neuron in the spindle to transmit an impulse to the spinal cord, where it synapses with alpha motor neurons. This causes activation of motor neurons that innervate the muscle. The muscle spindles determine the amount of contraction necessary to overcome a given resistance. When the resistance increases, the muscle is stretched further, and this causes spindle fibers to activate a greater muscle contraction.[11]

Golgi Tendon Organs

Golgi tendon organs (GTOs) are proprioceptors that are located in the tendon adjacent to the myotendinous

BOX 4-5

Home Exercise Program

The home exercise program should do the following:

1. Provide modified tension in the line of stress. Initially, this will be accomplished by performing light muscle contractions to move the joint through the full available pain-free range of motion.
2. Avoid reinjury. *Any exercise or activity that causes pain is an indication of tissue trauma.*
3. Provide the proper dosage. Give specific instructions about the number of repetitions, sets, breaks, positioning, and speed of exercises.
4. Indicate the frequency of exercise. This depends on healing time frames, intensity, volume, co-morbidities, and the tolerance to stress of the tissue. Be clear in the instructions to the client about the frequency of exercise. Initially this may be 3 or more times per day, but with increased exercise stress, there will be a decrease in frequency.
5. Supply adequate nutritional support. Explain the importance of eating a balanced diet and drinking a sufficient amount of water to stay hydrated. A well-balanced diet combined with exercise promotes healthy tissue.

junction. They are arranged in series with the extrafusal muscle fibers. They are sensitive to stretch but are activated most efficiently when the muscle shortens. The GTO transmits information regarding muscle tension as opposed to length. Neural input from the GTO causes an inhibition of muscle activation. This provides a protective mechanism to avoid development of excessive tension.[11]

Joint Mechanoreceptors

Four types of **mechanoreceptors** are found in the synovial joint capsules. Mechanoreceptors have a significant effect on muscle tone and pain sensation locally and distally along segmental innervations. The number of mechanoreceptors decreases with age. By age 70 the total number of receptors has decreased by about 50%, depending on factors such as genetics and activity level.[12]

Type I mechanoreceptors are found in the superficial layers of the joint capsule between the collagen fibers. A large percentage of the type I mechanoreceptors is found in the joints of the neck, hip, and shoulder. They have a great effect on the coordination of the tonic muscle

fibers. They are slow-adapting and inhibit pain. They fire during movement and for about 1 minute after movement stops. They provide postural and kinesthetic awareness (awareness of the position of the body or body part in space). They are active in the beginning and end-range of collagen tension.

Type II mechanoreceptors are found in deep layers of joint capsules. A high concentration of the type II mechanoreceptors is found in the joints of the lumbar spine, hand, foot, and temporomandibular joint. They are fast adapting and pain inhibiting. They fire during movement and continue to fire until about $1/2$ second after movement stops. They do not respond to stretch but are activated in beginning and midrange of collagen tension. They have more effect on the phasic muscle fibers and **kinesthesia.**

Type III mechanoreceptors are located in the deep and superficial layers of the joint capsules and ligaments. They are slow adapting and inhibit muscle tone in response to stretch at the extreme end-range of tension. They provide kinesthetic information, but their role is less understood than the type I and II mechanoreceptors.

Type IV mechanoreceptors are located in joint capsules, blood vessels, articular fat pads, anterior dura mater, ligaments of the spine, and connective tissue. They are not found in muscle. They fire when excessive levels of tension are reached in the collagen, and they warn of tissue trauma. They function as pain-provoking, nonadapting, high-threshold receptors. They fire continuously until the injurious stimulus is removed. They are provoked by excessive stretch, inflammation, high temperature (38° C to 42° C), or respiratory and cardiovascular distress.[12]

Pain has been defined by the International Association for the Study of Pain as an unpleasant emotional disorder evoked by sufficient activity in the **nociceptive** system and associated with real or potential tissue damage.[13] The irritation causing the pain may be due to immobilization, physical trauma, infection, or emotional tension.

Precaution. *Pain is a protective mechanism. Pain is NOT a warning that something is about to go wrong; it has already gone wrong! Pain is the way the body alerts the brain that an irritation to the tissue has occurred. For this reason, one must remember to exercise within a pain-free range of motion. In this case, feeling bad is a good thing because it is how your body communicates. Listen to the body.*

TRAUMATOLOGY

The response of the body to trauma is predictable and consistent, regardless of the tissue involved or the mechanism of injury. Trauma sets off a highly organized response involving chemical, metabolic, permeability, and vascular changes at a cellular level in preparation for tissue repair.

Phases and Time Frames of Healing

The initial response to a traumatic event is irritation. This lasts for 5 to 6 hours. Vasomotor constriction occurs in the first few seconds. An immediate release of chemical vasodilators occurs. These dilators are also transmitters for the nociceptive (pain) system. The vasodilation increases the hydrostatic pressure because of increased capillary permeability. Clinicians rarely can influence this phase because of its immediate occurrence.

The next stage of healing is the acute stage, which lasts for 1 to 3 days depending on the vascularity of the tissue. During this time frame, a migration of the larger cell bodies through the wall of the vessel occurs. Subsequently, blood flow increases to the area, increasing hydrostatic pressure and increasing bleeding. The large proteins leak out of the capillary, causing a shift in osmotic pressure with resultant pulling of fluid out of the capillary. Venous stasis occurs distal to the traumatized area, and edema results. (See Chapter 3.)

The third stage of healing is the subacute stage. The subacute stage begins with the settled stage, where muscle spasming occurs over the next 3 to 5 days. Bleeding is no longer present. Oxygen and macrophages are present. Walling off of the capillary occurs, which makes waste removal difficult. This leads to secondary healing or scarring. Externally applied heat in the settled stage promotes stasis and inflammatory exudates. The preferred method of heating tissue is internally. Initiating movement with low resistance exercise produces friction and naturally generates heat. This promotes increased blood flow.

The final stage is the chronic stage. Tissue becomes strongly chemical bonded (covalent bonds) and mature at 9 to 12 months. At this stage the tissue becomes non-elastic and cannot be deformed. Mature scar tissue may cause pain. Clinically, concentrate on increasing the tolerance of the tissue to tension about the scar by use of controlled stress through properly dosed exercises.

Tissue-specific exercise in the subacute stage provides the optimal stimulus for the removal of **metabolites,** which are products of metabolism, from the tissue. Muscle contraction is necessary to transport metabolites from the cell and provide oxygen/nutrition to the area. Increased vascularization accomplishes this goal. This is achieved through many repetitions of properly dosed exercise with minimal resistance while avoiding excessive tissue tension. In other words, the muscle contractions with proper exercise facilitate formation of capillaries, blood flow, and removal of metabolites.

Stages of Repair

The stages of repair can be categorized into three phases: inflammation, repair, and remodeling. During the inflammatory phase, the white blood cells/macrophages destroy cellular debris, synthesize fibronectin, and produce protein and fiber. During the repair stage, collagen is produced, and during the remodeling stage, the fibroblasts orient longitudinally within 28 days and repair is complete between 128 to 135 days. **Myofibroblasts** (involved in tissue reconstruction) are active from 5 to 21 days after trauma to up to 9 months. During the initial remodeling, a random configuration of collagen fibrils occurs. This arrangement provides minimal strength. During the maturation phase, the mechanical strength increases with remodeling and organization of fibers with modified tension in the line of stress.[14]

MUSCLE PHYSIOLOGY

CLINICAL *Pearl*

Strength is related to fiber diameter, not fiber type.

Type I muscle fibers are smaller in diameter than type II muscle fibers. Muscle recruitment progresses from smaller to larger diameter. **Tonic muscles** fire first because they are the primary dynamic joint stabilizers. Their nutrition mainly comes from the delivery of oxygen. They are predominantly type I or slow-twitch muscles and are responsible for sustaining proper joint **arthrokinematics** over time.[1]

Tonic versus Phasic Muscles

Tonic muscles initiate the easy work; they are better adapted for endurance exercise than **phasic muscles** because they have more capillaries, mitochondria, and metabolic enzymes (Table 4-2). With long-distance running the tonic muscles are primarily responsible for work because they are adapted for aerobic activity. The phasic muscles are recruited to participate if the load is too great or if it is increasing. They are better suited for short-duration activities that are of higher intensity. They also begin to participate if the light work has lasted for 2 to 3 hours, as seen with marathon runners who sprint when approaching the finish line. Phasic muscles are anaerobic and contract at a higher speed and with greater force of contraction; they fatigue more quickly than tonic muscles.

The tonic muscle fibers atrophy almost immediately when immobilized after injury because they depend pri-

TABLE 4-2

Comparison of Tonic and Phasic Muscle Fibers

TONIC	PHASIC
Red: High myoglobin concentration	White: Lower myoglobin concentration
Slow twitch: 10 to 20 impulses per second	Fast twitch: 30 to 50 impulses per second
Type I	Type II
Arthrokinematic	Osteokinematic
Bipenate	Fusiform
Antigravity	—

marily on oxygen for metabolism. Therefore exercise to improve vascularization provides the oxygen necessary to nourish the tonic system.

Habitually overloading a system will cause it to respond and adapt. The rate of protein synthesis in a muscle is related directly to the rate of amino acid transportation into the cell. Amino acids transported into the muscle are influenced by the intensity and the duration of the muscle tension. Conversely, muscle atrophies as a result of disuse, immobilization, guarding associated with pain, or starvation.[1]

Types of Muscle Work and Training Effects

Isometric muscle contraction is the production of muscle tension without a change in muscle length or joint angle. The tension in the **cross-bridges** (the portion of myosin filament that pulls the actin filaments toward the center of the sarcomere during muscle contraction) is equal to the resistive force, thereby maintaining constant muscle length.

Concentric muscle contraction is muscle shortening as the muscle produces tension while the insertion moves toward the origin. Movement occurs in the same direction as the tension and joint motion because the contractile force is greater than the resistive force. Based on the **sliding filament theory,** the cross-bridges on the myosin filament attach to the active site on the actin filament. When all of the cross-bridges in a muscle shorten in a single cycle, the muscle shortens by approximately 1%. Muscles have the capacity to shorten up to 60% of their resting length; therefore the contraction cycle must be repeated multiple times.[15]

Eccentric muscle contraction is muscle lengthing as the muscle produces tension and the insertion moves away from the origin. The net muscle movement is in the opposite direction of the force of the muscle because the contractile force is less than the resistive force. Eccentric contractions require less energy than concentric contrac-

tions and are thought to be responsible for some aspect of postexercise muscle soreness. The cross-bridges of myosin stay attached to the active sites while the resistance is lowered. It may be the actual "tearing" away of the cross-bridges while resisting the lowering of a heavy resistance that results in the delayed-onset muscle soreness.[15,16]

EXERCISE

Functional Qualities of Exercise

Coordination refers to quality of motion. With atrophy of the tonic system, coordination is the first functional quality to be lost because the tonic muscles are the primary dynamic stabilizers of the joints. Therefore coordination must be the first functional quality to be restored. With an increase in speed or an increase in resistance comes a need for increased coordination. Normalization of a **reflex disturbance,** which is abnormal action of the cell, tissue, organ, or organism caused by overstimulation or understimulation, requires 5000 to 6000 repetitions. The repetitions are necessary to regain optimal coordination of movements about a physiologic axis.[1]

Endurance is the capacity to maintain an intensity of exercise for a prolonged period. Endurance requires continuous restoration of energy sources. Tonic muscles primarily require oxygen from the vascular system for their nutrition. Phasic muscles require glucose and body fat for their nutrition. Because the tonic system is the first to atrophy, because of muscle guarding and decreased motor recruitment, endurance is the quality that will increase nutrition through vascularization. Endurance exercise also promotes removal of waste products and prevents continued firing of the type IV mechanoreceptors caused by an abnormal chemical environment. Exercise dosage for endurance and vascularization requires many repetitions (3 sets of 24) with low resistance.[1]

Speed is the time it takes to cover a fixed distance. Speed equals distance divided by time. With an increase

PART ONE *Fundamentals*

in speed of movement is an increase in inertia, and overcoming this inertia requires a higher level of coordination. Speed of movement ultimately must be functional. During the initial phases of healing, coordination is not sufficient to exercise safely at a fast/functional speed.[1]

Volume refers to the total amount of weight lifted in a workout. The weight per repetition determines the appropriate volume per set. Heavy weights cannot be lifted for many repetitions in a set. Volume can be determined by multiplying the number of repetitions by the number of sets times the weight lifted per repetition. Three sets of 25 repetitions with 5 lb would be calculated as $3 \times 25 \times 5\,lb = 375\,lb$ of volume. If other sets also are performed with different amounts of weight, the volumes per set are calculated and then all are added together to obtain the total workout volume.[17]

Strength is the maximal force that a muscle or group of muscles can generate against a resistance at a given speed. Strength can be tested a measure of **1 RM (resistance maximal;** see the following discussion for more on this topic). Strength training is performed at a percentage of 1 RM. For strength training, the number of repetitions decreases as the resistance increases. Increased resistance produces an increase in tissue tension and a decrease in blood flow to the capillaries during the muscle contraction, as well as an increase in blood flow when the exercise is over. Therefore only a few repetitions are performed. For pure strength gains, 85% of 1 RM (3 sets of 6 are performed). However, when there is muscle atrophy, after immobilization, strength gains are realized at 30% to 40% of 1 RM.[1,18,19]

Power is the ability to overcome resistance over a specific distance in a fixed time frame. Work equals force multiplied by distance. Power equals work divided by time. Power lifting is generally not a functional requirement for clients. However, increased power is necessary to perform a task at a faster rate. Power is therefore a critical component of exercise for clients.[20]

Dosing

Exercise initially is dosed based on the physiology of the type I muscle fibers and their depletion of nutrients in a state of guarding.

CLINICAL *Pearl*

Clinically, the first goal of dosing exercise is to deliver oxygen to the muscles, elicit no pain, and perform many repetitions.

Initially, focus on sustaining slow, coordinated movement around a physiologic axis. Ultimately, progress toward a fast/functional speed while maintaining coordination and providing optimal stimulus for regeneration of the specific tissue(s) in lesion.[1] Resistance should be objective and measurable, physiologic and adjusted to the tissues participating. (See later in the chapter for explanations of these concepts.) Training with free weights or a pulley system is easier to quantify and provides a more specific resistance throughout the entire range of motion than elastic bands.

Starting Positions

Determining a starting position depends on tolerance of the specific tissues to stress. Gravity assists, resists, or is eliminated, depending on what the tissue can tolerate while working in a pain-free synergy about a physiologic axis.

Precaution. *If there is pain while exercising against the force of gravity, position the limb in a posture that eliminates the effects of gravity.*[1]

If necessary, to complete a pain free arc of motion, the limb can be positioned so that the motion to be performed is assisted by gravity. This way, the **antagonists,** muscles that work in opposition to the prime movers, generate motion instead of the painful **agonists** or prime movers.

Range of Motion

Initially, localize motion to a specific joint in a specific direction with controlled range of motion maintained throughout the arc. Monitor the tension on noncontractile tissues. Watch for controlled, normal physiologic motion, and educate the client to avoid compensatory motion while exercising. Adjust the resistance to allow for acceleration toward maximal length-tension range and deceleration away from it. Quality of motion, while avoiding pain-provoking end-ranges, dictates quantity.[1]

Work Capacity/Effects of Aging

An individual's sustainable work capacity is approximately 30% of that person's available energy. The remaining 70% of the stored energy in the body is needed for protein synthesis and maintenance of tissue (Fig. 4-1). The amount of energy available for maintenance, repair, and regeneration of tissue decreases with age. With age, it takes less activity to dip into the 70% of energy reserve that is so necessary for tissue synthesis and repair (Fig. 4-2).

Precaution. *With an older client population, take care not to overexercise, or the risk for breakdown of collagen tissue and problems such as tendonitis will increase.*[1]

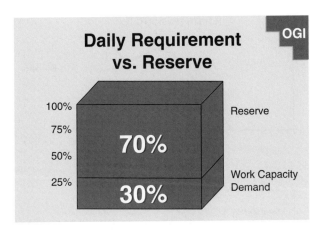

FIGURE 4-1 Total daily energy requirements. (Used with permission from the Ola Grimsby Institute.)

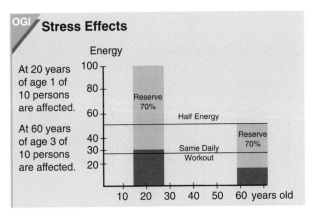

FIGURE 4-2 Effects of age on energy requirements. (Used with permission from the Ola Grimsby Institute.)

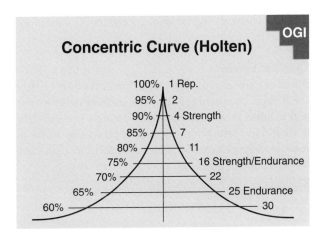

FIGURE 4-3 Holten diagram. (Used with permission from the Ola Grimsby Institute.)

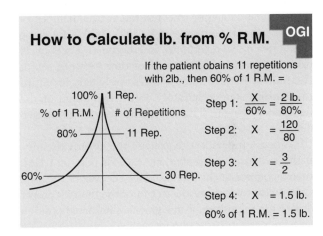

FIGURE 4-4 Example for calculating exercise dose. (Used with permission from the Ola Grimsby Institute.)

Calculating Dosage

In 1948, DeLorme defined the term *resistance maximal* (RM). This is the resistance that a group of muscles can overcome once. RM was used as a measure of strength. In the 1950s the Norwegian Oddvar Holten developed a curve that estimated guidelines for dosing repetitions/ resistance for concentric work (Fig. 4-3).[1,21]

Calculating Resistance by Percentage of 1 RM

Repetitions of Exercise
Because 1 RM is the maximum resistance that can be overcome once, this resistance has a high risk of causing further injury to the already compromised tissue. When dosing an exercise program initially, the first functional qualities desired are to promote vascularization and endurance while maintaining coordination. For this to be accomplished, according to the Holten diagram, the exercise should be dosed at 30 repetitions (Fig. 4-4).[1,21]

The client is given a weight that the therapist predicts will cause fatigue in less than 30 repetitions. The client then performs as many repetitions as possible before the onset of fatigue, pain, or loss of coordination. As an example, the client is provided with a 3-lb weight and is able to perform 16 repetitions with this weight before becoming fatigued or experiencing pain (16 repetitions correlates to 75% of 1 RM according to the Holten diagram).

Therefore

$$\frac{x}{60} = \frac{3}{75}$$

$$x = \frac{180}{75}$$

$$x = 2.4\,\text{lb}$$

This client should be able to perform 30 repetitions with 2.4 lb.

Speed of Exercise

Speed of exercise is another component that may change the dosage. Increased speed causes an increase in inertia and requires more coordination to execute. Oxygen debt is also important to avoid during exercising so as to provide the type I muscle fibers with nutrition while they are in a state of guarding.

Precaution. *If the client's respiratory rate is increasing during the exercise, then the speed of exercise must be decreased or there must be a longer break between sets or both.*

To increase the total number of repetitions while maintaining an accurate dose, increase the number of sets. It has been determined that to go from one set to 3 sets without changing the resistance, the number of repetitions must be decreased by 15% to 20%. By doing this, 1 set of 30 repetitions now becomes 3 sets of 24 to 25 repetitions. The amount of time between sets is determined by how long it takes the client to return to a **steady state respiratory rate** (equilibrium of the respiratory system). This is necessary to avoid oxygen debt.

When using pulleys to exercise the upper extremity, if the weight of the limb alone exceeds 60% of 1 RM, then a counterweight may be used to de-weight the arm. Other ways to decrease the weight of the limb for proper dosage are to position it in a gravity-eliminated position or even a gravity-assisted position.[1,21]

Length-Tension Relationship and Implications to Exercise

Blyx,[22] a Swedish physiologist, defined **muscle fiber length equilibrium** as the length the muscle will maintain when it is unaffected by outside forces. Muscle force production varies depending on the angle of the muscle in the arc of motion. The length/tension curve identifies the length at which a muscle generates the most contractile tension (Fig. 4-5). This length is influenced by histologic, biomechanical, and neurophysiologic factors. Histologically, the overlap of actin and myosin filaments is most extensive toward the midrange of motion. Biomechanically, the angle of the tendon insertion into the bone dictates where the greatest tensile strength will occur. The greatest amount of force is achieved when the moment arm for a muscular force is perpendicular to the lever arm. Neurophysiologically, the joint mechanoreceptors influence muscle facilitation around the joint. Type I and type II mechanoreceptors fire at the beginning of range. Type II alone fires at midrange, and type I fires at the end-range of capsular tension.[10]

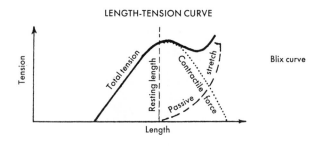
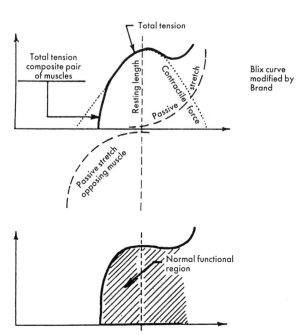

FIGURE 4-5 Length-tension curve. (From Brand PW, Hollister A: Clinical mechanics of the hand, St Louis, 1993, Mosby. In Trumble, *Principles of hand surgery and therapy*, St Louis, 2000, Philadelphia.)

The clinical importance of the length/tension concept can be discussed in terms of concentric and eccentric aspects.

Concentric Aspects

When working concentrically with pulleys, set the rope perpendicular to the lever arm at 20% into the lengthened range of the muscle that is going to do the work. If using free weights, position the limb where it is perpendicular to the force of gravity, when the lever arm is at 20% into the lengthened range of motion.

Eccentric Aspects

When working eccentrically, have the maximal resistance set perpendicular to the lever arm at 20% to 30% into the shortened range of the muscle that is going to do the eccentric work. The length/tension concept reveals that muscle produces the least amount of power at the beginning and end-ranges. When activated, the muscle contraction accelerates toward the midrange and decelerates away from it. The variability of speed is an important component of all activities of daily living. Because activity is task specific, the variables of speed and resistance throughout the range of a contraction are important for fiber recruitment and physiologic coordination.[1,21]

Formulation and Progression of an Exercise Program

When formulating an exercise program for treatment of hypomobility or hypermobility, you should start by identifying the specific problems that exist. Examples of these problems are the following:

- The complaint of pain
- Muscle guarding of the tonics (rotator cuff)
- Decreased endurance, and limited range of motion (external rotation [ER] > abduction [ABD] > internal rotation [IR])
- Articular compression
- Decreased synovium/decreased articular cartilage nutrition
- Decreased mechanoreceptor input in the capsule
- Compensatory motion.

Once an examination has been completed, establish functional or measurable goals that address the identified problems. The following suggestions are several possible goals for the client:

- Decrease pain with arm elevation (1 to 10 scale)
- Increase endurance with exercise (time and repetitions) and with functional work/avocation activities (time)
- Increase range of motion (specific planes of motion and to accomplish functional activities)
- Educate/improve posture to promote proximal stability and improved arthrokinematics of the glenohumeral joint (at work, with activities, time frames)
  Identify treatment approaches to resolve the goals:
  - Decrease pain and guarding: distraction of the joint to fire type I mechanoreceptors
  - Increase joint mobility: compression/decompression with gliding for cartilage, modified tension in the line of stress for joint capsule
  - Hydrate/lubricate cartilage: compression/decompression with glide
  - Increase proprioception: modified tension in the line of stress

Consider client and equipment needs before starting exercises. Box 4-6 outlines different aspects of an exercise program. Consider precautions and contraindications when implementing an exercise program.

BOX 4-6

Considerations for Exercise Program

Equipment: pulleys, benches, bolsters, and wedges for positioning; straps, free weights, and deweighting devices.

Ropes: Consider the range of motion, and set the rope perpendicular to the lever arm and parallel to the muscle fiber.

Pulley: single, double, concentric, or eccentric.

Starting positions: supine, prone, side-lying, sitting, standing, non–weight bearing, weight bearing, arm supported, or unsupported.

Movement range: full range of motion; inner, outer, or midrange of motion.

Weight: Consider the functional quality that is desired and what percentage of 1 RM is needed to accomplish that. (In this case the functional qualities most likely would be endurance and vascularization.) Also take into account the body/limb position, gravity, and quality of motion when determining weight.

Dosage: The number of repetitions and sets is determined by the desired functional qualities. These include coordination, vascularization, endurance, strength, and power.[7,23]

Speed: This will vary, but early in the rehabilitation, when working on vascularization and endurance, it is important to follow respiratory rate at steady state to avoid oxygen debt. Speed should increase as coordination and function increase.

Rest: Breaks between sets are determined by respiratory rate. As the client starts to increase strength (x resistance + x repetitions), the rest breaks will increase. As resistance increases, the frequency of exercise decreases as well (3 times per week).

Education: Instructions to the client must be specific. Demonstration of the exercise first or even guiding the client's limb through the arc of motion that is desired is often helpful. Use verbal, visual, and tactile cues as necessary.

Precaution. *Co-morbidities such as cardiac or pulmonary disease, specific physician protocol, and other medical/surgical considerations must dictate exercise decisions.*

Progressions of Hypomobilities

Progressions of hypomobilities has four stages (Table 4-3).

Stage I

Stage I begins with many repetitions to address coordination. Following the Holten diagram, 60% of 1 RM pro-

TABLE 4-3

Progression of Hypomobilities Stages I to IV

STAGE	PROCEDURES	GOALS
STAGE I		
	Many repetitions	Increase endurance
	Low speed	Increase circulation
	Minimal resistance	Increase exercise ability
	Outer range of motion	Avoid overexertion
STAGE II		
	Increase repetitions	Increase endurance
	Increase speed	Increase fast coordination
	Do not increase resistance	
STAGE III		
	Stabilizing exercise in the gained range of motion	Increase strength in the gained range of motion
	Concentric and eccentric	
STAGE IV		
	Coordinate tonic and phasic function throughout physiologic range of motion	Functional stability

motes vascularization. This is dosed at 3 sets of 25 repetitions. Fifty percent of 1 RM helps decrease joint edema. Beginning with 40% of 1 RM may be necessary when the amount of muscle fiber atrophy present is significant. Start at a slow speed with minimal resistance to maintain coordinated movement and help decrease inflammation. Work into the outer, pain-free range of motion to promote stimulation of fibroblasts and production of glycosaminoglycans. This stage of exercises stimulates joint mechanoreceptors and GTOs to inhibit pain and guarding. Begin with the joint in a resting position and provide support of bolsters or other equipment as needed to promote quality of motion around a physiologic axis. Start with concentric contractions initially to increase vascularity.[10]

Stage II

Have the client progress to stage II when the functional quality of coordination and vascularization is achieved. Signs for progressing to this stage are a decrease in complaint of pain, increased range of motion, increased speed of exercise, decreased muscle guarding, and less fatigue experienced by the client.

The goal of stage II is to increase endurance and speed. This is accomplished by increasing the number of sets and the number of exercises. With increased coordination, increase the speed of exercise. Do not increase resistance. At this point, remove the supportive bolsters so that the client can begin stabilizing proximally while improving the mobility of the hypomobile joint. Histo-

logic changes that take place in stage II are improved nutrition to the joint cartilage through decreased viscosity of synovial fluid associated with the increase in speed.[10]

Stage III

Have the client progress to stage III when pain has resolved, full range of motion is regained, and when speed and coordination have increased. For the newly gained range of motion there must be dynamic stability. This means that the musculotendinous units are strong enough to maintain controlled, physiologic mobility. Concentric and eccentric contractions in the newly gained range of motion promote functional stability. In stage III the resistance is increased to 60% to 80%, and the repetitions are decreased to 10 to 15 repetitions to promote strength/endurance. Begin triplanar motions by exercising in proprioceptive neuromuscular facilitation patterns. Add isometric contractions in the newly gained end-range of motion to promote strength.

Stage IV

Have the client progress to stage IV when the client is able to increase the speed of exercise and still maintain coordination. Absence of delayed-onset muscle soreness is also an indication that it is time to progress to the next level. Stage IV emphasizes functional exercises and retraining for activities of daily living, essential job functions, and sport-specific activities. Exercises are performed through a full range of motion at up to 80% to 90% of

TABLE 4-4

Progression of Hypermobilities Stages I to IV

STAGES	PROCEDURES	GOALS
STAGE I	Many repetitions Low speed Minimal resistance Beginning or midrange of motion	Increase endurance Increase circulation Increase exercise ability Avoid overexertion
STAGE II	Increase repetitions Include isometric contractions in inner range of motion	Increase strength Increase sensitivity to stretch
STAGE III	Submaximal (80% RM) resistance concentrically and eccentrically Include isometric contractions in the full range of motion (except the outer range)	Increase dynamic stability in the gained range of motion
STAGE IV	Coordinate tonic and phasic function throughout physiologic range of motion	Functional stability

1 RM at a functional speed in order to achieve the functional quality of power.[1]

Progressions of Hypermobilities

Exercise progressions for hypermobilities have four stages (Table 4-4).

Stage I

Stage I for hypermobilities is identical to stage I for hypomobilities, with one major exception. With a hypomobility the exercises are dosed to promote increased mobility, whereas with a hypermobility the goal is to increase stability. Therefore exercises for hypermobility are performed in the beginning and midrange of motion so that coordination can be maintained while developing stability.

Stage II

In stage II, increase repetitions, number of sets, and number of exercises. Add closed kinetic chain and slow plyometric exercises to increase sensitivity to stretch. Continue to perform exercise in a single plane of motion, and increase speed as coordination permits.

Stage III

In stage III, increase resistance to 80% of 1 RM and decrease the number of repetitions to promote strength. Perform concentric and eccentric contractions for increased stability in the physiologic range of motion.

Add a set of one isometric contraction at 75% to 85% of **1 IM (isometric maximum).** This contraction should be held for 15 seconds. Fast **plyometrics** (when an eccentric contraction is immediately followed by a concentric contraction) for recruitment of the muscle spindle helps increase sensitivity to stretch and aids in stability. Triplanar motion can start in stage III for promotion of functional stability.

Stage IV

Hypermobility progression in stage IV is equivalent to that for hypomobilities. The exercises become more functional, and you should focus more on retraining for a job, activities of daily living, and sport. Increase the resistance to improve the qualities of power and speed.[1]

Monitoring of Vital Signs

Monitoring of vital signs is a reliable, valid, and meaningful way of measuring clients' response to exercise. It takes practice to become accurate with monitoring vital signs and to understand the significance of these values. Taking a resting heart rate, blood pressure, respiratory rate, and oxygen saturation (SpO_2) only measures the body systems at rest. To get baseline measurements, take vital signs before, during, and after exercise. Doing this provides critical information about how the body is responding to the exercise loads placed upon it, as well as how well it recovers from the stress of exercise.

Precaution. *Proper dosing of exercise can improve the effi-ciency of the cardiovascular system, whereas overdosing may cause irreversible damage.*

Heart rate/pulse may be altered by many medications and diseases. When this is the case, as in clients who are taking beta-blockers or are in congestive heart failure, monitoring of the heart rate in response to exercise may provide inaccurate or misleading information. In such cases, one must use other forms of measuring the response of the body to exercise.[6]

Rate of Perceived Exertion

Gunner Borg established the Borg scale (rate of perceived exertion, or RPE) in 1962. The RPE is a subjective mea-surement of how hard clients think they are exercising. The RPE has been proved to be a valid and reliable way of measuring exertion during exercise and functional activities. The original scale was based on numeric values that ranged from 6 to 20, with 6 being a perception of minimal effort, as in relaxing in a chair, and with 20 describing maximal effort, as in running up a steep hill. Target RPE is between 11 and 13 (fairly light to some-what hard). This is a pace that could be maintained for at least a 15-minute workout. Breathing would be labored; one could carry on a conversation but likely would prefer not to do so. In more recent years, a modified RPE scale has become popular. This newer version is based on a 0 to 10 value system. Zero is equivalent to work at rest, and 10 is maximal exertion. Some find this modified scale easier to use. Table 4-5 gives the Borg rate of perceived exertion scales.[6]

Training Modes

Cardiovascular warm-up only gets the heart and lungs prepared for exercise, but it also is the healthy, natural way of preparing tissue for more vigorous, tissue-specific exercise. The warm-up may consist of 5 to 15 minutes of walking on the treadmill or riding on a stationary bike or upper body ergometer. This type of warm-up increases blood flow, heart rate, deep muscle/tissue temperature, and respiratory rate and decreases joint synovial fluid. This means of increasing circulation may be the wise choice as opposed to the passive hot pack application for tissue warming.

Core/proximal stabilization exercises are essential com-ponents of all phases of exercise and activities of daily living. For normal physiologic movement to take place, there must be distal mobility on proximal stability.

Precaution. *Increased mobility at the expense of proximal stability equates to compensatory or nonphysiologic movement.*

TABLE 4-5

Borg Rate of Perceived Exertion Scales

BORG SCALE	NEWER SCALE
6	0 Nothing at all
7 Very, very light	0.5 Very, very weak
8	1 Very weak
9 Very light	2 Weak
10	3 Moderate
11 Fairly light	4 Somewhat strong
12	5 Strong
13 Somewhat hard	6
14	7 Very strong
15 Hard	8
16	9
17 Very hard	10 Maximal
18	
19 Very, very hard	
20	

Therefore proper posturing and core stabilization exercises are an appropriate component of the hand therapist's repertoire.

Concentric exercise requires 3 times as much energy as does eccentric exercise. Most of the energy of the body is stored in muscle mass. Seventy percent of the stored energy is used to maintain all vital organ function. Thirty percent of the stored energy is used to carry out func-tional daily activities. If a person regularly exceeds the 30% of energy reserved for activities of daily living and dips into the 70% reserved for vital organs, pathologic conditions of the collagen will result. This may be mani-fested as a tendonitis, for example. To promote healing, when dosing initially for concentric exercise, it is best to require many repetitions with light resistance. Doing so will increase oxygen to the injured tissue by increasing its blood flow (Fig. 4-6).[1]

Isometric exercise occurs when a muscle contracts without joint motion. A strengthening effect for the muscle occurs at the angle the joint assumes during the contraction and at 20 degrees on either side of that angle. For example, if the biceps are isometrically contracted with the elbow at 90 degrees, a strengthening effect will result from 70 to 110 degrees. This is a safe way to begin strengthening after an injury if the isometric exercises are performed in a pain-free range. Isometric exercises can be performed at varying angles and can be dosed at different intensities. The amount of force that can be maintained by an isometric contraction for 1 second is

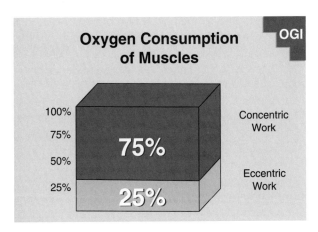

FIGURE 4-6 Oxygen consumption of muscles.

1 IM. In rehabilitation, therapists dose isometric contractions at a percentage of 1 IM. Percentage of isometric resistance is dosed in relation to holding time. For example, 60% of 1 IM can be held from 50 to 60 seconds; 80% of 1 IM can be maintained for 20 to 30 seconds.[1]

Open and closed kinetic chain exercises play an important role in rehabilitation of the upper extremity. Most functional activities of the upper extremity are **open chain.** Movement occurs from muscle origin to insertion, and the terminal joint is free. With **closed chain** exercises, movement occurs from muscle insertion to origin, and the terminal joint is constrained in a fixed position.[24]

Client Education

To increase compliance with exercise programs, it is essential to educate clients on why they are doing each component of the exercise program and what is being accomplished.

CLINICAL *Pearl*

Explain that the exercises that are dosed at high repetitions are to improve vascularization and endurance.

Movement is life, and conversely lack of movement will lead to tissue destruction. Many repetitions in a pain-free range of motion help to increase blood flow, which in turn brings more oxygen to the injured tissue. The body gets nutrition through the oxygen in the blood.

Precaution. *Avoid pain because pain indicates that the tissue is being irritated. With tissue irritation there will be more pain, which leads to muscle guarding, inflammation, and a decrease of blood flow/nutrition to the area.*

Emphasize quality of motion. The body responds to the stress placed upon it. Maintaining proper posture and body mechanics during exercises and throughout the day and night will result in optimal health. Encourage clients to keep a journal of their activities and home exercise program. This is often helpful for accountability and guidance for upgrades.

CASE Studies of Exercise Progressions

CASE STUDY 4-1: LATERAL EPICONDYLITIS

History

TP is a 36-year-old left-hand dominant female secretary who spends 8 hours a day working on the computer and talking on the telephone. She also is attending night school and studying nursing. Because of limited free time, she reports that she has not been participating in any regular exercise program. She admits that she has gained quite a bit of weight over the last year. TP often studies in bed at night, propped up by pillows, until she falls asleep. TP presents to therapy reporting that her right lateral elbow has been painful for approximately 3 months. She does not recall sustaining any injury. She notes that the pain in her elbow becomes more intense over the course of the work day. Upon questioning, she does recall that she often awakens during the night with numbness and tingling into the "whole hand."

Clinical Evaluation Findings

TP reports frustration because she has had 1 month of therapy for her elbow, and she feels that it has not improved but rather has gotten worse. She states that her therapy has consisted of hot packs, ultrasound, and stretching exercises. She also was provided with a wrist splint and tennis elbow strap.

Her evaluation was remarkable for rounded shoulder forward head posture, sixth cervical vertebra–facilitated segment (causing increased tone along the C6 distribution), pain to palpation at the insertion of the extensor carpi radialis brevis, pain at end-range elbow extension, decreased grip on the right (because of pain), and pain with resisted wrist extension. After explaining the findings and outlining the treatment plan, the therapist established goals for therapy with TP, and she agreed to comply.

An ergonomic evaluation of the work station was performed. Recommendations for computer monitor, keyboard height, and chair adjustments were made. New mouse placement and style were reviewed. A phone head set was ordered.

TP was instructed in some postural exercises including pectoralis stretches, chin tucks, neck stretches, and gentle brachial plexus/peripheral nerve glides. The postural strengthening exercises included wall letters and scapular retraction and depression exercises. TP agreed to perform these exercises during breaks at work and at home.

TP agreed to start walking daily, beginning with 15 minutes a day at a comfortable pace while maintaining good posture. Duration of the walks is to increase by 2 minutes a week over the next 2 months, as she is able. Speed of gait is also to increase as TP becomes more comfortable and acclimated to her walking program.

The first therapy treatment was spent evaluating TP, educating her on the different components of her present complaints. Explanations were provided on how posture, work, and exercise habits contributed to the elbow pain and how she could address this responsibly. She was provided with the foregoing home exercise program and was dosed for her clinical elbow exercise program.

The first stage of exercise was dosed with the physiology of the tonic muscle fiber of the elbow in mind. Three months of muscle guarding resulted in some tonic muscle atrophy, degeneration of collagen, and alteration in joint mechanics leading to a decrease in normal contact areas of cartilage. The optimal stimulus for regeneration of collagen is modified tension in the line of stress and the optimal stimulus for regeneration of cartilage is compression/decompression with glide. Following the stage I protocol for hypomobility, it was determined that TP could tolerate 21 repetitions of concentric wrist extension against gravity before pain set in.

On the second visit, treatment commenced. All exercises were dosed at 3 sets of 25 repetitions to promote vascularization and endurance while maintaining coordinated movement around a physiologic axis throughout a full pain-free arc of motion. TP warmed up on the upper body ergometer for 12 minutes at 120 rpm, forward and backward to avoid fatigue (please refer to the CD for illustrations of the following exercises).

1. Concentric wrist flexion, with forearm supported on a table (see CD for Fig. 4-7, A)
2. Concentric wrist extension, with forearm supported on a table (see CD for Fig. 4-7, B)
3. Pronation, with forearm supported on a table (see CD for Fig. 4-8, A)
4. Supination, with forearm supported on a table (see CD for Fig. 4-8, B)
5. Elbow flexion/extension, with forearm supported on a table (see CD for Fig. 4-9)

After finishing the foregoing 375 repetitions, the home exercise program was reviewed to ensure that the exercises were being performed correctly. Treatment concluded with an ice massage. TP reported fatigue but no pain.

TP returned to therapy 2 days later reporting that she had been compliant with her home exercises, walking program, and working on proper posture throughout the day/night. Her complaint of pain had decreased approximately 25%, and the "numbness and tingling" in the hand had resolved. TP went through the foregoing exercise program again and then was scheduled for one visit per week in therapy to make upgrades in the program as necessary. TP also agreed to add the dosed exercises to her current home exercise program.

One week later TP returned to the clinic and reported compliance and denied any problems with her exercises. She stated that the exercises were taking much less time now than they were originally. TP described minimal complaint of elbow pain during the work day and no more symptoms at night. The exercises were upgraded because she now could tolerate 30 repetitions (please refer to the CD for illustrations of the following exercises).

1. Wrist extension against gravity (see CD for Fig. 4-10)
2. Wrist flexion against gravity (see CD for Fig. 4-11)
3. Pronation with 1 lb (see CD for Fig. 4-12, A)
4. Supination with 1 lb (see CD for Fig. 4-12, B)
5. Elbow flexion—recumbent seated position flexion with 2 lb (see CD for Fig. 4-13)
6. Elbow extension in prone with 2 lb (see CD for Fig. 4-14)

TP agreed to continue with her home exercise program, adding the new upgrades with the 3 sets of 25 each.

Result of Care

On the following week, TP called to cancel her future therapy appointments. She reported that she had not had any elbow pain in the previous 4 days and that because of time constraints she felt that she could continue with her independent exercise program and make upgrades appropriately.

CASE STUDY 4-2: SHOULDER INSTABILITY

History

RJ is a 42-year-old right-hand dominant male carpenter who sustained an injury to his left shoulder 3 weeks before presenting for therapy. He reports that when unloading his truck at the job site early one morning, he lost his footing and started to fall backward off the truck. At the time, he was holding his tool box in his right hand. As he was falling he reached out with the left hand and grabbed on to a long 4 by 4 that was sticking out off the bed of the truck. He reports that "it happened so fast," but he is sure that he did not actually fall onto the shoulder or bump it on anything. Over the next 2 hours he found it difficult to do his job because of left lateral and posterior shoulder pain. He decided to go to the nearby urgent care facility when the pain did not resolve over the course of the day. X-ray films were taken, and no fracture was noted. Over the next 2 weeks RJ tried to persevere at work and apply ice to the shoulder whenever he could. He returned to the physician because his shoulder "just wasn't getting any better."

Clinical Evaluation Findings

Magnetic resonance imaging confirmed a near full-thickness tear of the supraspinatus and partial tear of the infraspinatus. Therapy evaluation ruled out any cervical spine involvement. Manual muscle testing of the left shoulder revealed 3+/5 grade strength of the supraspinatus and 4/5 grade strength of the infraspinatus. There was a positive sulcus test at zero degrees, positive Hawkins-Kennedy sign, and positive external rotation lag sign with the supraspinatus at greater than 10 degrees and with the infraspinatus at less than 10 degrees. The evaluation confirmed the magnetic resonance imaging findings, and it was determined that RJ had a right shoulder impingement with an underlying hypermobility because of the rotator cuff tear.

Goals of Therapy

The goals of therapy were as follows:

1. Decrease pain.
2. Resolve muscle guarding.
3. Restore functional range of motion around a physiologic axis.
4. Increase endurance/strength of the rotator cuff.

Initial Treatment

Exercises were selected for stage I hypermobilities:

1. Start with a warm-up exercise such as the upper body ergometer for 10 minutes at 120 rpm.
2. Dose with many repetitions initially to increase endurance and circulation to the type I muscle fibers of the rotator cuff (3 sets of 25).
3. Begin with slow speed to promote coordinated movement about a physiologic axis.
4. Choose starting positions that are in the inner range of motion to maintain stability from inner to midrange of motion.
5. Support the limb with equipment, as necessary, to aid with preserving proper joint arthrokinematics.

The following exercises were selected for RJ's shoulder rehabilitation (please refer to the CD for illustrations of the following exercises):

1. Scapular retraction (see CD for Fig. 4-15)
2. Internal rotation (see CD for Fig. 4-16)
3. External rotation (see CD for Fig. 4-17)
4. Abduction (see CD for Fig. 4-18)
5. Lateral pull downs (see CD for Fig. 4-19)
6. Triceps (see CD for Fig. 4-20)
7. Biceps (see CD for Fig. 4-21)

RJ's first treatment was spent evaluating and testing to determine the appropriate resistance to achieve the functional qualities of vascularization and endurance while maintaining coordination and quality of motion without eliciting pain. The outer range of motion initially was avoided because of instability. On return visits, RJ performed 3 sets of 25 repetitions for all of the foregoing exercises. He took rest breaks between sets. For each exercise the pulley rope was set perpendicular to the lever arm at 20% into the lengthened range of motion and parallel to the muscle fiber. Concentric contractions were performed initially, and between each repetition, the weight stack was let down to remove tension.

Continuing Care

RJ was scheduled for therapy 3 times per week for 4 weeks. On his third treatment he was noted to be moving through his exercise program more quickly, maintaining coordination, and reporting no pain with exercise and decreased pain overall. He then was dosed for four more exercises (please refer to the CD for illustrations of the following exercises).

1. Horizontal adduction (see CD for Fig. 4-22)
2. Horizontal abduction (see CD for Fig. 4-23)
3. Extension (see CD for Fig. 4-24)
4. Flexion (see CD for Fig. 4-25)

On the fifth visit, RJ began stage II for hypermobility. Slow plyometrics were added with a 1 lb ball tossed against a wall, catching it with the left hand. Closed chain exercises were initiated by performing wall pushups. He started to perform (2 sets of 25) concentric contractions and 1 set of isometric contractions in the inner to mid range of motion. The isometric contractions were dosed at 60% to 70% of 1 IM, which is a 40- to 60-second hold.

By the eighth visit, RJ was able to progress to stage III. Exercises were upgraded to include concentric contractions at 80% of 1 RM for 2 sets of 10 repetitions and 1 set of isometric contractions in the mid to outer (stable) range at 85% of 1 IM for a 10- to 15-second hold. Fast plyometrics were performed to recruit the muscle spindle. He started to incorporate diagonal (proprioceptive neuromuscular facilitation) patterns into his exercise routine as well.

Result of Care

In the fourth week, RJ's rehabilitation introduced some retraining of some of his essential job functions. At that time he was released back to full duty and was discharged from therapy. He decided to join a local gym and continue with his established exercise routine.

Acknowledgments

I would like to give special thanks to Ola Grimsby and the Ola Grimsby Institute for the invaluable education I received from them and the permission to share this knowledge with other clinicians and to Jeff Falkel for his support, knowledge, and critical thinking.

References

1. Grimsby O, Rivard J, Stensnes R et al: Physiological responses to exercise: exercise physiology. In Rivard J, Goodwin W, editors: *Residency course notes*, ed 3, San Diego, 1998, Ola Grimsby Institute.

2. Grimsby O, Rivard J: General principles of patient evaluation. In Rivard J, Goodwin W, editors: *Residency course notes*, ed 3, San Diego, 1998, Ola Grimsby Institute.

3. Goodman CC, Snyder TE: Overview of endocrine and metabolic signs and symptoms. In *Differential diagnosis in physical therapy*, ed 2, Philadelphia, 1995, WB Saunders.

4. Goodman CC, Snyder TE: Overview of immunologic signs and symptoms. In *Differential diagnosis in physical therapy*, ed 2, Philadelphia, 1995, WB Saunders.

5. Goodman CC, Snyder TE: Overview of gastrointestinal signs and symptoms. In *Differential diagnosis in physical therapy*, ed 2, Philadelphia, 1995, WB Saunders.

6. Mahler DA, Froelicher VF, Miller NH et al: *American College of Sports Medicine: guidelines for exercise testing and prescription*, ed 5, Philadelphia, 1995, Williams & Wilkins.

7. Goodman CC, Snyder TE: Overview of cardiovascular signs and symptoms. In *Differential diagnosis in physical therapy*, ed 2, Philadelphia, 1995, WB Saunders.

8. Carmona RH, Beato C, Lawrence A: *Bone health and osteoporosis: a report of the surgeon general*, Rockville, Md, 2004, Department of Health and Human Services.

9. Grimsby O, Grimsby K, Power B et al: Histology. In Rivard J, Goodwin W, editors: *Residency course notes*, ed 3, San Diego, 1998, Ola Grimsby Institute.

10. Grimsby O: Scientific therapeutic exercise progressions, *J Man Manipulative Ther* 2:94-101, 1994.

11. Dudley GA, Harris RT: Neuromuscular anatomy and adaptations to conditioning. In Baechle TR, Earle RW, editors: *Essentials of strength and conditioning*, ed 2, Omaha, 2000, Human Kinetics.

12. Grimsby O, Hinson B, Rivard J et al: Neurophysiology. In Rivard J, editor: *Residency course notes*, ed 3, San Diego, 1998, Ola Grimsby Institute.

13. *Classification of chronic pain*, Seattle, 1994, IASP Press.

14. Grimsby O, Cutchall L, Gray J: Pathophysiology of trauma. In Rivard J, Goodwin W, editors: *Residency course notes*, San Diego, 1998, Ola Grimsby Institute.

15. Falkel JE, Cipriani DJ: Physiological principles of resistance training and rehabilitation. In Zachazewski JE, Magee DJ, Quillen WS, editors: *Athletic injuries and rehabilitation*, Philadelphia, 1996, WB Saunders.

16. Cheung K, Hume P, Maxwell L: Delayed onset muscle soreness: treatment strategies and performance factors, *Sports Med* 33:145-164, 2003.

17. Baechle TR, Earle RW, Wathen D: Resistance training. In Baechle TR, Earle RW, editors: *Essentials of strength and conditioning*, ed 2, Omaha, 2000, Human Kinetics.

18. Peterson MD, Rhea MR, Alvar BA: Maximizing strength development in athletes: a meta-analysis to determine the dose-response relationship, *J Strength Cond Res* 18:377-382, 2004.

19. Wolfe BL, LeMura LM, Cole PJ: Quantitative analysis of single vs multiple set programs in resistance training, *J Strength Cond Res* 18:35-47, 2004.

20. Harman E: The biomechanics of resistance exercise. In Baechle TR, Earle RW, editors: *Essentials of strength and conditioning*, ed 2, Omaha, 2000, Human Kinetics.

21. *Medical exercise therapy*, Oslo, 1996, Norwegian MET Institute.

22. Blyx M: Blyx curve, *Scand Arch Physiol* pp 93-94, 1892.

23. Kraemer WJ, Adams K, Cafarelli E et al: Progression models in resistance training for healthy adults, *Med Sci Sports Exerc* 34:364-379, 2002.

24. Kibler B, Livingston B: Closed-chain rehabilitation for upper and lower extremities, *J Am Acad Orthop Surg* 9:412-421, 2001.

5

Evaluation of the Hand and Upper Extremity

LINDA J. KLEIN

KEY TERMS

Adhesion

Angiogenesis

Brawny edema

Cyanosis

Erythema

Eschar

Extrinsic tendon tightness

Exudate

Fibroplasia stage

Granulation tissue

Inflammatory stage

Innervation density

Intrinsic tightness

Macrophage

Pallor

Pitting edema

Referred pain

Secondary intention

Tonometer

Trophic

The client's initial evaluation sets the stage for successful rehabilitation. Evaluation establishes rapport, determines the areas of functional deficit, and serves as the foundation for treatment and recovery. Only with an accurate assessment can the therapist determine the best course of treatment for the client's condition. A number of assessment processes and clinical assessment skills are needed to perform a thorough evaluation (Fig. 5-1). The main areas of assessment for the injured hand include pain, wound and scar status, vascular status, range of motion (ROM), swelling, sensation, strength, current and previous use of splints, and functional limitations. Periodic reevaluations are necessary to show progress, identify new or remaining problems, and redirect goals.

Using an evaluation summary form is helpful (see Appendix 5-1 on the CD). The form will guide you through each step of the assessment, ensuring that you do not forget any areas. Defer areas of an evaluation when it is not appropriate to perform them at a certain time in the tissue healing process or if the client simply cannot tolerate these procedures. Sometimes an additional specific form is needed for an assessment. For example, the evaluation summary form should have an area listed as sensation even though a separate form is used for sensory tests including the Semmes-Weinstein monofilament test or two-point discrimination test. On the summary form,

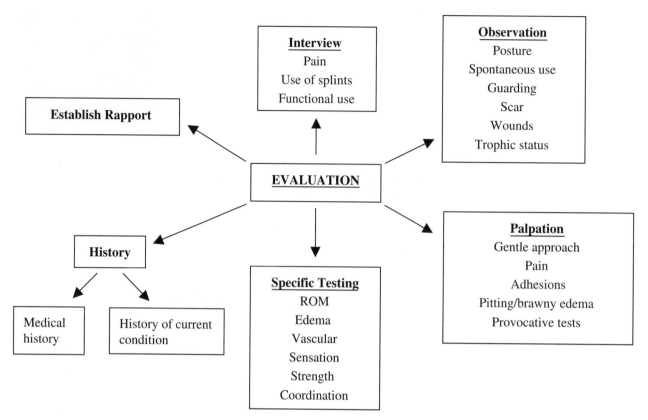

FIGURE 5-1   Summary of the evaluation process. *ROM,* Range of motion.

give a brief description that indicates where the client perceives altered sensation including numbness, tingling, burning, or hypersensitivity. Then use the Semmes-Weinstein monofilament, two-point discrimination, or other sensation forms for more specific and objective information. The evaluation summary form promotes clinical reasoning and assists the therapist's organization of thoughts and communication with a thorough and logical progression of categories.

INITIAL INTERVIEW

Obtaining a History

Before assessing the function of the client's hand, obtaining a history of the injury or symptoms that bring the client to the therapy clinic is essential. Understanding the onset of symptoms (e.g., trauma versus gradual) is essential. Next, ask about the prior medical intervention. Has there been surgery? An injection? X-ray films, magnetic resonance imaging, or computed tomography scan? Nerve study? Cast immobilization? Splinting? Medication? Manual tests by the physician? Or has there been no intervention by the physician except to send the client to therapy for the therapist's expertise in evaluation and treatment? Understanding what care the client

already had helps in a number of ways. It gives the client confidence that you understand what has been done, and it builds trust because you can explain in many cases what the physician was attempting to determine with various tests. Having clients develop trust in you leads to gaining their full cooperation and participation in the evaluation and rehabilitation process. In addition to the history of the injury or condition, you must understand the individual's pertinent medical history, because many medical conditions, such as diabetes or peripheral vascular disease, affect the healing process.

Observation

During the initial process of meeting new clients and discussing their history and symptoms, use your observation skills. Observe the client's nonverbal communication by facial expressions and body language, as well as how the client holds and uses the injured extremity and trunk. The client often guards the injured extremity at the time of initial evaluation, possibly as a subconscious protection from pain. I also have seen situations in which the client guards the extremity or exaggerates limitations such as strength or motion during the evaluation to be sure that the therapist recognizes and appreciates the extent of deficit. In these cases, it is sometimes possible to observe them move better during a spontaneous situation than during the formal assessment. For example, a client with an elbow injury who lacks 40 degrees of elbow extension during formal assessment may be seen extending the elbow significantly further while removing or putting on his or her coat. Another example is the client who guards the hand by holding it close to the body during the assessment but uses the hand more freely with gestures during informal discussion.

Observe differences in posture and use of the upper extremity in spontaneous situations compared with formal assessment. This gives clues regarding the client's comfort with the extremity. Use different approaches to elicit the best response from clients who are not comfortable moving freely (see Chapter 7). In my experience, most clients with abnormal posturing are unaware of their upper extremity positioning and are eager to change. In contrast, facilitation of positive involvement by clients who may be consciously controlling their responses in therapy is more challenging. I have had some success by reminding these clients that continued therapy is contingent on their showing progress. Use of a nonjudgmental approach, gently pointing out the inconsistency between formal testing and observation, is always best. Reinforcing that your goal is to work with the client toward recovery will maximize the client's positive involvement in the rehabilitation process.

In discussing each section of the evaluation, I will describe the tools and process of the evaluation, followed by inconsistencies and difficulties to be aware of, and when that portion of the evaluation should be deferred.

ASSESSMENT OF PAIN

Equipment

No equipment is necessary, but you may choose to use a pain scale during initial evaluation to summarize the client's overall perception of pain. Numerous pain scales are available (Box 5-1).

Methods

Obtain a verbal or written description by the client of the level of pain, location, type of pain, frequency or cause, and duration of pain. Also document when pain occurs during other parts of the evaluation, such as with active range of motion (AROM) or passive range of motion (PROM), strength testing, or palpation:

- Level of pain: Using a pain scale, have the client describe the pain at its worst on the scale and then at its best, and also obtain an average pain level. I use the 0-to-10 pain scale or the verbal rating scale

---

BOX 5-1

Evaluation of the Hand and Upper Extremity

- Numeric analog scales: A line with equal markings from 0 to 5, 0 to 10, or 0 to 20 is used to indicate the perceived level of pain at the initial evaluation compared with periodic reevaluations.
- Visual analog scale: Provide the client with a 10-cm line drawn vertically on paper, with one end labeled no pain and the other pain as bad as it could be. The client marks the location and level of pain, and the examiner later divides the line into 20 equal portions to determine the distance from 0 to the client's pain mark.
- Verbal rating scale: Client describes their pain with four to five descriptive words (e.g., mild, moderate, or severe).
- Graphic representation: The client marks his or her pain location and type on a body chart.
- Pain questionnaire: Written pain questionnaires are available that obtain more information about the client's pain, such as the McGill Pain Questionnaire.[2] These questionnaires are probably used most in specialty centers dealing with management of pain, but the knowledge of the content of specific questionnaires may be helpful to develop your skills in discussing pain during an evaluation.

---

of mild, moderate, or severe most often. Documentation then should be done accordingly; for instance, "Pain is described as varying from mild at best to severe at worst."

- Location of pain: Have the client point to the area(s) of pain. For clients with a more diffuse pain that may involve more of the upper extremity, I use a body chart on which the client can circle the areas that hurt and rate each area, if desired. When a client has **referred pain**—for instance, when palpation of one area results in pain in another area—this is best documented on a body chart as well. Referred pain can result from myofascial pain and may be treated best by a specialist trained in myofascial treatment.
- Type of pain: Ask the client to describe the pain as throbbing, aching, sharp, stabbing, shooting, burning, or hypersensitive to light touch.
- Frequency or cause of pain: Determine whether the pain is constant or intermittent. Have the client describe when the pain occurs and what seems to cause the pain. This information is helpful in determining a diagnosis if the physician has not provided a firm diagnosis.

- Duration of pain: Determine how long the pain has been present.

- Chronic pain often is associated with depression, anxiety, and other psychological involvement and may be helped best by a team approach with specialists in the area of chronic pain management.
- Also important is to note pain levels that occur during the evaluation, such as pain during AROM or PROM or strength testing. For instance, my evaluation might state "Strength: Grip strength right hand 100#, left hand 50# with moderate pain indicated in left volar wrist with grip." I may have a goal to reflect this in my initial evaluation note, such as "Increase left hand grip strength to 75# without pain." Tendonitis is associated more with pain on AROM than on PROM. Thus distinctions about pain during evaluation become part of the clinical reasoning and treatment process.

Discussion

I usually begin my assessment of a new client's injury by discussing the client's pain and reassuring the client that the evaluation is not intended to worsen the pain. As soon as the client has the opportunity to tell me about his or her pain, I see a level of relief develop. Many clients are apprehensive about attending therapy, concerned that the therapist may perform painful, provocative tests, might move the extremity beyond comfort, or simply may touch or grasp a sensitive or tender area. Knowing that the therapist is aware of the pain helps the client relax for and participate in the rest of the evaluation process.

Clinical Problem Solving

At times, the therapist is not given a firm diagnosis by the referring physician and simply may be instructed to evaluate and treat for hand pain, wrist pain, or elbow pain. The location of pain and whether pain occurs with active or passive motion can give the therapist clues as to the cause of the pain. Use provocative testing for specific conditions with the goal of reproducing the pain complaint for nerve compressions and tendonitis (see the

chapters on nerve compression and tendonitis for more information).

Consider the following:

- Pain with AROM that is not present with PROM most likely is caused by a problem with the muscle or tendon.
- Pain with PROM is more likely due to a joint problem, such as tightness of the joint structures, ligament injury, cartilage injury, or inflammation (pain may be present equally with AROM in these situations).
- When a joint is limited in motion because of pain, and pain is present with distraction of the joint but not compression of the joint, pain is most likely due to a ligament or joint capsule being stretched with distraction and relieved with compression.
- If pain is present with compression of the joint but is relieved with distraction, pain is more likely due to a problem at the joint surface, such as thinning or loss of cartilage, inflammation within the joint, or surface abnormality such as a bone spur.

Precaution. *Aggressive clinical problem-solving methods can be used safely only when the physician has allowed AROM and PROM as part of treatment. These methods are not appropriate following a tendon repair or tendon transfer.*

WOUND ASSESSMENT

Open wounds can be intimidating. Breaking the assessment down to wound size, depth, color, drainage, and odor is helpful. This assessment can be omitted if there are no wounds. When wounds are closed, it is appropriate to skip this section and go on to scar assessment.

Consider the following:

- Size: Measure length and width with a ruler. Make a tracing of the wound for future comparison, or use transparent calibrated grids. Do not touch the wound with the ruler or other measuring device unless the item is sterile.
- Depth: Wound depth may be measured with a sterile cotton swab if the client and therapist are comfortable with this procedure.
- Color: Open wounds are referred to as red, yellow, or black.[3,4] Many wounds have a combination of these colors, and wounds progress through stages of these colors.
  - Red wound: Wound may be a superficial wound, second-degree burn, acute fresh wound, surgical wound, or a wound left open to heal by **secondary intention** in the granulation process with new blood vessels forming.

- Yellow wound: Semiliquid to liquid slough (**exudate**) is present. Color ranges from cream to yellow. Pink or red **granulation tissue** usually is seen at the edges of or under the yellow tissue. Yellow tissue may facilitate infection. Yellow wounds are often in the late **inflammatory stage** or early **fibroplasia stage** and include exudates.
- Black wound: Wound characterized by necrotic black, brown, or gray tissue or thick **eschar.** Pus may form at the edges because of **macrophage** activity. New granulation tissue forms under the eschar. If bacterial infection forms under the eschar, the wound edges can become red, painful, and swollen. The wound may be in all stages of wound repair, with inflammation present while macrophages try to remove the necrotic debris, fibroblasts try to lay down new collagen under the eschar, **angiogenesis** is beginning to occur, and the wound is trying to contract despite being blocked by eschar.

CLINICAL *Pearl*

Wounds almost always have more than one color present at one time. Treat the worst stage first; that is, progress from treatment of black to yellow and then yellow to red.

- Drainage: Attempt to quantify the amount of drainage (mild, moderate, heavy) and color of drainage. Clear, pink, or white drainage does not indicate presence of infection. Exudate may have a yellow color and may or may not indicate infection.

CLINICAL *Pearl*

If there is any question of the possibility of infection, have the drainage examined by a physician.

- Odor: Odors often indicate infection. Note any odor emanating from the wound, and have the wound assessed by a physician for potential infection.
- Temperature: Surface thermometers or temperature tapes can be used to compare temperature of an area near the wound with an unaffected area.

SCAR ASSESSMENT

The characteristics to assess for scar status include color, size, whether it is flattened or raised, and the presence of **adhesion** (attachment) to underlying or surrounding tissue. Consider the following:

- Color: Scars usually begin as deep red and gradually become lighter as time progresses.
- Size: Use a ruler to measure the length and width of the scar.
- Flat/raised: Use observation and palpation to assess how far the scar is raised above the skin level, and describe it using terms such as *mild* or *moderate.* Sometimes the superficial scar may be flat, but there may be a lump under the skin. This happens most commonly on the dorsum of the hand or wrist, with a lump under the surface scar that is a thickening composed of a combination of scar and fluid. This lump of scar and fluid can be described by size and height (e.g., dorsal incisional scar is 3 cm in length along the third metacarpal, with a thickened area under the skin of 3 mm in height and 2 to 3 mm in width surrounding the scar).
- Adhesions: Assessment of adhesions of surface scars to underlying tissue is done by observation and palpation. Some adhesions can be seen during active motion. When the adhesion is on the dorsal hand or wrist or the volar wrist/forearm, the scar is often seen to dip deeper, or dimple, when active motion is attempted because of adhesions from the superficial scar to underlying fascia and tendons. Also assess adhesions of skin to underlying tissue by palpation. Attempt to slide or lift the scar tissue in a manner similar to the surrounding uninjured tissue, and describe the level of adhesion as mild, moderate, or severely adherent.

Precaution. *Respect the level of healing of a new scar and the tissue to which it may adhere. Avoid aggressively attempting to move scar tissue within the first week following suture removal, or when a portion of the wound is still open. Doing so may cause damage to fragile, healing tissue or possibly may reopen the wound. Avoid strong scar manipulation during assessment or treatment over a tendon in the early phase of healing.*

VASCULAR STATUS ASSESSMENT

A basic vascular evaluation of the hand can be done by observation (color or **trophic** changes, pain level), palpation (pulse, capillary refill assessment, modified Allen's test), and temperature assessment. Blood flow to the hand can be affected by proximal injury or diagnoses such as thoracic outlet syndrome, injury to the hand itself, or conditions such as Raynaud's phenomenon. Proximal conditions such as thoracic outlet syndrome are discussed in the chapter on shoulder disorders.

Observation

Observation includes assessment of color and trophic changes in the hand. Increased levels of white **(pallor)**, blue **(cyanosis)**, or red **(erythema)** coloration of the skin are the most common changes noted.

CLINICAL *Pearl*

Arterial interruption usually produces a white or grayish discoloration of the affected area (pallor), whereas venous blockage produces a congested, purple-blue color.[5] Dusky blue may indicate chronic venous insufficiency. Redness may indicate loss of outflow of blood from the hand or a venous problem, but it also may be an indication of a normal inflammatory phase of wound healing or the presence of infection.

Trophic changes refer to the texture of the skin and nail. Changes in the trophic status can occur from sympathetic nerve or vascular changes. Note the presence of increased dryness or moisture of the skin of the involved hand and the presence of open wounds or necrotic tissue at the initial evaluation. Reevaluate these items frequently for improvement.

Pain is present in two thirds of clients with upper extremity vascular disease.[6] Pain may be described as aching, cramping, tightness, or cold intolerance. Pain may be associated with activity that includes exposure to vibration, cold, or repetition.

Precaution. *Close monitoring of color and temperature change is important, and communication with the referring physician is recommended if abnormalities are worsening or not improving. Causes of vascular abnormalities are numerous, and in-depth evaluation and testing by the physician may be indicated.*

Palpation Tests of Vascular Status

Capillary Refill Test

For the capillary refill test, place pressure on the distal portion of the volar finger or over the fingernail of the digit until tissue turns white.[5,6] Capillary refill time is the number of seconds it takes for the color to return to normal after the pressure is released. Normal capillary refill time is less than 2 seconds, and the time can be compared with the same digit on the opposite hand or with uninjured digits.

Peripheral Pulse Palpation

With peripheral pulse palpation, placing light pressure over the radial artery or ulnar artery just proximal to the wrist crease provides information about the strength of the pulse or blood flow to the hand.[7] If the pulse is weaker in one wrist than the other, there may be a potential problem with blood flow proximal to the wrist. Palpation of peripheral pulse is used frequently for assessing for proximal vascular diagnoses such as thoracic outlet syndrome. Check the pulse before and after exercise in certain positions to determine whether position or exercise diminish blood flow to the distal upper extremity. Refer to the chapter on treatment of shoulder conditions for more information on specialized testing.

Modified Allen's Test

The modified Allen's test assesses the status of the blood supply within the hand through the ulnar and radial arteries of the wrist.[5-7] To perform the test, place firm pressure over the radial and ulnar arteries just proximal to the wrist crease. Instruct the client to make a tight fist and then open the fingers repeatedly until the palm turns white. Then instruct the client to relax the fingers to a partially opened position. Release the pressure from one side of the wrist, allowing blood flow through one of the arteries. Record the time it takes for the color to return to normal in the hand. Repeat the process, releasing pressure from the artery on the opposite side of the wrist. Record the time it takes for the color to return to normal in the hand. A normal response is 5 seconds or less and can be compared to the opposite extremity to confirm a normal response time for that individual.

Surface Temperature Assessment

Surface thermometers can be used to compare forearm temperature to fingertip temperature. If the forearm is at least 4° C (39° F) warmer than the fingertip surface, it may indicate vascular compromise. Assess Raynaud's phenomenon with a temperature assessment that measures the temperature of the involved fingertip(s) after being in a warm room (24° C [75° F]) for 30 minutes and then after being immersed in ice water for 20 seconds. Record the time it takes to return to the baseline temperature. The normal time for return to body temperature is within 10 minutes, but clients with Raynaud's phenomenon may take 20 to 45 minutes.[7]

RANGE OF MOTION ASSESSMENT

Assessment of ROM in this chapter is limited to the forearm, wrist, fingers, and thumb. A variety of ways to assess ROM are available and have resulted in the effort by the American Society of Hand Therapists to standardize this process.[8] This method is discussed later in this chapter; however, variations exist that are acceptable. All ROM of the forearm, wrist, and hand is performed with the client in the seated position. Clinical problem solving that interprets the cause of the limited ROM (e.g., joint stiffness, **intrinsic tightness,** and extrinsic tightness) is important for determining the most appropriate treatment.

Methods

Passive Range of Motion

PROM is the ability of a joint to be moved through its normal arc of motion while relaxed, with motion being performed by an outside source such as the therapist's hand, the client's opposite hand, or gravity. Limitations in PROM indicate a problem within the joint (e.g., stiffness caused by capsular or ligamentous tightness, decreased joint space, or bone spur). PROM also may be limited by tightness of the muscle/tendon group opposing the passive motion (e.g., a tight or adherent extensor muscle/tendon will prevent full passive or active flexion).

Precaution. *Traumatic injuries to the bone or joint in the acute phase of healing, or as determined by the physician, are limited to AROM, with no PROM allowed. PROM by an outside source may be performed too strongly, reinjuring the healing bone or ligament.*

Following a tendon repair in the early phases of tendon healing, PROM in the direction that would stretch the tendon is not allowed. PROM is begun only gently in the intermediate phase of tendon healing after medical clearance.

Active Range of Motion

AROM is motion of a joint caused by musculotendinous contraction, most often from a voluntary muscle contraction. Limitations in AROM can result from a number of causes. Some of these causes include weakness of the muscle, loss of tendon continuity, adhesions of the tendon preventing its motion, inflammation or constriction of the tendon, decreased tendon mechanical efficiency because of loss of pulley (bowstringing), and disrupted nerve supply to the muscle.

Precautions for Active Range of Motion

AROM using the repaired tendon (i.e., contracting the repaired tendon) is not allowed following a tendon repair or a tendon transfer in the acute phase of tendon healing. This restriction lasts approximately the first 4 weeks after the repair unless the type of repair performed by the surgeon allows use of an immediate active-motion protocol. Please refer to the chapter on tendon repair for specific guidelines.

You must recognize that AROM or PROM also may be limited by pain. If the client describes pain during ROM testing, note this on the evaluation form.

When there is no medical limitation regarding use of AROM and PROM, it is important to do the following:

- Measure passive and active motion for information that helps determine the cause of limitation.
- Compare ROM to the other hand to learn what is normal for that individual.
- Measure ROM at a consistent time or sequence in the treatment session (e.g., before or after exercise) for a more accurate reading of improvement.
- Be consistent in position of hand and proximal joints. For instance, it is more difficult to perform finger flexion when the wrist is flexed compared with when the wrist is extended. When the extensors are adherent, each individual joint measured alone or independently will flex further than when all three joints are flexed at the same time.

Total Active Motion

Total active motion (*TAM*) is used to describe the full arc of motion of the digit(s). TAM is measured as the total flexion of all three finger joints, subtracting any loss of full extension at all finger joints:

$$(MP + PIP + DIP \text{ flexion}) - (MP + PIP + DIP \text{ extension loss}) = TAM$$

where *MP* is metacarpophalangeal, *PIP* is proximal interphalangeal, and *DIP* is distal interphalangeal.

CLINICAL *Pearl*

Use of TAM when reporting ROM in situations where tendons limit motion and composite motion is more limited than individual joints is important.

Total Passive Motion

Total passive motion is the same process as TAM but is measured passively. This can be helpful to document the presence of adhesions.

CLINICAL *Pearl*

When flexor tendons are limited by adhesions, total passive motion will be better than TAM.

Standard plastic goniometers work well for measurement. Larger goniometers ($12^1/_4$ inches) are recommended for the larger elbow and shoulder joints. Standard goniometers (6 to 7 inches) are used for measuring the forearm

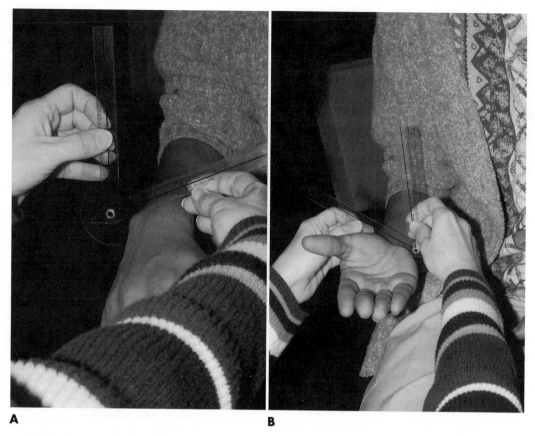

A   **B**

FIGURE 5-2   A, Pronation as measured with a standard 6-inch goniometer, demonstrating axis of motion on the dorsal distal ulna. **B,** Supination as measured with a standard 6-inch goniometer, demonstrating axis of motion on the volar distal ulna.

and wrist. They can be cut down in length to measure finger ROM. Metal finger goniometers are available at a higher cost and do not have the benefit of transparency when lateral placement is needed. Electronic and computer system goniometers are available at a much higher cost; however, they lack reliability and validity studies to support their use. For the wrist, I prefer the 6-inch goniometer with rounded ends because it allows dorsal placement on the wrist for flexion and extension (Fig. 5-2).

Hyperextension of the fingers is recorded with a plus sign (+), loss of full extension with a minus sign (−). When standard placement of the goniometer is not used because of scar, swelling, or wound, document the modified placement of the goniometer for future reference to allow for accurate comparative measurements.

Forearm Range of Motion

Consider the following for forearm ROM:

- Motions of the forearm are pronation and supination.

- Starting position is with the arm adducted at side, elbow flexed to 90 degrees, forearm and wrist neutral.
- Axis of motion is the ulnar edge of the forearm, dorsally for pronation, and volarly for supination.
- Placement of the goniometer is with both arms of the goniometer horizontally across the distal forearm, dorsally with axis placed at the lateral edge of the dorsal ulna for pronation, and along the volar surface of the distal forearm, with axis placed at the lateral edge of the volar ulna for supination.
- To measure pronation, one arm of the goniometer stays in place in the starting position (straight up), while the other arm of the goniometer stays in contact with the dorsal distal forearm as it moves into pronation. The stationary arm of the goniometer, which stays in the starting position, is now straight up and should be aligned with the humerus if the client has maintained the correct starting position of the trunk and arm. The moving arm of the goniometer is to stay flat on the dorsum of the distal forearm, flush

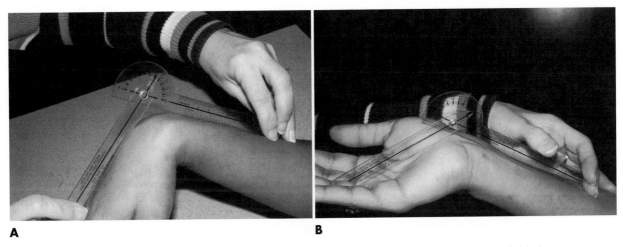

A   **B**

FIGURE 5-3 **A,** Wrist flexion measured dorsally over the central wrist with a standard 6-inch goniometer. **B,** Wrist extension measured volarly over the central wrist with a standard 6-inch goniometer.

with the center of the distal forearm, between the ulna and radius (Fig. 5-2, A).

- To measure supination, one arm of the goniometer stays in place in the starting position (straight up), while the other arm stays in contact with the volar distal forearm as it moves into supination. The stationary arm of the goniometer, which stays in the starting position is now straight up and should be aligned with the humerus if the client has maintained the correct starting position of the trunk and arm. The moving arm of the goniometer is flush on the center of the volar forearm on the flattest portion of the midvolar forearm (Fig. 5-2, B).

- Frequent errors are made when measuring pronation and supination by allowing the goniometer to overturn and measure more along the distal radius or underturn and measure more along the distal ulna, rather than correctly on the middle section of the distal forearm. Other common errors are to allow the client to lean or move the arm away from the starting position of humeral adduction against the side of the body. Feedback from an experienced therapist is helpful when one is learning to measure forearm motion.

Wrist Range of Motion

Consider the following for wrist ROM:
- Motions of the wrist are flexion, extension, radial deviation, and ulnar deviation.
- Starting position is with wrist neutral.
- Axis of motion is the center of the wrist.
- Placement of the goniometer according to American Society of Hand Therapists recommendations are

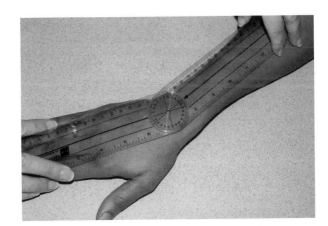

FIGURE 5-4 Wrist ulnar deviation measured dorsally.

volarly for extension, dorsally for flexion, and dorsally for radial deviation and ulnar deviation. Lateral placement is appropriate when scar or swelling make dorsal or volar placements inaccurate.

- To measure flexion, place one arm of goniometer along the dorsum of the forearm and the other arm along the third metacarpal on the dorsum of the hand (Fig. 5-3, A).

- To measure extension, place one arm of goniometer along the volar forearm and the other arm along the third metacarpal on the palmar side of the hand (Fig. 5-3, B).

- To measure radial and ulnar deviation, with hand flat on a table surface, place the goniometer flat on its side, one arm of the goniometer on the dorsum of the forearm, axis at the center of the wrist, and the other arm of the goniometer along the third metacarpal (Fig. 5-4).

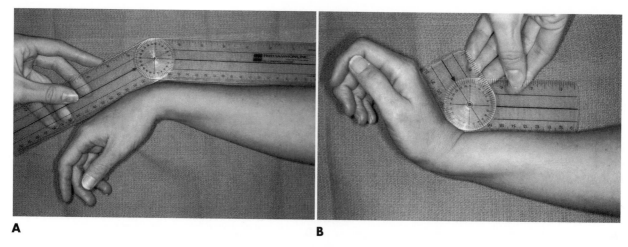

A   **B**

FIGURE 5-5 A, Alternate goniometer for wrist flexion, measured dorsally over the central wrist. **B,** Alternate goniometer, with rounded ends, used for wrist extension measured dorsally over the central wrist. Consistent dorsal skin contact compared with palmar placement with standard goniometer may decrease interrater variability when measuring over the curves of the palm.

Volar placement of the goniometer on the palm to measure extension is difficult because of the many curves in the palm and the goniometer does not lay flat in the palm. A goniometer with rounded ends (Fig. 5-5), available in many therapy supply catalogs, allows dorsal placement of the goniometer to measure flexion and extension of the wrist.

Digital Range of Motion

The metacarpophalangeal, PIP joints, DIP joints of the fingers, and metacarpophalangeal and interphalangeal joints of the thumb are measured with the same procedure and are described together next:

- Motions of the finger and thumb metacarpophalangeal and interphalangeal joints are flexion and extension. The metacarpophalangeal joints of the fingers also perform abduction and adduction, but this is not measured with traditional goniometric measurements. A tracing may be done to document finger abduction/adduction if a deficit is present in these motions.
- Starting position is extension. Neutral wrist is recommended for consistency in procedure.
- Axis of motion is central, directly over the joint being measured.
- Placement of the goniometer for all finger measurements is on the dorsal surface. The metacarpophalangeal joint is measured with one arm of the goniometer along the metacarpal, and the other arm of the goniometer along the proximal phalanx, with

the axis at the dorsal metacarpophalangeal joint (Fig. 5-6, *A*). Placement of the goniometer for the PIP joint is with one arm of the goniometer on the proximal phalanx and the other arm on the middle phalanx (Fig. 5-6, *B*). Placement for the DIP joints is with one arm of the goniometer on the middle phalanx and the other arm on the distal phalanx (Fig. 5-6, *C*). Alternate placement of the goniometer is laterally along the finger if there is a lump or other abnormality preventing dorsal placement.

- To measure motion, note the maximal extension at each joint, and when moving into flexion, move the distal arm of the goniometer to maintain its position on the dorsum of the finger section noted before. Note the degree of flexion attained. If loss of full extension is present, record it with a minus sign (–); for example, –25 to 50 degrees metacarpophalangeal motion means there was a loss of 25 degrees of extension and the joint was able to flex to 50 degrees of flexion. For hyperextension, use a plus sign (+): +25 to 50 degrees metacarpophalangeal motion means there is 25 degrees of hyperextension at the metacarpophalangeal joint and the joint was able to flex to 50 degrees of flexion.

Hyperextension is difficult to measure with the standard 6-inch goniometer or 6-inch goniometer cut down in length, and lateral placement is necessary for this measurement. The goniometer style with rounded ends described in the discussion section of wrist ROM (Fig. 5-2, *B*) can be used to measure hyperextension of the digit joints with dorsal placement.

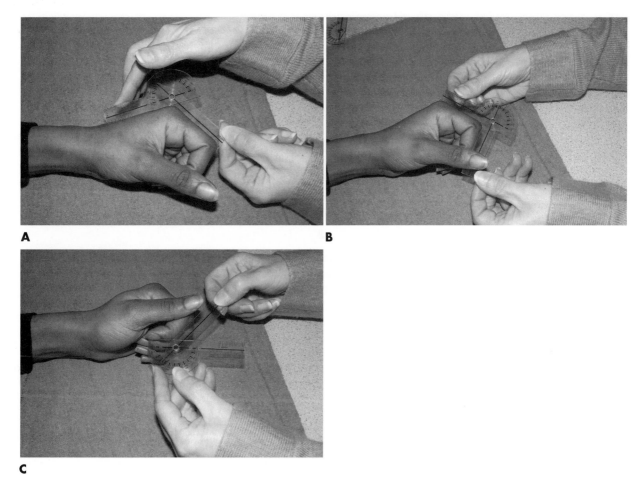

FIGURE 5-6   Finger flexion measured dorsally with a standard 6-inch goniometer that has been cut down in length. **A** demonstrates metacarpophalangeal flexion, **B** demonstrates proximal interphalangeal flexion, and **C** demonstrates distal interphalangeal flexion. Note the placement of the goniometer arms to allow distal interphalangeal flexion to be measured in a composite flexion position.

CLINICAL *Pearl*

Measurement of each digit in composite flexion and extension (TAM) is important during the initial evaluation.

Each joint may be near normal if measured in isolation, but significant limitation in ROM may be evident when total active flexion and extension are measured, because of tendon gliding or scar tissue limitations. The TAM of the digit measured in composite flexion and extension indicates the functional limitations of motion. Functional limitations of motion also can be demonstrated by measuring the distance, during a composite fist, from the fingertip pulp to the distal palmar crease of the hand.[9]

Thumb Carpometacarpal Joint

Consider the following:

- Motions include palmar abduction, radial abduction, and opposition.
- Axis of motion is the intersection of lines extending down the first and second metacarpals on the dorsal radial aspect of the hand.
- Starting position is with the forearm pronated with hand flat on table for radial abduction or with the ulnar side of the hand on the table, forearm neutral for palmar abduction or opposition. The thumb is adducted to be flat along the side of the index finger.
- Placement of the goniometer is with one arm placed along the second metacarpal and the other arm placed along the first metacarpal, dorsally for radial

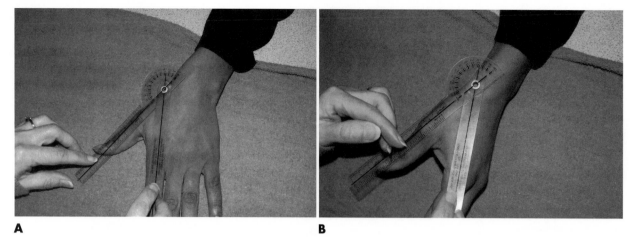

A   **B**

FIGURE 5-7   A, Thumb carpometacarpal radial abduction measured dorsally with a standard 6-inch goniometer. **B,** Thumb carpometacarpal palmar abduction measured radially with a standard 6 inch goniometer.

abduction and radially for palmar abduction. The axis of the goniometer then will be located over the carpals just proximal to the first and second metacarpals.

- To measure radial abduction, the goniometer arm placed over the second metacarpal is stationary, and the goniometer arm placed over the first metacarpal moves, staying in alignment over the first metacarpal as the thumb moves into radial abduction (Fig. 5-7, A).
- To measure palmar abduction, the goniometer arm placed on the radial side of the second metacarpal is stationary, and the goniometer arm placed on the dorsal first metacarpal moves, staying in alignment over the first metacarpal as the thumb moves into palmar abduction (Fig. 5-7, B).
- To measure opposition, use a ruler to measure the distance from the volar interphalangeal joint of the thumb to the third metacarpal with the nail parallel to the plane of the palm when the thumb is in opposition.[8] Other sources suggest measuring opposition as the distance between the thumb tip and the base of the small finger.[9] For this reason, it is important to define the method of measuring opposition in the documentation.

Thumb carpometacarpal joint ROM testing is difficult to perform consistently because placement of both arms of the goniometer is done using visual judgment of the therapist. Placing the goniometer arms correctly over the first and second metacarpal, with the axis at the carpometacarpal joint can be difficult, and practice with an experienced therapist is recommended.

Clinical Problem Solving

When ROM of the digits is limited, it is important to determine whether the limited ROM is due to joint stiffness, **extrinsic tendon tightness** or adhesions, or intrinsic tightness. Perform this type of assessment as soon as active and passive motion is allowed because it dictates the most appropriate type of treatment by determining the limiting structure(s).

Follow these steps:

- *Step 1:* Measure and record composite flexion and composite extension of the digits with the wrist in neutral to slight extension.
- *Step 2:* Compare composite flexion and extension of the fingers with the wrist fully extended and fully flexed (to determine whether extrinsic tendon tightness or adhesions are present).
- *Step 3:* Screen ROM of each finger joint separately, with the proximal joints supported in neutral (to determine whether the limited motion is isolated to the joint, regardless of the position of the proximal joints).
- *Step 4:* Perform passive motion of the digits. Comparison of passive motion to active motion provides information regarding tendon adhesions that may be limiting active motion.

The following is a description of the causes of finger joint motion limitations in each of the screened positions:

- If AROM of a joint is the same as PROM, and the motion is the same regardless of the position of proximal joints, the limitation is due to joint stiffness.

- If passive flexion is better than active flexion, the limited active flexion is due to flexor tendon adhesion.
- If passive extension is better than active extension, the limited active extension is due to extensor tendon adhesion.
- If active and passive flexion are equal and flexion is better with the proximal joint(s) in extension than with the proximal joint(s) in flexion, the limited flexion is due to extrinsic extensor tendon tightness or adhesions.
- If active and passive extension is equal and extension is better with the proximal joint(s) in flexion than extension, the limited extension is due to extrinsic flexor tendon tightness or adhesions.
- If the interphalangeal joints of the finger can be flexed passively further with the metacarpophalangeal joint flexed than when the metacarpophalangeal joint is extended, the limitation is due to intrinsic tightness.

Treatment choices can be made accordingly. For example, when limited flexion is due to tight or adherent extensor tendons, treatment should address the extensor tendon length and ability to glide, not the motion at individual joints. This type of situation occurs frequently following an open reduction and internal fixation of a metacarpal fracture, with scar tissue adhesions to underlying extensor tendons. My treatment choice would include applying heat over the hand that is placed in a composite flexion position with a wrap that supports the flexed fingers in a comfortable stretch. Following the heat treatment with the tissue in its lengthened position, manual techniques would include massage to the dorsal scar that is adherent to the extensor tendons and ROM exercises emphasizing composite flexion of the fingers distal to the site of adhesion. I would not choose to do joint mobilization or individual joint stretches, ultrasound, or heat to an individual joint. However, if the assessment shows individual joint stiffness, my treatment choice would include joint mobilization (when passive motion is allowed), modalities to the limiting joint structures, as well as AROM and PROM of the individual joint and composite motion to encourage functional use of the injured hand.

SWELLING

Swelling of the hand occurs after every surgery or injury to some extent and is the normal response of the body to injury, bringing cells that are important for healing to the injured area. Normal reduction of swelling begins within 2 weeks of the injury or surgery but may take a number of months to complete. Excessive edema or edema that is not decreasing gradually but instead remains in an area longer than 2 weeks can become problematic because it becomes more like gel, interfering with joint and tendon motion and functional use of the hand.

Precaution. *Concern about edema and assessment of the amount and characteristics of edema present are critical.*

As discussed in the chapter on edema, numerous types of swelling occur in the extremity. Inflammatory edema that occurs after injury, surgery, or other insult is initially fluid but over time may become spongy and eventually fibrotic and thus more resistant to methods aimed at reducing the swelling.

Amount of Swelling

The amount of swelling about the hand and wrist is assessed most often using circumferential and volumetric measurements. The characteristics of edema typically are evaluated by observation and palpation. When edema has become dense, it first must become less dense or "softer" before it can move out of the area. Thus to have a method to assess whether edema is becoming less dense is helpful because this change may be the first sign of improvement for firm edema. Fully standardized assessments of the denseness or firmness of edema are not yet available; however, some practical methods to measure the firmness are presented.

Volumetric Displacement

Equipment
The volumeter kit available in supply catalogues includes the volumeter tank, a collection beaker, and graduated cylinder for measuring the displaced water. A hand volumeter and arm volumeter are available.

Method
Always use the same level surface for each test. The client's hand must be free of jewelry or other objects. If jewelry cannot be removed, document such.[10]

Follow these steps:

Step 1: Fill the volumeter with room temperature water to the point of overflow, to allow an accurate starting point. Allow excess water to flow out into beaker, and then empty the beaker.

Step 2: Position the hand so the palm faces the client, and the thumb faces the spout of the volumeter. Keep the hand as vertical as possible; avoid contact with sides of volumeter (surfaces that are too high prevent the client from placing the arm straight down into the volumeter).

Step 3: Lower the hand slowly into the volumeter until the dowel in the volumeter is firmly seated between

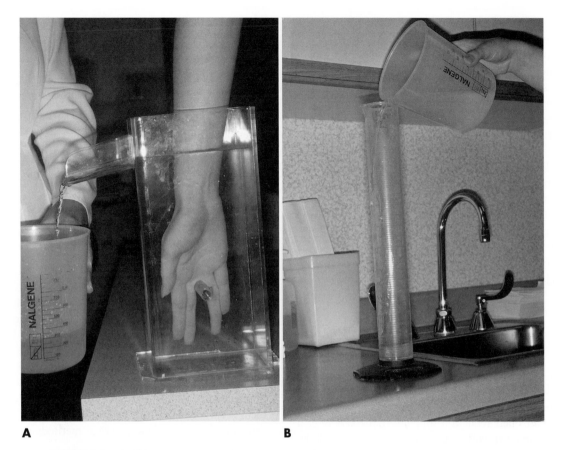

FIGURE 5-8 **A,** Edema measurement using the volumeter. The water that is displaced by immersion of the hand and distal forearm into the volumeter overflows into a collection beaker. **B,** Volumeter measurement is completed when the water from the collection beaker is poured into a graduated cylinder for accurate reading.

the middle and ring fingers. Collect the displaced water in the beaker. Hold the hand still in the volumeter until water stops dripping into the collection beaker (Fig. 5-8, A).

Step 4: Pour the displaced water from the beaker into the graduated cylinder for final measurement (Fig. 5-8, B).

Step 5: Repeat the foregoing step if you would like to average results for increased accuracy.

Step 6: Compare the volume to the other hand to determine a relative normal for the individual and to determine whether a systemic increase in volume is occurring. The difference between the two extremities is the most valuable information because there is a normal daily variance in volume, even in uninjured extremities. This test has been determined to be accurate to 5 mL, or 1% of the volume of the hand. Therefore a 10-mL difference is considered a significant change from one measurement to the next.[11]

Precaution. *Volumetric measurement should not be performed with open wounds, with an unstable vascular status, casts, external fixators, or other nonremovable supports or attachments to the extremity.*

Discussion

To increase reliability with retests, it has been helpful in my experience to use a waterproof marker to mark the spot on the forearm at the edge of the water when it is lowered into the water on the first trial. When swelling is reduced, it is possible for the hand and forearm to be lowered further into the volumeter because the web space between the fingers that is used as a stopping point against the dowel may deepen as swelling reduces. Thus there are times when I see a significant decrease in edema of the hand; however, because the forearm is lowering deeper into the volumeter, there is little if any change in the volumeter reading. Ensuring that the hand and forearm are lowered to the same depth on each repeat test minimizes this variable.

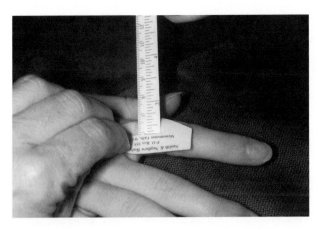

FIGURE 5-9 Edema measured using circumferential finger tape available in therapy supply catalogs. Application of the same amount of pressure when pulling the finger tape around the body part being measured is important.

Circumferential Measurement

Equipment

Tape measure or tape measure/loop for finger circumference is available in catalogs. When measuring circumference, identify the area being measured in relation to anatomic landmarks, and use the same amount of tension on the tape measure for each test.

Method

Follow these steps:

Step 1: Apply tape measure around area to be measured.
Step 2: Tighten lightly (Fig. 5-9).
Step 3: Record the circumference. Be sure to note exactly where tape was placed; for example, 4 cm proximal to radial styloid, around radial styloid and distal ulna, proximal phalanx, or PIP joint. Note positioning, such as elbow flexed or extended, wrist neutral, or fingers relaxed or extended.

Discussion

Consistency of repeat measurements with a tape measure is difficult because the tightness with which the tape measure is applied can vary with each application. Having the same therapist perform repeat measurements can help decrease variability of tightness.

Characteristics of Edema

Observation

The skin becomes shiny and more taut, with loss of wrinkles or joint creases when there is an increase in swelling. A description of the appearance of the skin may be documented. The evaluation form may have a checklist to choose from a variety of options, such as shiny, dry, and partial or full loss of joint creases. The color of the skin is also helpful to document and can be described as having increased redness (erythema), bluish tinge (cyanosis), or pallor (loss of normal color).

Palpation

Pressure with the examiner's finger into the swollen area may allow an indent into the swelling and may provide feedback as to the firmness of the swelling. If the examiner's finger is able to push into a soft edema fairly quickly, it is characterized as **pitting edema,** which is made up of large amounts of free fluid in the tissue that can be displaced by pressure, leaving a pit that slowly fills back up when the pressure is removed[12] (Fig. 5-10).

As the edema becomes more spongy and gel-like, it will refill more slowly than fluid edema. As time goes on, if the edema becomes very firm, it will decrease the ability of the fluid to move out of the way with pressure and no longer will be pitting. The more firm edema is characterized as **brawny edema** and usually is caused by the interstitial fluid becoming clogged, preventing it from moving easily.[12]

The terms *mild, moderate,* and *severe* can be used to quantify the extent of the pitting or brawny characteristic; however, this is a subjective observation made by the examiner. Objective measurement of the changes in firmness of the swelling is difficult, yet it is valuable information when measuring changes in edema. A helpful assessment for this characteristic to date is described by Artzberger[13] as an edema rebound test. This test measures the refill time or the time required for the indented tissue to return to its original shape. Consistency in the amount of time the examiner presses on the tissue and in the application force is important. The amount of force is simply the weight of the examiner's thumb placed on the tissue with no additional force and left there for 10 seconds (Fig. 5-10). When the examiner's thumb is removed, determine the time it takes for the tissue to return to its original shape. If it originally took 65 seconds to refill and on a retest it takes 40 seconds, this suggests that the edema has become more fluid. The more firm the edema, the more time the tissue will take to rebound. This can be measured for comparison with documented change as the edema becomes more or less firm. A device used in some lymphedema clinics to measure the compressibility of tissue is called a **tonometer.**[14] This device places pressure on tissue. The tonometer can measure changes in resistance of the tissue to pressure, but it has not been used widely outside of lymphedema clinics to date.

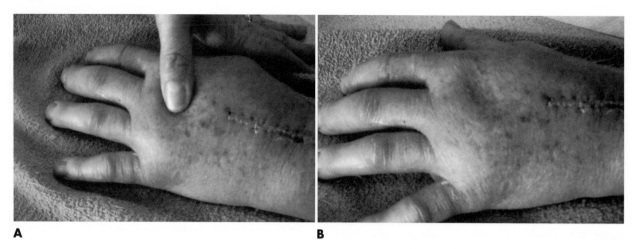

A   **B**

FIGURE 5-10 **A** and **B,** Pitting edema is seen when pressure from the examiner's finger leaves an indent or "pit" when removed.

SENSATION

Static Two-Point Discrimination

The static two-point discrimination test measures **innervation density** (the number of nerve endings present in the area tested). Flexor zones I and II are tested (the area between the distal palmar crease and the fingertips). Two-point discrimination determines the ability to discern the difference between one and two points and relates to clients' ability to determine not only *if* they can feel something but also *what* they are feeling.

Equipment
The device used for this test is the Disk-Criminator or Boley gauge, available in therapy supply catalogs.

Method
Follow these steps[15,16]:

Step 1: Instruct the client to respond to each touch, with vision occluded, by saying "one point" or "two points."
Step 2: Support the client's hand to avoid movement of fingers when touched by the point(s). Putty commonly is used as a support for the fingers.
Step 3: Occlude the client's vision. Begin at 5 mm. Touch the client's fingertip with one or two points, randomly applied (Fig. 5-11).
Step 4: The force of the touch pressure is just to the point of blanching, in a longitudinal direction, perpendicular to the skin.
Step 5: Increase or decrease the distance between the two points. If the client is unable to discriminate two points correctly at 5 mm, increase the distance between the points. If the client is able to discriminate

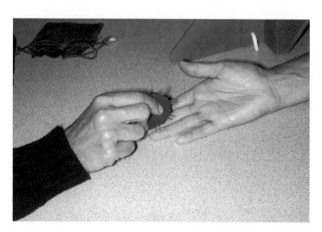

FIGURE 5-11 Two-point discrimination test is performed with the points placed longitudinally onto the skin of the fingertips, with pressure just to the point of blanching.

two points correctly at 5 mm, decrease the distance, and continue until you have determined the smallest distance the client can discriminate as two points.
Step 6: Begin distally and work proximally from fingertips to distal palmar crease.

Discussion
Seven out of 10 correct responses in one area are required for a correct response. Box 5-2 describes two-point discrimination scoring.

Moving Two-Point Discrimination

According to Dellon,[17] moving two-point discrimination always returns earlier than static two-point discrimination after nerve laceration and approaches normal 2 to 6 months before static two-point discrimination. This test is used to determine progress in return of sensation following nerve injury.

Equipment
The device used for this test is the Disk-Criminator or Boley gauge.

Method
Follow these steps[17]:

Step 1: Describe the test to the client.
Step 2: Fully support the client's hand.
Step 3: Occlude the client's vision.
Step 4: Instruct the client to respond with either "one" or "two" to the stimulus provided.
Step 5: Application is from proximal to distal on the volar distal phalanx of the fingertip. The points are longitudinal to the axis of the finger and are placed perpendicular to the skin. Move the points along the fingertip only, from proximal to distal. Speed has not been addressed.
Step 6: Begin with a distance of 5 to 8 mm, and increase or decrease as needed.
Step 7: Lift the points off the tip of the finger. Do not allow the points to come off the tip of the finger separately because this gives the client information that it was two points.

Discussion
Seven of 10 correct responses are needed for an accurate response. Two millimeters is considered normal moving two-point discrimination.

A common error is to press too hard during the testing process, and inconsistency in amount of pressure placed on the device and skin is the main problem with reliability of this test.

Touch/Pressure Threshold Test

This test determines light touch thresholds. The test is effective in identifying impairments in nerve compression injuries.

Equipment
The Semmes-Weinstein Pressure Aesthesiometer Kit is available in catalogs with 5 or 20 monofilaments. The 5-monofilament kit contains the largest monofilament in each category (normal, diminished light touch, diminished protective sensation, loss of protective sensation) and the largest monofilament of all (categorized as normal, diminished light touch, diminished protective sensation, loss of protective sensation, and untestable) (Table 5-1).

Method
Follow these steps[15,18]:

Step 1: Describe the test to the client.
Step 2: Support the client's hand in putty or on a rolled towel to prevent the fingers from moving with the touch.
Step 3: Occlude the client's vision.
Step 4: Instruct the client to respond with "touch" each time a touch is felt.
Step 5: Begin with the largest monofilament in the normal category (2.83). Proceed to larger monofilaments if there is no response.
Step 6: For the smaller monofilaments, sizes 1.65 to 4.08 (green and blue categories), the filament needs to be

---

BOX 5-2

Static Two-Point Discrimination Scoring[15]

1-5 mm = Normal
6-10 mm = Fair
11-15 mm = Poor
One point perceived = Protective sensation only
No points perceived = Anesthetic

TABLE 5-1

Semmes-Weinstein Monofilament Categories/Scoring[18]

COLOR CODE	DEFINITION	MONOFILAMENT SIZE RANGE
Green	Normal light touch threshold	1.65-2.83
Blue	Diminished light touch	3.22-3.61
Purple	Diminished protective sensation	3.84-4.31
Red	Loss of protective sensation	4.56-6.65
Untestable	Unable to feel largest monofilament	—

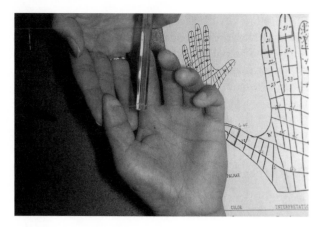

FIGURE 5-12 Semmes-Weinstein monofilament test measures touch force threshold.

applied for three trials. One correct response to the three trials is considered a correct response. All larger monofilaments are applied only one time for each trial.

Step 7: Begin testing distally and move proximally.

Step 8: Apply the monofilament perpendicular to the skin until the monofilament bends. Apply it slowly (1 to $1^1/_2$ seconds) to the skin and hold for $1^1/_2$ seconds and then lift slowly (1 to $1^1/_2$ seconds) (Fig. 5-12).

Step 9: Record on a hand map the monofilament size the client correctly perceives.

Localization of Light Touch

The localization of light touch test is used to determine functional ability to locate touch on the hand.[19] This is the last sensory stimulus to return and can cause significant problems following a nerve repair.

Equipment

The equipment needed is the Semmes-Weinstein monofilament (the smallest monofilament to be determined intact on threshold testing described previously) or a cotton ball.

Method

Follow these steps:

Step 1: Describe the test to the client. The client is to open his or her eyes and point to the location the touch was felt after the stimulus is given.

Step 2: Provide a light touch stimulus to an area. Place a dot on the hand map where the stimulus was placed.

Step 3: Following the client's response, if touch is felt in another place than given, draw an arrow pointing to the location the client felt touch from the location given. If the client did feel touch where given, draw the dot alone.

Additional Tests

Additional tests for determining sensation are the following[15,19]:

- Ninhydrin test: Used to evaluate sudomotor or sympathetic nervous system function. It does not require a voluntary response from the client and therefore can be used for children or the cognitively impaired. Ninhydrin (triketohydrindene hydrate) spray is a clear agent that turns purple when it reacts with a small concentration of sweat. The test identifies areas of distribution of sweat secretion after recent, complete peripheral nerve lesions. No sweat will be present after a complete laceration.
- O'Riain wrinkle test: Used to evaluate sympathetic nervous system function or recovery following a complete nerve lesion. Denervated palmar skin does not wrinkle when soaked in 42° C (108° F) water for 20 to 30 minutes, as normal skin will.
- Vibration: Helpful in determining threshold of touch and level of placement in a sensory reeducation program. Tuning forks of 30 and 256 cps are used. Sensory reeducation training has been initiated when a client could feel a 30 cps tuning fork but not moving touch to that same spot, or if the client could feel a 256 cps tuning fork but not constant touch to that same spot.
- Moberg's pick-up test: Used to determine tactile gnosis, or functional discrimination. Using specific small objects, the client picks the objects up with each hand and is timed, with vision and without vision.

Discussion

Although it is helpful to be aware of the battery of sensory evaluations described, a standard screening of sensation is limited to one or two assessments. I recommend use of the Semmes-Weinstein monofilaments for nerve compressions such as carpal tunnel or cubital tunnel syndrome, and monofilaments and two-point discrimination testing following a nerve injury or laceration. Following a nerve laceration, touch threshold (Semmes-Weinstein monofilaments) will show an improvement before the ability to discriminate touch (two-point discrimination).

COORDINATION

Coordination is the ability to manipulate items in the environment. This ranges from gross coordination to fine coordination tasks. A large number of standardized coordination tests are available, with methodology available for each test. Standardized coordination tests include O'Connor Dexterity Test, Nine-hole Peg Test, Jebsen-Taylor Hand Function Test, Minnesota Rate of Manipulation Test, Crawford Small Parts Dexterity Test, and the Purdue Pegboard Test.[20] A simple test for a quick screening of coordination is the Nine-hole Peg Test.[21] This test is standardized yet allows use of a low-cost homemade board and pegs. The Jebsen-Taylor Hand Function Test assesses functional tasks such as writing, as well as ability to manipulate large and small items.[22] The methodology is available with each test and will not be specified in this chapter because of the number of tests available. Use of a standardized test is helpful particularly for clients whose injuries might affect their coordination.

STRENGTH TESTING

Grip and Pinch Strength Testing

Grip and pinch strength testing is the standard method used for decades to determine functional grasp and pinch strength. The tests are used initially and in periodic retests to demonstrate improvement in the strength available to grasp or pinch. Contraindications are noted in the following discussion.

Contraindications

Do not perform these tests when resistance has not yet been approved by the referring physician. Grip and pinch strength testing are maximally resistive tests. Instruct clients to squeeze the dynamometer or pinchmeter as hard as they can. Testing is contraindicated before full healing, as determined by the referring physician, or following a fracture, ligament repair, tendon laceration, or tendon transfer of the forearm, wrist, or hand.

Precaution. *A sprain of a digital joint or wrist is also a contraindication for this test until resistive exercises are tolerated well.*

For any traumatic injury, I defer testing of grip or pinch strength until resistive exercises or strengthening have been approved by the referring physician. For a gradual-onset condition or injury, such as tendonitis or carpal tunnel syndrome, I will test strength at the time of initial evaluation, even though my initial treatment plan may not include strengthening until the level of pain decreases. At the time of initial evaluation for this type of condition, I instruct the client to stop grasping when mild pain occurs to prevent an increase in pain following use of the test, and I document when pain does occur with the test. Determination of initial grip and pinch strength for tendonitis or nerve compressions is important to allow future progress to be documented.

> **CLINICAL** *Pearl*
>
> The question always to ask yourself before performing strength testing is whether there are any healing tissues that can be damaged by this test.

Grip Strength Test

Equipment

To assess grip strength, the Jamar dynamometer is recommended by the American Society for Surgery of the Hand and the American Society of Hand Therapists.[20,23] The test has been determined to be accurate and reliable. Annual calibration is recommended and should be done more often in high-use settings. Do not ignore calibration. Pinchmeters are commercially available; however, no one specific type is endorsed by the aforementioned associations.

Method

The client is seated, with shoulder adducted, elbow flexed to 90 degrees, and forearm and wrist neutral. The therapist places the dynamometer in the client's hand and while gently supporting the base of the dynamometer, provides instruction to the client. Grip force should be applied smoothly, without rapid jerking motion. Allow the wrist to extend during the grip.[20,23]

Consider the following:

- Standard grip test: three trials on the second handle setting
- Five-level grip test: One trial on each of the five handle-width settings. This test is used to determine a bell curve when graphed. The strongest grip is almost always on the second or third handle-width setting. The weakest grips normally occur at the most narrow and widest settings, with scores on the middle three handle settings falling between the strongest and weakest scores, assimilating a bell curve. Lack of maximal effort may be a possibility when the five handle setting scores show a flat line when graphed, where readings at all handle settings are almost the same, or when there is an up/down/up/down type of curve.
- Rapid exchange grip test: The examiner rapidly moves the dynamometer, alternating from the client's right to left hands, for 10 trials to each hand. This test had been thought to prevent voluntary control of grip strength by the client, making it more difficult for a client to self-limit the grip response or provide less than maximal effort.[24] More recently, Schectman and colleagues[25-27] have articulated well-founded con-

cerns about the methods with which clinicians interpret sincerity of effort of grip tests. Their work provides some thought-provoking findings on the topic.

Discussion

Normative data exists for grip and pinch strength testing,[28] although none thus far are without problems. The American Society of Hand Therapists recommendations are to compare readings with the client's opposite extremity, if it is uninjured.

Pinch Strength Test

Equipment
The device used is the pinchmeter (styles vary).

Method
With the client seated, elbow flexed to 90 degrees with arm adducted at side, and forearm neutral, proceed as follows[20]:

- Lateral pinch (key pinch): Place the pinchmeter between the radial side of index finger and thumb, and instruct the client to pinch as hard as possible.
- Three-point pinch (three jaw chuck pinch): Place the pinchmeter between the pulp of the thumb and pulp of the index and middle fingers. Instruct the client to pinch as hard as possible.
- Two-point pinch (tip to tip pinch): Place the pinchmeter between the tip of the thumb and tip of the index finger, and instruct the client to pinch as hard as possible.

Discussion
Repeat each test 3 times and calculate an average. Calibrate equipment at least annually.

Manual Muscle Test

Manual muscle strength is essential to test and document for improvement when there is weakness related to a nerve injury or compression. Identifying the strength of various muscles along a specific nerve distribution helps determine the level of nerve injury and improvement over time. Measurement of manual muscle strength also is helpful in order to document improvement when weakness is present because of disuse, such as after prolonged immobilization.

Equipment
Manual muscle testing is a form of strength testing that measures the client's ability to move the body part being tested against gravity and, if able to move fully against

gravity, to maintain the end ROM against the examiner's resistance. Thus the only equipment needed is a reference book along with muscle action and placement of examiner resistance and a form on which to record the results.

Method
Manual muscle testing is performed according to methods documented in numerous sources. Strength is graded according to normal, good, fair, poor, and trace strength definitions, with fair strength defined as the ability to move the body part through its full available range against gravity, although not able to tolerate any additional resistance. Description of the method of applying resistance to each muscle of the hand, wrist, and forearm is beyond the scope of this chapter. An excellent reference for specific testing procedures for each muscle is found in *Muscles: Testing and Function* by Kendall et al.[29] I recommend use of a form designed for manual muscle testing with the muscles listed in relation to their nerve innervation, as described by Kendall et al.

Discussion
Manual muscle testing is contraindicated as for grip and pinch strength testing or when pain prevents full effort by the client. Because manual muscle testing is a maximally resistive test, any injury with healing tissues (bone, ligament, and tendon) that could be reinjured should not be tested until determined to be safe by the referring physician.

Precaution. *Finger or thumb tendon repairs are not sufficiently strong to test until 14 weeks after surgery.*

I use manual muscle strength testing mainly following nerve injuries or weakness because of disuse, not following a traumatic injury unless there is an unusual disuse pattern following the normal healing time.

USE OF SPLINTS

Many clients have obtained their own splints or have been given prefabricated splints by their primary or referring physicians. Determine the use of any splints and the amount of time and activities during which they are worn. This information is helpful in determining the client's functional limitations and allows you to offer insight into the appropriateness of splinting for the client's condition.

FUNCTIONAL USE

Functional use is an area that should be assessed as part of every evaluation. This portion of the evaluation is important to determine functional goals with the client and to document them for the insurance company. Determining difficulty in daily activities helps you set goals in conjunction with the clients' perception of their needs. This area often is forgotten or bypassed in a busy clinic situation. Discussing functional limitations and goals helps clients recognize that the therapist is aware of the ways in which their injury affects their life and gives them confidence that they are working together toward common and meaningful goals.

Equipment

A checklist to help the client think of areas in which they are successful or in which they have difficulty may be helpful. Categories such as self-care skills, home management (outdoor and indoor), and vocational tasks can be included. The evaluation summary form (see Appendix 5-1 on the CD) may include a list of common tasks, such as opening containers or performing fasteners. Some therapists use a writing device for the therapist to circle while interviewing the client. Some therapists prefer to take notes about specific functional tasks that the client describes as difficult. Please see the chapter on assessing functional outcomes for more about functional assessments.

Method

Functional use is assessed through discussion with the client or simulation of activities. Possibly the extremity is completely nonfunctional because of the presence of a cast, limitations by the injury such as a flexor tendon repair in the early stage of healing, a complex injury, inability to move the digits to grasp an object, loss of muscle innervation, or loss of sensation. In these cases, to list all the functional tasks that are limited is impossible, and it may be simpler generally to state the limitations such as, "Unable to use the right upper extremity for any functional tasks other than support of a light object using the forearm, as the hand is unable to grasp." At the other extreme may be a client with a single digit injured, with hypersensitivity that limits fine coordination. In this case, it may be possible to list specific task limitations. I prefer to include the category of functional use as the last section of the evaluation documentation. Following documentation of the status of pain, wounds/scars, ROM, sensation, and strength, the functional use statement becomes a reflection of the way in which the previously noted deficits affect the client's life daily.

In some situations, time limitations may preclude an in-depth assessment of all areas of the hand in one session. A screening of some sections may be done, with a full assessment deferred to the next session. For instance, I may screen the area of sensation by asking about the client's sensation and may defer monofilament or two-point discrimination testing to the next visit.

SUMMARY

Awareness of the areas to include in a thorough evaluation is enhanced by use of an evaluation summary form (see Appendix 5-1 on the CD), which facilitates the logical progression through the steps of the evaluation.

Precaution. *Awareness of situations in which it is unsafe to perform certain assessments is essential.*

Much evaluation is done by observation. Effectiveness as a therapist is enhanced when the therapist takes the time to communicate well with a new client during the evaluation. This occurs not only by describing the process of the assessments but also by listening as the client attempts to communicate verbally and nonverbally. The information gained during the assessment process is the foundation upon which treatment choices rest, and the connection the therapist makes with each new client is the foundation upon which the client's confidence in the treatment rests. Both are equally important.

References

1. Maurer GL, Jezek SM: Pain assessment. In *Clinical assessment recommendations*, ed 2, Chicago, 1992, American Society of Hand Therapists.
2. Melzack R: The short-form McGill pain questionnaire, *Pain* 30:191-197, 1987.
3. Ziegler Cuzzell J: The new red yellow black color code, *Am J Nurs* 10:1342, 1988.
4. Evans RB, McAuliffe JA: Wound classification and management. In Mackin EJ, Callahan AD, Skirven TM et al, editors: *Rehabilitation of the hand and upper extremity*, ed 5, St Louis, 2002, Mosby.
5. Seiler JG III: Physical examination of the hand. In *Essentials of hand surgery*, Philadelphia, 2002, Lippincott Williams & Wilkins.
6. Taras JS, Lemel MS, Nathan R: Vascular disorders of the upper extremity. In Mackin EJ, Callahan AD, Skirven TM et al, editors: *Rehabilitation of the hand and upper extremity*, ed 5, St Louis, 2002, Mosby.
7. de Herder E: Vascular assessment. In *Clinical assessment recommendations*, ed 2, Chicago, 1992, American Association of Hand Therapists.
8. Adams LS, Greene LW, Topoozian E: Range of motion. In *Clinical assessment recommendations*, ed 2, Chicago, 1992, American Association of Hand Therapists.
9. Cambridge-Keeling CA: Range-of-motion measurement of the hand. In Mackin EJ, Callahan AD, Skirven TM et al, editors: *Rehabilitation of the hand and upper extremity*, ed 5, St Louis, 2002, Mosby.

10. Jaffe R, Farney-Mokris S: Edema. In *Clinical assessment recommendations*, ed 2, Chicago, 1992, American Association of Hand Therapists.
11. Waylett-Rendall J, Seibly D: A study of the accuracy of a commercially available volumeter, *J Hand Ther* 4:10, 1991.
12. Villeco JP, Mackin EJ, Hunter JM: Edema: therapist's management. In Mackin EJ, Callahan AD, Skirven TM et al, editors: *Rehabilitation of the hand and upper extremity*, ed 5, St Louis, 2002, Mosby.
13. Artzberger S: Personal communication, Feb 2005.
14. Miller L: Management of breast related edemas. In Mackin EJ, Callahan AD, Skirven TM et al, editors: *Rehabiliation of the hand and upper extremity*, ed 5, St Louis, 2002, Mosby.
15. Stone JH: Sensibility. In *Clinical assessment recommendations*, ed 2, Chicago, 1992, American Association of Hand Therapists.
16. Dellon AL, Mackinnon SE, Crosby PM: Reliability of two-point discrimination measurements, *J Hand Surg* 12A:693-696, 1987.
17. Dellon AL: The moving two-point discrimination test: clinical evaluation of the quickly adapting fiber/receptor system, *J Hand Surg* 3:474-481, 1978.
18. Bell-Krotoski JA: Sensibility testing with the Semmes-Weinstein monofilaments. In Mackin EJ, Callahan AD, Skirven TM et al, editors: *Rehabilitation of the hand and upper extremity*, ed 5, St Louis, 2002, Mosby.
19. Callahan AD: Sensibility assessment for nerve lesions-in-continuity and nerve lacerations. In Mackin EJ, Callahan AD, Skirven TM et al, editors: *Rehabilitation of the hand and upper extremity*, ed 5, St Louis, 2002, Mosby.
20. Fess EE: Documentation: essential elements of an upper extremity assessment battery. In Mackin EJ, Callahan AD, Skirven TM et al, editors: *Rehabilitation of the hand and upper extremity*, ed 5, St Louis, 2002, Mosby.
21. Mathiowetz V et al: Adult norms for the nine-hole peg test of finger dexterity, *Occup Ther J Res* 5(1):25-37, 1985.
22. Jebsen RH et al: An objective and standardized test of hand function, *Arch Phys Med Rehabil* 50:311, 1969.
23. Fess EE: Grip strength. In *Clinical assessment recommendations*, ed 2, Chicago, 1992, American Association of Hand Therapists.
24. Hildreth DH, Breidenbach WC, Lister GD et al: Detection of submaximal effort by use of the rapid exchange grip, *J Hand Surg* 14A:742-745, 1989.
25. Shechtman O: Using the coefficient of variation to detect sincerity of effort of grip strength: a literature review, *J Hand Ther* 13:25-32, 2000.
26. Taylor C, Shechtman O: The use of rapid exchange grip test in detecting sincerity of effort. I. Administration of the test, *J Hand Ther* 13:195-202, 2000.
27. Shechtman O, Taylor C: The use of rapid exchange grip test in detecting sincerity of effort. II. Validity of the test, *J Hand Ther* 13:202-210, 2000.
28. Mathiowetz V et al: Grip and pinch strength: normative data for adults *Arch Phys Med Rehabil* 66:69, 1985.
29. Kendall HO, Kendall FP, Wadsworth GE: *Muscles testing and function*, ed 2, Baltimore, 1971, Williams & Wilkins.

APPENDIX 5-1

Evaluation Summary Form

<u>**History of Injury/Condition:**</u> _____
_____

Pertinent Medical History: _____

Pain Level   0 – 1 – 2 – 3 – 4 – 5 – 6 – 7 – 8 – 9 – 10   At best____Worst____
               (mild)   (intolerable)
Description (Circle all that apply):
    Sore Aching Throbbing Burning Sharp Stabbing Radiating
Location: _____
Frequency: Intermittent (Occasional   Frequent) / Constant
           At rest   With use   With exercise   Other_____

<u>Scar</u>   Location:_____
    Raised/Flattened   Color:_____
Adhesions (circle one):   Adherent   Partially adherent   Non-adherent

<u>**Wound**</u> (circle one):   Closed   Eschar   Sutured   Open
Wound color: Red   Yellow   Black   Combination   Size:_____
Location: _____
Drainage Amount and Color:_____

<u>**Vascular Status**</u>   Color (circle one):   Normal/Pink/Red/Blue/White/Mottled
Trophic: Normal Dry/Moist Shiny/Dull   Location: _____
Peripheral Pulse Strength/Quality: Right _____ Left _____
Capillary Refill Time: _____ Location: _____
Allen's Test: _____
Surface Temperature: Location/Degrees _____
Fingertip Pulp Changes: Narrowing/Thickened/Other: _____

<u>**Fixation Devices**</u>   Pins (Internal/Protrude through skin) _____
Screw(s) _____ Plate _____
External Fixation _____ Other _____

Use of Splints (Describe Splint and Times of Use) _____

Vascular Status   Color (circle one):   Normal/Pink/Red/Blue/White/Mottled
Trophic: Normal   Dry/Moist   Shiny/Dull   Location: _____
Peripheral Pulse Strength/Quality: Right _____   Left _____
Capillary Refill Time: _____   Location: _____
Allen's Test: _____
Surface Temperature: Location/Degrees _____
Fingertip Pulp Changes: Narrowing/Thickened/Other: _____

Swelling

Visual Inspection (circle one)
Not significant
Mild
Moderate
Moderate +
Severe

Volumetric Measurements (circle one)
Injured hand: _____ mL
Noninjured hand: _____ mL
Difference: _____ mL

Pitting/Brawny Location: _____

Circumferential Measurements (cm)

	Right	Left
Forearm (Location_____)		
Hand (MCP)		
Wrist		
Digit (Circle)	Thumb IF MF RF SF	Thumb IF MF RF SF
Proximal Phalanx		
PIP joint		
Middle Phalanx		
DIP joint		

Range of Motion

		Right	Left			Right	Left
Shoulder	Flexion			**Index Finger**	MP		
	Extension				PIP		
	Ext Rot				DIP		
	Int Rot			**Middle Finger**	MP		
Elbow	Flexion				PIP		
	Extension				DIP		
Forearm	Supination			**Ring Finger**	MP		
	Pronation				PIP		
Wrist	Extension				DIP		
	Flexion			**Small Finger**	MP		
	Radial Dev				PIP		
	Ulnar Dev				DIP		
Thumb MP				**Thumb CMC**	Radial Abd		
Thumb IP					Palmar Abd		

Sensation

Circle One: Intact   Hypersensitive   Tingling   Numb   Frequency: Intermittent/Constant

Occurrences: With use / At rest / Prolonged position / Repetitive use / At night

Semmes-Weinstein monofilament / Two-point discrimination / Other (see separate forms)

STRENGTH	Right	Left
Grip		
Lateral pinch		
2 point pinch		
3 point pinch		

Five-level or rapid exchange grip if indicated—see separate form

Manual muscle test if indicated—see separate form

Coordination

Observation: _____

Test Results (see separate form)

Functional Use Patient has difficulty with the following (circle all that apply):

Self-Care	*Home Management*
Dressing	Washing dishes
Fasteners	Meal preparation
Eating	Laundry
Bathing	Opening containers
Hygiene	Cleaning—light
Hair care	Cleaning—heavy (floors, tub)
Other	Lawn/outdoor maintenance
Driving/starting vehicle	Grocery shopping
Opening doors	Computer use
Writing	

Vocational (Describe)

Computer use,
assembly, heavy lifting

Other_____

Avocational (Describe)

Hobbies, gardening

Other_____

6

Assessment of Functional Outcomes

REBECCA VON DER HEYDE

Client-centered care is a high priority in the health professions. The commonly used subjective, objective, assessment, and plan (SOAP) note denotes the client's subjective discussion of recovery as our first priority. The problem, however, is the effective intake of the client's point of view and the consideration of this information from a **quantitative** and **qualitative** perspective. Quantitative aspects of evaluation and treatment include those variables that are measured in a standardized fashion and result in numeric data.[1] Typical quantitative tools include goniometric measurement, manual muscle testing, and sensory evaluations. These tests often are referred to using terms such as *objective* or *performance-based*.[2,3] Qualitative information, in comparison, is subjective and often consists of client narratives[1] (Box 6-1). Symptoms, abilities, and participation in daily activities are typical examples of *subjective* information. For client-centered care providers the challenge lies in attempting to measure and interpret qualitative information as a means of directing evaluation and treatment. Subjective information is considered to play a crucial role in maximizing therapeutic outcomes, and much research has been dedicated to this topic.

Literature pertaining to client outcomes is littered with terms such as *quality of life, emotional function, disability,* and *health status*.[4-6] Many researchers are pursuing measurement of these complex components in the form of **client self-report outcome measures.** These measures most often are found in questionnaire form using the **visual analog scale** (VAS) or **Likert scale** (Box 6-2). The development of these tools can be considered a conduit toward incorporating subjective data into evaluation and treatment planning and a means for analyzing and adding to the current evaluative repertoire.

As therapists, our goal is to evaluate our clients accurately and consistently with tools that are designed to detect changes in clinical status. Research terms for these expectations include **validity, reliability,** and **responsiveness.** As a group, these variables are known as **psychometric properties.** Validity is the degree to which an

BOX 6-1

Quantitative and Qualitative Aspects of Client Evaluation

QUANTITATIVE

Variables that are measured in a standardized fashion and result in numeric data[1]

Examples: goniometric measurement, manual muscle testing, and sensory evaluations

QUALITATIVE

Client narratives, self-report of symptoms or recovery, and subjective opinions

Examples: subjective section of a SOAP note and personal communication with therapist

BOX 6-2

Visual Analog and Likert Scales

Visual analog scale: *How much pain do you have at night?*

| No pain | | | | Extreme pain |

Ten-interval visual analog scale: *How much pain do you have at night?*

0   1   2   3   4   5   6   7   8   9   10

| No pain | | | | | | | | | | Extreme pain |

Likert scale: *How much pain do you have at night?*

?	?	?	?	?
No pain	Mild pain	Moderate pain	Severe pain	Extreme pain

instrument measures what it is intended to measure.[1] An outcome measure can be defined specifically as having construct, criterion, and/or content (face) validity. **Construct validity** refers to a comparison between a new measure and an associated measure, **criterion validity** compares a new measure with a gold standard, and **content validity** considers accurate measurement of a specific domain.[7] Reliability is the degree of consistency with which an instrument or rater measures a variable, and responsiveness is the ability of a test to demonstrate change.[1] Responsiveness often is referred to as *sensitivity to (clinical) change* and is established if change in scores accurately represents change in clinical status.[8] Similarities between measurement of responsiveness and validity have been addressed recently by researchers who question whether the two are distinct psychometric properties.[9]

The assessment of clinical outcomes from a qualitative and quantitative perspective is strongly encouraged in response to recent findings.[10] Clinical evaluation tools, such as range of motion, have been shown to demonstrate poor reliability[11] and decreased responsiveness when compared with client self-report measures.[12-14] Research also has shown a suboptimal relationship between client self-report of quality of life and ratings from health care providers.[15]

CLINICAL *Pearl*

Client perception of ability has been suggested as being more valuable than the therapeutic evaluation of independent function.[16]

In addition, it is recommended that the client is the one who ultimately should assess the importance of change in health status.[17] Despite these findings, incorporation of standardized, self-report outcome measures in treatment and/or clinical research is currently inconsistent.[18]

Over the past 20 years, client self-report outcome measures have been researched extensively and are becoming more readily available for use in clinical practice. These measures can be categorized as generic, regional, or disease-specific. **Generic measures** can be used to compare health conditions and therefore can assist in the analysis of policies and funds distribution. **Regional measures** are designed to demonstrate changes at the systems level, whereas **disease-specific measures** are intended to be highly responsive for individual diagnoses.[13] The purpose of this chapter is to introduce standardized, self-report outcome measures in each category as a means of facilitating their incorporation into evaluation and treatment.

GENERIC MEASURES

Canadian Occupational Performance Measure

The Canadian Occupational Performance Measure (COPM) initially was published in 1991 and is currently available in its third edition.[19-22] This measure uses individual activity limitation and goal setting as obtained through an open-ended, semistructured interview. The COPM is not diagnosis or age specific and asks clients to articulate concerns in areas of self-care, productivity, and leisure. The COPM is based on the model of human occupational performance and is designed for use by occupational therapists.[19,20]

The COPM is a clinical tool used to facilitate the client-centered evaluative process. During the standardized yet semistructured interview, clients identify five problems they would like to address during therapy sessions. These problems are rated by the clients in terms of their current performance and satisfaction. Ratings are given on a Likert scale ranging from 1 to 10, with higher scores indicating increased performance and satisfaction. Scores are totaled and averaged to give a final score that also ranges from 1 to 10. This measure is designed to be incorporated into the initial evaluation and repeated over the course of treatment as a means of reassessing clinical goals. The COPM is available in 20 languages.

Eighty-eight papers have been published with reference to the COPM, including analyses of psychometric properties, outcomes, and use in clinical practice.[22] This measure has been found to be valid, reliable, and responsive for multiple disease populations.[19-23] Validity was reinforced in two studies that included clients with hand injuries and rheumatoid arthritis.[16,23] The COPM was used to validate the Dutch form of the Disabilities of the Arm, Shoulder, and Hand (DASH) questionnaire[24] and was used in a study of evidence-based practice for radial nerve splinting.[25] Notable is that problems identified on the COPM by clients with upper extremity diagnoses have been used in multiple studies to analyze self-care, productivity, and leisure questions included in alternate measures.[16,23,24,26]

Health Assessment Questionnaire

Dr. James F. Fries established the Health Assessment Questionnaire (HAQ) at Stanford University in 1978. Despite its development in the field of rheumatology, the HAQ is considered a generic self-report outcome measure and has been used for clinical research in many disciplines. The HAQ was designed to assess the impact of chronic illness and accepts additional information when used in conjunction with alternate measures.[27]

The HAQ is used most commonly in its short, two-page format, which includes the HAQ Disability Index (HAQ-DI), the HAQ VAS pain scale, and the VAS client global health scale. The HAQ-DI consists of eight categories of functioning expressed through 20 questions. Activities are organized under the categories of dressing, rising, eating, walking, hygiene, reach, grip, and usual activities and are recalled over the past week. This section is presented in a Likert scale with answers from 0 (no disability) to 3 (completely disabled). An interesting feature of the HAQ-DI is found in the 2 questions that follow the 20 functional tasks. The first question asks about aids or assistive devices used to complete activities, and the second question addresses assistance from another person. This clarification is certainly an impor-

tant detail to consider during therapeutic intervention and is used in the scoring process in that it decreases the score to 2 (with much difficulty or limited). The average of all eight categories is used as the total score, and a score is not calculated unless questions are answered in six of the eight categories. Pain is reported on a VAS that ranges from 0 (no pain) to 3 (severe pain) or from 0 mm (no pain) to 100 mm (severe pain). The client global health scale is also a VAS, articulated as "how you are doing" and answered as a range from very well (0 mm) to very poor (100 mm). The HAQ is available in more than 60 languages.

More than 500 studies have included the HAQ, which has been established as valid and sensitive to change in many diagnostic categories, especially rheumatoid arthritis.[27] Validity and sensitivity to change were demonstrated in a study that considered independent living for elderly clients after upper or lower extremity fractures.[28] The HAQ also was used to validate the COPM for use with clients with rheumatoid arthritis.[16] The HAQ can be found in multiple forms in the literature, including the modified HAQ, upper extremity/upper limb HAQ (HAQUP/ULHAQ), and multidimensional HAQ (MDHAQ). The HAQUP/ULHAQ have yet to be validated formally, and the HAQ was found to have limited reliability and sensitivity in a study of measures for clients with osteoarthritis in the hand.[29] In addition, the modified HAQ was found to be less preferable than objective functional tests for physical assessment in a sample of clients with rheumatoid arthritis.[30]

Milliken Activities of Daily Living Scale

The Milliken Activities of Daily Living Scale (MAS) was developed with the goal of incorporating perceived task necessity into a client self-report measure.[31] A combined effort of the Washington University Program in Occupational Therapy and the Milliken Hand Rehabilitation Center in St. Louis, Missouri, this tool was completed in 1996 and published in 2005. The MAS aims to capture information regarding bilateral and unilateral tasks, gross and fine motor skills, and a variety of prehensile patterns and resistance levels.

The MAS is composed of 47 tasks in the areas of mobility (13 items), self-care (20 items), domestic life (13 items), and community/recreation (1 item). Clients are asked to complete the questionnaire by rating their current ability level on a Likert scale ranging from 1 (unable to do) to 5 (able to do as before injury). In addition, level of necessity for each item is considered on a Likert scale ranging from 1 (not necessary) to 3 (necessary). The client is instructed to answer the questions "regardless which hand you use." Scores are summed for each section, and a global activity score is attained by totaling scores for all sections. The authors suggest focusing on those items that are indicated as high-necessity/low-ability for treatment planning and clinical intervention. The publication of the MAS articulates two other studies that establish moderate criterion validity, good concurrent validity, and excellent reliability.[31]

Pediatric Musculoskeletal Functional Health Questionnaire

The Pediatric Musculoskeletal Functional Health Questionnaire (POSNA) is a combined effort of the American Academy of Orthopaedic Surgeons (AAOS), the Pediatric Orthopaedic Society of North America, the American Academy of Pediatrics, and Shriner's Hospitals. This group also is known as the Pediatric Outcomes Instrument Development Group. Published in 1998, the POSNA was developed to assess children and adolescents between the ages of 2 and 18. Measuring clinical outcomes in this population is considered a challenge because of normal developmental increases in function. Parental opinions of function, quality of life, and medical expectations were perceived as important factors in the assessment process.[32]

The POSNA consists of four tools: the pediatric-parent/child baseline and follow-up questionnaires for children ages 2 to 10 and the pediatric-parent/child baseline and follow-up questionnaires for adolescents ages 11 to 18. The tools include 117 items each, with 49 items specific to one of eight scales: upper extremity and physical function (8 items), transfer and basic mobility (11 items), sports/physical functioning (12 items), pain/comfort (3 items), treatment expectations (9 items), happiness (5 items), and satisfaction with symptoms (1 item). A global functioning scale also can be calculated via the first four scales, and raw scores on each scale are converted to standardized scores using the scoring algorithms as offered by the AAOS. Standardized scores range from 0 to 100, with a higher score indicating better function and decreased pain.[32] Scales are not scored unless at least 50% of the questions have been completed. Questions are formatted in yes/no, multiple choice, and Likert scales. Follow-up questionnaires are used 6 months after the baseline has been established.

In the original research article, more than 750 baseline and follow-up questionnaires were completed and analyzed. Good reliability, validity, and sensitivity to change were noted for the child and adolescent tools, with the tools for children ages 2 to 10 demonstrating slightly higher reliability. The authors state that the tools were discriminative to the upper and lower extremities and sensitive to clinical change for clients with moderate to severe diagnoses.[32] A second research article attends to the establishment of baseline scores with "normal" children and adolescents, setting baseline scores at the mid-80s to 90s.[33] The AAOS formally has established normative values, including means and standard deviations.[34] This tool also is referred to in the literature as the Pediatric Outcomes Data Collection Instrument (PODCI).[33]

Short Form 36

The Short Form 36 (SF-36) was standardized in 1990 as a self-report measure of functional health and well-being.[35] Version 2.0 was published in 1996 (SF-36v2), with copyright and trademark privileges belonging to the Medical Outcomes Trust, Health Assessment Lab, and QualityMetric Incorporated. The SF-36 was designed to be a brief yet comprehensive measure of general health status.

The SF-36 questionnaire consists of eight scales yielding two summary measures: physical and mental health. The physical health measure includes four scales of physical functioning (10 items), role-physical (4 items), bodily pain (2 items), and general health (5 items). The mental health measure is composed of vitality (4 items), social functioning (2 items), role-emotional (3 items), and mental health (5 items). A final item, termed *self-reported health transition*, is answered by the client but is not included in the scoring process. The SF-36 offers a choice of recall format at a standard (4 week) or acute (1 week) time frame. Likert scales and yes/no options are used to assess function and well-being on this 36-item questionnaire. To score the SF-36, scales are standardized with a scoring algorithm or by the SF-36v2 scoring software to obtain a score ranging from 0 to 100. Higher scores indicate better health status, and a mean score of 50 has been articulated as a normative value for all scales.[35] The SF-36 has been translated into more than 40 languages.

The SF-36 can be found in nearly 4000 publications, almost 400 of which are randomized controlled clinical trials and 225 of which are comparisons with alternate measures. The SF-36 has been found to be reliable, valid, and responsive for a variety of medical diagnoses.[35] The SF-36 has been chosen for many outcome studies that specifically address upper extremity function. Validity of the German version was demonstrated in a study that considered independent living after upper or lower extremity fractures in an elderly population.[28] The SF-36 has been shown to be valid and sensitive to clinical change when used as an outcome measure for workers with upper extremity disorders.[36,37] Notable is that the SF-36 has been found to be significantly responsive to change in physical components but not general health in studies of upper extremity function.[26] The SF-36 also has been demonstrated to be more sensitive to clinical change in the lower extremities compared with the upper extremities.[37,38] The SF-36 has been and continues to be used extensively as a foundational, quality-of-life measure in upper extremity outcomes research.[26,39-52]

Short Musculoskeletal Functional Assessment Questionnaire

The Short Musculoskeletal Functional Assessment questionnaire (SMFA) is an abbreviated version of the 101-item Musculoskeletal Functional Assessment questionnaire (MFA). The SMFA was published in 1999 and was funded by the National Institute of Child Health and Human Development, AAOS, and the Orthopaedic Trauma Association. The authors defined the purpose of the SMFA as "to detect differences in the functional status of clients who have a broad range of musculoskeletal disorders that are commonly seen in community practices."[39]

The SMFA has 46 questions in two parts: the dysfunction index and the bother index. The dysfunction index has 34 items in four categories of daily activities, emotional status, function of the arm and hand, and mobility. The bother index asks clients to rate how much they are bothered by problems during functional activities. Both indexes are answered reporting on the current week on a Likert scale ranging from 1 (good function/not at all bothered) to 5 (poor function/extremely bothered). A formula in the primary publication transforms raw scores to a total score ranging from 0 to 100, with higher scores indicating decreased function.[39] Unanswered items on the dysfunction scale are addressed by replacing them with the mean category score if 50% of the category is complete.

Swiontowski et al.[39] established excellent reliability, good validity, and very good responsiveness in a study of 420 clients with upper and lower extremity musculoskeletal diagnoses. Statistically significant correlation to the SF-36 also confirmed construct validity in the English and Swedish versions of this tool.[39,40] The dysfunction scale is recommended as having stability and consistency values suitable for individual client assessment,[39] and it has been suggested to have greatest value for those clients with chronic conditions or fractures in the late healing phase.[53] Means and standard deviations for this tool have been published by the AAOS.[34]

Table 6-1 provides information on the aforementioned assessment instruments.

REGIONAL MEASURES

Disabilities of the Arm, Shoulder, and Hand Index

The Disabilities of the Arm, Shoulder, and Hand (DASH) index was a joint effort of the AAOS, American Society

for Surgery of the Hand, American Association of Hand Surgery, the Council of Musculoskeletal Specialty Societies, and the Institute for Work and Health.[54] The DASH was conceptualized as a tool that would facilitate comparison of conditions throughout the upper extremity while considering it a single functional unit. Careful development of this tool, including an extensive literature review[54,55] and consideration of questions and attribution,[41] have made it a well-recognized and popular tool in upper extremity research and clinical practice.

Thirteen existing outcome measures were reviewed to create a pool of more than 800 possible items. These items were reduced to 30 through a process of expert opinion and group selection.[54,55] Two concepts of symptoms (9 items) and functional status (21 items) are addressed in the DASH, with functional status being classified further into domains of physical, social, and psychological status. A Likert scale format is used for assessment; options range from 1 (no difficulty, symptoms, or limitations) to 5 (unable to complete activities and extreme symptomatology). The DASH is scored when at least 27 items have been completed using a simple equation offered by the authors.[52] This equation anchors the score to a zero base; resultant scores range from 0 (no disability) to 100 (completely disabled). The DASH includes optional work and sports/performing arts modules (4 items each) and also has been offered as the Quick-DASH, which includes the 11 items that have been found to be the most responsive in clinical studies.[10] The DASH is available in more than 10 languages.

Psychometric properties of the DASH have been researched thoroughly. Studies in upper extremity clinics including a variety of diagnoses have demonstrated validity, excellent reliability, and responsiveness to clinical change.[24,26,42,52,56] The DASH also has been established as possessing the following attributes: content validity for clients with psoriatic arthritis[57]; responsiveness/sensitivity to clinical change for clients following carpal tunnel release[50,58]; responsiveness status after ganglion excision and distal radius fracture[43,59]; construct validity for clients with ulnar wrist disorders[44]; reliability for clients with pathologic conditions of the elbow[18,60]; and the ability to detect clinical change in clients with humeral fractures,[61] rotator cuff repairs,[62] and shoulder instability.[63] In addition, the DASH has been used to determine outcomes for clients with distal humeral fractures[45,46] and radial nerve palsy.[25] The DASH has been demonstrated to be comparable to, but slightly less responsive than, the COPM,[26] the Patient-Rated Wrist/Hand Evaluation,[56] the Boston Questionnaire,[50,58] and the Western Ontario Shoulder Instability Index.[63] The DASH was not found to be sensitive to differences in outcomes between clients following wrist arthroplasty or arthrodesis.[64] **Normative**

TABLE 6-1

Generic Measures

TITLE	DATE AND LOCATION	QUESTIONS	FORMAT	TO OBTAIN
COPM Canadian Occupational Performance Measure	1991, Canada	Five problems identified by client and rated in terms of performance and satisfaction	Likert scale	www.caot.ca/copm/
HAQ Health Assessment Questionnaire	1978, Stanford University	**HAQ-DI** 20 questions in eight categories **VAS pain scale** **VAS global health scale**	Likert scale and VAS	http://aramis.stanford.edu
MAS Milliken Activities of Daily Living Scales	1996, Washington University in St. Louis	Mobility: 13 Self-care: 20 Domestic life: 13 Community/recreation: 1 **Total: 47**	Likert scale	Mary Seaton seatonm@wustl.edu Washington University Program in Occupational Therapy
POSNA Pediatric Musculoskeletal Functional Health Questionnaire	1998, AAOS	Upper extremity and physical function: 8 Transfer and basic mobility: 11 Sports/physical functioning: 12 Pain/comfort: 3 Treatment expectations: 9 Happiness: 5 Satisfaction: 1 **Total scale items: 49** **Total tool items: 117**	Yes/no, multiple choice, and Likert scale	AAOS 6300 North River Road Rosemont, IL 60018
SF-36 Short Form 36	1990, Medical Outcomes Trust	**Physical health** Physical functioning: 10 Role-physical: 4 Bodily pain: 2 General health: 5 **Mental health** Vitality: 4 Social functioning: 2 Role-emotional: 3 Mental health: 5	Likert scale, yes/no	www.sf-36.com
SMFA Short Musculoskeletal Functional Assessment questionnaire	1999 University of Minnesota	**Dysfunction index: 34** Daily activities, emotional status, function of the arm and hand, mobility **Bother index: 12**	Likert scale	www.ortho.umn.edu

HAQ-DI, HAQ Disability Index; *VAS,* visual analog scale; *AAOS,* American Academy of Orthopaedic Surgeons.

data, including mean scores and standard deviations, have been published by the AAOS.[34]

Michigan Hand Outcomes Questionnaire

The Michigan Hand Outcomes Questionnaire (MHQ) was developed by Dr. Kevin Chung and colleagues[65] at the University of Michigan in 1998. The MHQ is defined as a hand-specific questionnaire; the authors specifically address function of each upper extremity separately as a means of analyzing independent use, hand dominance, and bilateral involvement.[10] Previously established tools and client input were used to create the MHQ.[65]

The MHQ consists of 67 questions including six domains, demographics, and work history. Domains of overall hand function, physical function with activities of daily living tasks, esthetics, and satisfaction with hand function are answered specific to each hand. Responses in the domains of pain and work performance are given regarding both hands. All domain items are formatted in Likert scales ranging from 1 to 5, with lower scores indicating higher function in all domains except pain. If less than 50% of a scale is complete, the scale is not scored, and if more than two scales are incomplete, a final score cannot be calculated. Raw scores are summed for each hand; bilateral scores are calculated by averaging scores from both hands. Summed and averaged scores are normalized from 0 to 100 according to the scoring algorithm as found in the original publication.[65] Scores closer to 100 on all scales indicate increased function and decreased pain.

The MHQ originally was found to be reliable and valid in a study including 200 clients with various upper extremity diagnoses.[65] Responsiveness as a function of significant clinical change was noted in a similar, diverse client group.[8] The MHQ has been established as valid and reliable for clients with rheumatoid arthritis[66] and as sensitive to clinical change for clients following carpal tunnel release.[67] The MHQ has been correlated to grip strength[68] and a standardized test of activities of daily living function,[69] and it was found to be sensitive to change in a long-term follow-up study of clients with metacarpophalangeal joint arthroplasties.[70]

Patient Evaluation Measure

The Patient Evaluation Measure (PEM) was introduced by Macey and Burke[71] in 1995. Developed in the United Kingdom, the PEM is novel in that it addresses client satisfaction as a primary component of outcome measurement.

The original PEM included three parts: treatment (5 items), "how your hand is now" (10 items), and overall assessment (3 items). A second version was published in

2001 that titled the second section as the Hand Health Questionnaire and added a question to this section addressing duration of pain. The PEM is presented in a seven-interval visual analog scale with lower scores indicating increased satisfaction and function. Parts two and three are summed and calculated as a percentage of the possible score. Part one is not included in the scoring process, and the authors suggest that clients should be given their previous answers when repeating this measure.[72] A cultural difference in language is noted in the use of the activity example "fiddly things," which is clarified as fine dextrous tasks.[73]

The PEM was found to be reliable, highly valid, and highly responsive in a study of 80 clients with scaphoid fractures.[72] Research including 35 clients with multiple diagnoses demonstrated very good reliability and validity as correlated to grip strength.[73] The PEM also was used for outcomes measurement in a follow-up study of clients with palmar wrist ganglia.[74]

Patient-Rated Evaluation Methods

Dr. Joy MacDermid and colleagues in Ontario, Canada, have carefully researched and developed four client-rated tools for outcome evaluation: the Patient-Rated Wrist Evaluation (PRWE), the Patient-Rated Forearm Evaluation Questionnaire (PRFEQ), the Patient-Rated Elbow Evaluation (PREE), and the Patient-Rated Wrist/Hand Evaluation (PRWHE). The PRWE was the first measure of the four to be developed; the process included a survey of the International Wrist Investigators for content and format. The goal in creating the PRWE was to capture client-rated measurement of impairment, disability, and handicap that could be used in clinical and research settings.[3] The three remaining tools were published as adaptations to the PRWE that more specifically could address measurement of outcomes for clients with lateral epicondylitis (PRFEQ), pathologic conditions of the elbow (PREE), and hand injuries (PRWHE).

All four tools include two scales of pain and function. The pain scales include 5 to 6 items that address magnitude and frequency of pain. Activities that might precipitate pain are specific to each tool. Function scales are divided further to specific and usual activities. Usual activities are identical for each tool and include personal care, household work, work, and recreation. Specific activities on PRWE, PRWHE, and PRFEQ consist of 10 items that pertain to the anatomic area under consideration. In comparison, the PREE lists 15 specific activities. Responses are marked on a scale ranging from 0 (no pain/difficulty) to 10 (worst pain imaginable/unable to do) as perceived over the past week. The authors present multiple scoring options; scales can be summed individually or combined with simple calculations to yield a total score of up to 100 points.[3,18] Higher scores on all scales indicate increased pain and decreased function.

The PRWE was published in 1996 in a study that established reliability and content, construct, and criterion validity.[3] These properties were reinforced in a group of clients with distal radius and scaphoid fractures, and the PRWE total score was found to demonstrate greater reliability than individual subscale scores.[47] Responsiveness of the PRWE was determined in a prospective study of 275 clients with distal radius fractures; this publication also offers means and standard deviations for the tool.[48] The PRWE was more responsive than the DASH and SF-36 for clients following distal radius fracture.[43,48] The PRWE was not sensitive to differences in outcomes between clients with wrist arthroplasty or arthrodesis[64] and was less sensitive than grip strength testing for clients with unstable wrist fractures.[75] The PRWE was chosen as an outcome measure in a publication that advocates low-level heat wraps for wrist pain.[76]

The PRFEQ was introduced in 1999 as a tool with excellent reliability for research groups.[77] The PREE followed in 2001 in a study that articulated excellent reliability for the total score, high reliability for the pain subscale, and moderate to high reliability for the function subscale.[18] The PRWHE differs from the PRWE only in introductory wording, changing "wrist" to "wrist/hand," and the addition of one appearance question. The PRWHE was found to be more responsive than the DASH in a study of 60 clients with a variety of hand injuries; however, the appearance question was less responsive than comparable scales.[56]

Table 6-2 provides information on the aforementioned assessment instruments.

DISEASE-SPECIFIC MEASURES

Arthritis Impact Measurement Scales 2 Short Form

The short form of the Arthritis Impact Measurement Scales 2 (AIMS2-SF) was established by Guillemin et al.[78] in France in 1997. The original Arthritis Impact Measurement Scales (AIMS) and Arthritis Impact Measurement Scales 2 (AIMS2) were published in 1980 and 1992, respectively, to measure quality of life for clients with rheumatoid arthritis. The new, shorter form was developed to reduce completion time and client/therapist burden. Contributors to this process included expert and client panelists.

The AIMS2-SF includes questions in five domains: physical components (12 questions), symptom components (3 questions), affect components (5 questions), social interaction components (4 questions), and role components (2 questions). These questions are answered on a Likert scale with options ranging from "all days" to "no days" in the past 4 weeks. Scores are summed and normalized when at least 50% of the domains have been completed; the role component is excluded for those clients who are unemployed, disabled, or retired. A composite score is given that ranges from 1 to 10, with a higher score indicating decreased status. This tool is available in English, Dutch, and French.

With the exception of the social interaction domain, the remaining components of the AIMS2-SF demonstrate acceptable levels of reliability, validity, and sensitivity to change for clients with rheumatoid arthritis[78] and osteoarthritis.[79,80] The AIMS2-SF also was found to be in agreement with and demonstrate responsiveness comparable to the AIMS2.[81] An interesting note is that multiple authors have recommended changes in the questions originally chosen from the AIMS2 to increase reliability, validity, and sensitivity to change of the social interaction and symptom domains.[81-83] With these changes, the AIMS2-SF was found to be preferable to the modified HAQ for detecting clinical change in clients with rheumatoid arthritis.[83]

Australian/Canadian Osteoarthritis Hand Index

Development of the Australian/Canadian (AUSCAN) Osteoarthritis Hand Index took place at two medical centers across the globe from one another: the University of Western Ontario in Canada and the University of Queensland in Australia. Dr. Nicholas Bellamy and colleagues[17] intended to create a disease-specific, self-report outcome measure for clients with osteoarthritis of the hand. Client interviews were used as an integral part of the development process.

The AUSCAN is a 15-item questionnaire that is available in Likert scale, VAS, or numeric rating scale response formats. The AUSCAN includes three subscales of pain (five items), stiffness (one item), and physical function (nine items). Clients consider items based on the past 4 weeks; Likert scale items include responses ranging from no days to all days. Scoring options include summation, normalization, pooling, or weighting as proposed in the user guide.[84] The Likert scale version of the AUSCAN results in a summed, total score ranging from 0 to 61. The VAS version ranges from 0 to 1500. A score of 0 on either version indicates that the client is asymptomatic. A lower score, therefore, indicates decreased pain and stiffness and increased physical function of the client with osteoarthritis of the hand. For the client who has not performed a task as listed on the AUSCAN, the authors recommend exchanging the item with a similar task.[66] This measure has been translated into more than 25 languages.

TABLE 6-2

Regional Measures

TITLE	DATE AND LOCATION	QUESTIONS	FORMAT	TO OBTAIN
DASH Disabilities of the Arm, Shoulder, and Hand	1996, AAOS, ASSH, AASH, COMSS, and Institute for Work and Health	Symptoms: 9 Functional status: 21 **Total: 30** Optional—Work: 4 Sports/performing arts: 4	Likert scale	www.dash.iwh.on.ca
MHQ Michigan Hand Outcomes Questionnaire	1998, University of Michigan	**Total: 67** Hand function, physical function with ADL, esthetics, satisfaction with hand function, demographics, and work history	Likert scale	www.med.umich.edu/surgery/plastic/ research/department/studies/ mi_hand_outcome.shtml
PEM Patient Evaluation Measure	1995, United Kingdom	Treatment: 5 Hand Health Questionnaire: 11 Overall assessment: 3	7-interval VAS	Dias et al.[72]
PRWE Patient-Rated Wrist Evaluation	1996, Ontario	Pain: 5 Function: 10 **Total: 15**	10-interval VAS	Dr. Joy MacDermid Hand and Upper Limb Centre St. Joseph's Health Centre 268 Grosvenor Street London, Ontario N6A 3AB
PRFEQ Patient-Rated Forearm Evaluation Questionnaire	1999, Ontario	Pain: 5 Function: 10 **Total: 15**	10-interval VAS	Dr. Joy MacDermid Hand and Upper Limb Centre St. Joseph's Health Centre 268 Grosvenor Street London, Ontario N6A 3AB
PREE Patient-Rated Elbow Evaluation	2001, Ontario	Pain: 5 Function: 15 **Total: 20**	10-interval VAS	Dr. Joy MacDermid Hand and Upper Limb Centre St. Joseph's Health Centre 268 Grosvenor Street London, Ontario N6A 3AB
PRWHE Patient-Rated Wrist/Hand Evaluation	2004, Ontario	Pain: 5 Function: 10 **Total: 15** Optional— Appearance: 1	10-interval VAS	Dr. Joy MacDermid Hand and Upper Limb Centre St. Joseph's Health Centre 268 Grosvenor Street London, Ontario N6A 3AB

AAOS, American Academy of Orthopaedic Surgeons; *ASSH,* American Society for Surgery of the Hand; *AASH,* American Association of Hand Surgery; *COMSS,* Council of Musculoskeletal Specialty Societies; *ADL,* activities of daily living; *VAS,* visual analog scale.

Construct validity and reliability were established primarily in a study including 50 clients with osteoarthritis[85] and secondarily in a study of 62 clients with rheumatoid arthritis.[66] Significant differences in pain, stiffness, and physical function were demonstrated in a group of 44 clients with osteoarthritis, supporting the responsiveness of this tool.[85] The AUSCAN also was found to be correlated to grip strength in a group of 522 subjects with osteoarthritis; such a result suggests criterion validity.[86] The AUSCAN is promoted as relevant to clinical and research applications.[84]

Boston Questionnaire

The Boston Questionnaire was developed by Levine et al.[87] at the Brigham and Women's Hospital as an assessment tool for clients with carpal tunnel syndrome. Consisting of an 11-item Symptom Severity Scale and an 8-item Functional Status Scale, the tool was not given a formal name in the initial publication. This outcome measure therefore has been referred to by these individual scales and multiple other names in the literature, including the Brigham and Women's carpal tunnel questionnaire,[13,50] the Carpal Tunnel Syndrome Assessment Questionnaire,[51,88] the CTS instrument,[14] the Brigham (carpal tunnel) questionnaire,[52] and the Boston Carpal Tunnel Questionnaire.[89]

Despite the confusing nomenclature, these scales include a reasonable number of questions and scoring that benefit client and therapist. The Symptom Severity Scale addresses pain, numbness, weakness, tingling, and difficulty with fine motor tasks on a typical day in the past 2 weeks. The Functional Status Scale considers the relationship between symptoms and function, including activities such as buttoning, writing, and activities of daily living tasks. These tasks also are evaluated for a typical day in the past 2 weeks. Questions are answered on a Likert scale with a score of 1 indicating a low level of symptom/difficulty and 5 indicating highly symptomatic or unable to complete functional tasks. The answers are averaged, with a higher score indicating decreased status, and questions that are not answered simply are not included in the scoring process.

The Boston Questionnaire has been demonstrated as reliable, valid, and sensitive to change in clients with carpal tunnel syndrome.[14,58,87,90,91] The Symptom Severity Scale has been found to be 4 times more sensitive to change and the Functional Status Scale 2 times more sensitive to change than standard measures of strength and sensibility.[13] In addition, this measure has been reported to be more sensitive to change in carpal tunnel syndrome than generic measures.[13,14,50,51] Copies of the Symptom Severity Scale and Functional Status Scale, as well as mean scores, can be found in the original publication.[87]

Rotator Cuff Quality of Life

The Rotator Cuff Quality of Life (RC-QOL) was introduced in 2000 by Dr. Robert Hollinshead and colleagues[49] at the University of Calgary Sports Medicine Center. The RC-QOL was conceptualized as a tool for measuring outcomes in clients with the "full spectrum of rotator cuff disease."[92] Clients with rotator cuff disease ranging from impingement to massive defects were included in the development of this measure.[49]

The RC-QOL consists of 34 questions measured by a 100 mm VAS. Individual questions ask the client to recall pain/difficulty over the past 3 months in the domains of symptoms/physical complaints (16 items),

sports/recreation (4 items), work-related concerns (4 items), lifestyle issues (5 items), and social and emotional issues (5 items). Items marked closer to 0 indicate increased pain, difficulty, and concerns; total scores range from 0 to 3400. Total scores can be converted to percentage scores for ease of comparison. The authors recommend the use of the RC-QOL in prospective, randomized clinical trials.[49]

In the pilot study of the RC-QOL, 70 clients (73 shoulders) were analyzed in a 6-year follow-up study. Excellent reliability was noted, as well as discriminant validity for clients with massive as opposed to large rotator cuff tears.[49] Sensitivity to clinical change has not been tested for this tool.

Western Ontario Shoulder Instability Index

Dr. Alexandra Kirkley has worked with colleagues in Ontario, Canada, to research and develop a set of three client self-report outcome measures for evaluation of shoulder-specific diagnoses.[92] The first measure offered was the Western Ontario Shoulder Instability Index (WOSI).[63] This tool was designed to consider those clients with combinations of traumatic and atraumatic anterior, posterior, or multidirectional shoulder instability, and clients were consulted during development and research.

The WOSI consists of 21 items, each measured on a 100 mm VAS. Four domains of physical symptoms (10 questions), sports/recreation/work (4 questions), lifestyle (4 questions), and emotions (3 questions) are framed to evaluate client perception during the past week. Clients are instructed clearly to make their "best guess" to questions that do not currently pertain to them. Raw scores range from 0 to 2100; scores closer to 0 indicate higher quality of life. Scores also can be converted quickly to percentage, with 100% designating normal function. The questionnaire is offered in the form of a packet including directions and scoring.

Reliability of the WOSI was established with a group of 51 symptomatically stable clients.[63] In addition, this tool was found to be valid and responsive in two groups of clients with anterior instability. The WOSI also was indicated to be more responsive to clinical change than generic, regional, and clinical (range of motion) measures for these clients.[63,93]

Western Ontario Osteoarthritis of the Shoulder Index

The second shoulder tool introduced by the Fowler Kennedy Sport Medicine Clinic was the Western Ontario Osteoarthritis of the Shoulder Index (WOOS). This tool was designed to measure disease-specific quality of life in clients with osteoarthritis of the shoulder,[6] and clients were included in development and research of this tool.

The WOOS includes 19 questions in four domains: pain/physical symptoms (6 questions), sports/recreation/work (5 questions), lifestyle (5 questions), and emotions (3 questions). Responses are considered for the past week and are marked on a 100 mm VAS; clients are instructed specifically to make their "best guess" to questions they have not experienced. Raw scores are calculated by measuring and totaling the data from each question. Raw scores range from 0 to 1900, with a higher score indicating decreased status. The score also can be translated to percent of normal with a simple equation offered in the questionnaire packet. If percent of normal is calculated, a higher percentage then would designate higher function. This tool is easy to obtain and offers clear directions, question explanations, and scoring instructions. The WOOS is available in French, Spanish, German, and English.

The WOOS has been demonstrated to be valid, reliable, and responsive in a randomized clinical trial of 41 clients. This tool also was found to be more responsive than generic, regional, and clinical measures for clients with osteoarthritis of the shoulder following operative procedures.[6]

Western Ontario Rotator Cuff Index

The third and most recent Western Ontario outcome measure is the Western Ontario Rotator Cuff Index (WORC). This questionnaire, published in 2003, is targeted for use with clients diagnosed with rotator cuff disease, including tendonitis, tendinosis with no tear, partial-thickness tears, full-thickness tears, and rotator cuff arthropathy.[94] Consistent with previous methodology, the authors included clients in each step of the development process.

Similar construction of the questionnaire, directions, and scoring compared with the WOSI and WOOS also were noted. The WORC has 21 items in four domains, including physical symptoms (10 questions), sports/recreation/work (4 questions), lifestyle (4 questions) and emotions (3 questions). Raw scores range from 0 to 2100, with a higher score indicating decreased quality of life because of pathological condition of the rotator cuff. Mathematic conversion yields a percentage score; higher percentages indicate proximity to normal function. The WORC can be found in English, French, and German translations.

The WORC was found to be reliable and valid in a study that included 110 clients being treated with operative and nonoperative interventions following rotator cuff injury.[94] This tool also was found to be responsive to clinical change in a group of 30 clients following subacromial decompression.[95]

Table 6-3 provides information on the aforementioned assessment instruments.

INCORPORATING SELF-REPORT MEASURES INTO CLINICAL PRACTICE

Choosing a Measure

With such a vast array of options for assessing functional outcomes, the task of choosing a measure for clinical practice or research may seem daunting. Dr. Peter Amadio,[96] who has had extensive experience in the development and research of client self-report outcome measures, offers a simple solution. His advice is to "define the job, then pick the tools." For a research study including multiple upper extremity diagnoses, a foundational, generic measure could be used along with a regional measure and objective assessments. For a research study specific to a diagnostic group, a specific measure could be added. Choosing a measure to assess individual outcomes daily requires analysis of multiple factors, many of which are based on therapist and clinic preference.

Time

Time as a function of client self-report outcome measures can be considered in two separate ways. The first is time taken to administer and score a questionnaire. The obvious preference would be toward shorter and more efficient tools; however, minutes in the waiting room or on a modality could become productive and proactive. Correct scoring takes practice and attention to detail, much like goniometric measurement, and becomes quicker over time. Simplicity of scoring systems leads to increased interrater reliability in the clinic. The second aspect of time is included in the instructions of each tool. A therapist must be confident that the client accurately can recall the past few days, the past week, or the past month.

Format

Format options include scale type, left-to-right organization and consistency, and question complexity. Likert scales and VASs are standard questionnaire formats (see Box 6-2). Likert scales have been discussed as difficult to construct in terms of meaning, consistency, and spacing,[6] and comprehension of VAS has been found to be challenging, especially for elderly clients.[3] Few tools offer choice in this area.

The English language includes a standard left-to-right reading format. With this in mind, it seems logical that numbers would increase from left to right. The problem that arises is that while we want function to increase, we want symptoms to decrease. In other words, a score of 10/10 for function is good, but 10/10 for pain is bad. Some scales attempt consistency of left and right as positive or

TABLE 6-3

Disease-Specific Measures

TITLE	DATE AND LOCATION	DIAGNOSIS/ POPULATION	QUESTIONS	FORMAT	TO OBTAIN
AIMS2-SF Arthritis Impact Measurement Scales 2 Short Form	1997, France	Rheumatoid arthritis	Physical: 12 Symptom: 3 Affect: 5 Social interaction: 4 Role: 2 **Total: 26**	Likert scale	www.hopkins-arthritis. som.jhmi.edu/mngmnt/ forms/aims2-sf.pdf
AUSCAN Australian/Canadian Osteoarthritis Hand Index	2002, Australia and Canada	Primary hand osteoarthritis	Pain: 5 Stiffness: 1 Function: 9 **Total: 15**	Likert scale (LK3.0) VAS* (VA3.0)	Professor Nicholas Bellamy nbellamy@medicine.uq .edu.au University of Queensland, Australia
Boston Questionnaire (Brigham & Women's Hospital; carpal tunnel syndrome assessment questionnaire)	1993, Boston	Carpal tunnel syndrome	Symptom Severity Scale: 11 Functional Status Scale: 8	Likert scale	Levine et al.[87]
RC-QOL Rotator Cuff Quality of Life	2000, Canada	Rotator cuff disease	Symptoms/physical complaints: 16 Sports/recreation: 4 Work-related concerns: 4 Lifestyle issues: 5 Social/emotional issues: 5 **Total: 34**	100 mm VAS	Hollinshead et al.[49]
WOSI Western Ontario Shoulder Instability Index	1998, Canada	Shoulder instability	Pain/physical symptoms: 10 Sports/recreation/ work: 4 Lifestyle: 4 Emotional: 3 **Total: 21**	100 mm VAS	Sharon Griffin stdshg@uwo.ca Fowler Kennedy Sports Medicine Clinic, London, Ontario
WOOS Western Ontario Osteoarthritis of the Shoulder Index	2001, Canada	Osteoarthritis of the shoulder	Pain/physical symptoms: 6 Sports/recreation/ work: 5 Lifestyle: 5 Emotions: 3 **Total: 19**	100 mm VAS	Sharon Griffin stdshg@uwo.ca Fowler Kennedy Sports Medicine Clinic, London, Ontario
WORC Western Ontario Rotator Cuff Index	2003, Canada	Rotator cuff disease	Pain/physical symptoms: 10 Sports/recreation/ work: 4 Lifestyle: 4 Emotional: 3 **Total: 21**	100 mm VAS	Sharon Griffin stdshg@uwo.ca Fowler Kennedy Sports Medicine Clinic, London, Ontario

VAS, Visual analog scale.

negative, whereas some maintain the standard left-to-right increase. Assessment of whether the client is confused by response options and intervention as necessary for clarification are important.

Complexity of questions also can lead to misinterpretation. Double-barreled questions ask clients to consider two variables at the same time, such as the effect of pain on function. Asking clients clearly to assess one variable facilitates reliability over time. It also has been suggested that the provision of previous answers decreases response variability,[97] but this was recommended only for one of the measures reviewed.[72]

Instructions

Questionnaire instructions should be clear and without room for error by the therapist or client. Individual clarifications and assumptions should be avoided because this decreases reliability in administration and completion. Instructions for scoring also should be used consistently and should be compared between clinicians.

Results and Goal Setting

Understanding what scores mean and how to interpret clinical change is a difficult yet necessary component of using self-report outcome measures as part of holistic therapeutic intervention. Simply writing down numbers in a chart would be comparable to performing manual muscle tests and noting results without application to treatment planning or short-term goals.

Dr. Joy MacDermid, a clinical epidemiologist and physical therapist, has made a concerted effort to develop, research, and assist in the everyday understanding and use of outcome measures in therapy practice. She advocates practice and, therefore, experiential learning as the best way to become versed in the use of these tools.[98] *Normative data,* **minimal detectable change,** and **minimally clinically important difference** are terms used to define analysis of client scores.

Normative data can be considered as average scores for large groups of clients with similar diagnoses and abilities. As clinicians, we are familiar with norms in objective measures such as grip and pinch strength. Normative values are helpful in providing a framework with which to compare client scores. With therapeutic progress or decline, we should expect to see a change in client-rated scores. The minimal detectable change is defined as a valid change in score that is not due to chance. Minimally clinically important difference (MCID), in comparison, goes beyond valid change to assess meaningful difference in client function.[98] Despite the fact that this information would be of great assistance, few publications were found to include normative values[33-35] or discuss MCID in scoring.[25,27,95] Dr. MacDermid clarifies equations that can assist with the

calculation of MCID using data retrieved from the literature and advocates the use of MCID for short- and long-term goal setting.[98]

Clinic Outcomes and Marketing

Once a tool has been chosen and the therapy staff is comfortable with administration, scoring, and analysis of scores for intervention and goal setting, data can be compiled to consider larger issues pertaining to clinic management. Outcomes for client groups, individual therapists, and surgeons can be used to reflect on quality of client care and treatment strategies. Positive trends can be used as tools for marketing and year-end reports. Quality of life and overall outcomes can make a significant impact on the justification currently needed for reimbursement in health care settings.

SUMMARY

Treatment of the client with a hand or upper extremity injury requires knowledge and attention to fine details. One of the most important details is the clients' perception of their abilities and health status. Current methods for client evaluation are moving toward a consistent and comprehensive assessment of quality of life and functional ability, and client self-report outcome measures have been developed and can be used clinically for this purpose. Consistent incorporation of these tools requires time for research, practice, and discussion, but ultimately results in a renewed focus on client-centered care and holistic evaluation.

References

1. Portney LG, Watkins MP: *Foundations of clinical research: applications to practice,* ed 2, Upper Saddle River, NJ, 2000, Prentice Hall Health.
2. Bindra RR et al: Assessing outcome after hand surgery: the current state, *J Hand Surg* 28B(4):289-294, 2003.
3. MacDermid JC: Development of a scale for client rating of wrist pain and disability, *J Hand Ther* 9:178-183, 1996.
4. Kirshner B, Guyatt G: A methodological framework for assessing health indices, *J Chronic Dis* 38(1):27-36, 1985.
5. Fienstein AR, Josephy BR, Wells CK: Scientific and clinical problems in indexes of functional disability, *Ann Intern Med* 105(3):413-420, 1986.
6. Lo IKY, Griffin S, Kirkley A: The development and evaluation of a disease-specific quality of life measurement tool for osteoarthritis of the shoulder: the Western Ontario Osteoarthritis of the Shoulder Index (WOOS), *Osteoarthritis Cartilage* 9(8):771-778, 2001.
7. Salerno DF et al: A review of functional status measures for workers with upper extremity disorders, *Occup Environ Med* 59:664-670, 2002.

8. Chung KC et al: The Michigan Hand Outcomes Questionnaire (MHQ): assessment of responsiveness to clinical change, *Ann Plast Surg* 42:619-622, 1999.

9. Lindeboom R, Sprangers MA, Zwinderman AH: Responsiveness: a reinvention of the wheel? *Health Qual Life Outcomes* 3(1):8, 2005.

10. Amadio PC: Outcome assessment in hand surgery and hand therapy: an update, *J Hand Ther* 14(2):63-68, 2001.

11. Koran LM: The reliability of clinical methods, data and judgments, *N Engl J Med* 293:642-646, 1975.

12. Katz JN et al: Responsiveness of self-reported and objective measures of disease severity in carpal tunnel syndrome, *Med Care* 32(11):1127-1133, 1994.

13. Amadio PC et al: Outcome assessment for carpal tunnel surgery: the relative responsiveness of generic, arthritis-specific, disease-specific, and physical examination measures, *J Hand Surg* 21A:338-346, 1996.

14. Atroshi I et al: Symptoms, disability, and quality of life in clients with carpal tunnel syndrome, *J Hand Surg* 24A:398-404, 1999.

15. Sprangers MAG, Aaronson NK: The role of health care providers and significant others in evaluating the quality of life of clients with chronic disease: a review, *J Clin Epidemiol* 45(7):743-760, 1992.

16. Ripat J et al: A comparison of the Canadian Occupational Performance Measure and the Health Assessment Questionnaire, *Can J Occup Ther* 68(4):247-253, 2001.

17. Bellamy N et al: Dimensionality and clinical importance of pain and disability in hand osteoarthritis: development of the Australian/Canadian (AUSCAN) Osteoarthritis Hand Index, *Osteoarthritis Cartilage* 10(11):855-862, 2002.

18. MacDermid JC: Outcome evaluation in clients with elbow pathology: issues in instrument development and evaluation, *J Hand Ther* 14(2):105-114, 2001.

19. Law M et al: The Canadian Occupational Performance Measure: an outcome measure for occupational therapy, *Can J Occup Ther* 57:82-87, 1990.

20. Law M et al: *Canadian Occupational Performance Measure*, ed 2, Toronto, 1994, CAOT Publications.

21. Law M et al: *Canadian Occupational Performance Measure*, ed 3, Ottawa, 1998, CAOT Publications.

22. Carswell A et al: The Canadian Occupational Performance Measure: a research and clinical literature review, *Can J Occup Ther* 71(4):210-222, 2004.

23. Dedding C et al: Validity of the Canadian Occupational Performance Measure: a client-centered outcome measure, *Clin Rehabil* 18:660-667, 2004.

24. Veehof MM et al: Psychometric qualities of the Dutch language version of the Disabilities of the Arm, Shoulder, and Hand Questionnaire (DASH-DLV), *J Hand Ther* 15(4):347-354, 2002.

25. Hannah SD, Hudak, PL: Splinting and radial nerve palsy: a single-subject experiment, *J Hand Ther* 14(3):195-201, 2001.

26. Case-Smith J: Outcomes in hand rehabilitation using occupational therapy services, *Am J Occup Ther* 57:499-506, 2003.

27. Bruce B, Fries JF: The Stanford Health Assessment Questionnaire: dimensions and practical applications, *Health Qual Life Outcomes* 1(1):20, 2003.

28. Wildner M et al: Independent living after fractures in the elderly, *Osteoporos Int* 13:579-585, 2002.

29. Dziedzic KS, Thomas E, Hay EM: A systematic search and critical review of measures of disability for use in a population survey of hand osteoarthritis (OA), *Osteoarthritis Cartilage* 13:1-12, 2005.

30. Arvidson NG, Larsson A, Larsen A: Simple function tests, but not the modified HAQ, correlate with radiological joint damage in rheumatoid arthritis, *Scand J Rheumatol* 31:146-150, 2002.

31. Seaton MK et al: Reliability and validity of the Milliken Activities of Daily Living Scale, *J Occup Rehabil* 15(3):343-351, 2005.

32. Daltroy LH: The POSNA Pediatric Musculoskeletal Functional Health Questionnaire: report on reliability, validity, and sensitivity to change, *J Pediatr Orthop* 18(5):561-571, 1998.

33. Haynes RJ, Sullivan E: The Pediatric Orthopaedic Society of North America Pediatric Orthopaedic Functional Health Questionnaire: an analysis of normals, *J Pediatr Orthop* 21:619-621, 2001.

34. Hunsaker FG et al: The American Academy of Orthopaedic Surgeons outcomes instruments: normative values from the general population, *J Bone Joint Surg* 84A(2):208-215, 2002.

35. Ware JE: *SF-36 health survey update*. Retrieved March 10, 2005, from http://www.sf-36.org/tools/sf36.shtml

36. Cheng MS et al: Employer, physical therapist, and employee outcomes in the management of work-related upper extremity disorders, *J Occup Rehabil* 12(4):257-267, 2002.

37. Beaton DE, Hogg-Johnson S, Bombardier C: Evaluating change in health status: reliability and responsiveness of five generic health status measures in workers with musculoskeletal disorders, *J Clin Epidemiol* 50(1):79-93, 1997.

38. Di Fabio RP, Boissonnault W: Physical therapy and health-related outcomes for clients with common orthopaedic diagnoses, *J Orthop Sports Phys Ther* 27(3):219-230, 1998.

39. Swiontowski M, et al: Short Musculoskeletal Function Assessment Questionnaire: validity, reliability, and responsiveness, *J Bone Joint Surg* 81A(9):1245-1260, 1999.

40. Ponzer S, Skoog A, Bergstrom G: The Short Musculoskeletal Function Questionnaire (SMFA): cross-cultural adaptation, validity, reliability, and responsiveness of the Swedish SMFA (SMFA-Swe), *Acta Orthop Scand* 74(6):756-763, 2003.

41. Marx RG et al: A comparison of clients' responses about their disability with and without attribution to their affected area, *J Clin Epidemiol* 54(6):580-586, 2001.

42. SooHoo NF et al: Evaluation of the construct validity of the DASH questionnaire by correlation to the SF-36, *J Hand Surg* 27A:537-541, 2002.

43. MacDermid JC et al: Responsiveness of the Short Form-36, Disability of the Arm, Shoulder and Hand questionnaire, Patient-Rated Wrist Evaluation and physical impairment

measurements in evaluating recovery after a distal radius fracture, *J Hand Surg* 25A(2):330-340, 2000.

44. Jain R, Hudak PL, Bowen CV: Validity of health status measures in clients with ulnar wrist disorders, *J Hand Ther* 14(2):147-153, 2001.

45. McKee MD et al: Functional outcome following surgical treatment of intra-articular distal humeral fractures through a posterior approach, *J Bone Joint Surg* 82A(12):1701-1707, 2000.

46. McKee MD et al: Functional outcome after open supracondylar fractures of the humerus, *J Bone Joint Surg* 82B(5):646-651, 2000.

47. MacDermid JC et al: Client rating of wrist pain and disability: a reliable and valid measurement tool, *J Orthop Trauma* 12(8):577-586, 1998.

48. MacDermid JC, Richards RS, Roth JH: Distal radius fracture: a prospective outcome study of 275 clients, *J Hand Ther* 14(2):154-169, 2001.

49. Hollinshead RM et al: Two 6-year follow-up studies of large and massive rotator cuff tears: comparison of outcome measures, *J Shoulder Elbow Surg* 9:373-381, 2000.

50. Gay RE, Amadio PC, Johnson J: Comparative responsiveness of the Disabilities of the Arm, Shoulder, and Hand, the carpal tunnel questionnaire, and the SF-36 to clinical change after carpal tunnel release, *J Hand Surg* 28A:250-254, 2003.

51. Bessette L et al: Comparative responsiveness of generic versus disease-specific and weighted versus unweighted health status measures in carpal tunnel syndrome, *Med Care* 36(4):491-502, 1998.

52. Beaton DE et al: Measuring the whole or the parts? Validity, reliability, and responsiveness of the Disabilities of the Arm, Shoulder and Hand outcome measures in different regions of the upper extremity, *J Hand Ther* 14:128-146, 2001.

53. Agel J et al: Administration of the Short Musculoskeletal Function Assessment: impact on office routine and physician-client interaction, *Orthopedics* 26(8):783-788, 2003.

54. Hudak P et al: Development of an upper extremity outcome measure: the DASH (Disabilities of the Arm, Shoulder, and Hand), *Am J Ind Med* 29:602-608, 1996.

55. Davis A et al: Measuring disability of the upper extremity: a rationale supporting the use of a regional outcome measure, *J Hand Ther* 12(4):269-274, 1999.

56. MacDermid JC, Tottenham V: Responsiveness of the Disability of the Arm, Shoulder and Hand (DASH) and Patient-Rated Wrist/Hand Evaluation (PRWHE) in evaluating change after hand therapy, *J Hand Ther* 17:18-23, 2004.

57. Navsarikar A et al: Validity assessment of the Disabilities of Arm, Shoulder and Hand questionnaire (DASH) for clients with psoriatic arthritis, *J Rheumatol* 26(10):2191-2194, 1999.

58. Greenslade JR et al: DASH and Boston Questionnaire assessment of carpal tunnel syndrome outcome: what is the responsiveness of an outcome questionnaire? *J Hand Surg* 29B(2):159-164, 2004.

59. Hwang JJ et al: The effect of dorsal carpal ganglion excision on the scaphoid shift test, *J Hand Surg* 24B(1):106-108, 1999.

60. Turchin DC, Beaton DE, Richards RR: Validity of observer-based aggregate scoring systems as descriptors of elbow pain, function, and disability, *J Bone Joint Surg* 80A(2):154-162, 1998.

61. Ring D, Perey BH, Jupiter JB: The functional outcome of operative treatment of ununited fractures of the humeral diaphysis in older clients, *J Bone Joint Surg* 81A(2):177-190, 1999.

62. Skutek et al: Outcome analysis following open rotator cuff repair: early effectiveness validated using four different shoulder assessment scales, *Arch Orthop Trauma Surg* 120:432-436, 2000.

63. Kirkley A et al: The development and evaluation of a disease-specific quality of life measurement tool for shoulder instability: the Western Ontario Shoulder Instability Index (WOSI), *Am J Sports Med* 26(6):764-772, 1998.

64. Murphy et al: Comparison of arthroplasty and arthrodesis for the rheumatoid wrist, *J Hand Surg* 28A:570-576, 2003.

65. Chung KC et al: Reliability and validity testing of the Michigan Hand Outcomes Questionnaire, *J Hand Surg* 23A:575-587, 1998.

66. Massy-Westropp N, Krishnan J, Ahern M: Comparing the AUSCAN osteoarthritis hand index, Michigan Hand Outcomes Questionnaire, and Sequential Occupational Dexterity Assessment for clients with rheumatoid arthritis, *J Rheumatol* 31(10):1996-2001, 2004.

67. Klein RD, Kotsis SV, Chung KC: Open carpal tunnel release using a 1 centimeter incision: technique and outcomes for 104 clients, *Plast Reconstr Surg* 3(5):1616, 2003.

68. Wahi Michener SK et al: Relationship among grip strength, functional outcomes, and work performance following hand trauma, *Work* 16(3):209-217, 2001.

69. Umraw N et al: Effective hand function assessment after burn injuries, *J Burn Care Rehabil* 25(1):134-139, 2004.

70. Goldfarb CA, Stern PJ: Metacarpophalangeal joint arthroplasty in rheumatoid arthritis: a long term assessment, *J Bone Joint Surg* 85A(10):1869-1878, 2003.

71. Macey AC, Burke FD: Outcomes of hand surgery, *J Hand Surg* 20B(6):841-855, 1995.

72. Dias JJ et al: Assessing the outcome of disorders of the hand: is the client evaluation measure reliable, valid, responsive, and without bias? *J Bone Joint Surg* 83B(2):235-240, 2001.

73. Sharma R, Dias JJ: Validity and reliability of three generic outcome measures for hand disorders, *J Hand Surg* 25B(6):593-600, 2000.

74. Dias J, Buch K: Palmar wrist ganglion: does intervention improve outcome? A prospective study of the natural history and client-reported treatment outcomes, *J Hand Surg* 28B(2):172-176, 2003.

75. Karnezis IA, Fragkiadakis EG: Association between objective clinical variables and client-rated disability of the wrist, *J Bone Joint Surg* 84B(7):967-970, 2002.

76. Michlovitz S et al: Continuous low-level heat wrap therapy is effective for treating wrist pain, *Arch Phys Med Rehabil* 85(9):1409-1416, 2004.

77. Overend TJ et al: Reliability of a client-rated forearm questionnaire for clients with lateral epicondylitis, *J Hand Ther* 12:31-37, 1999.

78. Guilleman F et al: The AIMS2-SF: a short form of the Arthritis Impact Measurement Scales 2, *Arthritis Rheum* 40(7):1267-1274, 1997.

79. Ren XS, Kazis L, Meenan RF: Short-form Arthritis Impact Measurement Scales 2: tests of reliability and validity among clients with osteoarthritis, *Arthritis Care Res* 12(3):163-171, 1999.

80. Taylor LF et al: Evaluating the effects of an educational symposium on knowledge, impact, and self-management of older African Americans living with osteoarthritis, *J Community Health Nurs* 21(4):229-238, 2004.

81. Haavardsholm EA et al: A comparison of agreement and sensitivity to change between AIMS2 and a short form of AIMS2 (AIMS2-SF) in more than 1000 rheumatoid arthritis clients, *J Rheumatol* 27(12):2810-2816, 2000.

82. Taal E, Rasker JJ, Riemsma RP: Psychometric properties of a Dutch short form of the Arthritis Impact Measurement Scales 2 (Dutch-AIMS2-SF), *Rheumatology (Oxford)* 42:427-434, 2003.

83. Taal E, Rasker JJ, Riemsma RP: Sensitivity to change of AIMS2 and AIMS2-SF components in comparison to M-HAQ and VAS-pain, *Ann Rheum Dis* 63:1655-1658, 2004.

84. Bellamy N: *AUSCAN Hand Osteoarthritis Index: user guide II*, Queensland, Australia, 2003, Centre of National Research on Disability and Rehabilitation Medicine.

85. Bellamy N et al: Clinimetric properties of the AUSCAN Osteoarthritis Hand Index: an evaluation of reliability, validity, and responsiveness, *Osteoarthritis Cartilage* 10(11): 863-869, 2002.

86. Jones G, Cooley HM, Bellamy N: A cross-sectional study of the association between Herberden's nodes, radiographic osteoarthritis of the hands, grip strength, disability, and pain, *Osteoarthritis Cartilage* 9(7):606-611, 2001.

87. Levine DW et al: A self-administered questionnaire for the assessment of severity of symptoms and functional status in carpal tunnel syndrome, *J Bone Joint Surg* 75A:1585-1592, 1993.

88. Bessette L et al: Prognostic value of a hand symptom diagram in surgery for carpal tunnel syndrome, *J Rheumatol* 24(4):726-734, 1997.

89. Giannini F et al: A new clinical scale of carpal tunnel syndrome: validation of the measurement and clinical-neurophysiological assessment, *Clin Neurophysiol* 113:71-77, 2002.

90. Mondelli M et al: Relationship between the self-administered Boston Questionnaire and electrophysiological findings in follow-up of surgically treated carpal tunnel syndrome, *J Hand Surg* 25B(2):128-134, 2000.

91. Heybeli N et al: Assessment of outcome of carpal tunnel syndrome: a comparison of electrophysiological findings and a self-administered Boston Questionnaire, *J Hand Surg* 27B(3):259-264, 2002.

92. Kirkley A, Griffin S, Dainty K: Scoring systems for the functional assessment of the shoulder, *Arthroscopy* 19(10):1109-1120, 2003.

93. Kirkley A et al: Prospective randomized clinical trial comparing the effectiveness of immediate arthroscopic stabilization versus immobilization and rehabilitation in first traumatic anterior dislocation of the shoulder, *Arthroscopy* 15:507-514, 1998.

94. Kirkley A, Griffin S, Alvarez C: The development and evaluation of a disease-specific quality of life measurement tool for rotator cuff disease: the Western Ontario Rotator Cuff Index (WORC), *Clin J Sport Med* 13:84-92, 2003.

95. Kirkley A et al: The use of the impingement test as a predictor of outcome following subacromial decompression for rotator cuff tendinosis, *Arthroscopy* 18(1):8-15, 2002.

96. Amadio PC: Outcomes measures: disease specific versus global instruments, AAHS Hand Therapy Day, Jan 2005, Fajardo, Puerto Rico.

97. Guyatt GH, Bombardier C, Tugwell PX: Measuring disease-specific quality of life in clinical trials, *CMAJ* 134:889-895, 1986.

98. MacDermid JC, Stratford P: Applying evidence on outcome measures to hand therapy practice, *J Hand Ther* 17:165-173, 2004.

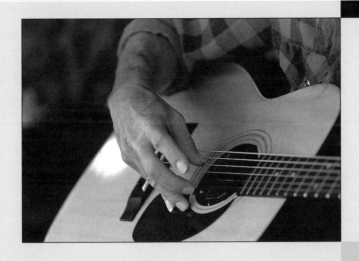

Part TWO

Professionalism

7

Clients with Functional Somatic Syndromes or Challenging Behavior

JOEL F. MOORHEAD AND CYNTHIA COOPER

CLIENTS WITH FUNCTIONAL SOMATIC SYNDROMES

A **functional somatic syndrome (FSS)** is defined as a physical illness that cannot be explained by an organic disease and that involves no demonstrable structural lesion or established biochemical change.[1] The distinction between *disease* and *illness* is particularly important. A **disease** is an anatomic or physiologic impairment of function in a structure or biochemical process. An **illness** is the client's personal experience of poor health. Clients frequently have illnesses that are not fully explained by available medical evidence of disease. Functional somatic syndromes can be classified as undifferentiated somatoform disorders, somatization disorders, factitious disorders, or malingering, depending on whether the client's actions are intentional or unintentional and whether motivation is conscious or subconscious.

The goal of giving clients satisfying and health-promoting rehabilitation care is particularly challenging for therapists treating clients with FSS. When the client's distress is disproportionate to the medical evidence of impairment, reducing the degree of impairment may not reduce the client's distress. The goal of this chapter is to

117

TABLE 7-1

Diagnostic Classification of Functional Somatic Syndromes

DIAGNOSIS	ICD-9 CODE	ICD-10 CODE
Undifferentiated somatoform disorders	300.82	F45.1
Hypochondriasis	300.7	F45.2
Body dysmorphic disorder	300.7	F45.1
Conversion disorder	300.11	F44.9
Psychogenic pain	307.8	F45.4
Unspecified psychophysiologic malfunction	306.9	F59
Somatization disorders	300.81	F45.0
Fibromyalgia	729.1	M79.0
Chronic fatigue syndrome	780.81	F48.8
Multiple chemical sensitivities	955.2	T88.7
Psychogenic tremor	306	F44.4
Factitious disorders	300.19	F68.1
Munchausen's syndrome	301.51	F68.11
Clenched fist syndrome	300.19	F68.1
Secretan's syndrome	300.19	F68.1
Malingering	V65.2	Z76.5

ICD, International Classification of Diseases.

help therapists become familiar with the types of FSS seen in clinical practice so that they can build a therapeutic relationship with even the most challenging client.

Undifferentiated Somatoform Disorders

Clients with symptoms that are out of proportion to impairments most often manifest one of the somatoform disorders, in which symptom magnification is subconscious and unintentional (Table 7-1).

Clients with **hypochondriasis** show excessive concern about minor health disturbances or intense worry over the possibility of future ill health. Clients with **body dysmorphic disorder** become preoccupied with imagined or innocent variations in appearance. Clients with **conversion disorder** have a bodily event (e.g., paralysis or seizure) that is psychologic in origin. Clients with psychogenic pain and unspecified psychophysiologic dysfunction have persistent symptoms without apparent organic origin and without other distinctive classifying features. Clients with medically unexplained pain may have other diagnostic features as well, which could lead to a diagnosis of one of the somatization disorders below.

Somatization Disorders

More controversial are the **somatization disorders,** in which clients experience persistent or recurrent symptoms without objective or measurable medical evidence of impairment. Although these disorders occur frequently, general agreement is lacking on the cause and

the treatment, and even on the status of some of them as legitimate diagnoses. However, questioning the validity of the diagnosis does little to help the client become more functional and may do irreparable harm to the therapeutic relationship. This chapter makes no judgment on the diagnostic legitimacy of the somatization disorders, but it recognizes the high level of distress in many clients diagnosed with these conditions.

Fibromyalgia

Fibromyalgia is perhaps the most common somatization disorder. The criteria for a diagnosis of fibromyalgia, established in 1990 by the American College of Rheumatology, include pain on both sides of the body, above and below the waist, accompanied by tenderness at 11 or more of 18 specific tender point sites.[2] Fibromyalgia affects approximately 2% of the population, although clients with fibromyalgia may account for 10% to 20% of visits to rheumatology clinics. The prevalence is inversely related to income and level of education, and females are affected more frequently than males at a ratio of up to 6 : 1. Fifty-nine percent of clients with a diagnosis of fibromyalgia rate their health as fair or poor.[3] Clients with this diagnosis commonly have other, associated symptoms, including nonrestorative sleep, fatigue, headaches, diarrhea or constipation, numbness, tingling, stiffness, a sensation of swelling, anxiety, and depression. Clients with rheumatoid arthritis and osteoarthritis report similar levels of distress, according to one measurement tool, the Rheumatology Distress Index[4]; however, clients with fibromyalgia report higher levels of

BOX 7-1

Criteria for Chronic Fatigue Syndrome

MAJOR CRITERIA
- Fatigue is unexplained by other diagnoses.
- Fatigue has been present longer than 6 months.
- Fatigue has a definite time of onset.
- Fatigue has resulted in decreased activity level not due to ongoing exertion.
- Fatigue isn't substantially relieved by rest.

MINOR CRITERIA
Four or more of the following symptoms are present:

- Impaired short-term memory or concentration
- Sore throat
- Tender lymph nodes
- Myalgias
- Arthralgias
- Headaches
- Nonrestorative sleep
- Postexertional malaise (lasting longer than 24 hours)

distress in the areas of anxiety, depression, sleep disturbance, global severity, and fatigue.[4] Fatigue is also prominent in another disorder in this classification, chronic fatigue syndrome.

Chronic Fatigue Syndrome

The case definition of **chronic fatigue syndrome (CFS),** or **chronic fatigue and immune dysfunction syndrome (CFIDS),** includes several important criteria: (1) the fatigue cannot be explained by other diagnoses; (2) it must persist for longer than 6 months; (3) it must have a definite time of onset; (4) it must result in a decreased activity level but cannot be the result of ongoing exertion; and (5) it must not be substantially relieved by rest.[5] This case definition, like that for fibromyalgia, was established primarily to identify subjects for clinical research. Salit[6] notes that these criteria "are not suitable for the determination of the presence and severity of illness, either in general medical settings or for medicolegal or insurance purposes" and that "clinical management should be based on an assessment of the client" (Box 7-1).

The case definitions for fibromyalgia and CFS overlap substantially. About 70% of clients with CFS meet the case definition for fibromyalgia, and 70% of clients with fibromyalgia meet the case definition for CFS.[7] Both disorders result in a high prevalence of work disability. Bombardier and Buchwald[8] found that 37% of clients with a diagnosis of CFS were unemployed. The prevalence of unemployment rose to 52% for clients diagnosed with CFS and fibromyalgia.[8]

Multiple Chemical Sensitivity Syndrome

A third somatization disorder that can affect perceived ability to work is **multiple chemical sensitivity (MCS) syndrome.** Clients with multiple chemical sensitivities, or **idiopathic environmental intolerance (IEI),** experience medically unexplained symptoms in response to low-level, identifiable environmental exposures.[9] Among the postulated mechanisms for MCS syndrome are **time-dependent sensitization (TDS)** and the development of **conditioned responses.** In TDS, repeated stressful episodes make an individual increasingly sensitive to low-level environmental stimuli.[10] With conditioned responses, cardiovascular, respiratory, gastrointestinal, or immunologic responses are triggered by heightened perception of environmental stimuli.[11]

Psychogenic Tremors

As with MCS syndrome, stress can be a factor in the development of **psychogenic tremors.** Psychogenic tremors of the hands and arms can manifest in unusual ways and have variable clinical characteristics. The severity of the tremor may be task specific, with the tremor often improving when the client is distracted.[12] Shaking of the limbs or body can appear exaggerated, whereas finger tremors often are absent. A twisting or ballistic component to the tremor can create the appearance of chorea.[13] Psychogenic tremor as a somatization disorder appears unintentionally and without conscious client awareness of motivation.

Factitious Disorders

Factitious disorders result from intentional client action, but without conscious client awareness of motivation. They more often arise from a psychologic need to be sick than from a conscious effort for material gain.[14] Clients with factitious disorders knowingly cause their own disease but are unaware of the underlying reason or reasons for their behavior. Several factitious disorders can affect clients' hands.

Munchausen's syndrome derives its name from Baron Karl Friedrich Hieronymous von Munchausen, an eighteenth century nobleman known for telling vivid but untrue stories. Clients with Munchausen's syndrome may cut, bruise, bite, or inject their hands and then give an untruthful history to the medical professionals who care for the resulting injuries.[15]

Clients with **clenched fist syndrome** have stiff, tightly curled fingers that resist extension.[15] The thumb and index fingers often are spared, enabling the client to maintain a level of function with the involved hand. Nerve block of the affected upper extremity or examination under anesthesia produces some relaxation of the hand, but often not full extension of the involved fingers.

Some edema of the hand may be present, but it is not as great as in a hand that is repeatedly traumatized. (See Case 7-1.)

Clients who repeatedly strike their hands on a wall or other hard surface eventually develop chronic dorsal hand edema, a condition that has been called *secretan's syndrome*.[15] The fibrotic changes that develop in a repeatedly traumatized hand eventually create an appearance similar to the brawny edema that develops in the lower legs of clients with chronic vascular insufficiency.

Malingering

Malingering can be defined as the intentional presentation of false or misleading health information for personal gain. This personal gain is described as *secondary gain*, distinct from the primary gain of recovery from illness. Some malingering clients are seeking financial gain, whereas others are consciously seeking social or interpersonal benefits.[16] Although malingering generally is recognized as an uncommon condition (prevalence 5% or less), Mittenberg and colleagues[17] estimate that 29% of personal injury cases, 30% of disability cases, 19% of criminal cases, and 8% of medical cases probably involve malingering and symptom exaggeration.[17]

Evaluation Tips: Findings Suggestive of Simulated or Exaggerated Upper Extremity Deficits

Inconsistent Force Generation

Manual muscle testing provides information to the examiner in several ways. First, normal strength through a joint's functional range of motion (ROM) reassures the examiner that no abnormalities have been identified on this screening test. Second, examination of a client with organic weakness, such as that caused by neuropathy or myopathy, will disclose a smooth, consistent inability to resist the examiner's opposition. For example, the examiner will be able to flex the client's extended wrist smoothly despite the client's full effort to maintain wrist extension. An experienced examiner takes into account the client's age, muscle mass, and overall medical condition when assessing the significance of such a finding. Third, a client with disease or injury may be unable to maintain consistent force generation because of pain or structural instability. This results in a sudden release of resistance to the examiner's opposition. The client can be expected to describe the reason for this release of resistance clearly, providing information that is helpful for diagnosis and management. Fourth, the client may release resistance inconsistently, without other organic signs of impairment and without reporting incapacitating pain or instability. This *cogwheel*, or *give-way, weakness* is one of the physical signs reported by Waddell and colleagues[18] as suggestive of nonorganic pain.[18]

Nonphysiologic Pain and Movement Patterns

Clients with simulated or exaggerated upper extremity deficits may exhibit additional **Waddell's signs,** including extreme reaction to light touch (overreaction), tenderness that does not conform to established myotomal or segmental patterns, and sensory disturbances that do not conform to established dermatomal or segmental patterns.[18] Other similar and easily observed tests include Mankopf's test and O'Donoghue's maneuver.

Mankopf's test relies on the observation that the pulse rate rises when a client experiences acute pain. The absence of a rise in heart rate of at least 5% on palpation of a reportedly painful area suggests symptom magnification. **O'Donoghue's maneuver** relies on the observation that passive ROM generally is greater than active ROM when structures in and around a joint are painful. The possibility of symptom magnification is raised when active ROM is greater than passive ROM.[19]

Associated Movements and Vicarious (Trick) Movements

Taking possibly simulated wrist extensor weakness as an example, several techniques can be used to assess the veracity of a client's complaints. A client simulating wrist extensor weakness may use the wrist normally when unaware that he or she is being observed. A client with a simulated wrist drop can be asked to make a fist while the examiner observes the actions of the wrist extensors. The wrist normally extends when a person makes a fist; only if the wrist extensors are truly paralyzed, as in a complete radial nerve injury, can the client make a strong fist without associated wrist extension.[16]

Even if the wrist extensors are truly paralyzed by radial nerve injury, a client with intact median innervation will be able to extend the interphalangeal joint of the thumb. This vicarious, or trick, movement is mediated by the abductor pollicis brevis and flexor pollicis brevis muscles, both of which insert onto the extensor expansion of the thumb.[20] Absence of this movement may be an indicator of symptom magnification.

Correct diagnosis of symptom magnification or an FSS is important for several reasons. First, an accurate anatomic or physiologic diagnosis for the client's complaints is an important step in determining what additional diagnostic tests, if any, are indicated. Second, the clinician becomes aware of the complexity of managing such a client and can plan to spend the needed additional time and mental energy to achieve a therapeutic alliance and a favorable outcome. Third, correct diagnosis is essential to designing a successful treatment plan.

Tips from the Field: Treatment of Clients with Functional Somatic Syndromes

As mentioned previously, the distinction between disease and illness is very important in the treatment of clients with FSS. To recap, disease is a demonstrable alteration in anatomy or physiology with unfavorable consequences for the client; illness is the client's perception and experience of poor health. Both disease and illness are valid and important concerns for clients and the health care professionals who treat them.

CLINICAL *Pearl*

Disease should be treated only when present; illness should always be treated.

Clients with a conversion disorder are unaware that their physical symptoms have a psychologic origin. Clients with somatization disorders feel unwell and can become truly convinced that they have a life-threatening or incapacitating disease or injury; this phenomenon has been called **dissimulation.**[16] Clients with factitious disorders have diseases or injuries that require treatment; in addition, to prevent future disease or injury, attention must be paid to the factors that caused these clients to harm themselves. As Hippocrates observed, "It is more important to know the person who has the disease, than the disease the person has."[21]

CLIENTS WITH CHALLENGING BEHAVIORS

Reaching Agreement on a Treatment Plan at Every Stage of Treatment

Treatment of clients with FSS requires attention to the biologic, psychologic, and social factors that influence a client's illness; that is, a *biopsychosocial* approach.[22] Kleinman[23] observes that clinicians tend to evaluate treatment success by improvement in signs of disease, whereas clients view success as healing of illness. The five-step strategy recommended by Kleinman recognizes the importance of the clinician and client finding enough common ground to reach agreement on a treatment plan (Box 7-2).

Not every client requires or wants the type of negotiated understanding produced by this five-step process. This is fortunate for the busy clinician, because the discussion can take a bit longer than the 10 to 15 minutes estimated by Kleinman. This is especially true when the client's and the clinician's models for explaining illness have little in common. The therapist often has the luxury

BOX 7-2

Five-Step Strategy for Reaching Agreement on a Treatment Plan

Step 1: The clinician develops an understanding of the client's explanatory model of his or her illness and the meaning of the illness to the client.

Step 2: The clinician presents his or her explanatory model for the client's illness in nontechnical terms.

Step 3: Clinician and client compare models.

Step 4: Clinician and client discuss illness problems.

Step 5: Clinician and client develop and agree upon specific interventions and elements of a plan for treating the client's illness.

From Kleinman A: Clinical relevance of anthropological and cross-cultural research: concepts and strategies, *Am J Psychiatry* 135:427-431, 1978.

of being able to work through these five steps gradually over two or three therapy visits, taking advantage of the natural rhythm and growing trust that develop between client and therapist over time. The experienced clinician is alert for opportune moments to explore psychologic or social factors that may contribute to a client's illness.

Windows of Opportunity

In their study on client interaction with five experienced physicians, Branch and Malik[24] described "windows of opportunity" as unique moments in which clients briefly discuss personal, family, or emotional issues with clinicians. Based on the findings from their study, they suggested the following four ways clinicians can explore important issues efficiently:

- Listen attentively.
- Ask open-ended questions, such as, "Is there anything else I can do for you today?"
- Listen for and recognize changes in the client's emotions, appearance, posture, or voice. These windows of opportunity often occur in the middle of the visit. Ask a second question in a softer, gentler tone. Use silence, nods, and small comments to encourage the client to talk while you listen.
- Know when to end the conversation. Summarize the discussion and convey understanding and empathy.

Other authors have offered additional suggestions for establishing therapeutic relationships with challenging clients; these are presented in Box 7-3.

BOX 7-3

Establishing Therapeutic Relationships with Challenging Clients

- Build trust. Positive client-therapist interactions require trust. Actions foster trust as much as words do. For example, return the client's phone calls and provide materials as promised.
- Provide good instructions. Focus on the client's agenda whenever possible. Clear instructions that fit with the client's agenda result in better client satisfaction and improved outcomes.
- Let the client talk without interruption at the beginning of the appointment. Identify which problems can be covered in the time available and which problems can be addressed at subsequent visits.
- Stay attuned to your sense of frustration, because this may be a sign that you find the client to be "difficult" (see Case 7-2).
- Be client centered. Use simple explanatory models that are easily understood. Avoid blaming the client; the therapeutic relationship can be harmed by the client's perception that he or she is being blamed (see Case 7-3).
- If a consensus cannot be reached with a challenging client despite compassionate listening, it may be best to refer the client elsewhere. Barriers to reaching a consensus include unexpected resistance from the client and communication mismatch. Noncompliance or oppositionality from a client is exemplified by denial of disease, conscious or unconscious

- sabotaging of the treatment, or a need to control every detail (see Case 7-4).
- Try to develop and convey unconditional positive regard for the client, family, and caregiver. Respect the client's autonomy and individuality and be willing to learn from clients' various backgrounds (see Case 7-5).
- Give your undivided attention to complaining clients. Dissatisfied clients tell 20 people, and satisfied clients tell three.
- Avoid dealing with difficult clients when you are too tired or busy.
- Don't downplay the client's perception of the seriousness of the complaints. Give each client time to describe his or her illness in its entirety. Listen responsively, but avoid interrupting.
- Make a statement that is empathetic. Work to establish a good rapport with the client and do not be defensive. Convey that you are working with, not against, the client.
- Ask additional questions and take control of the situation. Ask what clients would like to be done or how they believe the problem can be solved. Create an action plan and describe that plan in positive terms.
- Explain changes in treatment ahead of time. Fewer problems arise when there are fewer surprises.
- Follow up in a timely fashion and document the situation.

Modified from Levinson W, Stiles WB, Invi TS, et al: Physician frustration in communicating with patients, *Med Care* 31:285-295, 1993; Lin EHB, Katon W, Vo Korff M et al: Frustrating patients: physician and patient perspectives among distressed high users of medical services, *J Gen Intern Med* 6:241-246, 1991; Lerner AM, Luby ED: Error of accommodation in the care of the difficult patient, *J Psychiatry Law* 20:191-206, 1992; Kaplan CB, Siegel B, Madill JM et al: Communication and the medical interview: strategies for learning and teaching, *J Gen Intern Med* 12(suppl 2):S49-S55, 1997; and Baum NH: Twelve tips for dealing with difficult patients, *Geriatrics* 57:55-56, 2002.

The health care professionals most likely to be sued are those whose clients feel that they were rushed, that they were not given enough information, and that their complaints were ignored.[25] Physician traits associated with malpractice suits include aloofness, lack of good communication with the patient, and too great a desire to accommodate or please the patient even if the request is not rational. It is very important to document when the client does not participate in his or her care. It also is important not to overly accommodate inappropriate requests (see Case 7-6).[26]

Participatory Decision Making

Clients who have been encouraged to participate in decision making demonstrate better follow through on their decisions than those who have not been encouraged to participate. Clients with the best health outcomes are

those who express their opinions, who indicate their preferences about their treatment during appointments, and who ask questions. Physicians who regularly include their patients in treatment decisions are those who offer opinions and talk about the advantages and disadvantages of the options, who ask for input about patient preferences, and who pursue mutual agreement about treatment plans. These physicians demonstrate a *participatory* style. They elicit greater patient cooperation and better health outcomes than physicians who have more controlling styles of decision making.[27] This probably is also true for hand therapists.

Participatory decision making can be defined as the practice of offering clients choices among several treatment options and of giving them a sense of control and responsibility for their care.[27] Kaplan and colleagues[27] studied physicians' practice habits to determine the characteristics that promote participatory decision-making styles. They found that physicians who demonstrate participatory decision making are willing to spend extra time with patients and have lower volume practices.

Participatory physicians reported greater satisfaction with the autonomy they experienced in their personal lives. Short office visits in busier practices have demonstrated poorer outcomes. Medical office visits shorter than 18 minutes are associated with poor quality of information. Patients who had more time with their physicians rated the physicians more favorably. Physicians whose communication styles are less dominant receive higher satisfaction ratings than physicians who communicate in a more dominant manner.[27] In current practice, unfortunately, fiscal demands and business issues may challenge the ability of some physicians and hand therapists to provide participatory care.

Partnerships in Client Care

Quill[28] makes the following observations and recommendations:

- The relationship between the therapist and client is not obligatory, it is consensual. The therapist may speak with authority but should not be authoritarian. The client may ask questions, present alternatives, seek other opinions, or choose a different caregiver.
- The two parties must respect and trust each other.
- The client gets healed, cured, and/or relieved of pain. The provider derives enjoyment from being able to help, experiences personal or intellectual satisfaction from solving a problem, and receives financial compensation.
- The client's request may be incompatible with what the health care professional feels is the client's best interest, or it may conflict with the professional's personal beliefs. The caregiver should not compromise ethical, medical, or personal standards because of a client's request.
- Not all clients participate equally in their care. Caregivers may need to encourage clients to participate. It may be helpful, when appropriate, to request that clients participate more actively in their own treatment.

Case *Studies*

CASE 7-1

Factitious Disorders

A 58-year-old woman had tightly clenched long, ring, and small fingers on her nondominant left hand. This posture had persisted for 2 years and had been refractory to treatment by medications for dystonia and muscle relaxation. The client was able to use the thumb and index fingers to some degree. A diagnosis of clenched fist syndrome was made. Further discussion revealed that the condition began at the time of a stressful change at her workplace.

Treatment approach

Make sure the client understands that she has a condition that requires treatment and that the likelihood of improvement with treatment is excellent. Perform an examination under regional anesthetic block and fit the client for a custom wrist-hand orthosis while the arm is still under the effects of anesthesia. See the client daily for at least 2 weeks to reinforce wearing of the wrist-hand orthosis to preserve the ROM gained by the procedure. Perform and teach assertive passive, active-assisted and active ROM exercises with the goal of restoring full ROM. Consider a custom dynamic wrist-hand orthosis to speed restoration of full ROM. Consider the timing of recommending psychologic counseling. Often the time to suggest counseling is when the client reports feeling sad or anxious, as many clients naturally will do as they become more comfortable with the therapist. Work closely with the referring physician to achieve the best outcome from a mental health referral.

CASE 7-2

Windows of Opportunity

A female executive was seen after excision of a recurrent glomus tumor of the nondominant left small finger. She experienced a Code Blue that was narcotics induced. She stated at her next visit that her hand therapist had caused the code by upsetting her with a discussion of her therapy authorization status.

Treatment approach

Validate the client's concerns. Tell her that you recognize that discussions about therapy authorization can be upsetting and that you are sorry she was upset. Ask how she would like to be kept informed about authorization status in the future. Recommend that the client discuss the factors that led up to the Code Blue with her physician. Call the physician so that he or she is prepared to discuss the Code Blue with the client. Coordinate all care as a medical team and document the situation carefully.

CASE 7-3

Participatory Decision Making

A 60-year-old, right-dominant retired male executive suffered a radial collateral ligament injury to the small finger of his right hand while bicycling. He was shocked to learn that it would take longer than 2 weeks to recover from this injury. He could not accept this and demanded that he recover normal ROM and resolution of edema in 2 weeks' time.

Treatment approach

Supervise the client's home program closely. Provide good explanations of the typical recovery timeline at every visit and include the physician in this explanation. Offer encouragement and enthusiasm for the client's progress and explore ways he can pass the recovery time meaningfully.

CASE 7-4

Partnerships in Client Care

An elderly female underwent open reduction and internal fixation with volar plating for a left nondominant distal radius fracture. At follow-up, she had shoved long black strings from her holiday ham into her postoperative dressing; she claimed that these were her sutures, which had "fallen apart."

Treatment approach

Make sure to notify the physician, who can explain to the client that the black threads are not her sutures. Also, document the situation carefully. Focus therapy on functional needs and positive aspects of the client's recovery.

CASE 7-5

Partnerships in Client Care

An elderly right-dominant female underwent excision for recurrent sarcoma of the right forearm, with radiation and multiple tendon transfers. She had had 11 previous surgeries on the involved extremity and was a well-informed client who had realistic expectations of her functional prospects. She followed her home program very well and often suggested appropriate upgrades. She and her therapist had a seemingly compatible and effective relationship. Near the end of one therapy session, she voiced an ethnic slur that was personally hurtful and offensive to the therapist.

Treatment approach

Try to strike a balance between sincerity and professionalism. Focus on the client's clinical picture and use the situation as an opportunity to practice professionalism.

CASE 7-6

Partnerships in Client Care

An operating room nurse was treated nonoperatively for a boutonniere deformity of the dominant long finger. She refused to make appointments and frequently arrived at hand therapy unscheduled. She was unwilling to wait to be seen even though she had no scheduled appointment. She called and interrupted the department director to complain, wrote letters of complaint, and also complained to the hand surgeon about being told she needed to make appointments to be seen in hand therapy.

Treatment approach

Provide a nonemotional, factual explanation to the department director and the physician and be consistent in requiring all clients to have appointments for therapy. Offer the client the option of seeking care elsewhere if she prefers to do that.

SUMMARY

Ideally, the hand therapy client and the hand therapist will have similar goals. Also ideally, the client will attend therapy as scheduled, describe his or her illness honestly and accurately, make clinically appropriate requests, participate actively in treatment, and follow the treatment plan. When the therapist-client relationship does not benefit from these positive attributes, the relationship can deteriorate.

Through their recognition of the various patterns of FSS and the characteristics of challenging clients, hand therapists can more effectively shape rewarding therapeutic relationships. These positive relationships can favorably affect the clinical outcome for even the most challenging clients. Challenging client situations are opportunities for professional growth and can bring out the best care we have to offer.

References

1. Manu P: *Functional somatic syndromes*, Cambridge, 1998, Cambridge University Press.
2. Wolfe F, Smythe HA, Yunus MB et al: The American College of Rheumatology 1990 criteria for the classification of fibromyalgia: report of the Multicenter Criteria Committee, *Arthritis & Rheumatism* 33:1863-1864, 1990.
3. Wolfe F, Anderson J, Harkness D et al: Health status and disease severity in fibromyalgia: results of a six-center longitudinal study, *Arthritis & Rheumatism* 40:1571-1579, 1997.
4. Fukuda K, Straus SE, Hickle I et al: Measuring the epidemiology of distress: the rheumatology distress index, *J Rheumatol* 27:2000-2009, 2000.

5. Fukuda K et al: The chronic fatigue syndrome: a comprehensive approach to its definition and study, *Ann Intern Med* 121:953-959, 1994.

6. Salit IE: The chronic fatigue syndrome: a position paper, *J Rheumatol* 23:540-544, 1996.

7. Aaron LA, Buchwald D; A review of the evidence for overlap among unexplained clinical conditions, *Ann Intern Med* 134(9 pt 2):868-881, 2001.

8. Bombardier CH, Buchwald D: Chronic fatigue, chronic fatigue syndrome, and fibromyalgia: disability and health-care use, *Med Care* 34:924-930, 1996.

9. Cullen MR: The worker with multiple chemical sensitivities: an overview, *Occup Med* 2:655-661, 1987.

10. Sorg BA, Prasad BM: Potential role of stress and sensitization in the development and expression of multiple chemical sensitivity, *Environmental Health Perspectives* 105(suppl 2):467-471, 1997.

11. MacPhail RC: Evolving concepts of chemical sensitivity, *Environmental Health Perspectives* 105(suppl 2):455-456, 1997.

12. Koller W, Lang A, Vetere-Overfield B et al: Psychogenic tremors, *Neurology* 39:1094-1099, 1989.

13. Deuschl G, Koster B, Lucking CH et al: Diagnostic and pathophysiological aspects of psychogenic tremors, *Movement Disorders* 13:294-302, 1998.

14. Iverson GL, Binder LM: Detecting exaggeration and malingering in neuropsychological assessment, *Journal of Head Trauma Rehabilitation* 15:829-858, 2000.

15. Kasdan ML, Stutts JT: Factitious disorders of the upper extremity, *J Hand Surg* 20A(3 part 2):S57-S60, 1994.

16. Green LN: Malingering, dissimulation, and conversion-hysteria, *Trauma* 6:3-21, 2002.

17. Mittenbert W, Patton C, Canyock EM et al: Base rates of malingering and symptom exaggeration, *J Clin Exper Neuropsychology* 24:1094-1102, 2002.

18. Waddell G, McCulloch JA, Kummel E et al: Nonorganic physical signs in low back pain, *Spine* 5:117-125, 1980.

19. Kiester PD, Duke AD: Is it malingering or is it real?: eight signs that point to nonorganic back pain, *Postgrad Med* 106:77-84, 1999.

20. Parry CBW: Trick movements, *Proc Royal Soc Med* 63:674-676, 1970.

21. Novack DM, Epstein RM, Paulsen RH: Toward creating physician-healers: fostering medical students' self-awareness, personal growth, and well-being, *Academic Medicine* 74:516-520, 1999.

22. Goldberg RJ, Novack DH, Gask L: The recognition and management of somatization: what is needed in primary care training, *Psychosomatics* 33:55-61, 1992.

23. Kleinman A: Clinical relevance of anthropological and cross-cultural research: concepts and strategies, *Am J Psychiatry* 135:427-431, 1978.

24. Branch WT, Malik TK: Using "windows of opportunity" in brief interviews to understand patients' concerns, *JAMA* 269:1667-1668, 1993.

25. Eisenberg L: Medicine: molecular, monetary, or more than both? *JAMA* 274:331-334, 1995.

26. Lerner AM, Luby ED: Error of accommodation in the care of the difficult patient, *J Psychiatry Law* 20:191-206, 1992.

27. Kaplan SH, Greenfield S, Gandek B et al: Characteristics of physicians with participatory decision-making styles, *Ann Intern Med* 124:497-504, 1996.

28. Quill TE: Partnerships in patient care: a contractual approach, *Ann Intern Med* 124:228-234, 1983.

8

Fundamentals of Client-Therapist Rapport

TERI BRITT PIPE

IMPORTANCE OF THE THERAPUTIC RELATIONSHIP

Holistic, client-focused care is a unifying goal among client care professionals. Holistic care involves viewing clients as complex, dynamic beings with evolving, developing personas, needs, and strengths. Developing and nurturing the therapeutic relationship are the keys to understanding clients from a holistic perspective. The client-therapist relationship then can serve as the foundation for assessment, prioritization, mutual goal setting and shared decision making.

Creating and maintaining rapport are essential first steps in coming to know and understand the client. Much more than simply being nice or acting respectful, truly knowing the client is part of effective clinical care and has important implications for client outcomes. **Knowing the client** means comprehending the client's physical, emotional, cognitive, spiritual, and social sense of personhood and connecting to it as one human being to another within the boundaries of a professional therapeutic relationship.

Research and theory provide evidence that knowing the client is crucial to one of the most important yet basic aspects of clinical care: ensuring the client's safety. Learning more about clients, understanding their unique perspectives, listening to what is and is not said, and accurately reading behaviors to formulate a correct clinical impression are all vital steps in keeping clients aligned with their therapeutic program and keeping them from harm. For instance, research indicates that the clinical behaviors of knowing and connecting with clients provide protection against untoward events and promote early recognition of client problems.[1] Serving as a client advocate and guarding clients' best interests are professional responsibilities that are deeply rooted in the therapeutic relationship.

In addition to having implications for the client's safety and well-being, meaningful therapeutic relationships also have implications for professionals. At times therapists may not be fully aware of the impact on clients of "simple" interventions, such as listening, being present, and offering encouragement. Behaviors such as these lead to knowing the client. Perhaps if therapists understand the depth of caring that can be conveyed by a simple gesture or by listening to clients talk about their experiences, they themselves can find renewal and healing in their practice.

DEVELOPING A SUCCESSFUL THERAPEUTIC RELATIONSHIP

Developing a therapeutic relationship is fundamental to working well with clients. The most effective approach is guided by a theoretical context, so that thoughts and behaviors can be seen in a broader, systematic perspective of caring for the client as a comprehensive whole. A theoretical perspective helps the therapist perceive, recognize, and process clinical information in a systematic way and can help bring order out of chaotic clinical data. The theoretical perspective that provides a framework for this part of the chapter is Watson's theory of human caring.[2] This model is not simply "applied to" a situation; rather, it lends itself to being experienced, so that the elements of the model come alive for the participants in caring relationships and encounters.

WATSON'S THEORY OF HUMAN CARING

Watson's model has gained international recognition and has been used by a variety of disciplines since its origin in nursing. For the purposes of this chapter, the therapist is the "self," and the client is the "one being cared for." The theory of human caring is also sensitive to the changing realities of society and health care. (http://www2.uchsc.edu/son/caring/content/jwbio.asp) This chapter presents an overview of some of the theory's major concepts, as well as examples based on clinical experience. The three major components used to frame the discussion are caritas, transpersonal caring healing relationships, and the caring moment.

Caritas

Caritas derives from the Greek word meaning "to cherish, appreciate, and give special attention, if not loving attention, to; it connotes that something is very fine, that indeed it is precious." Caritas characterizes how hand therapists may choose to approach their clients.

Whether they meet clients in the home, hospital room, office, or other setting, therapists' extension of a positive *caritas* regard for clients and their personal environment sets the stage for the development of therapeutic rapport. The ideal way to begin is to spend a moment or two mentally settling down and reaching a clear state of mind before meeting the client. This centering approach need not take a great deal of time; it requires merely the time it takes to inhale and intentionally clear one's focus in preparation for the client encounter. It is a way of cultivating mindfulness about one's practice.

Mindfulness is simple but not easy; it requires effort and discipline to "pay attention in a particular way: on purpose, in the present moment and nonjudgmentally."[3] The purposes of this centering moment are (1) to bring therapists awareness and understanding of their own minds; (2) to teach them how this can influence perceptions and actions; and (3) to show them how perceptions and actions influence the clinical environment, the client-therapist relationship, and the clinical encounter. The essence of mindfulness is to cultivate self-awareness through self-observation, self-inquiry, and mindful action. The overall attitude is one of gentleness, gratitude, and nurturing.[3] From this point of inward clarity, the therapist can progress to the therapeutic relationship with the client. Again, this practice of focused attention need not take a great deal of time; it can be done in a moment. Yet the effects can be quite powerful because of the intention and focus this approach brings to the clinical encounter.

Watson's theory of human caring delineated 10 caritas processes,[2,4-8] which are used to explore the development of the therapeutic relationship. The discussion of each process includes common pitfalls and ways the therapist can avoid them.

Caritas Process 1: "Practice of Loving-Kindness and Equanimity within Context of a Caring Consciousness"

The word *practice* in the definition of caritas process 1 is a reminder that the attitude of loving-kindness and equanimity is not something that can be accomplished quickly or permanently; therapists practice it not with the goal of achievement, but rather with the objective of becoming more conscious of how they approach clients. **Equanimity** is the quality of being calm and even tempered. It is an evenness of mind characterized by calm temper or firmness of mind, reflected as patience, composure, and steadiness of mind under stress. For the hand therapist, cultivation of this mindful, caring approach to the therapist-client relationship translates into reflections such as, "Who is this person? Am I open to participating in his or her personal story? How ought I be in this situation? What are the client's priorities?" The client's response is also affected and may include the person's perceptions of how the interaction and relationship will be part of the healing process and how the client will choose to participate in the therapist-client relationship.

Common Pitfalls and How to Avoid Them

1. Allowing yourself to be distracted: When you find yourself thinking about something other than the client in the present moment, gently refocus your attention. Try not to scold or reprimand yourself, because this is a fairly common occurrence, particularly early on in the development of a reflective practice.
2. Forgetting to take a moment to focus: Generally, once you notice how much more productive your focused encounters are, the reward will reinforce the practice of taking the small amount of time required.
3. Letting your mind say, "This client is just like that other client I had last week . . .": Remember that just as you are different from any other person and your reactions are unique, so is this client different from any other, and his or her reactions are unique.

Caritas Process 2: "Being Authentically Present and Enabling and Sustaining the Deep Belief System and Subjective Life World View of Self and One Being Cared for"

Authenticity requires that hand therapists know who they are and how they can contribute to their clients' care. Although authenticity sounds very simple, it can be counterintuitive in the context of modern standardized health care practice to remember that each therapist and each client brings something unique to the therapeutic relationship; unless therapists know their individual talents and gifts, those talents and gifts can't be shared. Discovering one's unique sense of authenticity involves taking the time to reflect on how experiences, clinical learning, personal knowledge, culture, belief system, aspects of personality, and a vast array of other factors unique to each individual can be cultivated to help in the current clinical situation. During this phase of the therapist-client relationship, the therapist is using his or her sense of self to be intentionally present with the client. This means being able to focus on only the client for this time. It means turning attention to what it is the client is experiencing in order to support the client in his

or her belief system and discovering the things that will sustain and inspire hope or faith for that client.

In this phase of rapport building, helpful questions therapists might ask themselves include, "What information is needed to care for this person? Can I imagine what this experience is like for this client and what it means in his (or her) life?" Likewise, the client can contribute to the clinical relationship by sharing stories of his or her past as it relates to the person's current health status, exploring sources of strength and meaning that can be used in the work of hand therapy.

Common Pitfalls and How to Avoid Them

1. Thinking that a diagnosis (e.g., a fractured wrist) has the same meaning to every client: Remember that this client will formulate a personal meaning from this condition and about the therapy.
2. Failing to assess or understand the client's sources of strength and meaning: It is refreshing for clients to be reminded that they have overcome challenges in the past and that they have a reservoir of strengths to use in the present and future.

CLINICAL *Pearl*

Clients often are pleased and relieved to be asked about the strengths they bring to a situation, because health care providers generally ask instead about weaknesses or problems.

Caritas Process 3: "Cultivation of One's Own Spiritual Practices and Transpersonal Self, Going Beyond Ego Self"

This element of caring requires a delicate balance. Caring involves tapping into one's own source of strength according to a personal belief system while taking care not to assume that the client shares those values. In order to use the **transpersonal self,** the therapist must sustain healthy personal boundaries and put aside personal concerns, worries, and needs to care for the client. This part of the rapport-building process involves supporting the client in his or her **spiritual** beliefs and source or sources of strength and meaning, even when those differ from the therapist's own beliefs. Going beyond the **ego self** means acknowledging the uniqueness of each individual while recognizing that the connections between individuals can be used for healing.

In this phase, the therapist may reflect on a question such as, "How am I attending to this person's spiritual needs and soul care?" The client can assist in building this part of the relationship by identifying the aspects of his or her life style that the client feels "feed my spirit."

Common Pitfalls and How to Avoid Them

1. Assuming the client shares the therapist's belief system: Ask the client; don't presume to know, even if seemingly obvious signs are present (e.g., religious symbols).
2. Failing to clarify and uphold professional boundaries: Clients can feel vulnerable and may say things to please the therapist. Always keep in mind the influence of the healer on the client and use it responsibly.
3. Neglecting to call in resources: The trust between client and therapist is strengthened if limitations are communicated and arrangements or referrals are initiated for social workers, community providers, and other sources of help.
4. Neglecting to devote the time and energy to "feed one's own soul," leading to a professional sense of eroded spirit and diminished effectiveness: This is perhaps the most common pitfall among health care professionals. The remedy is to cultivate activities and recreational pursuits that strengthen the sense of self. Find a source of restoration and recreation that builds your self-confidence and self-respect. Your clients will benefit, because you will be much more effective in your professional role.

Precaution. *Remember to use your own personal sources of strength but not to overstep professional standards regarding relationship boundaries.*

Caritas Process 4: "Developing and Sustaining a Helping-Trusting Authentic Relationship"

Participating with a client in a caring, healing relationship is a choice. The therapist can "go through the motions" and still deliver safe, effective care; however, a much higher standard is set when the therapist deliberately creates the potential for the development of a healing relationship. Within this framework, the professional must cultivate a caring consciousness that is integral to the healing process, requiring self-development and ongoing personal growth.

The therapist's thinking about the therapeutic relationship should include questions such as, "What significance does this illness or injury have for this client and how can I honor that meaning? What are the specific forms of caring and hand therapy that will best acknowledge, affirm, and sustain this client?"

From the client's perspective, this phase of the relationship means choosing and showing a degree of trust and openness with the hand therapist. The client may show signs of willingness to relate to the therapist by sharing experiences and deeper meanings, past occurrences, and validating the therapist's understanding of concerns, needs, and priorities.

Common Pitfalls and How to Avoid Them

1. Getting caught in the routine and distracted by time constraints and schedules. Keep your attention and focus on what is happening with *this* client, in *this* moment. Verbally set realistic and positive expectations about time with your client by saying something such as, "Mr. Smith, we have 15 minutes together to accomplish our work. This will be ample time, so let's get started."
2. Rushing into a client's space before considering the best approach: Try to imagine what it would be like to have to ask for help from someone and then having that person disrespect your sense of privacy and your need for personal space.
3. Overlooking the significance that illness, injury, and therapy have for clients: The hand therapist represents a significant source of hope, repair, and return to function for the client.
4. Failing to recognize that trust is a changing characteristic: Be patient and allow the trusting relationship to develop. Once it does, diligently guard that trust.

CLINICAL *Pearl*

Keep in mind that your time will be better spent if you slow down and focus.

Caritas Process 5: "Being Present to and Supportive of the Expression of Positive and Negative Feelings as a Connection with a Deeper Spirit of Self and the One Being Cared for"

The hand therapist recognizes that within a trusting relationship, the client will feel more comfortable if he or she can share negative as well as positive aspects and can voice disagreements and deeper feelings than might not otherwise be exchanged. The hand therapist's role is to listen to what is said and to understand what is left unsaid (i.e., read between the lines). It is a good idea to confirm or validate verbally what you understand from the client's expression. This is crucial with expressions of pain or discomfort, which is highly subjective and open to interpretation.

What is perceived becomes reality. However, two realities, the client's and the therapist's, operate within the relationship. Clients may be trying to assimilate what their injury, disease, symptoms, diagnosis, or treatment means within their culture or personal relationships. Clients also are often trying to get a clear picture of what the current health situation means for their life and future.

Common Pitfalls and How to Avoid Them

1. Feeling offended when the client expresses negative emotions or behaviors: Remember that if the client

didn't trust you, he or she would not reveal these feelings to you. Demonstrating that you accept the negative as well as the positive is one way of showing a caring attitude.

2. Forgetting to validate meanings: Verbally acknowledge the behavior or expression and verify the meaning of what you observed. For example, "You are crying and seem upset right now. I wonder if you are physically tired or maybe you are frustrated that you aren't completing this activity as well as you'd like, or maybe it is something else. Can you help me understand?"

3. Dismissing the client's stories as irrelevant to the current clinical situation: Remember that for the client, the story may be connected to the client's view of his or her health condition and therapy.

Caritas Process 6: "Creative Use of Self and All Ways of Knowing as Part of the Caring Process; to Engage in Artistry of Caring-Healing Practices"

In many cases, standardized methods of structuring client care serve as guidelines for a certain diagnosis or treatment approach. The art of caring involves a spirit of willingness to explore and discover other approaches to care that build on the unique aspects of the particular client and on situations that might lend themselves to creative or artistic healing methods.

The hand therapist might choose to address the following reflections to support the artistry of caring: "What are the unique attributes of this client and this situation? How can I use the environment to support healing for this client?"

Clients' perspectives included determining the degree to which they feel comfortable disclosing their uniqueness as individuals and their ways of expressing themselves. Clients may also be coming to new levels of understanding about their pattern of response to the health situation, changes in roles and responsibilities, and how their life style may change.

Creative innovations can be very simple, and many hand therapists incorporate artful insight into their practice with each client. Such innovation could involve simply finding out the kind of food the client likes to cook or eat and then facilitating some aspect of that food preparation as part of hand therapy, or finding out the kind of music the client enjoys and incorporating that into the practice environment. If the client enjoys writing, the hand therapist may ask the client to keep a journal of what the recovery process means to him or her, describing important milestones and setbacks along the way.

Common Pitfalls and How to Avoid Them

1. Failing to consult the client regarding preferences about artful ways of caring: Remember that some clients are more willing than others to incorporate nontraditional approaches. The client's comfort level is always the guide.

2. Becoming disappointed or discouraged if an artful approach does not work: Role model the qualities of persistence and optimism for the client.

3. Forgetting to ask about role changes and significant issues: Take the time to figure out what this illness or injury means to the client as you go about designing an artful approach. For example, if a pianist is working to recover from a hand injury, the significance of using music in the therapy will rest on whether the client finds this approach motivating or if it is a source of despair.

4. Moving too quickly into the artful approach without building a sense of rapport: Wait until you can gauge the types of approaches to which the client might respond and then share the ideas with the client at the appropriate time.

Caritas Process 7: "Engaging in a Genuine Teaching-Learning Experience That Attends to Unity of Being and Meaning, Attempting to Stay within the Other's Frame of Reference"

Teaching and learning are key activities in the hand therapist-client relationship. The hand therapist's role is to create a teaching-learning environment that supports the client's progression through healing.

CLINICAL *Pearl*

Although the primary outward activities of hand therapy involve the body, a significant part of treatment also involves the client's mind and spirit.

Teaching requires attending to the client's ways of learning and preferences for information exchange and decision making. The hand therapist may ask, "Is this person able to understand what he or she is experiencing? How can I share knowledge and expertise with this client in a way that is relevant and meaningful for facilitating self-healing?"

It is very important to ascertain the client's definition of health, healing, and wholeness so that the therapist can incorporate this into the teaching-learning plan. The hand therapist also must assess the client's understanding of self-care needs, limitations, resources, and strengths.

Common Pitfalls and How to Avoid Them

1. Focusing only on the physical aspects of treatment and overlooking the cognitive, emotional, and spiritual impact hand therapy can have. Bring an intentional awareness to how the treatment may be influenced by the client's thoughts, attitudes, beliefs, and experiences. It may be beneficial to ask the client

to help you understand what questions or concerns he or she is having about therapy and what it means for the healing process.

2. Failing to use the client's strongest learning style: People usually find it easiest to teach in the style in which they learn best; take care that you don't always choose the teaching approach that best suits *you*. Some clients prefer multiple approaches (e.g., visual, auditory, kinesthetic), therefore offer a variety of activities.

Caritas Process 8: "Creating a Healing Environment at All Levels, Physical as Well as Nonphysical, a Subtle Environment of Energy and Consciousness Whereby Wholeness, Beauty and Comfort, Dignity, and Peace Are Potentiated"

The hand therapist can work with the client to create the best environment, physical and nonphysical, to promote healing. Manipulation of the environment can range from basic methods to more complex approaches. The treatment environment should be well lighted, ventilated, and clean. Beyond that, the hand therapist can incorporate elements of beauty, including sources of color, movement, texture, and form, to enhance the healing environment. When possible, a view of the outdoors, a change in surroundings, paintings, flowers, plants, and music can also be included. It is important to eliminate or reduce unnecessary noise, clutter, and other distractions from the environment during the clinical interaction.

The hand therapist can focus on questions such as, "What is important to this person to make his or her experience comfortable? How can healing art be incorporated into this space and time? How can I use creativity in managing institutional imperfections, constraints, contingencies, and scheduling issues while sustaining the context of a healing environment?" The client's role is to participate with the therapist in the creation of an environment that is most suitable. It is very important that the client is honest and forthcoming in discussions of how the environment can be adapted to be more pleasing to the senses.

Common Pitfalls and How to Avoid Them

1. Trying to do everything yourself: Hand therapists are probably more aware of the environmental aspect of care than many of their professional counterparts. Ask for help from the client or family in creating a healing environment, or talk with others on the healthcare team to share ideas and insights. This type of collaborative work will enhance the client-therapist relationship and can promote teamwork among members of the interdisciplinary team.

2. Neglecting the physical and psychologic environment: Remember that a link exists between the

physical environment and how a person feels emotionally and physically. Change the physical environment as much as possible to support the healing process; when this is impossible, do your utmost to create a positive psychologic environment.

CLINICAL *Pearl*

A positive attitude conveyed by the hand therapist can make a significant difference in the client's immediate surroundings.

Caritas Process 9: "Assisting with Basic Needs, with an Intentional Caring Consciousness, Administering Human Care Essentials That Potentiate Alignment of Mind/Body/Spirit Wholeness and Unity of Being in All Aspects of Care, Tending to Both Embodied Spirit and Evolving Spiritual Emergence"

It is essential to the building of a therapeutic relationship that the therapist take care to notice the client's very basic needs for safety, comfort, nutrition, clothing, cleanliness, privacy, and the need for relationships with others. Until these basic needs are attended to, the goals of hand therapy cannot be fully addressed. These facts seem self-evident, but many clients start hand therapy when they are hungry, weak, in pain, or not fully clothed (e.g., hospital gowns), or they are experiencing alterations in their normal patterns of personal hygiene. All these factors can leave clients feeling eroded in spirit and "less" than they could be. By putting the client in the best condition possible for therapy and acknowledging the impact of basic human needs, the therapist can more effectively accomplish the goals of the therapeutic session, and the client probably will be more confident about trying new approaches. As a result, the client-therapist relationship operates on a higher level.

The hand therapist can reflect on questions such as, "Am I process focused or outcome focused? Can I let go of the need to fix things? Am I honoring this person in my actions? What is the practice I can use now that will honor caring as a moral ideal?" The client's role is to provide honest and timely information about his/her own experience of how well basic needs are met. For instance, the client can be as prepared as possible for the therapy experience by having toileting needs met prior, eating a small meal or snack prior as appropriate, and being open about telling the therapist when needs are unmet. Also, the client can share with the therapist the approaches that will help the client feel most cared for. The therapist can work to set this expectation with the client in the initial meeting.

Common Pitfalls and How to Avoid Them

1. Overlooking basic needs: To the extent that you can, make sure the client comes to the clinical encounter with basic needs met.
2. Forgetting to honor the process: Remember that outcomes are very important, but the journey is, too.
3. Focusing only on the "broken" body part: Remember and remind clients that they are more than this part of their body and that many aspects of the body and spirit remain strong, even in times of illness or injury. Avoid using terminology such as "the bad arm"; instead use "the affected arm." A small semantic difference may help the client reframe the injury and see the body as an integrated whole rather than made up of "good" and "bad" parts.

CLINICAL *Pearl*

Bring honor to the process of your work with clients by developing an unhurried presence, one that reassures clients that their individual treatment journey is an essential part of arriving at the outcome.

Caritas Process 10: "Opening and Attending to Spiritual-Mysterious and Existential Dimensions of One's Own Life-Death; Soul Care for Self and the One Being Cared for"

During times of illness or injury, clients often have questions about their future and what the health event means for them personally. At this juncture, clients often confront issues of loss and mortality, even if the injury or illness is not considered life-threatening. Clients may experience heightened emotions as they consider these existential questions.

In this phase the hand therapist focuses on how the client views the future for himself or herself and others, how the client can find meaning in the current experience, and how he or she can make good decisions about life and death. Therapists may ask themselves, "What are the life lessons in this situation for the client and for me? What soul care is useful for this client at this time?"

The client can consider his or her openness to deeper self-exploration and soul care and what that means in relation to healing. Key existential questions may arise during this time of illness or injury. The hand therapist's role is not to provide answers to these questions, but rather to support clients as they ask the questions and then realize that they simply may have to live with uncertainties. Clients may be facing critical life decisions that require deep reflection, and this may affect their physical stamina and motivation.

Common Pitfalls and How to Avoid Them

1. Feeling fearful or uncomfortable about bringing up difficult issues: Remember that your role is to walk along with this client through a difficult time in the person's life. Sometimes the most helpful thing you can do for clients is not to do anything, but simply to "be"; that is, be present with them, listen to them and, if they ask questions or express deep spiritual needs beyond your comfort level or professional preparation, ask them for permission to arrange a referral to others trained in these areas.
2. Failing to recognize the limitations of hand therapy: Work within the scope of professional practice and consult others for assistance and referral as needed.

CLINICAL *Pearl*

You are not charged with meeting all the client's needs, but you can be instrumental in arranging the right combination of resources to do so.

Transpersonal Caring Healing Relationships

The second major element of Watson's theory of human caring is transpersonal caring healing relationships. Transpersonal caring "conveys a concern for the inner life world of another . . . seeking to connect with and embrace the soul of the other through the processes of caring and healing and being in authentic relation, in the moment." (http://www2.uchsc.edu/son/caring/content/transpersonal.asp) A **transpersonal caring relationship** connotes the sharing of authentic self between individuals and within groups in a reflective frame. All parties are changed within the relationship.

Care is founded on transpersonal caring relationships and is built on moral commitment, intentionality, and caritas consciousness. It is a vehicle for healing through the auspices of the relationship. The hand therapist recognizes and connects with the inner aspect of the other through presence, being centered in the caring moment, and through actions, words, intuition, body language, cognition, thoughts, senses, and other ways of interacting and connecting with others. (http://www2.uchsc.edu/son/caring/content/transpersonal.asp)

An assumption of transpersonal relationships is that "ongoing personal and professional development and spiritual growth, and personal spiritual practice assist the [therapist] in entering into this deeper level of professional healing practice." (http://www2.uchsc.edu/son/caring/content/transpersonal.asp) The hand therapist learns how to build and expand transpersonal caring relationships based on his or her own life history and previous experiences or conditions or by having imagined others' feelings in various circumstances.

The Caring Moment

The third component of Watson's theory of human caring is the caring moment or occasion. The **caring**

moment happens when the therapist and the client come together with their unique life histories and enter into the human-to-human transaction in a given focal point in space and time. (http://www2.uchsc.edu/son/caring/content/transpersonal.asp)

There is awareness that the moment in time is transient; one makes choices about how to spend the time, occasion, or opportunities that transcend the moment itself. If the caring moment is characterized by transpersonal relationship and caritas consciousness, a connection develops between the therapist and the client at a spiritual level, transcending time and space and creating the potential for healing and human unity at deeper levels. (http://www2.uchsc.edu/son/caring/content/transpersonal.asp) On a more global plane, "We learn from one another how to be human by identifying ourselves with others, finding their dilemmas in ourselves. What we all learn from it is self-knowledge. The self we learn about . . . is every self. It is universal—the human self. We learn to recognize ourselves in others, [it] keeps alive our common humanity and avoids reducing self or other to the moral status of object."[7]

NONVERBAL ASPECTS OF COMMUNICATION

Personal Space, Body Language, and Gestures

The first impression a client gets is often the nonverbal communication that begins before the conversation ever starts. Hand therapists' posture and use of personal space often are clues to how they feel about themselves and their practice. *Personal space* can be thought of as an invisible bubble or zone that varies from person to person and depends on the circumstances. Studies of personal space generally describe four zones: *intimate distance,* for embracing or whispering (6 to 18 inches); *personal distance,* for conversations among good friends ($1^1/_2$ to 4 feet); *social distance,* for conversations among acquaintances (4 to 12 feet); and *public distance,* for public speaking (12 feet or more). With most clients, the personal zone becomes the territory of the health care team for the purposes of assessments, treatments, and therapies. However, by always maintaining an awareness of personal space and its influence on client comfort, therapists can more easily comply with the client's preferences and take care not to compromise communication by violating this space.

CLINICAL *Pearl*

A person's space becomes his or her safety zone, and people feel varying degrees of ownership and territoriality about their personal space.

The position and posture of clients (and of hand therapists, too) can convey relevant information about physical and emotional health, comfort with communication strategies, and general attitude. Clearly, nonverbal communication can be an important source of clinical information for the hand therapist, but it is a subjective means and can be misinterpreted. Therefore a very important part of therapy is validating the meanings of nonverbal communication with the client.

Therapists also must take special note of how they use space, body language, speech tone, and volume when engaging in activities with clients. Much of the work of hand therapy is performed within personal boundaries that would be considered socially uncomfortable in another context.

Studies of physician nonverbal behaviors have indicated that behaviors such as increased facial expression, frequent eye contact, smiling, leaning forward, open body posture, and nodding correlate with client satisfaction in a variety of clinical scenarios.[9] Also, in the most favorably rated clinical encounters, the clinician's behaviors often mirror or are patterned after the client's behaviors. Two people in conversation usually tend toward this mutual behavior when they are on good terms and relating well. This is **interactional synchrony,** a term used to describe the extent to which behaviors in an interpersonal interaction are patterned or synchronized. The patterning can take place in the way movements and behaviors are timed or in the actual behaviors themselves, such as scratching one's nose or leaning forward.[10] This model of rapport includes three elements: mutual attentiveness, positivity, and coordination. Although the hand therapist may not consciously try to match the client's behavioral conversational responses, the natural unfolding of this mutual conversational pattern may positively affect the sense of rapport reported by the client.

Nonverbal communication can provide valuable clinical information and can serve as a tool for enhancing the therapeutic relationship. However, the therapist must always use caution in interpreting nonverbal cues. Culture, health issues, context, and the social situation are just a few of the many variables that can alter the meaning of nonverbal communication. Therapists should always confirm their understanding of nonverbal behaviors with the client.

Reading Between the Lines

Sometimes the hand therapist must call attention to something that is not said or a gesture that is not made. At times the verbal message conflicts with the nonverbal message. Some clients are very reluctant to open up to the health care team, even about health-related issues such as pain or functional status. Pain is one of the most difficult factors to assess because of its subjective nature;

some people have a very high tolerance, whereas others have a very low threshold. An effective approach to dealing with this is to continue to ask verbal questions while assessing nonverbal cues until the client verifies that the therapist understands what the client means. For example, you might say, "You are rating your pain as a 3, yet we aren't seeing the movement in your finger that we did yesterday. Can you tell me more about your discomfort or stiffness so that I can understand it better?"

Empathy is a strong component of an ability to understand what might be missing from a conversation. By truly trying to put oneself in the client's place, the hand therapist may gain further insight into what is not part of the conversation. For example, if the hand therapist is working with a young farmer who recently had an upper extremity amputation, yet the subject of farming and role change has not yet been introduced, the hand therapist may surmise that the client might like to talk about this issue but does not know how to begin—it is the proverbial pink elephant in the middle of the room. Unspoken concerns such as this one require a sensitive approach because they usually represent very difficult issues. In most cases, giving the client the chance to express concerns opens up new possibilities. The energy that was spent worrying about the issue now can be spent addressing it.

The ability to figure out what is left unspoken or unexpressed is a high-level clinical skill that therapists develop after experiencing several similar client care scenarios. Patterns of expected behaviors and issues usually begin to make sense after the therapist sees clients in similar circumstances. Then, when a client's specific communication does not fit with the basic pattern, the therapist may conclude that something unspoken warrants attention.

Listening

In our fast-paced culture of information overload, people often are forced to triage information rather than truly listen. Paying attention can mean skimming through the bulk of the material present to pick out what is really useful. "Sound bites," text messaging, digital images, and executive summaries are the norm. Listening is more difficult and takes longer.

CLINICAL *Pearl*

Listening requires one to stop, put an end to personal internal chatter, and fully attend to what the other person is saying, how he or she is saying it, what the person's behavior shows, and what the environment is like.

Listening means perceiving the words and creating meanings or interpretations for them. Listening also means mentally capturing the concrete message the client is sending while at the same time exploring deeper meanings that might be part of the message. For example, if a client says, "My hand is killing me," it probably means the client is in physical pain. The deeper meaning may also be true; this statement may also send a message of loss and grief that would not be discerned if the listener only hears the text of the concrete message.

For therapists, listening requires more than sorting through information to decipher which data are clinically meaningful. It means incorporating what the client is saying into the therapist's perception of that person as a whole. For instance, if a client starts talking about the quilt she hoped to make for her new grandson and this expression is dismissed as irrelevant to the clinical encounter, the hand therapist might miss an important opportunity, such as the chance to learn what is meaningful to the client and to work with the client on skills that would allow her to regain this function and restore her sense of role competency.

Listening takes time. Listening with the focused intention of caring and concern is a therapeutic technique in its own right. Often when clients are asked which interventions they find most meaningful, they report that when therapists listen to their concerns, they feel understood and cared for. Listening can be a means to the desired result of a productive therapist-client relationship, and it can also be an outcome in and of itself. Listening provides a chance to connect with the client in a meaningful way, and it also can be very rewarding for the therapist.

Even when the client cannot communicate verbally, listening is still an important skill. Listening can be accomplished with more than the ears and through means other than sound. Consider how attention might be turned to the client in a meaningful, silent way, supporting and accepting the person's sense of being without words.

CLINICAL *Pearl*

Some of the most stunning listening takes place in silence.

HOPE

Hope is a positive attitude or orientation toward the future. It has cognitive aspects (such as when the client thinks about how treatment will affect outcomes) and affective components (such as the emotional excitement a client feels when thinking about regaining abilities).

Scientists also are investigating the physiologic aspects of hope, such as how hope may affect neurologic and immunologic function.

CLINICAL *Pearl*

Hope can be present even in the most desperate circumstances.

Individuals can simultaneously feel hopeful about one thing and hopeless about another. Sometimes hope extends beyond the constraints of the physical world; that is, sometimes, in the face of impending death, clients express hope for a future beyond death or describe hope in the people or things they will leave behind. Hope can be vested not so much in extending the quantity of life, but rather the quality. Clients look for signs of hope in the faces of those who care for them. The simple words, "The body has an amazing capacity for healing," can provide clients with a foundation for believing hand therapy can and will work for them.

Hope plays an important role in health and healing and in adjusting to serious injury, illness, and death.

CLINICAL *Pearl*

Providing realistic hope is a crucial aspect of care.

Taking away hope can have devastating effects. Hope can be viewed conceptually as requiring four critical attributes: a time-focused future orientation, energized action, the existence of a goal or desired outcome, and a feeling of uncertainty.[11] Hope is both a universally important construct and a very individualized experience.

Statements that clients can rate to indicate their level of hope are found in Herth's Hope Index,[12] an instrument used to measure hope in research settings (Box 8-1).

Hope is an attitude that can be affected by clinical interventions; to some degree, an outlook of hope can be taught. Important work is emerging that focuses on specific, scientifically based interventions designed to inspire hope[13] and to teach people thought patterns and behavioral competencies that enhance personal happiness and meaning.[14]

How should clinicians approach the issue of supporting realistic hope while not making unwarranted positive predictions or statements? In his book, *The Anatomy of Hope*, Jerome Groopman[15] addresses this question from the point of view of a medical oncologist caring for clients with life-threatening illness. He explores the dangers of taking away psychologic hope by providing only survival statistics and factual summaries, as well as the perils of

BOX 8-1

Herth Hope Index

1. I have a positive outlook toward life.
2. I have short-range and/or long-range goals.
3. I feel all alone.
4. I can see possibilities in the midst of difficulties.
5. I have a faith that gives me comfort.
6. I feel scared about my future.
7. I can recall happy/joyful times.
8. I have deep inner strength.
9. I am able to give and receive caring and love.
10. I have a sense of direction for my life.
11. I believe that each day has potential.
12. I feel my life has value and worth.

Herth K: Abbreviated instrument to measure hope: development and psychometric evaluation—the Herth hope index, *J Adv Nurs* 70:1251-1259, 1992.

giving too much hope or unrealistic hope. The approach he finds most therapeutic is to balance a straightforward appraisal of the worst-case scenario with realistic optimism. He finds that clients are very appreciative when practitioners show an awareness of their diagnosis and predicted course and that these clients make the most beneficial personal strides in building a sense of meaning and hope when they have a realistic picture combined with emotional support and reinforcement of hope.

The hand therapist can assume an important role in assessing hope and providing clients with realistic hope for the progress and outcomes of hand therapy. Hope can be conveyed in words, through encouraging remarks or by reminding clients how far they have progressed. Helping clients to identify their individualized sources of support and to build on past successes are two approaches that go a long way in sustaining hope. Clients are much more likely to reach the physical and functional goals of hand therapy when they participate with a sense of hope intact.

CREATING A MOTIVATING ENVIRONMENT

One function of the therapeutic relationship is to create an environment in which the client can reach the very best possible clinical outcome. Motivation plays a key role in how much effort, dedication, and resilience a client will have in the therapeutic regimen. Naturally motivating factors and ways the therapist can enhance that motivation include the following:

1. Significant contributions: Identify the efforts clients are making; help them see the work they are accomplishing.

2. Goal participation: Take the time and effort to achieve mutual goal setting.
3. Positive dissatisfaction: When clients are not comfortable with their current status, help them use this dissatisfaction as a positive motivator for change.
4. Recognition: Create ways of acknowledging progress.
5. Clear expectations: Clarify reasonable goals, strategies, and regimens with the client; be a leader, encouraging and inspiring the client to reach beyond current abilities.

Clients often need help learning how to be successful in their treatment; they must realize that knowledge alone does not necessarily get them to the goal. The most effective rewards usually are those that are positive, valued by the individual client, and intermittent.

Clients become motivated when therapists help them find meaning in their therapeutic regimen. Point out the link between the activities or exercises and the way they will help the client got about daily life, especially the activities most important to the client. Share your observations with the client, such as, "Your range of motion is much better today." Even the simplest observation conveys to the client that you are paying attention to the person's progress (or lack thereof), and this feedback itself provides motivation. Also use any available nonverbal means of feedback (e.g., chart, graph, or journal for keeping track of progress) for motivation.

Certain strategies do not work as motivational tools and can even set back motivational success. These include belittling clients, treating them in childlike ways, drawing attention to weaknesses or calling clients lazy, showing insensitivity to cultural or age-related norms, and in general behaving disrespectfully. Negative reinforcement should not be used. Sometimes confronting people about their negative behaviors or lack of focused effort is a reasonable tactic, but it should be done with care and respect.

CLINICAL *Pearl*

Clients find it easier to be motivated if the hand therapist also is motivated or energized.

Clients are keenly aware of the authenticity of encouragement. Therefore the therapist must find ways to maintain a personal sense of energized optimism. Clearly this is tied to self-care strategies; for example, taking good care of your own health and well-being has some of its clearest implications for professional success when it comes to providing motivation. A tired, depleted, "burned out" hand therapist finds it very difficult to support clients in the motivational domain. Find and engage in personal strategies that provide opportunities for healthy growth and development so that these strengths can be shared with your clients.

Working with clients who have little motivation can be particularly frustrating for the therapist. Clients have differing levels of readiness for adopting the changes required by hand therapy. Patience, gentle persistence, and time generally are the most effective strategies for managing weak motivation.

A motivating hand therapist provides the client with clear direction about goals, how therapy will progress, what to expect along the way, how long it will take, and the results. Providing honest, constructive feedback during each session and about the whole course of therapy is the most effective way to maintain motivation for most clients. Reinforcing a client's "can do" spirit and conveying an attitude of "I knew you could do it" are excellent ways to boost motivation. Such encouragement leaves clients better prepared to draw from this motivation as a resource in the future, when they are discharged from therapy. The hand therapist can make the impossible become possible and can give the client the courage to turn a possibility into a reality.

TERMINATING THE THERAPEUTIC RELATIONSHIP

It is important that the therapist take the time and opportunity to acknowledge the end of the therapeutic relationship, if at all possible. The client may be discharged from the hand therapy program for a variety of reasons. At this juncture, the therapist should note the progress that was made, not only in terms of functionality, but also in terms of the process of therapy. The therapist may want to share some thoughts with the client about the goals accomplished, the strengths or characteristics that most obviously helped on the journey, and any reflections about humorous, meaningful, or important moments the therapist and client shared.

Clients often feel a great deal of gratitude to the hand therapist for the work that has been accomplished, and they may have difficulty expressing this gratitude in a way that is fitting within the professional culture of the therapist. For instance, clients may offer gifts or tokens of appreciation. As a rule, it is best to thank the client and explain that you really can't accept personal gifts. Maintaining professional boundaries is very important, even as the therapist-client relationship is coming to a close.

Some of the most difficult good-byes can arise when a client enters a phase in treatment in which hand therapy is no longer relevant because of the client's declining condition or impending death. It is important not to ignore the transition. Instead, tell the client good-bye. You might take the chance to say how much you enjoyed working with the client and spending time together.

Other situations also can create difficulty in maintaining social and professional roles. For instance, in a large health care organization, some of the hand therapist's clients may be fellow employees. In rural settings, clients may also be neighbors. In these situations it is helpful to acknowledge that the professional therapeutic relationship is ending but that the social role will continue. If this transition in roles is acknowledged verbally, the former client is far less likely to ask a therapy question in the hospital elevator or request advice in the grocery store.

The end of the therapeutic relationship sometimes can cause emotions the client may be feeling about the hand therapist to bubble up. These can range from gratitude for reaching a therapy goal to frustration that goals were not accomplished. A client may even have just stopped therapy abruptly without giving notice. Most health care professionals develop a personal method of managing these thoughts and emotions, such as talking to colleagues, journaling (using no client names or identifiers), and finding ways to "let go" of clients when they leave. After you have been in practice for a while, you will have many client stories, some of them good memories, some not. Your expertise will be deepened by the complicated parade of clients that comprise an active clinical practice.

CASE *Studies*

CASE 8-1

An 80-year-old, right-dominant woman arrives for hand therapy accompanied by her 54-year-old son, who recently lost his job and now lives with his mother, "working" as her caregiver. The client was referred with a diagnosis of stiff fingers of both hands secondary to disuse after right shoulder surgery to repair the rotator cuff. The physician's notes explicitly state that the son aggressively debated the issue of surgery with the physician and that he had been argumentative at office visits. He also had "pestered" the physician to the extent that the physician suggested that the client and son find another doctor with whom they might be happier. The client and son have decided to stay with this physician, but they make derogatory remarks about the doctor to the hand therapist. At the first hand therapy visit, the son challenges every recommendation the therapist makes and is reluctant to let his mother participate in the conversation. The son also makes numerous recommendations that are clinically contraindicated.

1. What is your first client/family relationship priority?
2. What is your clinical priority?
3. How do you plan the therapeutic interventions so that they will have the greatest effect?

Suggested Approach

The physician's notes make it clear that this will be a psychosocially complex case. The initial priority is to establish a trusting professional relationship with the client and her son. The clinical priority is safety for the client, followed by the formulation of clear working relationship roles and responsibilities that support the physical work of therapy.

Before initiating the client encounter, the hand therapist might take a moment to clear his or her mind of other distracting thoughts and to bring into focus a "fresh start" perspective for this client/family visit. A first step here might be to request and arrange for separate time with the client and the son and to arrange a physical setting that is conducive to privacy. Reassure both that they will have an adequate opportunity to voice concerns and questions. Recognizing that the son may have a lot of emotional investment in his caregiving role, since he is otherwise unemployed, the therapist may find it beneficial to comment on his strengths in this area. It will be important to draw clear lines about how the hand therapist will treat the family as a unit, but the primary therapeutic recommendations and work will be focused on the client's priorities. Building a positive rapport with the son will facilitate the care of the client. The hand therapist might ask what the son's priorities are, if he feels that his priorities match the client's goals, and what the barriers have been up to this point. When talk turns to complaints about the physician, the hand therapist could refocus the son, saying, "Let's focus on what we can accomplish for your mother here today." After rapport is established, it will be more feasible to discuss therapeutic recommendations with the son. If he continues to suggest things that are clinically contraindicated, the therapist can explain the reasons for the contraindication. If rapport is not well established, the son is likely to dismiss the therapist's recommendations.

In the client encounter, it is important for the therapist to notice nonverbal communication and to do an unobtrusive assessment for possible elder abuse. In scenarios in which the caregiver expresses a lot of anger and blame, the elderly individual sometimes is at risk for verbal, physical, or financial abuse. If signs of abuse are present and the client seems comfortable talking with the therapist, the therapist can assess the situation verbally to discern whether the client feels vulnerable. If so, a referral to social services and/or the elder abuse hotline is in order. If no signs of abuse are noted, the therapist proceeds with assessing the client's goals for therapy and her readiness to begin.

The private consultation with the client focuses on gaining trust, establishing priorities, and clarifying everyone's roles: client, son, hand therapist, and physician. Once the part each person plays in the client's therapy is clearly understood, realistic goals can be established. In this situation, establishing trust and rapport may take longer, but without these elements hand therapy probably will be unsuccessful. The time spent "up front" in establishing a positive working relationship will pay benefits by fostering a more productive therapeutic progression.

The hand therapist must be very careful to document the findings in this case thoroughly because of the son's issues with anger and hostility. It also is important for the therapist to have an opportunity to debrief and reflect about his or her time with this client and son. Progress probably will take time, and this case has the potential to be discouraging if the therapist focuses only on physical gains. The first major accomplishment in this case will be creating rapport with and establishing realistic expectations for all those involved; these outcomes are more difficult to see. After each visit, the therapist should take a few moments to reflect on the strategies that did and did not work in this particular situation and to envision how things might be more successful in future encounters.

CASE 8-2

A precocious 9-year-old arrives for hand therapy with her mother, a pediatric nurse. The child has been referred with a diagnosis of bilateral wrist tendonitis. She is in gifted classes at school and is an avid reader. She is quite active and has trouble sitting in one place for longer than 5 minutes. She does not make eye contact with her mother or the therapist unless the mother specifically commands her to do so; she then makes eye contact for less than 30 seconds. Her hand therapy examination does not reveal any isolated structures that fit the criteria for tendonitis. She is hypermobile in numerous joints, including her wrists, and she has a habitual practice of forcefully passively stretching her wrists into extremes of flexion and extension. She does this often and states that it both "hurts and feels good." The mother is concerned that the physical problem causing the child's painful wrists has not been properly diagnosed, and she hopes that therapy will correct the condition.

1. How can rapport be gained?
2. What are the competing clinical priorities?
3. What referrals would be appropriate?

Suggested Approach

Presenting a focused, calm, accepting demeanor will be particularly helpful in this case, therefore the hand therapist might want to spend a few moments getting focused and clearing the mind of distractions before initiating this encounter. This client will be particularly sensitive to anxiety carried by the therapist. Maintaining a calm presence will be challenging, given the client's many movements and lack of eye contact, as well as the mother's presence. A very simple, yet effective, way therapists can remain focused and serene is to be aware of their own breathing, focusing on making the exhalation longer than the inhalation. This means of slowing down can have a positive effect on the client, who typically will slow her own breathing in response. Getting the client to slow down and focus is a critical first step in establishing rapport.

The hand therapist probably suspects that this child is experiencing anxiety or attention deficit characteristics. Further assessment of these suspicions warrants a complete history and may involve referrals to other professionals and perhaps school personnel. Competing clinical priorities include clarification of the behavioral issues that seem to be exacerbating the tendonitis, discerning medical versus psychologic etiologies for the behaviors, and identifying social or academic issues that might be compounding the condition. The fact that the child is academically precocious may mask her other developmental needs, which may be more in line with those of the average 9-year-old. Although there may be interventions the hand therapist can recommend for the tendonitis, the picture is complicated by the child's repeated behaviors. Treating the underlying psychosocial conditions extends the effectiveness of hand therapy. Referrals to developmental specialists, social workers, psychologic and medical care providers, and the school counselor may also be appropriate. Again, the referral process can be facilitated if the therapist develops a sound, trusting relationship with the client and her mother, particularly if this is their first encounter with the health care system regarding this constellation of issues.

As in the first case study, the hand therapist should evaluate the client out of the mother's presence, if at all possible. The mother's presence may be interfering with the daughter's ability to focus. Also, the girl may have goals for therapy that are different from those of her mother, which will be important to discern. The therapist can capitalize on the client's love of reading by giving her age-appropriate books or pamphlets about her tendonitis and its treatment. The therapist also should work with the client to identify ways of creating a soothing environment for her treatment, techniques that may extend to her living and academic activities. For example, the therapist might help the client identify music she finds relaxing or activities that help her unwind before therapy.

The hand therapist must work to gain an understanding of the significance of the client's repeated flexion and extension of her wrists. Is this action symbolic of a desire for flexibility? Is the client's "hurts and feels good" statement symbolic of what it is like for her to be academically gifted, given the social realities of her school setting. These symbolic meanings can greatly influence the client's desire to quit the behaviors if the movements themselves are comforting psychologically.

Working separately with the mother, the hand therapist must first establish rapport and then gauge the mother's understanding of her daughter's underlying anxiety or attention-related condition. If no workup has been done on these issues, it is important that the therapist address the possibility of referrals. It is essential that the therapist make no assumptions about the mother's cognitive understanding of her daughter's condition; just because the mother is a pediatric nurse does not mean that she can objectively identify issues in her own family. The hand therapist must verify the mother's understanding and her concerns verbally, in addition to assessing her nonverbal communication. Working with the mother to identify priorities for diagnosis and treatment comes after this basic assessment of her understanding the larger picture of her daughter's condition. Supporting the mother and helping her accept the possible psychosocial diagnoses for her daughter also strengthens the therapeutic rapport and places the client in a better environment for improvement in overall well-being.

CASE 8-3

A 61-year-old, right-dominant teacher is referred for hand therapy after repair of a fracture of the right distal radius with plating. The referral is for pain management, edema, and stiffness that limit functional use of her hand. She tells the therapist that she is an overachiever and is highly motivated to recover. The therapist provides the woman with written instructions for gentle exercises; she also instructs her to stop or modify the exercises if they cause pain or do not feel good. When the client arrives for the next therapy session, the pain, swelling, and stiffness are all worse. She states that she had tripled the recommended exercise regimen, although she realized immediately that it increased her pain, swelling, and stiffness. She explains that she did this because she was eager to recover. The client is developing a highly guarded posture of the painful right upper extremity that is contributing to the worsening of all symptoms, and she is at risk for complex regional pain syndrome (CRPS).

1. How can you sustain this client's high level of motivation, yet convince her that she has overdone her exercises?
2. How can you best approach this client about the worsening symptoms and pain?

Suggested Approach

The hand therapist can draw on the client's many strengths to optimize treatment. First, the woman is highly motivated to get better. Second, she clearly understands the link between treatment and outcomes. Third, she must have a high level of trust in the hand therapist, as evidenced by her wanting to follow the recommendations, if not the level of gentleness, recommended by the therapist.

The therapist's first step is to capitalize on the rapport already established. The therapist should acknowledge the client's hard work and then gently but firmly remind her that in her case, "less is more." The link between exercise and rest should be explained, as well as how pain affects mobility. The teacher is highly motivated to learn and likely will respond to logical, clear, and multifaceted explanations of why vigorous or repeated exercise is causing her pain. In this case it probably will be beneficial to give the physiologic explanations of overuse, edema, and pain. These explanations will appeal to the client's sense of reason, and this is likely to increase her motivation to be slower and gentler in her approach.

The hand therapist should not scold the client or trivialize the time and work she has already invested in her recovery. Shaming this client would be very detrimental to her overall well-being and to her progress in therapy. However, the hand therapist might want to gently inquire about other reasons the client overdid her therapy. Are there underlying reasons for her not to want to regain function, or was the overexertion truly related to wanting to get better faster? Such questions may help the client come to a better understanding of herself and her motives. If her sole motive is a speedy recovery, helping her discover that the most beneficial method is a gently paced approach that respects tissue tolerances may give her a deeper insight into other areas of her life.

References

1. Minick P: The power of human caring: early recognition of client problems, *Sch Inq Nurs Pract* 9:303-317, 1995.
2. Watson J: *Postmodern nursing and beyond*, Edinburgh, 1999, Churchill-Livingstone/Harcourt-Brace.
3. Kabat-Zin J: *Wherever you go, there you are: mindfulness meditations in everyday life*, New York, 1994, Hyperion.
4. Watson J: Watson's philosophy and theory of human caring in nursing. In Riehl-Sisca J, editor: *Conceptual models for nursing practice*, ed 3, Norwalk, CT, 1989, Appleton & Lange.
5. Watson J: A meta-reflection on reflective practice and caring theory. In Johns C, Fleshwater D, editors: *Trans-*

forming nursing through reflective practice, London, 1998, Blackwell Science.

6. Watson J: New dimensions of human caring theory, *Nurs Sci Q* 1:175-181, 1988.
7. Watson J: *Nursing: human science and human care*, New York, 1985, Appleton-Century.
8. Watson J: *Nursing: the philosophy and science of caring*, Boston, 1979, Little, Brown.
9. Griffith C, Wilson J, Langer S et al: House staff nonverbal communication skills and standardized client satisfaction, *J Gen Intern Med* 18:170-174, 2003.
10. Bernieri F, Rosenthal R: Interpersonal coordination: behavior matching and interactional synchrony. In Feldman R, Rime B, editors: *Fundamentals of nonverbal behavior*, London, 1991, Cambridge University Press.
11. Haase J, Britt T, Coward D et al: Simultaneous concept analysis of spiritual perspective, hope, acceptance, and self-transcendence, *Image J Nurs Sch* 24:141-147, 1992.
12. Herth K: Abbreviated instrument to measure hope: development and psychometric evaluation—the Herth hope index, *J Adv Nurs* 70:1251-1259, 1992.
13. Herth K: Development and testing of a hope intervention program, *Oncol Nurs Forum* 28:1009-1016, 2001.
14. Foster R, Hicks G: *How we choose to be happy*, New York, 1999, Perigee Books.
15. Groopman J: *The anatomy of hope: how people prevail in the face of illness*, New York, 2004, Random House.

9

Roles of Therapy Assistants in Hand Therapy

CYNTHIA COOPER

The managed care system affects all health care fields, including hand therapy. One result of this change in the approach to health care is the increasing amount of treatment provided by occupational therapy assistants (OTAs) or physical therapy assistants (PTAs). This trend is likely to persist, and higher caseloads, shorter treatment times, and budget constraints will mean staffing patterns in which more assistants perform therapy. A knowledgeable, well-trained assistant can improve the care provided in a hand therapy program. This chapter discusses the roles of therapy assistants and suggests ways to develop and maximize an effective team. For clarity, the chapter uses the term *assistant* to mean an OTA or a PTA and the term *therapist* to mean an occupational therapist (OT) or a physical therapist (PT). It is understood that all are professionals who are therapy practitioners, and that semantics vary.

In some states, therapy assistants need a license to practice. The fields of occupational therapy and physical therapy have separate practice acts and different licensing agencies, which can affect the staffing options of hand therapy programs. Typically, OTAs must work under the supervision of OTs and follow an OT plan of care,[1] and PTAs must work under the supervision of PTs and follow a PT plan of care. A PTA with hand experience can be added to a hand therapy program only if the assistant reports to a PT. However, more OTs practice hand therapy than do PTs. These types of considerations affect staffing decisions.

The therapist sets the standard of care for the program. The assistant is responsible for adhering to these standards. Ideally, therapists and assistants work collaboratively. The term *collaboration* has more than one definition; in this sense, it means "working together, especially in a joint intellectual effort."[2] By definition, collaboration implies a hierarchy, with the assistant reporting to the therapist. The hand therapist is responsible for the care the client receives; the therapist also determines the level of supervision an assistant requires. The assistant aids in the client's goal setting and contributes ideas for the client's program.[1] Assistants' responsibilities are increased as appropriate, depending on their clinical skills. All therapists and assistants are responsible for learning about and following their state laws concerning supervision and scope of practice.

HAND THERAPY EXPERIENCE MATRIX

The hand therapy experience matrix (Fig. 9-1) is a model of collaborative roles for therapists and assistants.[3] The x axis represents the therapist's level of experience in hand therapy. The y axis represents the assistant's level of experience in hand therapy. The hand therapy team's goal is to move to a higher quadrant through supervision and training, with competencies demonstrated in a manner consistent with state and facility guidelines.

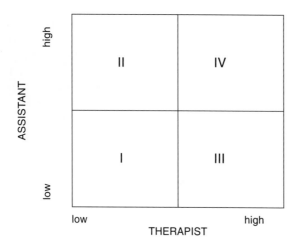

The Hand Therapy Matrix

FIGURE 9-1 Hand therapy matrix.

In quadrant I, both the therapist and the assistant are inexperienced in hand therapy. In such cases, you, as the therapist, should study as much as possible about the diagnosis and arrange for mentoring from and close communication with experienced hand therapists. If you have hand therapy colleagues in the area, phone calls may be helpful. Also, keep in close touch with the physician's office about the client's status. Be honest with the referring physician and communicate well; this style of interaction can build trust and lead to a close working relationship, with a strong likelihood of future referrals.

In quadrant II, an inexperienced therapist is paired with an experienced assistant. The therapist must supervise the assistant but may not even know what is clinically wrong with the client. The assistant cannot fully evaluate the client and cannot and should not supervise the therapist. In this case, the therapist and the assistant, working as a team, should pool their knowledge, read as much as possible about the diagnosis, and follow the suggestions for a quadrant I situation. Special care must be taken in these cases to avoid any role reversal of therapist and assistant.

In quadrant III, an experienced therapist is working with an inexperienced assistant. The therapist can help train the assistant, and competencies can be achieved in accordance with the facility's guidelines, maximizing the assistant's potential to broaden clinical skills. In this team, it is important for the therapist to supervise the assistant closely. The therapist should create a structured learning program with the assistant's assistance, identifying reading assignments, reviewing cases, and sharing resources from conferences and journals. This enrichment is more meaningful if it is shaped to match existing

Clinical Reasoning Tool for Hand Therapy Case Reviews

Client: _____
Diagnosis: _____
Date: _____

Wounds	
Drainage	
Edema	
Pain	
Scar	
AROM limitations	
PROM limitations	
Intrinsic tightness	
Extrinsic extensor tightness	
Extrinsic flexor tightness	
Joint tightness	

Joint end-feel
  Hard
  Spongy
  Soft	

Precautions	
Structures to treat	
Interventions	

clients. For example, if a client has just been referred to you and your assistant for therapy after repair of the flexor pollicis longus, try to make that diagnosis your topic of study, so that it is relevant to your case. If you have a client with adhesions, study scar management with your assistant and ask the OTA or PTA how the knowledge gained can be applied to the client's treatment. Box 9-1 presents a tool that can help assistants develop their clinical reasoning capabilities in reviewing hand therapy cases.

Quadrant IV is the best of both worlds. In this situation, both the therapist and the assistant are experienced in hand therapy. This team can continue to grow professionally and clinically by discussing cases, studying review articles, and keeping up with professional journals.

In all quadrants, it is very important that the assistant know when to ask the therapist for input about the client; this comes closest to a truly collaborative relationship.

An inexperienced therapist practicing hand therapy faces increased risk and a reduced likelihood of a favorable outcome. Inexperienced therapists should always use extra caution and should keep striving to learn. They should seek out all possible avenues for obtaining mentoring from other hand therapists and physicians. It strengthens, rather than weakens, your credibility and authority as a therapist if you are willing to ask questions and admit you do not know something, rather than pretending to be more knowledgeable than you are. Most professionals will respect you more for this approach. Even the most experienced therapists do not know everything; there is always more to learn in hand therapy. The knowledge will come if you apply yourself, follow the suggestions made previously, and stay committed to reading and studying. The knowledge base for hand therapy is very broad; in fact, it can be overwhelming. It takes time to learn all this material and to see all these clients, who will continually teach you more. Pacing yourself through this learning process is far better than overdoing it, which can result in burn-out.

Diagnoses that ideally should be referred to more experienced hand therapists include the following:

- Flexor tendon injury
- Extensor tendon injury
- Rheumatoid reconstruction
- Replantation/revascularization
- Complicated crush injury
- Nerve injury
- Complex regional pain syndrome (CRPS, also RSD)
- Dupuytren's release
- Significant or infected wound

DEVELOPING A RESPECTFUL AND EFFECTIVE TEAM RELATIONSHIP

Clients are sensitive to the subtleties of communication among coworkers, and they often comment on their perception of a team's work relationships. In a professional environment, the therapist explicitly shows respect for and appreciation of the assistant's work in front of clients. If the assistant reciprocates, all the better. Clients may remark on the friendly flow they notice among team members; this type of collaborative arrangement is very favorable to a successful clinical experience. Conversely, clients can tell if tension exists among coworkers; this situation affects the quality of care and reduces clients' comfort and satisfaction with the program.

Promoting a Learning Experience for Assistants

When all team members have a high level of clinical skills, the result is a better program. Supervising thera-

pists should serve as role models and foster continual learning for the entire staff. For example, the staff could hold a journal club meeting once a month at lunch, sharing information from conferences that team members have attended and encouraging assistants to attend courses and read about hand therapy.

An awkward situation can arise if a team member feels that a therapist or an assistant is using outmoded treatment techniques. Some such techniques might include treating subacute hand edema with string wrap or retrograde massage instead of manual edema mobilization (MEM); failing to recognize or ignoring obvious and objective clinical signs of tissue intolerances (flare reaction); or performing hands-on treatment (e.g., passive range of motion [PROM]) that is painful, aggressive, and/or injurious. In such cases it may help to challenge that practitioner to bring in evidence from the literature supporting that choice of treatment. At the same time, recommend and provide reading that supports MEM or explains flare reactions.

What to Say to Clients

Hand therapists and assistants should explain their roles when they introduce themselves to clients. This should be done in a way that conveys both the concept of teamwork and the fact that the assistant's contributions are a valued component of therapy. Team members must have a thorough understanding of their different roles if they are to explain them well to clients.

The hand therapist and OTA or PTA might introduce themselves to a client as follows:

Hand therapist: "Hello, my name is Jane. I will be your hand therapist, and today I will evaluate you. This is Sam, who is an [occupational or physical] therapy assistant. We will be your hand therapy team, and both of us will be working with you."

OTA or PTA: "Hello, my name is Sam. I will be working with you today. I am an [occupational or physical] therapy assistant. Jane is your hand therapist. We are your hand therapy team, and we both will be involved with your care."

TIPS FROM THE FIELD

- When a physician calls about a client, the therapist should take the call if available. If the assistant handles the call, the assistant should inform the therapist. Also, if the therapist is not available and the assistant takes the call, the assistant should ask the physician if he or she would like to discuss the case further with the hand therapist. If so, this should be arranged.

- Therapists should show respect for assistants' knowledge and their desire to learn. Hand therapy assistants with good experience can be more knowledgeable in some areas than relatively new hand therapists. Assistants who have just attended a conference have educational material to share; they should be allowed to do so without awkwardness, because this will help to improve client care.
- Team members should have as much clinical and philosophic compatibility as possible.
  - The therapist should know about tissue tolerances. If the assistant is being too aggressive on a client, this must be corrected with instruction and hands-on practice. Conversely, if a therapist is not well versed in tissue tolerances, the assistant should not be overly aggressive just because the therapist orders it.
- The therapist makes the final decisions about treatment, including modalities. The assistant can provide input and suggestions, but the therapist is responsible for the decision.
- The therapist and assistant should meet regularly to review their client cases, including cases in which the clinical needs seem to be minor. The therapist is responsible for ensuring that clients' therapy programs are appropriate and are upgraded regularly. For this and other reasons, the hand therapist should see each client approximately every third or fourth visit if possible. Some state licensing agencies stipulate how often the therapist must be directly involved with care that is provided by an assistant.
- Assistants should always feel that they can question or ask about the treatment a therapist prescribes. However, any discussions should take place in private.
- The therapist should try to avoid correcting or reprimanding an assistant in front of a client. Instead, the therapist and assistant should use an agreed-upon set of signals that convey specific messages that may mean, for example:
  - Stop doing that immediately. What you are doing is not safe or appropriate for the client.
  - We need to go down the hall immediately to discuss what you are doing before continuing treatment.
  - This client needs both of us now to reinforce an instruction or a precaution.
  - Please come help with this splint or dressing.

CASE *Studies*

CASE 9-1

An assistant was trained by a relatively new, inexperienced hand therapist. The assistant was not taught to

instruct clients with wrist fractures to isolate the wrist extensors when they performed wrist active range of motion (AROM) exercises during the home exercise program. The assistant had more years of experience than the new therapist had.

An experienced hand therapist subsequently was hired, and he identified wrist extensor isolation as an important clinical priority. This therapist began his discussion with the assistant by complimenting her for her hard work and acknowledging her clinical strengths. The therapist then said, "I know you have many years of clinical experience. As we develop our work relationship, I will be identifying things I want us to do more similarly. Feel free to ask me more about these topics. I will be happy to recommend reading on these subjects. It is very important to teach clients how to isolate the wrist extensors when they are learning AROM after wrist fracture so that they do not substitute this motion using the extensor digitorum communis [EDC]. Let's practice this together, and I will tell you what I like to say to clients so that they learn this motion well. Clients find it much harder to learn this motion if they have already learned to extend the wrist with the EDC; that is why I prioritize this technique and want you to practice it with clients quite a bit, so that they learn it thoroughly."

CASE 9-2

An inexperienced hand therapist worked on a team with an experienced assistant who was excellent at making splints. The therapist acknowledged her need for more practice making splints. The assistant shared her expertise, and they practiced together. The assistant made it clear that she enjoyed splinting and did not want to lose the opportunity to be involved in that work. The therapist improved her splinting skills and made sure that the assistant continued to have rewarding opportunities to make splints.

SUMMARY

Much of hand therapy probably falls into quadrants I and II of the hand therapy matrix. Be careful with this; *a well-intended but inexperienced therapist or assistant can do permanent harm to a hand client.* For this reason, it is critical that the hand therapy team recognize clinical limitations and improve competencies. Therapists and assistants who are inexperienced in hand therapy but are treating these clients should consult or network with more experienced hand therapists while advancing their clinical skills through reading, workshops and conferences, professional networks, and self-study. The rewards are well worth the effort. At the same time, therapists and assistants should work to maximize their team effectiveness, because this enhances personal satisfaction and improves client care.

Acknowledgments

I wish to thank Michelle Robin Abrams, MS, OTR/L, CEAS; and John L. Evarts for their thoughtful reviews of this chapter and valuable suggestions.

References

1. Brayman SJ, Clark GF, DeLany JV et al: Guidelines for supervision, roles, and responsibilities during the delivery of occupational therapy services, *Am J Occup Ther* 58:663-667, 2004.

2. American Heritage Dictionaries, editor: *The American heritage dictionary of the English language,* ed 3, Boston, 1996, Houghton Mifflin.

3. Cooper C, Zarbock P, Zondlo JW: OTR and OTA collaboration in hand therapy, AOTA Physical Disabilities Special Interest Section Quarterly 23:2-4, 2000.

APPENDIX TO PART TWO

Some Thoughts on Professionalism

CYNTHIA COOPER

"Sincerity is the most important thing . . . learn to fake that, and you've got it made". From
The Human Stain, by Philip Roth, New York: Vintage International, 2000.

WHAT IS PROFESSIONALISM?

Professionalism is a combination of maturity and effectiveness. In the workplace, professional behavior is demonstrated by being the best you can be and doing the best you can, even if you are not in the mood to do so. Professionalism has been described as being a "class act," with emotionality being replaced by focus and responsibility. Instead of making decisions based on emotion, the professional relies on intellect and experience. Although professionalism implies treating others with respect, it does not imply elimination of empathy. While behaving professionally, we should still wonder what it is like to be in the client's shoes. In other words, we should try to understand our clients' subjective experiences.

WHY IS PROFESSIONALISM IMPORTANT IN HAND THERAPY?

Lack of professionalism contributes to low morale, which reduces our job satisfaction and also negatively affects our clients' experiences. Professional behaviors foster team work, which is advantageous for meeting clients' needs. Opportunities for advancement and success are associated with being perceived as a professional. Additional benefits of professional behavior include receiving the trust of clients and the admiration of colleagues and co-workers.

COMMUNICATION SKILLS RELATED TO PROFESSIONALISM

Professionalism is exemplified by polite and respectful styles of communication, efficient use of time, punctuality, and integrity. These behaviors help convey the message that the client comes first. Minimizing interruptions, answering questions, smiling, having a friendly or open facial expression, and providing eye contact are examples of effective communication. Projecting a sense of confidence and staying calm during difficult situations are additional examples of professionalism.

EXAMPLES OF NON-PROFESSIONAL BEHAVIOR

Example One

AA is an attractive female hand therapist who is single. She would like to meet a doctor at work. She wears low-cut tops and skimpy clothes to work, eliciting the attention of male clients and physicians. She has conversations in front of clients about her dates from previous nights. She is asked by doctors in front of clients if she would like to be fixed up with their single friends.

Questions: How does AA's behavior affect the professionalism of the clinic? What can be done to help correct this situation?

Example Two

BB is a hand therapist who feels she has excellent splinting skills. When a co-worker's client returns to clinic after not showing for appointments for 3 weeks, BB assesses the client's splint and notices that it no longer fits well due to clinical changes in the client's forearm and hand over the 3-week absence. BB states to the client: "This splint was made poorly and does not fit well. In fact, it is causing damage to your tissues. I will fix it for you and will make sure the other therapist is informed of the poor quality of her splint."

Questions: How could she have worded this more professionally?

Example Three

DD is a therapist who believes that hand therapy should be painful. She imposes painful forces on delicate finger joints during PROM and tells clients that this will help them. Her clients frequently have flare responses with pain, edema, and stiffness. She yells at her clients to "Relax" while she performs painful PROM on their digits.

Questions: Is this an issue of professionalism or is it a lack of clinical understanding? What type of communication skills would be more effective in helping a client relax? For example, before removing sutures, what could you say to your client and how would you say it?

Example Four

EE is a hand therapist who is hoping to find a new career. She treats a client who is self-employed. She begins a business relationship with the client, exploring prospects to start a business together while still treating him. She uses the work computer on this project while her scheduled clients wait to be seen late by her.

Questions: What problems in professionalism do you see here? What solutions do you suggest?

Example Five

FF is an experienced hand therapist who has a very busy home life. She talks to her clients more about her own home life than about their lives or their hand therapy. She often receives presents from clients.

Questions: What changes in behavior would improve FF's professionalism with her clients?

CHARACTERISTICS OF PROFESSIONAL BEHAVIOR

- Arrive at work on time and start your first clients on time.
- Notify clients who are waiting if you are running late.
- Listen to your clients.
- Take pride in your work.
- Take initiative by identifying and implementing changes that improve efficiency and clinical care.
- Be open to constructive feedback.
- Ask for help if you need it.
- Admit it if you do not know something.

- Be trustworthy.
- Be pleasant.
- Be aware of your facility's policy about receiving gifts from clients.

TIPS FROM THE FIELD

- Start the day with a pleasant expression on your face, even if you are not feeling that way. Doing so may actually make you feel better.
- Be hopeful with clients and pleasant with colleagues.
- Present a harmonious team front to clients, even if there are differences to be ironed out in private. Be as professional as possible.
- Do not discuss politics or religion with clients.
- Do not have any business activity with clients.
- Be open to suggestions from colleagues and give positive feedback for good suggestions.
- Do not feel obliged to become friends with or socialize with team members. Prioritize a good working relationship that focuses on clients' needs. If your clients feel well-cared for, you will become close with your team members on a professional level.
- If the workload is skewed, try to help each other as appropriate.

SUMMARY

Our profession is hurt by therapists who are competent in hand therapy if they are incompetent in professionalism. We probably all recognize acquaintances or colleagues in the examples sited above. In truth, we may even recognize ourselves there a little bit. These thoughts and case examples remind readers that therapists and clients alike can benefit from ongoing efforts to improve our professionalism.

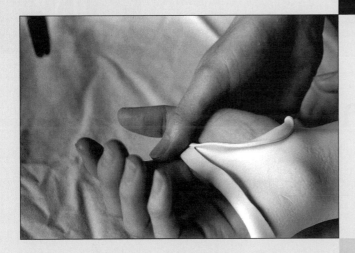

Part THREE

Treatment Guidelines for Common Diagnoses of the Upper Extremity

10

Common Shoulder Diagnoses

MARK W. BUTLER

KEY TERMS

Adhesive capsulitis

Annulus fibrosis

Autonomic instability

Axial skeleton

Bankart lesion

Bifocal

Capsular plication

Closed chain exercises

Close packed position

Concentric

Degrees of freedom

Directional preference

Disk herniations

Eccentric

Elevated Arm Stress Test

Extraarticular

Facet joints

Force couple

Gold standard

Hemiarthroplasty

Hill-Sachs lesion

Impingement

Intervertebral foramen

Intraneural scarring

Mechanoreceptors

Negative intracapsular pressure

Neural mobility

Neurolysis

Nociceptors

Nucleus pulposus

Open chain exercises

Open packed position

Perineural scarring

Plane synovial joint

Plyometric exercises

Premorbid

Roos Test

Rotator interval

Scaption

Scapular kinematics

Sensitivity

Specificity

Spurling's Test

Supraclavicular scalenectomy

Tinel's sign

Trigger point

Uncinate processes

Unifocal

Positioning the hand in space to allow for interaction with the environment is the primary function of the shoulder. Accordingly, dysfunction of the shoulder complex often results in profound impairment of the entire upper extremity (UE).[1] The shoulder will compensate for decreased mobility of the wrist and elbow, which can lead to shoulder dysfunction as the individual tries to perform normal activities of daily living (ADL).

CLINICAL *Pearl*

When treating a client with elbow or wrist dysfunction, the therapist needs to monitor the health of the shoulder. Therefore a thorough understanding of the shoulder is imperative for therapists treating clients with UE dysfunction.

The shoulder has the greatest range of motion (ROM) of any joint in the body. This ROM is the result of the aggregate movement of a series of articulations that make up the shoulder complex. These articulations work in concert to provide a unique balance between mobility and stability, with the emphasis on mobility. A shift in this balance often results in (or can be caused by) the pathologic processes we review in this chapter.

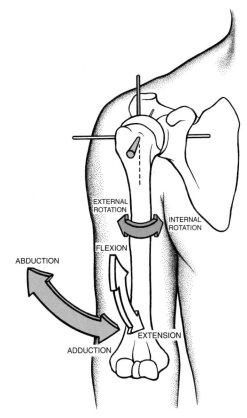

FIGURE 10-1   The three degrees of freedom of the glenohumeral joint: flexion/extension, abduction/adduction, and internal/external rotation. (From Neumann DA: Shoulder complex. In Neumann DA, editor: *Kinesiology of the musculoskeletal system*, St Louis, 2002, Mosby.)

ANATOMY

The shoulder complex consists of the following:

*   Three bones: the humerus, the clavicle, and the scapula
*   Three joints: the glenohumeral, acromioclavicular, and sternoclavicular
*   One pseudojoint: the scapulothoracic articulation.

Glenohumeral Joint

The glenohumeral joint is a multiaxial, synovial, ball-and-socket joint that moves around three axes of motion: internal/external rotation around a vertical axis, abduction/adduction around a sagittal axis, and flexion/extension around a frontal axis (Fig. 10-1). The humeral head forms roughly half a sphere with the glenoid fossa, forming the socket component of the joint. The glenoid fossa covers only one third to one fourth of the humeral head (Fig. 10-2). The glenoid labrum, a ring of fibrocartilage, surrounds and deepens the glenoid socket by about 50% and increases joint stability by increasing humeral head contact 75% vertically and 56% transversely.[2,3]

The **open packed position** (joint position in which the capsule and ligaments are most lax and separation of joint surfaces is greatest) of the glenohumeral joint is 55 degrees of abduction and 30 degrees of horizontal adduction. The **close packed position** (joint position in which the capsule and ligaments are under the most tension with maximal contact between joint surfaces) of the joint is full abduction and lateral rotation. At rest, the humerus sits centered in the glenoid cavity; with contraction of the rotator cuff (RC) muscles, the humeral head translates anteriorly, posteriorly, superiorly, inferiorly, or any combination of these movements. These translations are small, but full motion of the glenohumeral joint is impossible without them. The motion of the glenohumeral joint contributes the most to shoulder movement.

Acromioclavicular Joint

The acromioclavicular joint is a **plane synovial joint** (joint with a synovium-lined capsule and relatively flat surfaces) that augments the ROM of the glenohumeral

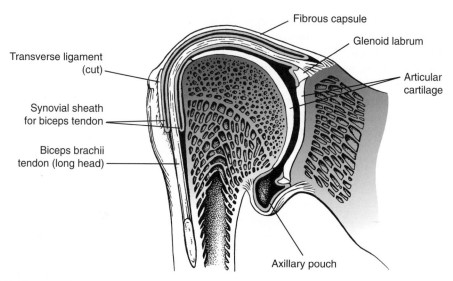

FIGURE 10-2 Anterior view of a frontal section through the right glenohumeral joint. (From Neumann DA: Shoulder complex. In Neumann DA, editor: *Kinesiology of the musculoskeletal system*, St Louis, 2002, Mosby.)

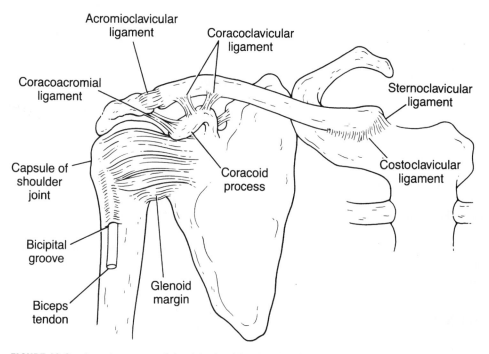

FIGURE 10-3 Anterior aspect of the right shoulder showing the joint capsule and acromioclavicular ligaments. (From O'Donoghue DH: *Treatment of injuries to athletes*, Philadelphia, 1984, WB Saunders.)

joint, as this is the joint around which the scapula moves. The bones that compose the acromioclavicular joint are the acromion process of the scapula and the distal end of the clavicle. The acromioclavicular joint moves around three axes: pure spin around a longitudinal axis for abduction/adduction of the shoulder, a vertical axis for

protraction/retraction of the shoulder, and a horizontal axis for shoulder elevation/depression.

The acromioclavicular and coracoclavicular ligaments support the acromioclavicular joint (Fig. 10-3). The acromioclavicular ligaments contribute the least to joint stability; they function mainly to support the joint capsule and check anterior/posterior translation of the clavicle on the acromion. The acromioclavicular ligaments are damaged in grade I shoulder separations. The coracoclavicular ligaments have no attachment to the acromion and consist of the conoid and trapezoid ligaments. They transmit scapular motion to the clavicle and check superior clavicular displacement.[4] Complete rupture of these ligaments represents a grade III separation resulting in a step deformity at the acromioclavicular joint (Fig. 10-4).

The open packed position for the acromioclavicular joint is with the arm by the side. The close packed position is at 90 degrees of shoulder abduction.

Sternoclavicular Joint

The sellar-shaped (saddle-shaped) sternoclavicular joint is the only direct articulation between the shoulder complex and the **axial skeleton** (skeletal components consisting of the skull, rib cage, spine, and pelvis). The articulations of the sternoclavicular joint are between the medial end of the clavicle, the clavicular notch of the sternum, and the cartilage of the first rib. Interposed between the clavicle and the sternum is an articular disk that enhances stability of the joint (Fig. 10-5, A). Movement between the disk and clavicle is greater than movement between the disk and sternum. The joint is stabilized further by the joint capsule and ligaments that primarily check superior and anterior translation. In fact, the ster-

noclavicular joint is stabilized so well by the disk and ligaments that trauma to the clavicle usually results in fracture instead of dislocation.[5] The three **degrees of freedom** (direction or type of motion at a joint) at the sternoclavicular joint are elevation/depression, protraction/retraction, and rotation (spin) (Fig. 10-5, *B*). The open packed position for the sternoclavicular joint is with the arm by the side. The close packed position is full UE elevation.

Scapulothoracic Articulation

Because the scapula has no direct bony or ligamentous connections to the thorax, the scapulothoracic articulation cannot be considered an anatomic joint.[6] Scapular movement results in movement of the shoulder girdle. These movements are described as elevation/depression, abduction (protraction)/adduction (retraction), upward rotation, and upward tilt.[7] The bony articulation of the scapula is with the acromioclavicular joint, but the sta-

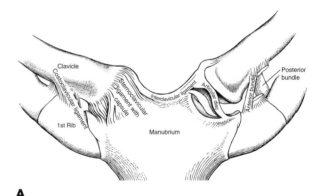

A

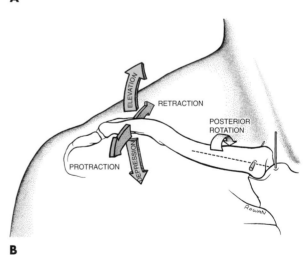

B

FIGURE 10-5 A, Sternoclavicular joints. **B,** The right sternoclavicular joint showing osteokinematic motions of the clavicle. (From Neumann DA: Shoulder complex. In Neumann DA, editor: *Kinesiology of the musculoskeletal system,* St Louis, 2002, Mosby.)

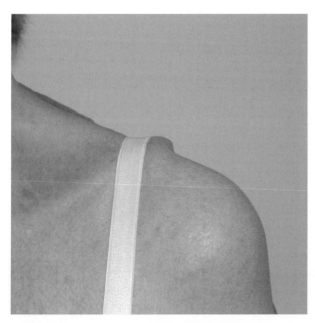

FIGURE 10-4 Chronic grade III acromioclavicular separation showing step deformity indicating disruption of the coracoclavicular ligaments.

bility of the scapulothoracic joint comes from muscular attachments to the scapula.

Much like a street performer balancing a ball on the end of a stick, the scapula must change position during shoulder elevation to keep the humeral head balanced in the glenoid fossa. With shoulder elevation, the majority of motion occurs at the glenohumeral joint during the initial (0 to 60 degrees) and final (140 to 180 degrees) phases of motion. During these phases, the scapulothoracic articulation plays a more subtle balancing or stabilizing role. Throughout the middle or critical (60 to 140 degrees) phase of shoulder elevation, the ratio of glenohumeral to scapulothoracic motion shifts, with more emphasis on scapulothoracic movement.[6]

This movement of the scapula is the result of force couples between groups of muscles that run from the thorax to the scapula (Table 10-1). A **force couple** is defined as two resultant forces of equal magnitude in opposite directions that produce rotation of a structure. The upward rotation of the scapula that occurs during shoulder elevation primarily results from the **concentric** (muscle contraction resulting in approximation of the origin and insertion) actions of the upper and lower trapezius and the lower portion of the serratus anterior muscles. **Eccentric** (muscle contraction to stabilize movement resulting in increased distance between the origin and insertion) actions of the levator scapulae, rhomboids, and pectoralis minor produce smooth motion.

In the normal resting position the scapula sits angled 20 to 30 degrees forward relative to the frontal plane and 20 degrees forward in the sagittal plane, with the medial boarder angled at 3 degrees top to bottom from the spinous processes. This position, combined with the orientation of the glenoid fossa, results in elevation of the arm in a plane that is 30 to 45 degrees anterior to the frontal plane. This motion is termed *scapular plane abduction* or **scaption**.[7] The scapula extends from the level of the T2 spinous process to the T7 or T9 spinous process based on size. Because the scapulothoracic articulation is not an anatomic joint, there is no close packed position.

PROXIMAL (CERVICAL) SCREENING

Because of the proximity of the cervical spine to the shoulder, the cervical spine must be screened for contribution to the client's symptoms. A basic understanding of cervical anatomy and of the structures that refer symptoms to the shoulder and UE is essential to the screening process.

Anatomy

The cervical structures that refer symptoms to the shoulder and entire UE that are cleared via cervical screening are the following:

- Cervical nerve roots
- Cervical disks
- Cervical facets

TABLE 10-1

Scapular Force Couples

MOVEMENT	CONCENTRIC FORCE COUPLE	ECCENTRIC STABILIZERS
Upward rotation (glenohumeral elevation)	Upper trapezius Lower trapezius Serratus anterior	Levator scapulae Rhomboid muscles Pectoralis minor
Retraction	Trapezius Rhomboid muscles	Serratus anterior Pectoralis major Pectoralis minor
Protraction	Serratus anterior Pectoralis major Pectoralis minor	Trapezius Rhomboid muscles
Elevation	Upper trapezius Levator scapulae	Serratus anterior Lower trapezius
Depression	Serratus anterior Lower trapezius	Upper trapezius Levator scapulae
Downward rotation	Levator scapulae Rhomboid muscles Latissimus dorsi Pectoralis minor	Upper trapezius Lower trapezius Serratus anterior

- Cervical intrinsic soft tissue (muscles, ligaments, joint capsules)
- Cervical extrinsic musculature

Cervical Nerve Roots

The C4 to C7 nerve roots supply structures that overlie or compose the shoulder complex (Fig. 10-6). The C5 and C6 nerve roots innervate most of the glenohumeral joint structures, with the C4 nerve root innervating the acromioclavicular joint.

Because of their location and path of travel, the cervical nerve roots are susceptible to injury. **Disk herniations** (damage to the annular wall of the disk resulting in disk deformity as the nucleus displaces into the lesion) can entrap the nerve root against the vertebral lamina and encroach upon the dorsal root ganglion. Hypertrophy of the **facet joints,** spurring of the vertebral end plates, and spurring of the **uncinate processes** (winglike projections from the superior portion of the cervical vertebrae that articulate with the inferior portion of the vertebrae above) will narrow the **intervertebral foramen** (bony canal that contains the spinal nerve), resulting in compression of the cervical nerve roots. Degenerative loss of cervical disk height further enhances this process.

Cervical Disks

The cervical spine contains five disks, with the most superior disk located between C2 and C3, and the most inferior disk located between C7 and T1. The disk con-

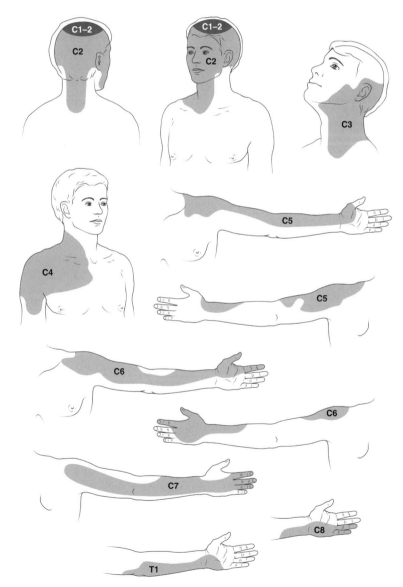

FIGURE 10-6 Cervical dermatomes affecting the shoulder. (From Magee DJ: *Orthopaedic physical assessment,* ed 4, Philadelphia, 2002, Saunders.)

sists of three parts: the **annulus fibrosis** (multilayered ligamentous exterior of the disk), the *vertebral end plate* (cartilaginous interface between the vertebral disk and the vertebral body), and the **nucleus pulposus** (pulpy semiliquid center of the disk). The cervical disks are morphologically different from lumbar disks because they essentially lack a posterior annular wall. That role mainly is supplied by the posterior longitudinal ligament. Also, the cervical disk develops horizontal annular clefts or tears in the lateral portion by age 15 that progressively extend across the back of the disk.[8] Likely because of these differences, the cervical disks degenerate more quickly than the lumbar disks.[9]

CLINICAL *Pearl*

The onset of neck and arm pain with cervical disk herniation is usually insidious and often starts in the neck and medial scapular border before radiating to the shoulder and arm.

Symptoms can spread as far as the hand, depending on the involved nerve root.

Cervical Facets
The facet joints of the cervical spine are paired synovial joints with fibrous capsules. The capsules are heavily innervated by **mechanoreceptors** (specialized nerve endings that transmit information regarding position and motion) and **nociceptors** (specialized nerve endings that transmit pain signals) that likely modulate protective muscle reflexes that are important in preventing joint instability and degeneration.[10]

Studies on normal individuals and clients with neck pain demonstrated pain referral patterns from the cervical facets to the cervical and shoulder regions.[11,12] These studies demonstrated a consistent pain referral pattern to the top and lateral parts of the shoulder, extending to the inferior border of the scapula from the C6-C7 facet joints.

Cervical Intrinsic Soft Tissue
The intrinsic soft tissue structures of the cervical/thoracic region include the muscles that do not originate or insert on the clavicle or scapula. Of these muscles, the scalene muscles demonstrate **trigger point** (palpable taut muscle bands that refer pain when compressed) pain referral patterns to the shoulder (see Fig. 10-20 on the CD). Substantial anatomic variations in the attachments of the scalene muscles exist. In general, the proximal portions attach to the transverse processes of the cervical vertebrae. The distal attachments of the anterior and

medial scalene muscles are the first rib; the distal attachment of the posterior scalene muscle is the second rib. The trigger points refer pain to the anterior lateral aspect of the shoulder and medial scapular border.[13]

Cervical Extrinsic Muscle
The extrinsic muscles are those that have attachments to the shoulder structures (scapula and clavicle) and cervical spine. Of these, the trapezius and levator scapulae demonstrate trigger point pain referral patterns to the shoulder.

The trapezius extends down the midline from the occiput to T12, laterally to the acromion, anteriorly to the clavicle, and posteriorly to the scapular spine. Six trigger points with distinctive pain patterns are located in the upper, middle, and lower fibers. The trigger point located in the lower trapezius refers pain to the mastoid area and the posterior acromion[13] (see Fig. 10-21 on CD).

The levator scapulae attaches proximally to the transverse processes of the first four cervical vertebrae and distally to the superior angle of the scapula. The trigger point refers pain to the angle of the neck and often projects to the posterior aspect of the shoulder[13] (see Fig. 10-22 on CD).

Diagnosis and Pathology

The primary goal of the cervical screening examination is to screen efficiently for pathologic cervical conditions that may be contributing to or causing shoulder symptoms. If screening indicates a pathologic cervical condition, the examiner must perform further testing of the cervical spine. Numerous examination procedures are described in the literature that are beyond the scope of this chapter.

Precaution. *The following screening procedures are not a substitute for a complete examination of the cervical spine.*

Range of Motion Testing: Intrinsic versus Extrinsic Restrictions
Having the client perform active movements of the cervical spine is an excellent beginning point for your screening examination. By changing the relative position of the shoulder and cervical spine during testing, you can begin to differentiate between intrinsic and extrinsic restrictions to cervical motion.

The client performs the basic motions of the cervical spine (flexion/extension, rotation, lateral flexion) from a corrected neutral seated posture with the arms unsupported. Next, the client performs the same motions in a crossed-arm position (see Fig. 10-23 on the CD). The client grasps as close to the acromioclavicular joints as possible and then relaxes the arms and shoulders, letting the arms rest against the chest wall.

This position effectively elevates the scapulae, and by having the client grasp the shoulders, the scapular elevators are allowed to relax. An improvement in ROM in this position implicates the extrinsic cervical structures as contributing to motion loss. No change in motion implicates the intrinsic structures. However, the extrinsic structures still may be limiting motion. The test is designed to rule out intrinsic restrictions if a difference exists between the two test positions.

Repeated Motion Testing: The Search for a Directional Preference

Repeated motion testing is the basis of the McKenzie model of examination. By having the client perform the cervical motions of protrusion, retraction, retraction and extension, flexion, lateral flexion, and rotation in groups of 5 to 10 repetitions, the therapist looks for a **directional preference**.

A directional preference exists if any of these movements centralize or decrease the client's symptoms. An important note concerning centralization is that the client's proximal pain levels may intensify.

CLINICAL *Pearl*

Worsening or peripheralization of the client's distal symptoms with repeated cervical motion indicates a pathologic cervical condition.[14]

Intervertebral Foramen Closing/Facet Loading Testing: Spurling's Test

Although the use of **Spurling's Test** as a screening tool to detect radiculopathy has been questioned[15] because of a **sensitivity** (few if any clients with the disease will have negative test results) of 30% compared with electromyogram findings, its **specificity** (all persons who do not have the disease will have negative test results) was high at 95%. The use of electromyogram as a **gold standard** (the best available test to diagnose a condition) for detecting radiculopathy is questionable because the American Academy of Electrodiagnostic Medicine[16] estimates a sensitivity of 50% to 71%. By accurately applying a test with high specificity, clients without a confirmed pathologic condition should test negative. Therefore in ruling out the cervical spine as a possible source of shoulder pain, the Spurling's Test is clinically relevant.

Spurling and Scoville[17] described the test as positive with provocation of the client's symptoms when the

client's neck was flexed laterally to the painful side, extended, and with axial loading of the client's spine added by the examiner after rotation toward and away from the painful side. With the cervical spine in this position the intervertebral foramen diameter closes down, decreasing the available space for an inflamed nerve root. The presence of a space occupying lesion such a disk herniation or osteophytic spur intensifies the test result. Axial loading at end-range of extension and rotation also stresses the facet joints, provoking symptoms if a pathologic condition is present.

THORACIC OUTLET SYNDROME/BRACHIAL PLEXOPATHY

The term *thoracic outlet syndrome* (TOS) encompasses an assortment of clinical entities involving the shoulder region. The thoracic outlet provides the pathway for the neural and vascular structures to the upper limb; therefore a pathologic condition of this area has profound and often disabling results. Because vascular presentations of TOS are relatively uncommon (3% to 5%), the great majority of clients with TOS have brachial plexopathies.[18]

Anatomy

Thoracic Outlet

The thoracic outlet can be divided into four regions: the sternocostovertebral space, the scalene triangle, the costoclavicular space, and the pectoralis minor (coracopectoral) space. Each region has distinct boundaries, contents, and potential pathologic conditions that result in neurovascular compression and/or entrapment (Fig. 10-7).

Sternocostovertebral Space

The sternocostovertebral space is bordered anteriorly by the sternum, posteriorly by the spinal column, and laterally by the first rib. The contents are the roots of the plexus, the subclavian artery and vein, jugular vein, and neck lymphatic vessels. Compression of the contents usually is caused by tumors of the lung (Pancoast's), thymus, parathyroid glands, and lymph nodes.

Scalene Triangle

The scalene triangle is bordered anteriorly by the anterior scalene muscle, posteriorly by the middle scalene muscle, and inferiorly by the first rib. The contents are the roots and trunks of the plexus and subclavian artery. Compression and entrapment of these structures are caused by variations in scalene anatomy and the presence of congenital fibrous bands that may interdigitate with the plexus.[19]

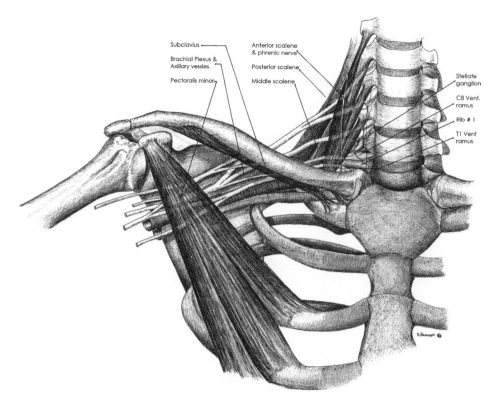

FIGURE 10-7 The thoracic outlet. (From Edgelow PI: Neurovascular consequences of cumulative trauma disorders affecting the thoracic outlet: a patient-centered treatment approach. In Donatelli RA, editor: *Physical therapy of the shoulder*, ed 4, St Louis, 2004, Churchill Livingstone. Courtesy Peter Edgelow.)

Costoclavicular Space

The costoclavicular space is bordered superiorly by the clavicle and inferiorly by the first rib. The contents are the divisions of the plexus and the subclavian artery and vein. Compression of these structures between the clavicle and first rib occurs as a result of postural deficits resulting in shoulder girdle depression, clavicular and first rib fractures, and the presence of a cervical rib.

Pectoralis Minor (Coracopectoral) Space

The coracopectoral space is bordered superiorly by the coracoid process, anteriorly by the pectoralis minor, and posteriorly by the chest wall. The contents are the cords of the plexus and the subclavian artery and vein. Compression of these structures is caused by hypertrophy and contracture of the pectoralis minor and hyperabduction of the arm as they are pulled up against the pectoralis minor tendon.

Brachial Plexus

The brachial plexus is netlike, which allows for the individual neurons from the spinal nerves eventually to reach their respective peripheral nerve. The brachial plexus also serves as a force distributor to dissipate traction

forces from the peripheral nerve, helping to prevent traction injuries of the lower cervical nerve roots.

Although anatomic variations exist, the brachial plexus is fairly consistent in its organization (Box 10-1). Moving proximal to distal, the plexus is organized into roots (C5 to T1), trunks (upper, middle, lower), divisions (anterior, posterior), and cords (medial, lateral, posterior). Trunks are supraclavicular and cords are infraclavicular, with the divisions occurring under the clavicle.

Diagnosis and Pathology

Vascular Component

The diagnosis of TOS versus brachial plexopathy is somewhat controversial. TOS, being a syndrome, by definition is a collection of symptoms related to a pathologic condition of an anatomic space (the thoracic outlet). Brachial plexopathy by definition is a pathologic condition of a specific anatomic structure (the brachial plexus). A wide range of criteria are used as to what symptoms make up TOS. To simplify the diagnosis, true TOS should include a component of vascular compression and brachial plexus compression and/or entrapment. The vascular component of TOS ought to be diagnosed via

BOX 10-1

Organization Highlights of the Brachial Plexus

- Of the five nerve roots that supply the plexus, the top two make up the upper trunk, the bottom two make up the lower trunk, and the middle root makes up the middle trunk
- Upper trunk supplies the scapular musculature and scapular stabilizers
- Lower trunk supplies the hand intrinsics
- Anterior division of the lower trunk supplies the medial cord
- Anterior divisions of the upper and middle trunk supply the lateral cord
- Anterior divisions supply the elbow and wrist flexors with the exception of the brachioradialis, which is supplied by the posterior cord
- Posterior divisions of all trunks supply the posterior cord
- Posterior cord supplies the elbow and wrist extensors

vascular studies because there is often a sympathetic nervous system component to the brachial plexopathy that presents clinically with vascular symptoms.

Unfortunately, the clinical tests advocated in the literature to look for vascular compromise—such as the Adson's and Wright's Tests, which rely on obliteration of the radial pulse while in the test position—have a high incidence (as high as 87%) of positive results in normal persons.[20-23] Therefore, drawing conclusions based on the results of these tests in the clinic is questionable.

Neural Component: Brachial Plexopathy

Because of the paucity of diagnostic tests that detect mild to moderate brachial plexopathies, the best way to identify a brachial plexopathy is through careful and thorough evaluation. This should include a detailed history as to the onset of symptoms and mechanism of injury. Onset of symptoms is often traumatic, with trauma involving forced lateral cervical flexion with the shoulder held in a fixed position (as in a seat belt injury), or forced depression of the shoulder combined with forced lateral cervical flexion (as in a sports injury such as "burner" syndrome), or even dislocation of the shoulder. Symptoms may be delayed for months as adhesions form between the neural tissue and surrounding nerve bed. This leads to restricted **neural mobility** (the ability of the neural structures to adjust to changes in the nerve bed length through a combination of gliding and elongation), ultimately resulting in loss of UE motion and function.

Onset can be insidious, with genetic and morphologic predisposition combined with poor postural and movement habits leading to the development of the condition. During the growth phase into adolescence, the scapulae gradually descend down the posterior thorax, with the descent being greater in women. A strain with resulting weakness of the scapular suspensory muscles that lengthen during this process is associated with the development of brachial plexopathy. This helps to explain the rarity of insidious-onset brachial plexopathy before puberty and the increased incidence of the disease in women.[24]

Clients with brachial plexopathy often complain of unilateral headaches in the occipital region, with facial pain from the angle of the jaw to the zygomatic region to the ear. They may complain of shoulder and chest wall pain from the trapezius ridge down the medial border of the scapula, in the supraclavicular/infraclavicular fossa, and from the sternum to the axilla to the epigastric region. These clients often are seen in the emergency room for a suspected heart attack but are misdiagnosed with costal chondritis or gastritis.[25]

Arm and hand involvement often includes complaints of pain, paresthesia, and weakness.

CLINICAL *Pearl*

A strong clue that the plexus is involved is that these symptoms do not follow dermatomal or peripheral nerve distributions. Other strong indications that the plexus is involved are intolerance to overhead activities, reports of dropping objects, cramping of the hand intrinsics while writing, waking with a "dead arm," and intolerance of straps across the top of the shoulder.

Timelines and Healing

Full recovery from a brachial plexus injury is rare. However, clients often can achieve enough of a reduction in symptoms to allow for a return to restricted activity. The level of restriction is related to the severity of the original injury and the amount of **intraneural scarring** (contained within the nerve) and/or **perineural scarring** (between the nerve and the nerve bed). This is a lifelong injury, and the client must be instructed in management of the condition. Unfortunately, the condition is characterized by periods of high and low neural irritability based on the client's activity level and the degree of pathology. Reirritation of the injured plexus leads to further scarring and pathology as a result of inflammatory reaction.

Nonoperative Treatment

The most important step to begin healing is to teach the client how not to irritate the injured plexus. Through neural mobility assessment, clients can be taught where the safe boundaries of motion are. If the client is able to follow these movement restrictions and plexus irritation drops to a stable level, the client can attempt to regain plexus mobility through gliding and stretching exercises. As plexus mobility improves, the safe boundaries of motion increase, resulting in improved ADL function.

Clients must be taught how to breathe using the diaphragm, minimizing the use of the scalene muscles; and they must be instructed in safe sleeping positions to avoid stretching or compressing the plexus. Most importantly, the client must be taught to maintain a posture that minimizes stress on the brachial plexus while maximizing the apertures of the thoracic outlet.

Precaution. *Clients with brachial plexopathy rarely tolerate weight training at the gym, but guided exercises to strengthen the scapular stabilizers and elevators are essential.*

With direct supervision, clients can use resistance bands to strengthen the upper, middle, and lower trapezius, as well as the levator scapulae, rhomboid muscles, and serratus anterior. Doing the exercises in sets of 3 repetitions allows the therapist and client to assess for signs of increased plexus irritation between sets, thereby avoiding overstressing of the thoracic outlet contents.

Clients can regain scapular proprioception through visual feedback exercises. The client stands facing the mirror while performing scapular motions, targeting points of the clock. With 12 o'clock being superior, 9 o'clock anterior, and 3 o'clock posterior, the client symmetrically elevates the shoulders to the 12, 1, and 2 o'clock positions. These exercises are performed in straight lines of motion as smoothly as possible. After each cycle the client assesses the level of irritation and adjusts the exercise accordingly.

The client performs gliding and stretching exercises in front of the mirror as well. The client begins the glide exercise with the arms against the side, elbows flexed to 90 degrees with the palms facing up. Next, the client elevates the shoulders while slowly extending the elbows. To bias the medial and lateral cords of the plexus, the client maintains supination while extending the wrists (see Fig. 10-24 on the CD). To bias the posterior cord of the plexus, the client pronates the forearms and flexes the wrists (see Fig. 10-25 on the CD).

The client begins the stretch exercise with the palm of the hand brought to eye level in front of the face, elbow held close to the body. While maintaining the hand at eye level, the client moves the shoulder into abduction and external rotation, with the wrist held in supination. Again keeping the hand at eye level, the client slowly extends the elbow just until a stretch is felt or a slight increase in symptoms occurs. At this point the client backs off slightly on the elbow extension and flexes and extends the wrist 3 times (Fig. 10-8). The client attempts to straighten the elbow further with each cycle of the exercise. The glide and stretch exercises are performed in sets of 3 as well.

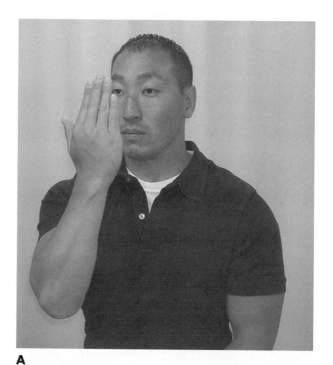
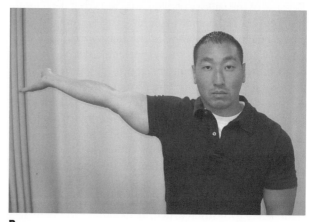

FIGURE 10-8 The brachial plexus nerve stretch. **A,** Starting position and ending position. **B,** Maximal stretch position.

The client performs all exercises from a neutral posture. The client achieves this by lifting the sternum through increasing the lumbar lordosis and elevating the rib cage. This effectively corrects the forward-head–rounded-shoulders posture, relieving stress from the thoracic outlet contents. From this position, the client performs a posture exercise combined with a proximal nerve glide by elevating the shoulders to the 12 o'clock position and then doing the posterior half of a shoulder roll, ending at the starting point. Instruct the client to perform these exercises hourly for 5 to 10 repetitions to reinforce proper posture.

Precaution. *These clients are not to be instructed to "chin tuck" and retract their shoulders to correct their posture, for this often aggravates their condition.*

Clients who demonstrate tight scalene muscles and pectoralis minor muscles must be taught stretching exercises.

Precaution. *Because these muscles lie against the brachial plexus, the therapist must watch for an increase in the client's symptoms during stretching.*

The rule of threes works in this situation as well: sets of three stretches held for 3 seconds. As your client demonstrates good tolerance to the stretch, the stretch can be held for longer periods, or the number of sets can be increased.

Precaution. *The scalene muscle stretches described in the literature and in exercise card kits bias stretch the brachial plexus and therefore should be avoided.*

The literature usually instructs the client to depress the shoulder while stretching, often causing further irritation to the injured plexus (Fig. 10-9). The scalene muscles, having no attachment to the shoulder and being intrinsic to the cervical and thoracic regions, should be stretched with the shoulder held elevated, thereby relieving tension from the brachial plexus during stretching.

Operative Treatment

The primary goal of TOS surgery is decompression of neurovascular contents or **neurolysis** (the removal of scar tissue from the nerve) of the entrapped brachial plexus. Clients who fared the best were those with confirmed vascular or neurologic compromise in the thoracic outlet via diagnostic testing.[26] Unfortunately, surgical outcomes have been disappointing; therefore surgery is reserved as a last resort.[27] The most common procedures are transaxillary first rib resection and **supraclavicular scalenec-**

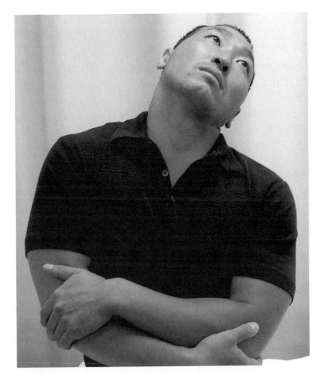

FIGURE 10-9 Scalene muscle stretch of the right scalene muscles. Note shoulder elevation to avoid stretching the plexus.

tomy (surgical removal of the anterior scalene muscle) with neurolysis.

CLINICAL *Pearl*

Maintaining postoperative neural mobility is imperative because the formation of perineural scarring will entrap the plexus, leading to poor surgical outcome.

Neural mobilization exercises are begun as soon as the client is stable, often within the first 3 postoperative days.

Questions to Ask the Doctor *(for the Postoperative Client)*

- *How soon can range of motion exercises begin?*
- *Are there any restrictions to movement of the neck or shoulder?*

What to Say to Clients

About the Condition

"Here is a drawing of your thoracic outlet. You can see that the nerves and blood vessels that supply the arm travel through here. The areas of possible damage are here in your neck (the scalene muscles), between the collar bone and first rib, or under the muscles of your chest wall (pectoralis minor)."

About the Home Exercise Program

"In order for you to move your arm comfortably, your nerves must be able to slide through the thoracic outlet smoothly. You may have developed restrictions that prevent this from happening. Maintaining good posture is critical because you place excessive strain on the nerves with poor posture habits. Your exercises are designed to reinforce proper posture and help the nerves slide through the thoracic outlet, much like sliding a string through a straw."

"Your postural exercises are to be performed hourly to help reinforce good postural habits. Purchase and wear a cheap digital watch you set to 'beep' on the hour to remind you to exercise. Your gliding and stretching exercises are to be performed a minimum of three times a day. Tie these exercises to mealtimes so you will remember to do them."

Evaluation Tips

- Assess the client's ability to achieve the corrected posture position described before.
- Check for asymmetry of scapular/shoulder position.
- Look for swelling over the supraclavicular fossa.
- Monitor the client's UE for evidence of **autonomic instability** (sympathetic nervous system irritation) during testing; for example, reticular mottling, color changes, or temperature changes.
- Palpate along the course of the brachial plexus and peripheral nerves for tenderness and evidence of a **Tinel's sign** (production of tingling or paresthesia with percussion over the nerve)
- Neural mobility testing of the brachial plexus can be graded as follows:
  - 0/5: Shoulder in internal rotation, elbow flexed to 90 degrees with arm across stomach, wrist and fingers in neutral (see Fig. 10-26, A, on the CD)
  - 1/5: Shoulder in neutral, elbow flexed to 90 degrees, wrist and fingers in neutral (see Fig. 10-26, B, on the CD)
  - 2/5: Shoulder in approximately 100 degrees of abduction, neutral rotation, elbow flexed to 90 degrees, wrist and fingers in neutral (see Fig. 10-26, C, on the CD)
  - 3/5: As with the shoulder in approximately 90 degrees of external rotation, forearm in supination, wrist in extension, and fingers in neutral (see Fig. 10-26, D, on the CD)
  - 4/5: As with the elbow flexed to 45 degrees (see Fig. 10-26, E, on the CD)
  - 5/5: As with the elbow to 0 degrees (see Fig. 10-26, F, on the CD)
  - Use the plus or minus signs (+/−) for positions between each grade; or for more specific documentation, list the last grade achieved followed by the goniometric measurement of the shoulder or elbow position, such as 1/5 with 45-degree shoulder abduction or 3/5 with 60-degree elbow flexion.
  - Record position at provocation of symptoms to grade the test.
  - Block shoulder elevation during testing; *do not depress the shoulder.*
- Use the **Elevated Arm Stress Test** (EAST; or Roos Test), and record time to provocation of symptoms. The test is described as a 3 minute test[28]; in my experience, clients with plexopathy will not tolerate more than 1 minute (Fig. 10-10).
- During myotomal screen, focus on scapular elevators for upper trunk lesions and hand intrinsics for lower trunk lesions.
- Using a safety pin flagged with tape as pictured in Fig. 10-11 to check for sensitivity to sharp sensation keeps the level of pressure applied during testing constant. Clients with brachial plexopathy show differential sensation of the middle finger versus sensation of the ring finger for clients with carpal or cubital tunnel syndrome. Decreased sensitivity along the medial half of the ring finger and hand indicates medial cord involvement; decreased sensitivity along the lateral half of the ring finger and hand indicates lateral cord involvement.[25]

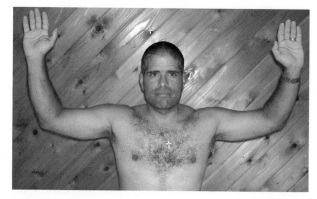

FIGURE 10-10   Test position for the Elevated Arm Stress Test, or Roos Test.

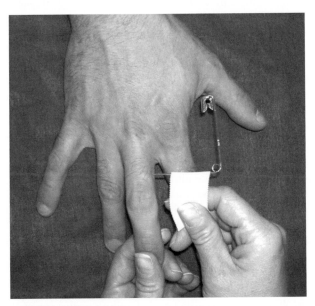

FIGURE 10-11 Example of the use of a flagged safety pin to maintain constant pressure to check for differential of sensation between the medial and lateral aspect of the long finger.

Diagnosis-Specific Information That Affects Clinical Reasoning

CLINICAL *Pearl*

Clients who cannot tolerate the corrected posture position have a positive EAST result in less than 30 seconds or who have neural mobility of the plexus lower than 3/5 have a poorer prognosis, for they easily aggravate their condition during ADL.

Achieving these basic parameters listed in the *Clinical Pearl* section above should be the initial goal of treatment. Base the speed and intensity of the rehabilitation program on the client's level of symptom irritability/stability. Inform your clients with chronic restrictions that they may experience increased symptoms for up to 48 hours after treatment.

Precaution. *If the client's level of posttreatment irritation persists for more than 48 hours, the intensity of the treatment needs to be decreased.*

Tips from the Field

Constantly stress proper posture when your clients are in the clinic. Instruct them to notice the poor posture of others they encounter during their day and to use these observations as a reminder to correct their own posture.

Precaution. *The inability of your client to achieve stable symptoms at correct posture is one of the best predictors of treatment failure.*

Clients often complain that their home exercises are increasing their symptoms. Have them demonstrate their home program regularly and correct any modifications they have made. Adjust the amount of movement during the home exercises to keep symptoms stable.

The application of heat before exercise helps to calm symptoms. Riding the stationary bike for 10 to 15 minutes using proper posture with the involved arm supported is an excellent warm-up exercise.

Precautions and Concerns

- *Avoid overstretching the brachial plexus during treatment.*
- *Be careful with overhead exercise such as wall pulleys.*
- *Use of an upper body ergometer is not recommended for these clients.*
- *Advance the progress of strengthening exercises cautiously.*
- *Watch exercise positions to avoid overstressing the brachial plexus.*

PROXIMAL HUMERUS FRACTURE

Anatomy

Proximal humerus fractures are the most common fracture of the humerus and may involve the articular surface, greater tuberosity, lesser tuberosity, or the surgical neck. These four regions are described as the four major fracture fragments that occur and are the basis of the classification systems for proximal humerus fracture.[29]

Diagnosis and Pathology

The majority of proximal humerus fractures occur as a direct result of a fall on the involved shoulder in the elderly population or a direct blow to the humeral region and are stable one-part or A2 fractures involving the surgical neck of the humerus.[30]

One-part fractures as classified by the Neer system are described as no fracture fragments being displaced more than 1 cm and no more than 45 degrees of angulation. Two-part fractures exceed these position limits and can involve the humeral head and surgical neck or the humeral head and greater tuberosity. Three- and four-part fractures involve the humeral head, greater tuberosity, and lesser tuberosity.[29]

An alternative classification system is that of AO North America (*www.aona.org*) and is predicated on disruption of blood supply to the articular segment. Type A fractures are **extraarticular** (outside the joint capsule) and **unifocal** (one fracture line). Type B fractures are extraarticular and **bifocal** (two fracture lines). Type C fractures are articular. Each of these types then is subdivided into three groups. A1 classified fractures have the least severity and best prognosis; C3 classified fractures have the greatest severity and worst prognosis.

Timelines and Healing

One-part and A2 fractures are treated by sling immobilization initially for 1 to 3 weeks. Clients can start passive movements when the humeral shaft and head move as a unit, which can be as early as 2 weeks. Type B and C or two- to four-part fractures, being more complex, usually require 4 to 6 weeks of immobilization, except in clients with hemiarthroplasties, who begin passive range of motion (PROM) exercises on postoperative day 1.

Nonoperative Treatment

The client begins treatment while still in the immobilizer by performing gripping exercises and active ROM of the elbow and wrist to prevent edema and joint stiffness. Once clinically stable, the client starts PROM exercises in the clinic and pendulum and tabletop PROM exercises at home. The client should continue to wear the sling immobilizer in public and while sleeping for support and protection the first 6 weeks after injury or surgical repair.

The therapist can start more aggressive stretching and the client begins active ROM exercises around 4 to 6 weeks. The focus at this time should be on proper glenohumeral and scapulothoracic movement to prevent the substitution patterns of early scapular elevation and trunk leaning to achieve UE elevation.

Precaution. *Substitution patterns discourage proper recruitment of the RC muscles, so they need to be avoided at all costs.*

The therapist plays a significant role by having the client perform hand-to-hand active-assisted ROM progressing to active ROM mirroring exercises in a seated position while the therapist prevents early scapular elevation (see Fig. 10-27, A, on the CD). Once the client understands the movement concept, the client can perform the same exercise through self-scapular stabilization and wall walking (see Fig. 10-27, B, on the CD). These motions are performed in the scapular plane initially to provide the RC muscles the best length-tension relationship to encourage coordinated activity. At 8 to 12 weeks after injury/repair the client can begin resisted strength training. The focus is on the RC muscles and scapular stabilizer/force couple muscles. Therapist-provided manual resistance in diagonal planes of motion are essential at this stage of the program to encourage functional movements and to discourage substitution movements.

A mixture of open and closed chain exercises must be included at this stage because the shoulder functions in both situations. **Open chain exercises** are defined as working against resistance where the extremity is free to move in space resulting in movement of the distal segment. **Closed chain exercises** are defined as working against resistance with the extremity working against a stationary or mobile but motion-constrained object or surface. Closed chain exercises impart a degree of stability during the exercise motion.

Closed chain exercises include wall push-ups, seated press-ups, weight shifting in quadruped, or prone resting on elbows. Variations include ball rolling against the wall and use of a tilt board for weight bearing in quadruped (see Fig. 10-28 on the CD).

If at 12 weeks after injury/repair the client has achieved functional ROM and normal movement patterns, the client can begin **plyometric exercises** (which link strength and speed of movement to produce an explosive-reactive type of muscle response) and sport-specific activities to prepare them for return to full function. Therefore one must understand the client's goals of rehabilitation and the **premorbid** (before injury) activity level.

Operative Treatment

Proximal humeral fractures graded as two- to three-part or type B usually require surgical intervention of open reduction and internal fixation to reduce the displaced fracture fragments. **Hemiarthroplasty** (prosthetic replacement of one joint surface) usually is indicated to replace the avascular humeral head in four-part and type C fractures.

Questions to Ask the Doctor

Operative Clients

- *What structures were repaired? (Ask for a copy of the operative report.)*
- *How soon can active motion start?*
- *When can I begin lifting weights?*

Nonoperative Clients

- *When can I begin to take off the sling?*
- *How much longer do I need to wear the sling to sleep?*

- *How soon can I begin moving my shoulder?*
- *When can I begin lifting weights?*

What to Say to Clients

About the Injury

If the fracture is classed as one part or A2, say, "Your fracture is considered stable, so you are allowed to begin moving your arm while the healing process continues. In fact, the motion will help the healing process. All motions must be passive, meaning motion provided by the therapist, by gravity, or on a supported surface such as a tabletop. You are not to attempt to raise your arm by itself for the next couple of weeks because this could affect the healing fracture."

If the fracture has been repaired surgically or if it is a two-part or type B and now is considered stable, say, "Your doctor has determined that the fracture is healed enough to begin motion exercises. Movement will make a big difference in how quickly you recover and is critical to your recovery."

About Exercise

"You need to move your arm as often and as much as possible. The motion helps to lubricate the joint and keeps it healthy." If the client is doing tabletop exercises, say, "By using your fingers to pull your arm forward, you will avoid stressing your shoulder during this exercise. Keep your shoulder relaxed while moving; at the end of tolerable motion, rest your hand flat on the table surface while you sit back upright, dragging your arm back to the starting position." If the client is doing pendulum exercises, say, "Do your exercises next to a table or counter. Using the table for support with your uninjured arm, bend at the waist as far as you can and let your injured arm swing forward as if it were a piece of rope. Now rock your body side to side and in circles to get your arm swinging just as you would do with your hand to swing a rope side to side or in a circle."

For all ROM exercises, say, "It is not how hard you push your stretches, but how often you stretch and how much cumulative time you spend at the end of motion that counts. Try for a minimum of fifteen minutes of total end-range time by doing fifty stretches a day, each held for twenty seconds."

Evaluation Tips

Take PROM measurements with the client seated. Make sure motions are slow and gentle because the client will be apprehensive about moving the arm. Often, when you attempt to return the client's arm to neutral after full elevation, the client will experience sharp pain as the deltoid and humeral head elevators reflexively contract, causing sharp pain. By having the client actively lower the arm against your resistance, this reflex is inhibited and the motion will be considerably more comfortable.

Measure functional internal rotation (IR) by seeing which bony landmark on the pelvis or spinous process the client can touch with the thumb (e.g., anterior superior iliac spine, iliac crest, posterior superior iliac spine, or L5).

Diagnosis-Specific Information That Affects Clinical Reasoning

CLINICAL *Pearl*

The type of fracture directly affects how aggressively you may rehabilitate your client.

Obtaining this information from the doctor is crucial. This information is also available from radiology and operative reports.

Alignment of the humeral head to the shaft will affect how much ROM the client ultimately will recover with a minimum of one degree of motion loss in the opposite direction for each degree of deformity. For example, if the shaft is in 45 degrees of extension relative to the humeral head, the client's expected flexion ROM will be 135 degrees (180 degrees − 45 degrees = 135 degrees). The same holds true for rotational deformities.[29]

Tips from the Field

Clients presenting to therapy a few weeks after a one-part or type A proximal humeral fracture usually will be apprehensive about moving the arm because of fears about fracture instability. You have two ways to calm their fears. First, tell them that as you rotate their arm, the humeral head will not move with unified motion if the fracture is unstable. Have them place their hand over their injured humeral head while you gently rotate the arm from IR to external rotation (ER); they should feel the humeral head move. The second and rather novel technique involves using a stethoscope. Explain to the client that sound will not travel well across an open fracture. Next, have the client listen through the stethoscope placed on the humeral head of their healthy shoulder while you tap on their lateral epicondyle. Do the same to their injured shoulder, where the intensity of sound should be the same. This often will decrease their apprehension about moving their shoulder and will speed recovery.

Scapular position and posture have a direct affect on shoulder ROM. Clients must be given postural exercises as previously described for brachial plexus clients.

Precautions and Concerns

- *RC injuries often are overlooked at the time of injury. Watch for evidence of RC tear during rehabilitation.*
- *Clients are at a high risk of developing* **adhesive capsulitis** *(frozen shoulder). Movement must be the basis of any therapy program.*
- *Many of these clients have a concurrent axillary nerve or brachial plexus injury. Screen for this during the initial examination by checking sensation over the deltoid (axillary distribution) and by asking if the client is experiencing paresthesias in the hand or arm (possible brachial plexus involvement).*

FROZEN SHOULDER/ADHESIVE CAPSULITIS

Anatomy

The fibrous capsule that envelopes the glenohumeral joint is lined with synovial tissue. The capsule is attached medially to the glenoid margin and encompasses the glenoid labrum and long head of the biceps. Laterally, the capsule attaches to the anatomic neck of the humeral head near the articular surface. The inferior portion attaches laterally about 1 cm distal to the articular surface on the humeral shaft. The capsule is slack enough that distraction of the glenohumeral joint surfaces up to 3 cm can occur.[5]

The capsule has three distinct thickened areas known as the glenohumeral ligaments (superior, middle, and inferior) that help stabilize the glenohumeral joint. These ligaments become taut at various portions of glenohumeral motion as their fibers run in radial and circular directions. During abduction and rotation, the capsule becomes shortened, producing a compressive and centering force of the humerus on the glenoid.[31] During abduction and rotation, the inferior glenohumeral ligament forms a sling providing anterior, posterior, and inferior stability to the joint. With the arm at rest, this portion of the capsule forms the dependent axillary pouch, which often is obliterated with frozen shoulder (Figs. 10-2 and 10-12).

The coracohumeral ligament extends from the base of the coracoid process as two bands that blend with the capsule running to the greater and lesser tuberosities. Parts of the ligament form the tunnel for the biceps tendon and reinforce the **rotator interval** (the region between the superior edge of the subscapularis and anterior edge of the supraspinatus tendons).

The tendons of the subscapularis, supraspinatus, infraspinatus, and teres minor fuse with the lateral part of the joint capsule forming the RC. With contraction of the RC muscles, the lax capsule is pulled away from the movement path of the humeral head, preventing capsular **impingement.**[5]

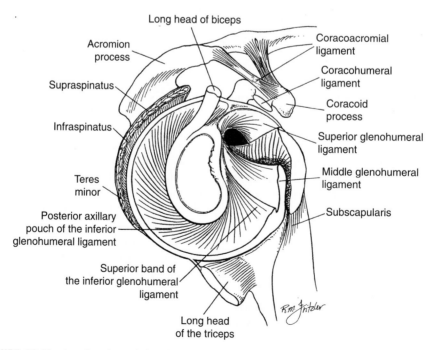

Labels (clockwise):
Long head of biceps
Acromion process
Coracoacromial ligament
Coracohumeral ligament
Supraspinatus
Coracoid process
Infraspinatus
Superior glenohumeral ligament
Middle glenohumeral ligament
Teres minor
Subscapularis
Posterior axillary pouch of the inferior glenohumeral ligament
Superior band of the inferior glenohumeral ligament
Long head of the triceps

FIGURE 10-12 Interior view of the right shoulder joint, looking into the glenoid fossa and joint capsule. (From Canale ST: *Campbell's operative orthopaedics,* ed 10, St Louis, 2003, Mosby.)

Diagnosis and Pathology

The terms *adhesive capsulitis* and *frozen shoulder* are used interchangeably in the literature.

CLINICAL *Pearl*

> Frozen shoulder is characterized by a progressive loss of glenohumeral ROM usually in the capsular pattern of ER being most limited followed by abduction and IR.

Magnetic resonance imaging (MRI) studies demonstrate capsular thickening with loss of the axillary recess.[32] The disease appears to be periarticular, with most authors finding little to no capsular adhesions during arthroscopic examination.

The condition is found in 2% to 3% of the U.S. population, most commonly in the fourth through sixth decades of life. Frozen shoulder is more common among women, with one study reporting women making up 70% of the frozen shoulder clients.[33] Frozen shoulder usually is classified as primary or secondary adhesive capsulitis, with the course of the disease following three phases: the freezing phase, the frozen phase, and the thawing phase.[34]

Primary Adhesive Capsulitis

Primary frozen shoulder is idiopathic. Considerable debate has occurred over the pathogenesis of frozen shoulder, with possible causes being inflammatory, immunologic, endocrine alterations, or biochemical.[34] This form of the disease is overrepresented in clients with diabetes, with rates 3 times that of the normal population.[35]

Histologic findings in a group of clients with primary frozen shoulder revealed active fibroblastic proliferation of the coracohumeral ligament and rotator interval with the absence of inflammation or synovial involvement, much like that of Dupuytren's disease (disease process resulting in thickening and contracture of the palmer fascia).[36] In examining the hands of 58 clients with frozen shoulder, Smith et al.[37] found 30 clients had a pit, nodule, or band of Dupuytren's contracture.

Secondary Adhesive Capsulitis

Secondary frozen shoulder is characterized by a precipitating event such as surgery, trauma to the shoulder, or specific pathologic condition of the shoulder such as bursitis, impingement syndrome, or tendonitis. Although the same pattern of motion loss occurs, these clients may not go through all the stages of freezing, frozen, and thawing.[34]

Freezing Phase

The freezing phase is characterized by shoulder pain interrupting sleep, pain with ADL such as brushing one's hair or tucking in one's shirt, and often pain at rest. Distinguishing frozen shoulder from pathologic conditions such as RC tendonitis, shoulder bursitis, or impingement syndrome is difficult.

Examination of the client during this phase reveals ROM to be close to full with pain occurring often before the end of motion. Palpation reveals nonspecific tenderness at the anterior, lateral, and posterior aspects of the shoulder. Strength is often normal or slightly decreased with pain on resisted testing.

Clients tend to limit the use of the affected extremity because all movements are painful, leading to further loss of motion. Over the next 2 to 9 months, the pain subsides and the client is left with the typical frozen shoulder with pain occurring at the end of motion.

Frozen Phase

The frozen phase may last up to a year. This phase is characterized by distinct pathologic movement patterns as the client attempts to substitute scapulothoracic motion to compensate for the lack of glenohumeral mobility. In this phase, pain occurs with stretching of the joint capsule at the end of motion.

Thawing Phase

The thawing phase is characterized by a gradual return of motion and lasts on average up to 26 months. The idea that full motion will return is a misconception. Thirty percent of clients with primary frozen shoulder exhibited some degree of motion loss compared with the uninvolved shoulder at an average follow-up of 7 years after surgery.[38]

Timelines and Healing

As noted before, there are average timelines for each phase of the disease. The majority of clients complete the thawing phase within 18 months to 3 years from onset.[39]

Nonoperative Treatment

No evidence suggests that therapeutic modalities such as ultrasound or interferential electric stimulation affect the outcome of the disease. Treatment should be directed at the process occurring during each phase of the disease.

Precaution. *Overstretching the capsule during the freezing phase may enhance the inflammatory process, stimulating further capsular fibrosis.*

When the joint has achieved the frozen and thawing phases, the stretching exercises can be more aggressive.

However, avoid pushing to the point that reinitiates the inflammatory process.

The role of the occupational therapist in assisting clients with bilateral frozen shoulder in ADL modifications or adaptive equipment for grooming, bathing, and dressing cannot be overestimated. Clients with unilateral frozen shoulder may benefit from workstation modification to help them remain productive during the protracted course of the disease.

The use of corticosteroids intraarticularly in the freezing phase of the disease may be helpful in stabilizing the synovial tissue, allowing for better tolerance to stretching exercises.[33]

Operative Treatment

For frozen shoulder cases that fail to progress after protracted conservative treatment, manipulation under anesthesia and arthroscopic release are two of the most common surgical interventions. Of the two, arthroscopic release of the anterior glenohumeral ligament and coracohumeral ligament currently has the most promising outcome.[40]

Questions to Ask the Doctor

Operative Clients

- *What was the intraoperative range of motion?*

What to Say to Clients

About the Injury

"Here is a diagram of your shoulder, and this is the joint capsule. Normally, the capsule is loose and develops a redundant pouch at the bottom when your arm is at your side. Having this extra capsule space allows you to raise your arm above your head. Think of your shoulder capsule as an accordion with its folds glued together. That accordion would be unusable since it could not expand; your shoulder is restricted in motion and function as well."

About Exercises/Activities of Daily Living

"Moving your shoulder regularly to the end of comfortable motion helps to prevent motion loss. Avoid positions and activities that cause your shoulder to hurt for more than a few minutes afterward. Sleeping on your back is the best position. If you must sleep on your side, keep your arms to your sides if possible to prevent shoulder irritation. Using a body pillow may help you find a comfortable sleeping position."

"You have to watch your posture. Having your shoulders rounded will place more stress on the supportive tissue and will slow the healing process."

Evaluation Tips

- Take careful baseline and follow-up ROM measurements with the client supine to stabilize the trunk and scapula. This will allow for careful tracking of the progress of the condition.
- If all passive and resisted motions are painful throughout the ROM, the client is still in the freezing stage.
- If resisted motion is pain free and pain occurs only at end ROM, the client is in the frozen or thawing phase.

Diagnosis-Specific Information That Affects Clinical Reasoning

The intensity of the therapy program is directly proportional to the phase of the condition. The primary treatment goal of the freezing phase is to prevent motion loss. The primary treatment goal of the frozen and thawing phase is to restore functional ROM.

Tips from the Field

CLINICAL *Pearl*

Proper posture and normal **scapular kinematics** (scapular movement in sequence and proportion to humeral movement) must be stressed during exercise at all times.

Clients with frozen shoulder quickly develop the pathologic motion of early scapular elevation to raise their arm. This movement pattern can lead to secondary cervical problems, further complicating the recovery process.

Precautions and Concerns

- *Do not push ROM during the freezing phase to the point of pain that lasts more than a few minutes. This will only enhance the inflammatory and fibrosing process.*
- *These clients must avoid self-imposed immobilization.*

GLENOHUMERAL INSTABILITY
Anatomy

Glenohumeral instability could be considered the antithesis of adhesive capsulitis. However, laxity of the glenohumeral joint is a quality that allows full ROM; laxity is not synonymous with instability. When laxity leads to pain with loss of power and shoulder function, then glenohumeral instability exists.

The concepts and structures that contribute to glenohumeral stability can be categorized as static and dynamic. The static stabilizers have a larger role when the shoulder is at rest, whereas the dynamic stabilizers play a larger role when the shoulder is in motion.

The static restraints include **negative intracapsular pressure** (air pressure inside the joint capsule being lower than pressure outside the capsule), the suction effect of the glenoid labrum acting on the humeral head like a plunger, and cohesion-adhesion between the wet smooth surfaces of the humeral head and glenoid fossa. The orientation of the humeral head and glenoid fossa contribute to the static stability of the glenohumeral joint as well. With proper postural positioning of the scapula, the dynamic stabilizers need minimal effort to maintain glenohumeral congruency.[41]

The dynamic restraints include the RC that provides a compressive and positioning force and to a certain degree the long head of the biceps tendon. Although the glenohumeral ligaments are passive structures, they are under relatively little tension with the shoulder at rest. These ligaments serve as a restrictive leash to check force and limit ROM at various positions of the glenohumeral joint during movement. Of these ligaments, the inferior glenohumeral ligament is the most crucial to dynamic glenohumeral stability. The role and functions of this ligament are described in the anatomy section of the discussion of frozen shoulder.

Diagnosis and Pathology

Two major categories are useful in understanding shoulder instability. They are known by the acronyms of AMBRII and TUBS. The major points of each are summarized in Table 10-2. The pathology and treatment of AMBRII and TUBS shoulders are different.

AMBRII shoulders have no history of dislocation or subluxation. The client's major complaint is pain with activity, usually in overhand-throwing motions. This pain often results from impingement (compression of soft tissue between bony structures) that is related to the client's inability to adequately stabilize the scapulothoracic and/or glenohumeral joint because of a pathologic condition of the RC, capsular laxity, and altered proprioception (awareness of joint position). Budoff et al.[42] described this condition as primary instability leading to secondary impingement.

Primary instability is often a combination of global capsular laxity and pathologic imbalances of the RC and shoulder muscles. Weak and/or proprioceptively compromised RC muscles cannot effectively oppose the upward pull of the deltoid muscle during UE elevation. The result is superior migration of the humeral head and impingement of the greater tuberosity and RC against the underside of the acromion and coracoacromial ligament (Fig. 10-13).

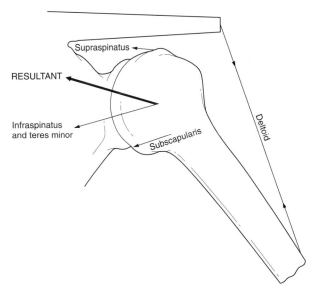

FIGURE 10-13 Force couple between the rotator cuff and deltoid muscle resulting in inferior glide of the humeral head during elevation of the arm. (From Greenfield BH et al: Impingement syndrome and impingement-related instability. In Donatelli RA, editor: *Physical therapy of the shoulder*, ed 4, St Louis, 2004, Churchill Livingstone.)

TABLE 10-2

TUBS versus AMBRII

TUBS OR "TORN LOOSE"	AMBRII OR "BORN LOOSE"
Traumatic etiology	Atraumatic or microtrauma with no specific episode
Unidirectional instability	Multidirectional instability may be present
Bankart lesion is the pathology	Bilateral: asymptomatic shoulder is also loose
Surgery is required	Rehabilitation is the treatment of choice
	Inferior capsular shift and
	Interval between the supraspinatus and subscapularis closed surgically if conservative measures fail

TUBS shoulders have a history of dislocation, usually in the anterior direction. The mechanism of injury is a fall or blow to the arm while in the position of abduction and ER. Recurrent subluxation or dislocation results when the client places the arm in the position of injury, leading to apprehension and dysfunction. These clients often have a resulting **Bankart lesion,** which consists of damage to the anterior glenohumeral capsule and glenoid labrum, and a **Hill-Sachs lesion,** which consists of an osseous defect of the posterolateral portion of the humeral head caused during traumatic anterior dislocation. Both conditions usually require surgery to restore stability to the glenohumeral joint.

Between these categories of shoulder instability are a group of shoulder pathologies related to asymmetric capsular tightness.[43] This occurs from the excessive distraction force on the glenohumeral joint during the deceleration phase of throwing, leading to thickening and contracture of the posterior-inferior portion of the capsule.[44] The sequela of this asymmetric capsular tightening is a loss of glenohumeral IR resulting in a cascade of events that may lead to pathologic conditions of the biceps tendon and labrum.

The long head of the biceps tendon helps stabilize the glenohumeral joint during the overhand throwing motion.[45] The unstable and asymmetrically tight shoulder places extra stress on the biceps tendon, leading to bicipital tendonitis and superior labrum anterior to posterior (SLAP) lesions. The SLAP lesion is hypothesized to result from increased torsional force from the biceps tendon that "peels back" the biceps and posterior labrum from the glenoid rim.[46] The SLAP lesion then enhances the dynamic and static instability of the already unstable shoulder.

Timelines and Healing

For the client with an unstable shoulder not surgically corrected, 4 to 8 weeks of rehabilitation is common. The length of rehabilitation depends on the client's ability to gain control of the instability. Once stable, the client is released to a sustained home exercise program to continue indefinitely. Surgically corrected unstable shoulders require more time for rehabilitation. After a period of immobilization lasting 2 to 4 weeks, 3 to 6 months of rehabilitation is common. These clients also require a sustained home exercise program. Most postoperative clients report that it takes 6 months to a year before their shoulder feels "normal."

Nonoperative Treatment

Treatment focuses on strengthening the RC and scapular stabilizers. Strengthening starts with shoulder isometric exercises in the safe position of the arm at the side. The motions resisted include shoulder flexion/extension, IR/ER, and abduction/adduction, as well as elbow flexion and extension. While performing isometric exercises, clients must "set" their scapula against their rib cage in a corrected posture position to engage the scapular stabilizers.

The next step in the rehabilitation program, once the client demonstrates fair to good control of the instability, is progression to isotonic exercises in a subimpingement range using light resistance and a high number of repetitions. For clients with anterior instability the focus is on strengthening the internal rotators, adductors, and biceps. For clients with global instability, the focus is on the RC, scapular stabilizers, deltoid, biceps, and triceps.

An essential at this stage is incorporation of open and closed chain exercises as previously described for proximal humeral fractures. The intensity of the closed chain exercises can be increased by using weighted medicine balls against the wall; by moving the body into a more horizontal position, or even working off the exercise ball while in prone UE weight-bearing.

Therapist-applied manual resistance can be used throughout each phase of the rehabilitation process. Starting with isometric exercises and active-assisted ROM and then progressing to concentric and eccentric exercises, the therapist controls the speed of movement and amount of force. The major benefit of manual resistance is the immediate feedback the therapist receives from the client during rehabilitation.

For the clients with posteroinferior capsule restrictions, stretching exercises to restore IR are critical. Use of towel behind back stretches and the sleeper stretch (Fig. 10-14) work well.

Operative Treatment

Surgical correction of the multidirectionally unstable shoulder should be considered only after a minimum of 3 months of conservative therapy has failed.[47] Two surgical procedures most often recommended in the literature are the open inferior capsular shift (surgical detachment and superior advancement of the inferior glenohumeral ligament)[48] and thermal capsulorraphy (selective heating of portions of the joint capsule, resulting in capsular shrinkage).[49] Each of these procedures has advantages and disadvantages.

Greater surgical morbidity occurs with the open capsular shift, and the repair has good and predictable outcomes. This procedure often is augmented by surgical closure of the rotator interval.

Thermal capsulorraphy can trace its origins to Hippocrates' time. He describes inserting a hot iron into the axilla to cauterize the unstable joint. Treatment

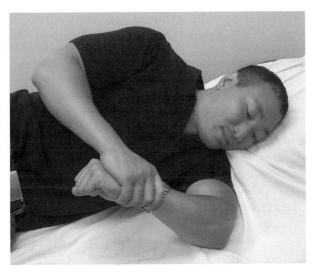

FIGURE 10-14 Example of the sleeper stretch. Gentle pressure applied in the direction of internal rotation while the body weight stabilizes the scapula.

has improved much since then, and this is now an arthroscopic procedure. However, there is a paucity of long-term studies about surgical outcomes. Complications include return of the instability, axillary nerve damage, and adhesive capsulitis.[50] Because of these complications and less than promising long-term outcomes, this surgery as a stand-alone procedure is becoming less popular because it is used increasingly in combination with, or is being replaced by, arthroscopic **capsular plication** (suturing folds into the joint capsule).

Precaution. *Great care must be taken in the rehabilitation of these clients to avoid* attenuating *(weakening, stretching) the healing capsule.*

The client can initiate ROM exercises earlier because the RC structures are left intact, but the therapist needs to supervise carefully the return of motion.

For clients with traumatic anterior dislocation, the need for surgical repair of the Bankart lesion varies based on the client's age range and the physical demands on the shoulder. Rates of recurrent dislocation were highest in clients younger than 30 years old,[51] with rates ranging from 79% to 100%. Conservative therapy had little effect on reducing rates of recurrence.[52] Therefore, clients younger than 30 and those over 30 who perform UE labor-intensive jobs should consider surgical repair.

Questions to Ask the Doctor

Nonoperative Clients

- *What is the nature and direction of the instability?*
- *Are there any secondary pathologies that need to be addressed (such as rotator cuff tear or SLAP lesion)?*
- *Is this client a surgical candidate?*

Operative Clients

- *What type of repair was performed? Ask to see an operative report.*
- *What are the range of motion restrictions?*
- *How soon can the client begin strengthening exercises?*
- *Do you have a specific postoperative protocol for rehabilitation?*

What to Say to Clients

About the Injury

"Your shoulder is a ball-and-socket joint with the ball much larger than the socket. This design allows for a lot of motion, but your shoulder must rely on the muscles and ligaments to keep the joint stable."

For the AMBRII client, say, "Because the ligaments that support your joint are so loose, your rotator cuff muscles need to work much harder to keep the joint stable. When they fatigue, the ball is able to slide up and pinch the tendons of the rotator cuff against the bony roof of your shoulder during throwing and overhead activities."

For the TUBS client, say, "When you fell with your arm out to the side, the ball was forced from the socket, which likely caused damage to the rim of the socket and the supportive ligaments in the front of the shoulder. As a result, your shoulder is unstable, and the ball can slip out of the socket easily if you raise your arm out to the side as if you are going to throw a ball. While your shoulder heals, you must avoid this position or the problem will keep occurring. There is a chance that even if you avoid this position during your recovery, the damage is great enough that your shoulder will remain unstable."

For the client with the tight posterior capsule, say, "Because of the way your shoulder has adapted to the stress of throwing, you have developed tightness in a portion of the ligaments that support the shoulder joint. As a result, your joint has a decreased ability to rotate internally. This restriction causes abnormal motion of the ball in the socket when your shoulder is under the stress of throwing, resulting in your pain and loss of function."

About Exercises

For the AMBRII client, say, "Your exercises are designed to compensate for your unstable shoulder by increasing the strength, coordination, and endurance of your rotator cuff and scapular stabilizing muscles. This exercise program is a lifelong commitment, because if the weakness returns, your shoulder problems will return as well."

For the TUBS client, say, "Your exercises strengthen the muscles in the front of your shoulder to support the damaged part of the joint. You must follow the motion restrictions carefully during exercise to avoid disrupting the repair process."

For the client with the tight posterior capsule, say, "You need to regain the internal rotation motion of your shoulder to restore the normal function. The stretches work best if performed frequently. Three sets a day is not enough. You should try for a minimum total of thirty minutes of stretch time each day. Remember, it is not how hard you push the stretch, but how much time you spend at the end of motion that counts."

Evaluation Tips

- For the unstable shoulder, the goals are to find the direction(s) of instability and to reproduce the client's symptoms. Their feedback during examination is critical.
- The client must be as relaxed as possible during examination because muscle guarding will hide the degree of instability.
- Various tests are described in the literature to test for shoulder instability. Basic tests to check for the direction of instability are as follows:
  - *Anterior and Posterior Drawer Test:* With the client seated, the therapist grasps the humeral head with one hand while stabilizing the scapula and clavicle with the other. Next, the therapist applies an anterior and then a posterior translation pressure tangential to the glenoid surface while assessing the amount of humeral head movement. The therapist then compares the amount and quality of movement to the opposite side.
  - *Sulcus Sign Test:* With the client seated and the client's arm supported in 20 to 50 degrees of abduction, the therapist pulls inferiorly on the client's arm. A depression of more than a finger width resulting between the acromion and humeral head indicates a positive test. This test indicates multidirectional instability.[48]
  - *Apprehension Test:* With the client supine the therapist moves the client's shoulder into 90 degrees of abduction and end-range ER. If with the application of overpressure the client experiences apprehension but not pain, the test is considered positive for anterior instability.[53]
  - *Relocation Test:* With the client positioned as at the end of the Apprehension Test, the therapist applies posteriorly directed pressure from the anterior aspect of the humeral head. The test is positive if the client's apprehension disappears. This test helps to confirm anterior instability.[54]

Diagnosis-Specific Information That Affects Clinical Reasoning

The direction of the instability dictates the course of treatment as described before. Consequently, you must have a clear understanding of the client's instability pattern.

Precaution. *Applying an incorrect exercise and stretching program may aggravate the client's condition.*

Many of these clients have impingement and/or SLAP lesions as well. If a SLAP lesion is present, your client may need to avoid rotary exercises with the arm above shoulder height. In these cases, overhead throwing exercises are contraindicated.

Tips from the Field

- Proprioception exercises (activities to enhance position and movement sense/control of the scapula and shoulder complex) need to be stressed with these clients.
- Manual resisted exercises in diagonal patterns at various speeds using concentric and eccentric force are a valuable component of the rehabilitation program.
- Have your client perform UE exercises to strengthen the RC while concurrently working on balance while in quadruped, sitting, kneeling, and standing positions.
- Stress proper posture as described before.

Precautions and Concerns

- *Do not perform joint mobilization or stretches on the client with multidirectional instability.*
- *Clients with anterior instability require that their posterior capsule be mobilized. Avoid stretching the anterior capsule.*
- *Pay close attention to ROM restrictions for postoperative clients.*

ROTATOR CUFF DISEASE

Anatomy

After neck and back pain, shoulder pain is the third most common musculoskeletal disorder. *Up to 70% of shoulder disorders are related to RC disease.*[55]

The structures of the shoulder that are involved in RC disease include the muscles of the RC, the long head of the biceps tendon, the subdeltoid-subacromial bursa, and coracoacromial arch.

The supraspinatus, infraspinatus, and teres minor make up the greater tuberosity attachments of the RC.

The subscapularis attaches to the lesser tuberosity. All the RC muscles work together to stabilize the head of the humerus in the glenoid fossa during shoulder motion while their tendons form a cuff that surrounds the humeral head.

Along with their primary role of stabilizing the glenohumeral joint, each muscle of the RC imparts specific motion to the humeral head. The supraspinatus is an abductor, the infraspinatus is an external rotator, the teres minor is an external rotator and weak adductor of the humerus, and the subscapularis is an internal rotator (see Figs. 10-12 and 10-15).

The stabilizing role of the long head of the biceps tendon is reviewed in the section on glenohumeral instability. As the arm elevates overhead, the head of the humerus glides along the biceps tendon as it sits in the bicipital groove between the greater and lesser tuberosities. The long head of the biceps plays a role in shoulder flexion and in forearm flexion and supination.

The subdeltoid-subacromial bursa is a smooth serosal sac that sits between RC tendons and the coracoacromial arch. Above, the bursa is adherent to the underside of the deltoid, coracoacromial ligament, and the acromion. Beneath, the bursa is adherent to the RC and greater

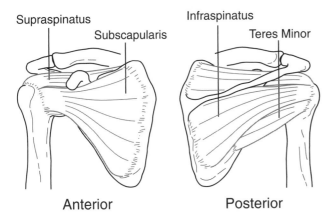

FIGURE 10-15 Rotator cuff muscles consist of the supraspinatus, infraspinatus, teres minor, and subscapularis. (From Budoff JE: Examination of the shoulder. In Trumble TE, Cornwall R, Budoff J, editors: *Core knowledge in orthopaedics: hand, elbow, and shoulder,* St Louis, 2006, Mosby.)

tuberosity. This structure provides a cushioning and low-friction interface between the convex humeral head and RC as they rotate below the concave coracoacromial arch during arm elevation.

The coracoacromial arch consists of the anteroinferior aspect of the acromion process, the inferior surface of the acromioclavicular joint, and the coracoacromial ligament. This structure forms a roof over the RC and humeral head.[56] The coracoacromial arch not only serves as an attachment site for the deltoid and subdeltoid-subacromial bursa but also provides superior stability and protection to the glenohumeral joint.

Diagnosis and Pathology

Two major hypotheses have been proposed about the cause of RC disease. One is based on extrinsic causes and the other is based on intrinsic causes. Current evidence demonstrates that both contribute to the disease process and are affected by age, postural habits, movement quality, and activity level.

Extrinsically caused lesions result from the repeated impingement of the RC tendon against different structures of the glenohumeral joint. Neer[56] describes impingement between the long head of the biceps and supraspinatus tendons and the coracoacromial arch during UE elevation, resulting in lesions on the bursal side of the RC. His three-stage classification of impingement syndrome is still used today (Table 10-3). Bigliani et al.[57] described three types of acromion morphology (Fig. 10-16) with cadaver studies demonstrating a 70% incidence of RC tears in subjects with a type III acromial shape and a 3% incidence in subjects with a type I acromial shape. Walch et al.[58] described a type of impingement between the supraspinatus and infraspinatus tendons in the late cocking phase of throwing on the glenoid rim, resulting in lesions on the articular side of the RC.

Intrinsically caused lesions result from age-related degeneration of the RC tendon. These lesions are related to the vascularization of the RC cuff and are on the articular side of the tendon.[59,60] Lindblom[61] was the first to describe an area of hypovascularity of the supraspina-

TABLE 10-3

Neer's Three-Stage Classification of Impingement Syndrome

STAGE	AGE RANGE	PATHOLOGY
I	<25 years	Reversible edema and hemorrhage from excessive overhead use
II	25–40 years	Irreversible fibrotic changes to the rotator cuff following repeated episodes of mechanical inflammation
III	>40 Years	Bone spurs and tears (complete and incomplete) of the rotator cuff and long head of the biceps tendon

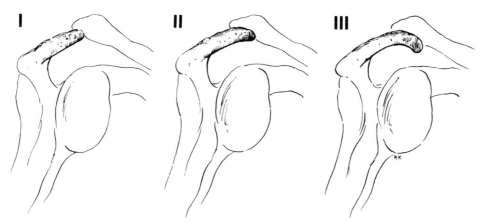

FIGURE 10-16 Acromion morphology types I (smooth), II (curved), and III (hooked). (From Jobe CM: Gross anatomy of the shoulder. In Rockwood CA, Matsen FA III, editors: *The shoulder,* Philadelphia, 1990, WB Saunders.)

tus tendon where it attaches to the greater tuberosity. Codman[59] referred to the same area as the "critical zone" because it appeared to be at greater risk of developing a tear.

Because most RC tears are partial-thickness tears,[62] the condition is often progressive and can lead to a full-thickness lesion. As tendon fibers fail, they retract because the RC is under constant tension. This process leads to at least four adverse effects[63]:

- Increased load on intact neighboring fibers, leading to their potential failure
- Loss of muscle fibers attached to bone, leading to decreased strength and function of the RC
- Blood supply of intact tendon placed at risk by distorted anatomy from fiber failure, leading to progressive ischemia and tendon degeneration
- Loss of tendon repair potential as the tendon is exposed to joint fluid containing lytic enzymes, which inhibit hematoma formation that would facilitate healing

Usually beginning in the supraspinatus tendon, the tear may progress to involve the infraspinatus tendon. Once this occurs, the ability of the RC to stabilize the humeral head in the glenoid fossa is compromised severely, leading to superior migration under the unopposed pull of the deltoid. Humeral head superior migration loads the long head of the biceps tendon, leading to tendonopathy and potential failure. Traction spurs develop at the coracoacromial ligament attachment on the acromion through repeated loading from the upward displacement of the humeral head, leading to further RC damage. This damage allows the RC tendon to slide down below the axis of joint rotation. Much like a boutonniere deformity of the finger, the buttonholed RC becomes a humeral head elevator instead of a depressor. The RC is then ineffective as a humeral head stabilizer,

and the client is unable to elevate the arm above a horizontal position.

Timelines and Healing

Recovery from pathologic conditons of the RC varies greatly because of multiple presentations of the disease. If the case is uncomplicated, such as a tendonitis, the condition can stabilize in 2 to 6 weeks. If secondary pathologic conditions are present—such as frozen shoulder, impingement, instability, and RC tear—recovery time lengthens considerably. Complex cases may take up to a year to resolve with or without surgical intervention.

Nonoperative Treatment

Initial treatment focuses on rest and antiinflammatory modalities to stabilize the disease process. Early ROM exercises such as pendulum and wand-assisted elevation in the scapular plane to avoid impingement help to moderate pain through the analgesic effect of mechanoreceptor stimulation.

CLINICAL *Pearl*

Maintaining full, pain-free IR and ER is critical to preventing frozen shoulder.

Strengthening of the healthy portion of the RC and scapular stabilizer muscles, usually in the motions of shoulder IR, adduction, and extension, is safe and encourages the stabilizing function of the RC. The use of isometric exercises and resistance band exercises are effective during this portion of the program. As pain levels decrease and RC function improves, the next step is to strengthen the UE elevators and external rotators.

Throughout this process, you must stress muscle balance and proper scapular kinematics. Incorporating open and closed chain and manual exercises, as described for proximal humerus fracture and for glenohumeral instability, complete the exercise program.

You should focus on strengthening the scapular force couples once your client demonstrates good control of the RC muscles. The addition of sport/activity-specific exercise is usually the final phase of your client's rehabilitation program.

Operative Treatment

Indications for RC surgery are the presence of a full or partial tear that has not responded to a course of conservative care and that interferes with the client's ADL. RC surgery is evolving rapidly as more and more physicians perform complex repairs through the arthroscope.

Arthroscopic debridement for freshening of the frayed, partially torn RC tendon stimulates healing. For full-thickness tears, the surgeon debrides the tear edges and then closes the defect to provide a foundation to regain RC strength and shoulder function. The surgeon often performs an acromioplasty at the time of RC repair to decompress the subacromial space and to prevent impingement of the repaired structures.

Most postoperative therapy programs include a 2- to 4-week period of immobilization while the tissue stabilizes. The client then starts therapy to regain ROM. For the next 2 to 3 weeks, ROM progresses from passive to active motion exercise. At approximately 8 weeks postoperative, the client begins strengthening exercises and follows the program for the nonoperative client listed before.

Questions to Ask the Doctor

Nonoperative Clients

- *Are there any concurrent pathologies (such as instability or impingement)?*
- *Is surgery a possibility?*

Operative Clients

- *What structures were repaired? Try to obtain an operative report.*
- *Do you have a specific rehabilitation protocol?*
- *Are there any range of motion restrictions or precautions?*
- *How soon can strengthening begin?*

What to Say to Clients

About the Injury

"Your shoulder relies on the rotator cuff muscles to stabilize the head of the humerus in the socket and to prevent the humeral head from being pinched against the roof of your shoulder when you raise your arm. Your rotator cuff is damaged, so this protective function has been interrupted, placing your shoulder at risk. If the problem progresses, you may lose the ability to raise your arm."

About Exercise

"By strengthening the healthy portions of your injured rotator cuff, there is a good chance you can regain the ability to use your arm for your daily needs. The exercises are specific and need to be performed regularly."

"When you perform the range of motion exercises, you should not experience sharp sudden pain when raising your arm up. To prevent this from occurring, you must lead the motion with the thumb side of your hand while keeping the point of your elbow facing the ground throughout the motion. Before raising your arm, you must correct your posture [as described in the section on thoracic outlet syndrome and brachial plexopathy]. By following these movement precautions, you will minimize the chance of pinching the rotator cuff under the bony roof of your shoulder."

Evaluation Tips

A multitude of tests are used to detect RC disease. The following tests are included because they are easy to perform and research indicates they have reasonable sensitivity and specificity:

- A quick screening test to detect an RC tear involving the supraspinatus and infraspinatus is to resist ER with the client's shoulders in neutral and the elbows flexed to 90 degrees. In the presence of an RC tear, the unopposed deltoid will abduct the arm while the hand dips into IR (Fig. 10-17).
- Client positioning to palpate the RC insertions are as follows[64]:
  - Supraspinatus: With the client's dorsum of the hand resting on the posterior iliac crest, palpate just inferior to the anterior aspect of the acromion (see Fig. 10-29, A, on the CD).
  - Infraspinatus: With the client's shoulder in ER and the elbow brought to the navel, palpate just inferior to the posterior aspect of the acromion (see Fig. 10-29, B, on the CD).
  - The long head of the biceps tendon: With the client's arm held in IR and the forearm resting on a pillow in the client's lap, the tendon should lie in the deltopectoral interval (the sulcus formed by the medial border of the deltoid and the lateral edge of the pectoral muscle belly) (see Fig. 10-29, C, on the CD).
  - Subscapularis: With the client positioned as previously, bring the shoulder to neutral rotation. Palpate the lesser tuberosity and tendon in the deltopectoral interval (see Fig. 10-29, D, on the CD).

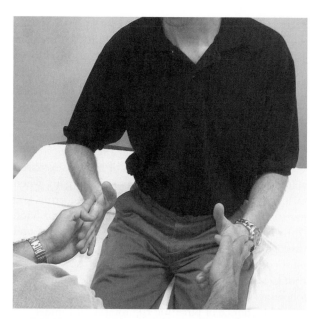

FIGURE 10-17 Quick screening position test for full-thickness rotator cuff tears involving the supraspinatus and infraspinatus. A positive test is pictured. The right shoulder moves into abduction and internal rotation on resisted external rotation because the deficient rotator cuff cannot stabilize against the action of the deltoid.

- Shoulder impingement is a sign of RC disease. The Hawkins-Kennedy Test and Neer Impingement Test are useful in detecting this pathologic condition.[65]
  - Hawkins-Kennedy Test: With the client's shoulder flexed to 90 degrees, bring the shoulder into full IR. This drives the greater tuberosity under the coracoacromial arch and will elicit pain if impingement is present (Fig. 10-18, A).
  - Neer Impingement Test: Passively flex the client's shoulder to end ROM. Positioning the shoulder in IR at the start of the test enhances the impingement of the RC on the underside of the anterior third of the acromion and coracoacromial ligament (Fig. 10-18, B).
- Isometric testing of the specific muscles of the RC and the long head of the biceps aids in detecting tendonopathy. These tests include the Jobe or "Empty Can" Test, the Patte Test, the Gerber Liftoff Test, and the Speed's Test.
  - The Jobe or "Empty Can" Test: Bring the client's arms to horizontal in the scapular plane with the shoulder in IR. Next, apply downward pressure while the client provides isometric resistance. Weakness or the inability to hold this position implicates the supraspinatus[66] (Fig. 10-19, A).
  - The Patte Test: The client's arm is positioned in 90 degrees of abduction with neutral rotation in

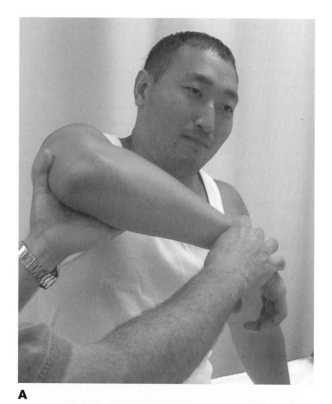

A

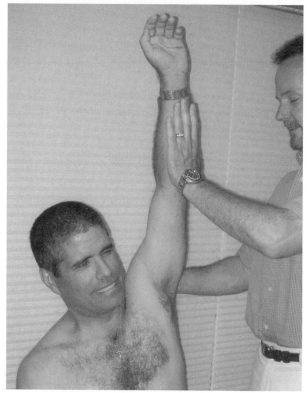

B

FIGURE 10-18 Tests to determine shoulder impingement in rotator cuff disease. **A,** End test position of the Hawkins-Kennedy Impingement Test. **B,** End test position of the Neer Impingement Test.

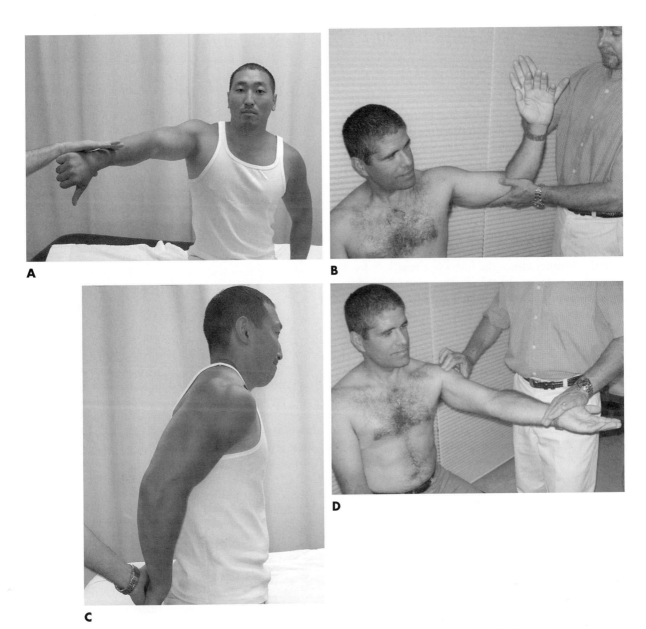

FIGURE 10-19   Isometric testing of muscles of the rotator cuff. **A,** Test position for isometric testing of the supraspinatus or the "empty can" test. **B,** Test position for the Patte Test for isometric strength of the infraspinatus and teres minor. **C,** Test position for the Gerber Liftoff Test for isometric strength of the subscapularis. **D,** Speed's Test for pathologic conditions of the long head of the biceps tendon and superior glenoid labrum.

the scapular plane. Apply pressure at the client's wrist to resist shoulder ER while stabilizing the arm at the client's elbow. Weakness and/or pain implicates the infraspinatus[66] (Fig. 10-19, *B*).

- The Gerber Liftoff Test: Position the client's arm so the dorsum of the hand rests against the posterior iliac crest. Have the client actively raise the hand 2 to 5 inches from the back while you apply resistance (Fig. 10-19, *C*). The client's inability to apply pressure or hold the hand in this position implicates the subscapularis.[67]

- The Speed's Test: Position the client's shoulder in 90 degrees of flexion with the elbow in extension and the forearm in supination. Resist shoulder flexion while palpating the long head of the biceps tendon in the bicipital groove. A painful response implicates the long head of the biceps[68] (Fig. 10-19, *D*).

- No resistance test is specific to isolating the teres minor.

- While performing these tests, watch for patterns that support specific locations of RC lesions.

Diagnosis-Specific Information That Affects Clinical Reasoning

The existence of an RC tear does not always lead to a surgical repair. Clinical experience shows that many clients function well with RC deficits confirmed via MRI. Clients who are unable to regain pain-free shoulder function are the best candidates for surgical repair.[69]

Tips from the Field

Good palpation skills aid substantially in differentiating subacromial-subdeltoid bursitis from RC tendonitis. The bursa lies beneath the therapist's finger as well when palpating the supraspinatus and infraspinatus insertions as described earlier. Since the bursa is a relatively fixed structure, its position changes little during arm movement. Conversely, the palpation locations for the RC tendons change with arm movement. A pain response with palpation implicates both structures.

CLINICAL *Pearl*

By maintaining constant pressure on the palpation points listed for the supraspinatus and infrapinatus while the client returns the arm to the resting position, the pain will remain constant if the bursa is the source and will decrease if the RC tendons are the source.

Precautions and Concerns

- *Watch for a tight posterior capsule with these clients and treat accordingly.*
- *In clients showing impingement signs, take care to avoid impinging the shoulder during overhead exercise.*
- *Monitor for excessive scapular elevation during UE elevation. Abnormal movement patterns must be avoided.*
- *Discourage clients from sleeping on their involved side, for this often increases the chance for impingement.*

The Role of Therapy Assistants

- *Supervision and set up of clients' exercise programs established by the therapist*
- *Application of manual therapy to help with pain control, ROM gains, and strengthening*
- *Supervising and reviewing of the clients' home exercise programs as established by the therapist*
- *Instruction in ADL modification and adaptation*
- *Assisting the therapist in obtaining measurements of performance (e.g., ROM, strength, and functional capacity) to track clients' progress*

CASE *Studies*

CASE 10-1

J.S. is a 48-year-old right dominant stock broker, non-smoker, who received a diagnosis of mild brachial plexus stretch injury. He reported symptoms of headache in the C2 distribution, anterior chest wall pain on the left, and pain in the left anteriolateral neck extending to the angle of his jaw and to the anterior aspect of his shoulder. He noted occasional swelling with flushing of the left side of his face, extending to his ear. This symptom became more prevalent when his left upper quarter pain was high. He was experiencing slight numbness of the thumb, index, and long finger, and arm pain on the inside of the proximal humerus of the left UE while sitting at his desk and with overhead activities. He reported difficulty combing his hair because of arm pain.

Symptoms began 2 months ago when he decided to return to surfing after a 15-year hiatus. He stopped surfing about 1 month ago because his face, chest wall, and arm symptoms would increase dramatically during and for days after time spent on his board.

He had a thorough cardiac workup and was cleared. X-ray films and MRI of the cervical spine were unremarkable. He is in excellent physical shape, with an unremarkable medical history.

On exam, he demonstrated a drooped left shoulder with a forward-head–rounded-shoulders posture. Cervical ROM was limited 25% only for rotation and lateral flexion to the right. Crossed-arm cervical ROM testing showed no improvement in motion. Shoulder ROM was limited in flexion to horizontal by arm pain, with IR and ER being full. RC strength was at 5/5 bilaterally and pain free on testing. Muscle spasm occurred in the suboccipital region, across the trapezius ridge and along the medial scapular border.

Palpation at the left supraclavicular fossa was tender with spread of pain into the side of the face to the ear. Palpation at the left infraclavicular fossa and neurovascular bundle was painful with an increase of left UE symptoms. Tinel's sign was positive in the same areas.

Decreased sensitivity to pin prick of the thumb, index, and radial side of the long finger on the left was noted. The Roos (EAST) Test was positive immediately. Neural mobility of the brachial plexus was at 2–/5 on the left with increase of left upper quarter symptoms and 5/5 on the right.

Impressions

Based on clinical presentation, J.S. demonstrated evidence of an upper trunk–lateral cord brachial plexopathy with decreased plexus mobility restricting UE elevation. Cervical motion loss implicated scalene muscle tightness.

Facial symptoms with headache combined with shoulder droop implicate the upper trunk. Decreased sensitivity to pin prick on the radial side of the long finger continuing to the index finger and thumb implicate the lateral cord as well. No change in cervical motion with the crossed-arm position combined with the pattern of cervical motion loss implicates the scalene muscles.

Because J.S. has full shoulder IR and ER, his limited UE elevation likely was not due to a capsular restriction. A pathologic condition of the RC is unlikely as well because RC strength was 5/5 and he was pain free on testing.

Treatment

Treatment on the first visit consisted of instruction in posture correction exercises, modification of computer placement to encourage proper posture while working, and to limit all overhead activities. J.S. was instructed in nerve gliding exercises to be performed 3 times a day in sets of 3, with his posture correction exercises to be performed hourly in sets of 10.

J.S.'s work schedule only allowed for weekly visits, so his treatment program was designed accordingly. On his second visit, J.S. demonstrated excellent technique with his home program. He had avoided all overhead activity and modified his work station to encourage proper posture. He reported a 50% improvement in symptoms, with no headache for the past week.

Brief exam revealed neural mobility at 3+/5, good postural awareness and less left shoulder drooping.

Treatment consisted of pectoral minor and scalene muscle stretching with nerve glides. Neural mobility improved to 4+/5 by the end of treatment. J.S.'s home program was modified to include scalene muscle stretching and pectoralis minor doorway stretches. He was allowed to perform nerve glide and stretching exercises as long as his symptoms remained stable in sets of 3 for 3 times a day. Scapular clock exercises were added to work on proprioception on an hourly basis.

On J.S.'s visit 1 week later, he again demonstrated excellent compliance with his home program. He had full neural mobility and his cervical ROM was full. Shoulder position was equal bilaterally. The EAST was positive at 45 seconds of testing.

Treatment consisted of home program modification with the addition of scapular strengthening with focus on the upper, middle, lower trapezius, and serratus anterior using resistance bands. All exercises were performed daily in sets of 3 once through each exercise before starting the next set. J.S. was instructed to stop exercising if symptoms returned.

Results

On the fourth visit 2 weeks later, J.S. had been symptom free for 1 week. Exam was normal except for a positive

EAST Test at 1 minute of testing, leading to paresthesia into the thumb and index finger. Because his condition was stable and he had excellent understanding of his home program, J.S. was discharged from therapy with instruction to call as needed for program progression or if his status changed. He was instructed to avoid surfing.

Because J.S. was in excellent shape before his injury and he was compliant and motivated, he quickly stabilized and returned to a functional baseline. Many clients have difficulty modifying their lifestyle to avoid further injury to their brachial plexus, resulting in a protracted recovery period.

CASE 10-2

F.B. is a 75-year-old right dominant female who tripped over her cat and sustained an A2 fracture of the proximal humerus. Three weeks after injury, she came to therapy in a simple sling for immobilization. Therapy orders were for ROM exercises with no strengthening for the next 3 weeks. F.B. was apprehensive about moving her arm because she felt that the break was still unstable since not enough time had passed from her injury date.

Before moving F.B.'s right shoulder, I explained that sound will not travel across an open fracture and used a stethoscope at the humeral head while tapping on the lateral epicondyle to demonstrate to her there was no difference in the sound level. Next, I showed her that the head of her humerus was moving as I rolled her arm from IR to ER, again indicating that she was ready to begin ROM exercise.

Exam revealed severe ecchymosis in the axilla and around the elbow. I explained that when she fractured her arm, there was a lot of bleeding from the bone and that blood had run down her arm along the interior tissue planes to collect around her elbow and distal axilla.

Shoulder elevation was 50 degrees, abduction was 40 degrees, IR was arm across the abdomen and thumb to the iliac crest while attempting arm behind back position. ER was neutral. ROM of the elbow was 20 to 110 degrees with wrist and hand ROM normal. Strength testing was deferred at that time.

Treatment

I instructed F.B. in pendulum and tabletop ROM exercises that she was to perform hourly in sets of 3 to 10, up to 3 sets each exercise session. She started ROM exercises for her elbow that she was to perform whenever sitting.

F.B.'s treatment over the next 2 weeks focused on scapulothoracic stabilization via manual resistance applied to the scapula along with scapular mobilization and proprioception scapular clock exercises. PROM of the shoulder also was stressed, focusing on avoidance of substitution patterns of excessive scapular elevation and protraction.

Reevaluation 2 weeks later revealed ROM of elevation at 110 degrees, abduction at 90 degrees, and ER to 30 at 75 degrees of abduction and 40 degrees at neutral shoulder abduction. IR was at thumb to L5 reaching behind the back.

Treatment continued to focus on ROM, stressing active motion in normal movement patterns as F.B. mirrored my UE elevation while I stabilized her shoulder to prevent early scapular elevation. F.B. then added wall walking to her program incorporating self-stabilization of the scapula with her left hand.

At 6 weeks after injury, F.B.'s shoulder elevation was 150 degrees, abduction was 135 degrees, ER at 90 degrees of abduction was 50 degrees, ER at shoulder neutral was 60 degrees, and IR behind the back had progressed little at thumb to L3. Elbow, hand, and wrist ROM were full.

Because F.B. then was allowed to begin strengthening, isometric exercises for all planes of shoulder movement and resistance band exercises of the elbow flexors and extensors were added. Behind the back stretches with good scapular position and upright posture were stressed as well. At this point the therapy program included joint mobilization and more aggressive stretching to focus on gaining end ROM.

Results

F.B. attended therapy for 6 weeks. She had 160 degrees of elevation, 150 degrees of abduction, and 70 degrees of ER at 90 degrees of abduction and with the shoulder at neutral. IR behind the back remained restricted with the thumb reaching the L2 spinous process. F.B. was fully independent in self-care with her right arm, and she was pain free. Shoulder strength was 4/5 except for abduction and ER, which were 4–/5. She never regained full IR because there may have been a rotary component to her fracture as she healed, limiting the potential for normal IR ROM.

CASE 10-3

T.B. is an 18-year-old high school football player who sustained a traumatic anterior dislocation of his right (dominant) shoulder. MRI demonstrated a Bankart lesion with anterior glenoid labrum and capsule tear. Because T.B. was a heavily recruited athlete, he opted to have arthroscopic shoulder surgery 4 weeks after injury.

T.B. presented to therapy 2 weeks after surgery with his arm in a sling immobilizer.

Active motion was contraindicated to avoid disrupting the surgical repair. PROM of the right shoulder was 90 degrees of flexion, 40 degrees of abduction, and 10 degrees of ER. IR was arm across stomach. Strength testing was deferred.

Treatment

Treatment initially focused on protecting the surgical repair by following ER ROM restrictions to 40 degrees. Scapular proprioception exercises were issued for home program to get a head start on preventing poor scapular kinematics. These consisted of half shoulder rolls in the posterior direction only and clock shoulder elevation to the 12, 1, and 2 o'clock positions performed in front of a mirror for feedback.

Over the next 4 weeks treatment consisted of submaximal isometric exercises of the internal and external rotators with ER limited to 40 degrees to avoid disrupting the repaired anterior structures. Scapular stabilization exercises continued during this period. PROM manual therapy was the primary component of treatment.

At 8 weeks, T.B. had 145 degrees of flexion with active flexion at 135 degrees and ER at 40 degrees. ER safe zone was now to 60 degrees. The protocol allowed for resistance band exercises of the external and internal rotators. Active shoulder elevation by T.B. while mirroring the therapist with the therapist preventing early scapular elevation was started.

During the next 4 weeks, the resistance band exercises progressed to include shoulder elevation and abduction as long as scapular substitution patterns were avoided. Strengthening of the triceps and scapular depressors/stabilizers by doing seated press-ups were added. Manual resistance exercises in diagonal planes supine and seated with focus on normal kinematics also were started. Throughout all phases, ROM exercises were stressed.

By 12 weeks, flexion was 170 degrees, abduction was 165 degrees, and ER was 60 degrees with IR at 70 degrees. Strength of the shoulder was 5/5 for extension, with flexion and IR at 4+/5; ER and abduction was at 4/5. By then, all motion restrictions were removed. The focus of the next 4 to 6 weeks was to gain full ROM and full strength and to start sport-specific training. Plyometric drills with two-hand throw-catch activities using weighted balls were started.

Results

By 18 weeks, T.B. had full ROM, and scapular kinematics/shoulder mechanics were normal. He had returned to work out at the gym using a custom program designed to strengthen the anterior shoulder structures and globally strengthen the RC, deltoid, serratus anterior, pectoral, and back muscles. Because of his successful rehabilitation, T.B. went on to play collegiate football.

References

1. Burkart SS: A 26-year-old woman with shoulder pain, *JAMA* 284:1559-1567, 2000.
2. Saha AK: Dynamic stability of the glenohumeral joint, *Acta Orthop Scand* 42:491-505, 1971.
3. Howell SM, Galiant BJ: The glenoid-labral socket: a constrained articular surface, *Clin Orthop* 243:122-125, 1989.
4. Dempster WT: Mechanism of shoulder movement, *Arch Phys Med Rehabil* 46A:49, 1965.
5. Johnson D, Ellis H: Pectoral girdle, shoulder region and axilla. In Standring S, editor: *Gray's anatomy*, ed 39, Edinburgh, 2005, Churchill-Livingstone.
6. Donatelli RA: Functional anatomy and mechanics. In Donatelli RA, editor: *Physical therapy of the shoulder*, ed 4, St Louis, 2004, Churchill Livingstone.
7. Dutton M: The shoulder complex. In *Orthopaedic examination, evaluation, & intervention*, New York, 2004, McGraw-Hill.
8. Mercer SB, Bogduk N: The ligaments and anulus fibrosus of human adult cervical intervertebral discs, *Spine* 24(7):619-626, 1999.
9. Boden SD, McCowen PR, Davis DO et al: Abnormal magnetic resonance scans of the cervical spine in asymptomatic subjects: a prospective investigation, *J Bone Joint Surg* 72A:1178-1184, 1990.
10. McLain RF: Mechanoreceptor endings in human cervical facet joints, *Spine* 19:495-500, 1994.
11. Dwyer A, Aprill C, Bogduk N: Cervical zygapophyseal joint pain patterns. I. A study in normal volunteers, *Spine* 15(6):453-457, 1990.
12. Fukui S, Ohseto K, Shiotani M et al: Referred pain distribution of the cervical zygapophyseal joints and cervical dorsal rami, *Pain* 68(1):79-83, 1996.
13. Travell JG, Simmons DG: *Myofascial pain and dysfunction the trigger point manual*, vol 1, Baltimore, 1983, Lippincott Williams & Wilkins.
14. McKenzie RA: *The cervical and thoracic spine mechanical diagnosis and therapy*, Waikanae, New Zealand, 1990, Spinal Publications.
15. Tong HC, Haig AJ, Yamakawa K: The Spurling test and cervical radiculopathy, *Spine* 27(2):156-159, 2002.
16. American Association of Electrodiagnostic Medicine: Guidelines in electrodiagnostic medicine, *Muscle Nerve Suppl* 8:S209, 1999.
17. Spurling RG, Scoville WB: Lateral rupture of the cervical intervertebral discs: a common cause of shoulder and arm pain, *Surg Gynecol Obstet* 78:350-358, 1944.
18. Whitenack SH, Hunter JM, Jaeger SH et al: Thoracic outlet syndrome: a brachial plexopathy. In Hunter J, Macklin E, Callahan A, editors: *Rehabilitation of the hand: surgery and therapy*, St Louis, 1995, Mosby.
19. Roos DB: Congenital anomalies associated with thoracic outlet syndrome, *Am J Surg* 132:771-778, 1976.
20. Gergoudis R, Barnes R: Thoracic outlet arterial compression: prevalence in normals, *Angiology* 31:538, 1980.
21. Costigan DA, Wilbourn AJ: The elevated arm stress test: specificity in the diagnosis of thoracic outlet syndrome, *Neurology* 35(suppl 1):74, 1985.
22. Warrens A, Heaton J: Thoracic outlet compression syndrome: the lack of reliability of its clinical assessment, *Ann R Coll Surg Engl* 69:203-204, 1987.
23. Rayan G, Jensen C: Thoracic outlet syndrome: provocative examination maneuvers in a typical population, *J Shoulder Elbow Surg* 4:113-117, 1995.
24. Leffert RD: Thoracic outlet syndrome, *J Am Acad Orthop Surg* 2(6):317-325, 1994.
25. Schwartzman RJ: Brachial plexus traction injuries, *Hand Clin* 7(3):547-556, 1991.
26. Degeorges R, Reynaud C, Becquemin JP: Thoracic outlet syndrome surgery: long-term functional results, *Ann Vasc Surg* 18(5):558-565, 2004.
27. Cherington M, Happer I, Machanic B et al: Surgery for thoracic outlet syndrome may be hazardous to your health, *Muscle Nerve* 9(7):632-634, 1986.
28. Roos DB, Owens C: The thoracic outlet syndrome, *Arch Surg* 93:71, 1966.
29. Neer CS 2nd: Displaced proximal humeral fractures. I. Classification and evaluation, *J Bone Joint Surg* 52A(6):1077-1089, 1970.
30. Palvanen M, Kannus P, Parkkari J et al: The injury mechanisms of osteoporotic upper extremity fractures among older adults: a controlled study of 287 consecutive clients and their 108 controls, *Osteoporos Int* 11(10):822-831, 2000.
31. Gohlke F, Essigkrug B, Schnitz F: The pattern of the collagen fiber bundles of the capsule of the glenohumeral joint, *J Shoulder Elbow Surg* 3:111-128, 1994.
32. Emig EW, Schweitzer ME, Karasick D et al: Adhesive capsulitis of the shoulder: MR diagnosis, *AJR Am J Roentgenol* 164(6):1457-1459, 1995.
33. Hannafin JA, Chiaia TA: Adhesive capsulitis: a treatment approach, *Clin Orthop* pp 95-109, March 2000.
34. Beyers M, Bonutti P: Frozen shoulder. In Donatelli RA, editor: *Physical therapy of the shoulder*, ed 4, St Louis, 2004, Churchill Livingstone.
35. Bridgman JF: Periarthritis of the shoulder and diabetes mellitus, *Ann Rheum Dis* 31(1):69-71, 1972.
36. Bunker TD, Anthony PP: The pathology of frozen shoulder: a Dupuytren-like disease, *J Bone Joint Surg* 77B(5):677-683, 1995.
37. Smith SP, Devaraj VS, Bunker TD: The association between frozen shoulder and Dupuytren's disease, *J Shoulder Elbow Surg* 10(2):149-151, 2001.
38. Shaffer B, Tibone JE, Kerlan RK: Frozen shoulder: a long-term follow-up, *J Bone Joint Surg* 74A(5):738-746, 1992.
39. Grey RG: The natural history of "idiopathic" frozen shoulder, *J Bone Joint Surg* 60A:564, 1978.
40. Ogilvie-Harris DJ, Biggs DJ, Fitsialos DP et al: The resistant frozen shoulder: manipulation versus arthroscopic release, *Clin Orthop* pp 238-248, Oct 1995.
41. Matsen FA III, Thomas SC, Rockwood CA: Glenohumeral instability. In Rockwood CA, Matsen FA III, editors: *The shoulder*, Philadelphia, 1990, WB Saunders.

42. Budoff JE, Nirschl RP, Guidi EJ: Debridement of partial thickness tears of the rotator cuff without acromioplasty, *J Bone Joint Surg* 80A(5):733-748, 1998.

43. Harryman DT, Sidles JA, Clark JM et al: Translation of the humeral head on the glenoid with passive glenohumeral motion, *J Bone Joint Surg* 72A(9):1334-1343, 1990.

44. Cooper J, Donley PB, Morgan CD: Throwing inuries. In Donatelli RA, editor: *Physical therapy of the shoulder,* ed 4, St Louis, 2004, Churchill Livingstone.

45. Rodosky MW, Harner CD, Fu FH: The role of the long head of the biceps muscle and superior glenoid labrum in anterior stability of the shoulder, *Am J Sports Med* 22(1): 121-130, 1994.

46. Burkhart SS, Morgan CD: The peel-back mechanism: its role in producing and extending posterior type II SLAP lesions and its effect on SLAP repair rehabilitation, *Arthroscopy* 14(6):637-640, 1998.

47. Zazzali MS, Vad VB, Herrera J et al: Shoulder instability. In Donatelli RA, editor: *Physical therapy of the shoulder,* ed 4, St Louis, 2004, Churchill Livingstone.

48. Neer CS 2nd, Foster C: Inferior capsular shift for involuntary inferior and multidirectional instability of the shoulder: a preliminary report, *J Bone Joint Surg* 62A:897-908, 1980.

49. Hayashi K, Markel M: Thermal capsulorraphy treatment of shoulder instability: basic science, *Clin Orthop* 390:59-72, 2001.

50. Ritzman T, Parker R: Thermal capsulorraphy of the shoulder, *Curr Opin Orthop* 13:288-291, 2002.

51. Rowe CR: Acute and recurrent anterior dislocations of the shoulder, *Orthop Clin North Am* 11(2):253-270, 1980.

52. Wilk K, Arrigo C: Current concepts in the rehabilitation of the athletic shoulder, *J Orthop Sports Phys Ther* 18:356-378, 1993.

53. Mok DW, Fogg AJ, Hokan R et al: The diagnostic value of arthroscopy in glenohumeral instability, *J Bone Joint Surg* 72B(4):698-700, 1990.

54. Speer KP, Hannafin JA, Altchek DW et al: An evaluation to the shoulder relocation test, *Am J Sports Med* 22:177-183, 1994.

55. Matsen FA III: Rotator cuff. In Rockwood CA Jr, Matsen FA III, editors: *The shoulder,* ed 3, Philadelphia, 1998, WB Saunders.

56. Neer CS 2nd: Anterior acromioplasty for the chronic impingement syndrome in the shoulder: a preliminary report, *J Bone Joint Surg* 54A(1):41-50, 1972.

57. Bigliani LU, Morrison D, April EW et al: The morphology of the acromion and its relationship to rotator cuff tears, *Orthop Trans* 10:228, 1986.

58. Walch G, Boileau P, Noel E et al: Impingement of the deep surface of the supraspinatus tendon on the glenoid rim, *J Shoulder Elbow Surg* 1:239-245, 1992.

59. Codman EA: *The shoulder,* ed 2, Boston, 1934, Thomas Todd.

60. Rothman RH, Parke WW: The vascular anatomy of the rotator cuff, *Clin Orthop* 41:176-186, 1965.

61. Lindblom K: On pathogenesis of ruptures of the tendon aponeurosis of the shoulder joint, *Acta Radiol* 20:563-567, 1939.

62. Fukada H, Mikasa M, Yamanaka K et al: Incomplete thickness rotator cuff tears diagnosed by subacromial bursography, *Clin Orthop* 223:51-58, 1987.

63. Matsen FA III, Arntz CT: Rotator cuff tendon failure. In Rockwood CA Jr, Matsen FA III, editors: *The shoulder,* vol 2, Philadelphia, 1990, WB Saunders.

64. Mattingly GE, Mackarey PJ: Optimal methods for shoulder tendon palpation: a cadaver study, *Phys Ther* 76:166-174, 1996.

65. Frieman BG, Albert TJ, Fenlin JM Jr: Rotator cuff disease: a review of diagnosis, pathophysiology and current trends in treatment, *Arch Phys Med Rehabil* 75:604-609, 1994.

66. Leroux JL, Thomas E, Bonnel F et al: Diagnostic value of clinical tests for shoulder impingement syndrome, *Rev Rhum Engl Ed* 62(6):423-428, 1995.

67. Gerber C, Krushell RJ: Isolated rupture of the tendon of the subscapularis muscle: clinical features in 16 cases, *J Bone Joint Surg* 73B(3):389-394, 1991.

68. Calis M, Akgun K, Birtane M et al: Diagnostic values of clinical diagnostic tests in subacromial impingement syndrome, *Ann Rheum Dis* 59(1):44-47, 2000.

69. Itoi E, Tabata S: Conservative treatment of rotator cuff tears, *Clin Orthop* pp 165-173, Feb 1992.

Common Elbow Diagnoses

MICHAEL J. STAINO

The elbow is important in placing the hand in various functional positions. The elbow is the vital link between the hand and the shoulder. Motions at the elbow joint include flexion/extension and forearm rotation.

The elbow is critical in functional hand use for activities of daily living and work and leisure activities. Disruption in elbow function limits one's ability to reach forward, groom hair, and rotate the forearm to hold money and open door knobs.

In addition to fracture, associated nerve, tendon, or ligament injury can complicate recovery and rehabilitation. This chapter highlights distal humeral, proximal ulnar, and radial head fractures and associated elbow trauma. The chapter also addresses distal biceps tendon injury.

ANATOMY

The elbow is classified as a hinge joint but actually consists of three joints. The articulations are the **distal humerus** and ulna **(ulnotrochlear joint),** the distal humerus and the radial head (the **radiocapitellar joint**), and the **proximal radioulnar joint.** The distal portion of the humerus articulates with the radial head on the lateral side and the ulna on the medial side of the elbow.

The distal humerus consists of two **condyles** that form the articular surfaces of the **trochlea** and the **capitellum.** The trochlea articulates with the ulna, and the capitellum articulates with the radial head (Figs. 11-1 and 11-2).[1] Two fossae or divots are in the distal humerus. The **olecranon fossa** is on the dorsal surface and houses the **olecranon,** and the **coronoid fossa** is on the anterior surface. The coronoid process of the ulna articulates with the coronoid fossa of the humerus.

A single and continuous joint capsule covers the articulations. In normal conditions the elbow joint capsule is extremely thin. With trauma, the joint capsule thickens, contributing to elbow stiffness.[2] Complex traumatic elbow injuries can involve bone, ligament, and nerve tissue and frequently lead to a great deal of stiffness, pain, and loss of function.

A natural anatomic **valgus** orientation to the elbow occurs at 0 degrees of extension and full forearm supination. This also is called the **carrying angle of the elbow.** In males the normal valgus orientation is 5 to 10 degrees; in females it is 10 to 15 degrees (Fig. 11-3).[3] When the carrying angle is lost following elbow trauma, you may observe a **varus** presentation of the elbow joint. This presentation sometimes is referred to as a **gunstock deformity.** In this abnormal varus position, the elbow angles away from the side of the body, and the hand and forearm angle toward the hip.

The lateral and medial collateral ligaments act as important stabilizers of the elbow joint. The anterior joint capsule provides varus and valgus stability when the elbow is in full extension. The capsule folds when the elbow is flexed, which decreases stability (Table 11-1).

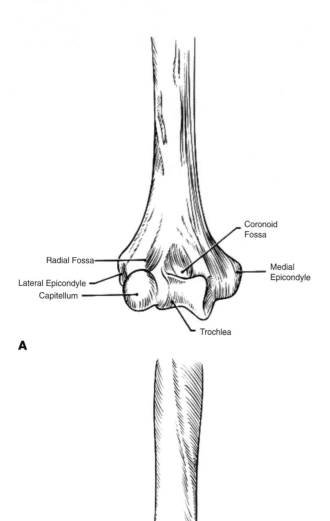

A

B

FIGURE 11-1 Anterior **(A)** and posterior **(B)** topical anatomy of distal humerus. (From Veneziano CJ, Nofzger MJ, Nirschl RP: Elbow anatomy and physical examination. In Trumble TE, Cornwall R, Budoff J, editors: *Core knowledge in orthopaedics: hand, elbow, and shoulder,* Philadelphia, 2006, Mosby.)

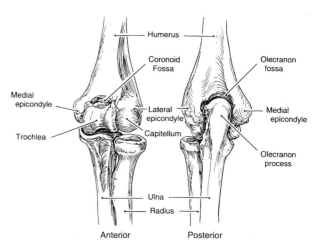

FIGURE 11-2 Anterior and posterior view of the topical anatomy of an elbow joint. (From Schmidt JI: Elbow fractures and dislocations. In Burke SL, Higgins J, McClinton MA et al, editors: *Hand and upper extremity rehabilitation: a practical guide,* ed 3, St Louis, 2006, Churchill Livingstone.)

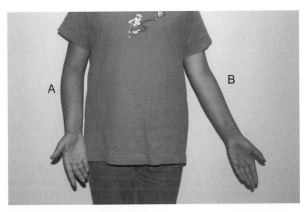

FIGURE 11-3 A, Abnormal varus carrying angle of the patient's right elbow. **B,** Normal carrying angle of the patient's left elbow in the valgus position.

ELBOW KINEMATICS

The elbow is a **trochoginglymoid joint,** having two planes of motion—extension/flexion and supination/pronation. The normal arc of elbow motion is 145 degrees with full extension at 0 degrees and full flexion at 145 degrees. Up to 60% of the compressive forces on the elbow are transmitted through the radiocapitellar joint, with 40% through the ulnotrochlear joint. The range of elbow extension/flexion needed to complete most activities of daily living is 30 to 130 degrees of motion.[4] Table 11-2 describes the muscles that act on the elbow.

The motions of supination and pronation are referred to as forearm rotation. The normal arc of motion for forearm rotation is 180 degrees, with 90 degrees of pronation and 90 degrees of supination. The functional range of motion needed to complete most activities of daily

TABLE 11-1

Collateral Ligaments and the Support Provided at the Elbow Joint

COLLATERAL LIGAMENTS	STABILITY
Radial collateral and annular ligaments	Provide stability to the radial head
Lateral collateral ligament	Connects the lateral epicondyle to the supinator crest of the proximal ulna. It is taut throughout elbow range of motion.
	This is the primary stabilizer on the lateral side of the elbow joint.
Anterior fibers of the medial collateral ligament	Taut in flexion and extension; primary constraint in valgus stability throughout the arc of motion
Posterior fibers of the medial collateral ligament	Taut only in flexion; a stabilizer of the ulnohumeral joint during flexion

TABLE 11-2

Muscles that Produce Motion about the Elbow Joint and the Specific Elbow Motions

ELBOW MUSCULATURE	MOTIONS
Brachialis	Primary elbow flexor
Brachioradialis	Secondary elbow flexor with forearm neutral
Biceps	Secondary elbow flexor when forearm is supinated
Triceps	Primary elbow extensor
Anconeus	Secondary elbow extensor. May be active during elbow flexion/extension arc and provides elbow stabilization.
Pronator teres and pronator quadratus	Pronation of the forearm
Supinator and biceps	Supination of the forearm

living is 50 degrees each of pronation and supination for a total arc of 100 degrees of motion.[5]

Although the osseous structures and ligaments compose the deep portions of the elbow joint, other structures surrounding the joint capsule are important to hand function. The distal humerus is the origin for wrist and finger extensor and flexor muscles. The median, ulnar, and radial nerves carry motor and sensory information to and from the hand. Arteries also travel to the hand via the elbow joint. All of these structures can be affected by traumatic elbow injuries.

DISTAL HUMERAL FRACTURES

CLINICAL *Pearl*

Approximately one third of all elbow fractures involve the distal humerus.[5]

Elbow fractures are classified in three categories that are subdivided based on their location and type. **Extraarticular fractures** involve the medial/lateral epicondyles and **supracondylar regions**. Fig. 11-4 shows a displaced supracondylar fracture. Some extraarticular distal humeral fractures extend distally along the supracondyles and become **intracapsular**. These fractures are classified according to the direction of the fracture fragment. **Intraarticular fractures** have multiple classifications based on location of the fracture within the capsule and the pattern of fractures. Capitellar and trochlear fractures are examples of intraarticular fractures (Table 11-3).

Anatomy

The median, ulnar, and radial nerves are susceptible to trauma associated with distal humeral fractures. Pressure from extensive swelling may cause clients to experience distal numbness, tingling, and motor loss in the wrist and hand.

CLINICAL *Pearl*

The median nerve passes on the anterior aspect and is prone to injury with displaced radial head or distal humeral fractures. The radial nerve passes dorsal to anterior in the region of the distal third of the humerus, which makes it susceptible to injury with distal humeral fractures. The ulnar nerve courses dorsal to the medial epicondyle and is subject to injury with distal humeral medial condylar fractures.

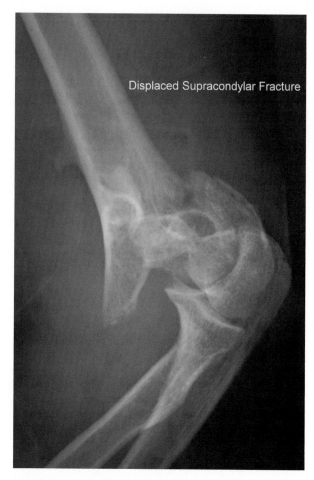

Displaced Supracondylar Fracture

FIGURE 11-4 Lateral radiograph of a supracondylar distal humeral fracture.

Diagnosis and Pathology

Standard anteroposterior and lateral radiographs typically are used to detect most distal humeral fractures. Like most fractures, distal humeral fractures generally occur as a result of high-energy force from a fall. Some fractures may occur from a direct blow to the elbow. Fractures that are comminuted may result in associated neurovascular trauma or ligament injury. A complete neurologic evaluation is important to assess distal motor and sensory function. With a concurrent collateral ligament injury, early active range of motion guidelines and splint positioning should be modified to protect the injured structures (Fig. 11-5). Table 11-4 identifies stages of healing and general treatment guidelines.

Nonoperative Treatment

Extraarticular or intraarticular fractures may be treated using closed reduction and cast immobilization with the elbow supported in flexion and the forearm in neutral

TABLE 11-3

Types of Distal Humeral Fractures with ASIF Descriptive Classification

REGIONS OF THE DISTAL HUMERUS	LOCATION AND TYPE OF FRACTURES
Supracondylar	Epicondylar avulsion fracture
Extraarticular	Simple fracture
	Comminuted fracture
Unicondylar occurring in the frontal or sagittal planes	Lateral condylar, including the capitellum
	Medial condylar, including the trochlea
Transcondylar, bicondylar, or intercondylar	Simple articular, simple metaphyseal
	Simple articular, comminuted metaphyseal
	Comminuted articular

ASIF, Association for Study of Internal Fixation.

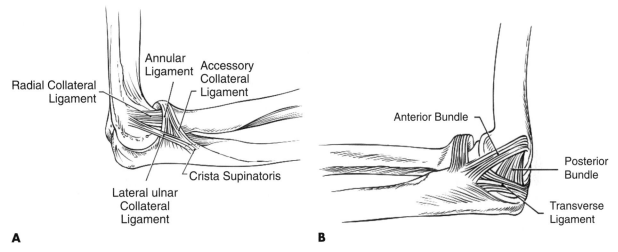

FIGURE 11-5   A, Schematic drawing depicting the lateral ligaments of the elbow. **B,** Schematic drawing depicting the medial ligaments of the elbow. (From Veneziano CJ, Nofzger MJ, Nirschl RP: Elbow anatomy and physical examination. In Trumble TE, Cornwall R, Budoff J, editors: *Core knowledge in orthopaedics: hand, elbow, and shoulder,* Philadelphia, 2006, Mosby.)

TABLE 11-4

Stages of Healing

PHASES OF HEALING	TREATMENT GUIDELINES
Inflammatory phase	Treatment is focused on protecting, maintaining stability, controlling pain, reducing edema, and light active range of motion throughout the range of motion.
Fibroblastic phase	Tensile strength of the healing tissue is minimal and progressively increases with time. Increased collagen density contributes to contractures. Treatment focuses on gentle passive and active range of motion to influence the collagen remodeling. Patients can begin heat modalities, light activities of daily living, and static progressive splinting.
Remodeling phase	Treatment focuses on heat modalities, passive/active range of motion, and progressive strengthening to enhance collagen orientation and plastic elongation of musculotendinous and capsular tissues. Low-grade joint mobilizations and static progressive splinting can be initiated. The final aspect of this phase is endurance training and work hardening.

position. This immobilization typically is maintained for 2 weeks for stable fractures and for 4 to 6 weeks for displaced unstable fractures.[2]

Precaution. *The elbow joint is notorious for developing flexion contractures from prolonged immobilization. This is worsened when swelling is persistent.*

Operative Treatment

Recent advances in open reduction and internal fixation (ORIF) permit sufficiently stable fixation and allow early active range of motion.[6] ORIF for distal humeral fractures may include column plate placement with multiple screw fixation through each fracture fragment. This stable fixation allows the client to start early active motion to reduce distal swelling, to avoid frozen shoulder, and to prevent/correct elbow flexion contractures. An olecranon osteotomy may be performed to repair a comminuted distal humeral fracture. This posterior approach minimizes trauma to anterior structures including nerves.

Closed reduction and percutaneous pinning of the fracture fragment under fluoroscopy for **low transcolumn** (involving the condyles of the distal humerus) or supracondylar fractures may be an option in the elderly, those with advanced osteopenia, and those who are not candidates for ORIF.

Precaution. *Percutaneous pins are susceptible to pin tract infections.*

Another method of pin fixation is the use of traction with pin placement through the olecranon for 2 weeks. With this method, the client is immobilized for an additional 2 to 3 weeks (Fig. 11-6).

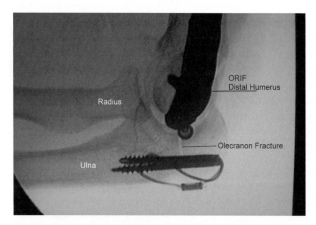

FIGURE 11-6 Lateral radiographic view of an open reduction and internal fixation of the distal humeral fracture pictured in Fig. 11-4.

Questions to Ask the Doctor

- *Is there an associated nerve or vascular injury?*
- *Is the fracture stable?*
- *What type of fixation was used?*
- *Was there an associated ulna/radius fracture?*
- *Was there collateral ligament injury?*
- *Were there associated procedures that involved the triceps and olecranon?*

What to Say to Clients

About the Injury

"This is a diagram of your elbow. The bone that was fractured is the distal humerus. Your physician wants to start active range of motion exercises. It is important to start these exercises to minimize elbow stiffness. You can bend and straighten your elbow with your forearm in neutral (thumb up), supination (palm up), and pronation (palm down).

"Following operative fixation with plates and screws, your goals are to be able to start early active range of motion, monitor your operative site for signs of infection, and control swelling. Observe your scar in the mirror. Look for redness and liquid discharge or fluid seeping from the scar. *Note the color and quantity of the liquid. Also, touch the area for increased warmth. These are signs of possible infection, and if you notice these, you should contact your physician immediately.* Following an elbow injury, swelling is common. It is important to minimize swelling to promote range of motion. You can help to reduce swelling by keeping your arm elevated."

"Your median, radial, and ulnar nerves travel past the elbow. Occasionally, these nerves are injured, causing numbness, tingling, and reduced motor function in the hand and wrist. The recovery time for the nerve condition depends on the amount of injury and the cause. We will check the motor function and sensation of the hand at regular intervals to monitor progress."

About Splints

"There are a variety of splints used during the course of rehabilitation for distal humeral/elbow fractures. Static long arm splints commonly are used to support and protect the elbow joint. They are volar or dorsal and may be custom-molded. Other long arm splints are hinged, which allow for limited movement of flexion/extension while protecting the collateral ligaments. A hinge splint can be locked in a position or set to allow active motion within certain parameters established by the physician."

"Your physician prescribed a long arm splint for you to wear for protection. This splint is designed to position your arm to prevent stress and pressure on the healing elbow ligaments and fractured bones. It is important to follow the splint guidelines to maximize the healing, minimize the swelling, and improve comfort for sleeping."

"There are splints that improve functional range of motion using constant gentle pressure or force. These are dynamic or static progressive splints. The concept of dynamic splinting is called creep, which is the process of realigning the soft tissue by providing a low-load prolonged stretch to increase range of motion. Static progressive splints position your elbow joint at comfortable end range of motion. The end-range is progressively increased to improve joint range of motion and tissue alignment."

If there has been a nerve injury, say, "Some splints can assist with function. For example, following a radial nerve injury, dynamic extension splints increase your ability to open your hand to release objects (Fig. 11-7). You may need to use this type of splint for a number of months. You also will use a resting hand splint at night

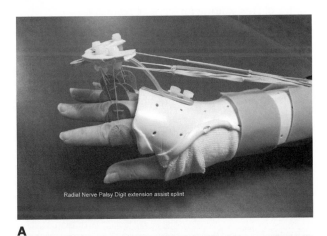

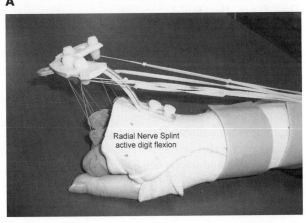

FIGURE 11-7 A, Profile radial nerve splint assisting digit metacarpophalangeal (MP) extension to allow this patient the ability to open the hand when releasing objects. **B,** Patient making a full fist while wearing a radial nerve splint.

to prevent wrist and finger flexion contractures or stiffness."

About Exercise

In the initial stage of rehabilitation, say, "Reducing swelling and improving active range of motion are the goals for the initial phase of hand therapy. We will focus on active range of motion of the shoulder, elbow, wrist, and hand. It is important that you understand that active range of motion of the entire upper extremity will assist in the reduction of swelling in the hand and promote normal hand motion.

"As you attempt to bend your elbow, try to keep your wrist and shoulder stationary. To prevent substituting the wrong motions, place a towel roll under the upper arm at the elbow. This will encourage the shoulder to remain neutral. While holding the towel and keeping your elbow bent at ninety degrees, hold your hand so the thumb is pointing straight to the ceiling. This is the twelve o'clock position or neutral forearm. Turn your palm up facing the ceiling (supination) and hold for three to five seconds. Now turn your palm down to the floor (pronation) and hold for three to five seconds. Generally, full pronation of the right hand points the thumb to the nine o'clock position, and full supination points to the three o'clock position. The hours are reversed for the left hand. Use the clock positions as a visual guide to monitor improvement. It may be difficult to achieve full motion at first, so use the two and ten o'clock positions as goals for the initial phases of therapy."

"The elbow flexes and extends in three forearm positions, which are with the forearm neutral, palm up, and palm down. The neutral position is similar to a 'karate chop' with the thumb pointing to the ceiling. This is typically the easiest position for you to bend and straighten your elbow. Straightening and bending your elbow with the palm up or down is more difficult following traumatic elbow fractures. Always keep your elbow at your side when you perform forearm range of motion. Lock your elbow at your side, and then turn your palm up and down, and then bend and straighten the elbow."

In the second stage of rehabilitation, say, "As you heal, you will be cleared medically to begin weaning from the splint and to use your hand for light activities during the day. At this stage, continue to avoid heavy lifting. We are going to initiate isometric strengthening of the shoulder, wrist, and hand. Isometric exercises are exercises that allow you to use force without moving the joint that is exercising. Force with repetitive movement is more strenuous and can cause your elbow, forearm, wrist, and fingers to swell, leading to increased discomfort and loss of motion."

In the third stage of rehabilitation, say, "You now are entering the third phase of rehabilitation, and your elbow

TABLE 11-5

End-Feel When Assessing End Ranges of Motion at the Elbow Joint

TYPE	DESCRIPITIVE TERMINOLOGY
Bone block	Hard end-feel with bone on bone that is sensed at the end-range of normal elbow extension
Capsular	Leathery feel with resistance at the end-range motion; similar to that which is sensed with normal end-ranges of supination and pronation
Soft tissue approximation	Soft end-feel similar to end-range elbow flexion
Spasm	Tight feel where muscle spasm limits motion
Springy block	Intracapsular (rebound feel)
Empty	No feel

is stable enough to begin progressive resistive strengthening, short periods of return to work, and sports training. We have designed a strengthening program to include resistive exercise to improve your strength and endurance for the heavy loads of your job/sport. You should expect to have muscle fatigue and some possible soreness related to muscular use. Please report any local joint pain, swelling, or numbness that may occur during this phase of your rehabilitation."

Evaluation Tips

- Investigate the mode of injury for insight into possible associated conditions.
- Assess sensory and motor function of the forearm, wrist, and hand.
- Assess edema of the extremity from elbow to the fingers using circumferential measurements taken every 2 inches starting at the elbow crease, including one measurement 2 inches proximal to the elbow crease.
- Perform a wound assessment for seepage and signs of infection following ORIF/pin fixation. Note color, odor, and location of drainage.

Precaution. *If you detect signs of possible infection, contact the physician.*

- Assess active elbow range of motion in forearm neutral, supination, and pronation.
- Assess levels of wrist and shoulder pain.

Diagnosis-Specific Information That Affects Clinical Reasoning

- Radial nerve palsy may occur with humeral shaft fractures with lateral dorsal displacement of the fracture fragments. Provide wrist and digit extension

support with static splint for night use and dynamic extension splint for day use to assist hand function. Radial nerve palsy can continue for up to 21 months following injury, with 6 months being the average time to full recovery.[7] This time can be frustrating for clients waiting for signs of recovery.

Precaution. *A possible complication of ORIF is adherence of the ulnar nerve with subsequent ulnar neuritis.*

- If an olecranon osteotomy was performed, consult the physician for exercise precautions and protection of the triceps.
- Aggressive stretching of the elbow joint can promote **ectopic bone formation** (pathologic bone growth).[8]
- End ranges of motion of the elbow and forearm have specific "end-feels." This information is important in determining splinting needs (Table 11-5).

Tips from the Field

Splinting

Splints or immobilizers for distal humeral fractures typically support the dorsal aspect of the upper arm and forearm. Some clients may be immobilized in a sling for support. When the wrist is unsupported in the immobilization device, the hand may swell as it drapes over the distal edge of the device. The therapist should consider adding wrist support for client comfort. In such instances, a volar wrist splint may be fabricated under the long arm or sugar tong splint.

Custom molded thermoplastic long arm splints provide the rigid support but can cause irritation to the olecranon and epicondyles. Blue T-foam padding used during splint fabrication can be inserted permanently into the splint to avoid areas of skin pressure. The splints can be removed easily for exercise and can be remolded to accommodate changes in swelling. Have clients return to the clinic weekly for assessment of pressure areas, appropriate fit, and repairs of mechanical parts/straps.

The purpose of the splint determines the style of the splint. Clients with collateral ligament injuries who are permitted limited elbow flexion and extension may benefit from a hinge splint that has range of motion blocks. This splint will protect varus/valgus stress. The range of motion blocks serve to limit the amount of flexion and extension as dictated by the surgeon, thus protecting the tissues from stress.

For clients with stable fractures, try night extension splinting for protection. During the waking hours, these clients could use a collar sling holding the elbow at 90 degrees. The collar sling allows the client easy access to active range of motion exercise.

Exercises

Help guide patient motion during the early weeks of rehabilitation following traumatic elbow fractures. Early on, start the client with elbow and forearm active and active-assisted range of motion exercise in the supine position. Support the distal humerus on a towel roll, avoiding pressure over sutures, scars, pins, and plates. This helps prevent compensatory motions of the shoulder and allows focus on isolated elbow motion. As the client demonstrates accurate uncompensated elbow motion, the client can progress to exercising in seated or standing positions.

Instruct the client in the progression of treatment starting with the initial goals of restoration of motion, followed by light resisted activity and return to light functional activity and ultimately ending with heavy resisted/work/sport simulation.

Precaution. *Passive range of motion and joint mobilizations should be avoided until the fracture is healed per the physician's determination.*

Early motion starts at 40 to 60 degrees of flexion and progresses each week by 10 degrees. You can use range of motion blocking splints to keep clients from flexing or extending beyond the prescribed safe ranges of motion. The strengthening phase should begin between 8 and 10 weeks after injury with medical clearance.

Precautions and Concerns

- *The elbow will develop stiffness and flexion contractures with prolonged immobilization.*
- *Early range of motion should be active only to avoid the possibility of chronic instability related to loss of collateral ligament support, fracture orientation, and bony defect, all of which cause pain.*
- *Ectopic bone formation as a result of dislocation can cause stiffness and pain. Do not use passive range of*

motion and dynamic/static progressive splinting until the fracture is stable.
- *Early motion for clients with lateral collateral ligament injury should start with the elbow at 90 degrees of flexion and the forearm pronated. From this position, when the client is medically cleared, have the client perform 10 degrees of flexion and extension actively for the first week (from 80 to 100 degrees arc of motion). Increase active range of motion 10 degrees in flexion and extension each week until the client is medically cleared for full motion. The physician should establish the goals regarding end range of motion.*

PROXIMAL ULNAR FRACTURES

Fractures of the ulna include olecranon fractures, coronoid fractures, and **Monteggia's fractures.** These fractures rarely occur in isolation and usually include associated radial head fractures/dislocations. The olecranon is vulnerable to direct impact trauma. Coronoid fractures commonly are associated with radial head fractures and dislocations. Monteggia's fractures are fractures of the proximal third of the ulna with anterior dislocation of the radial head. Multiple classifications of these fractures are based on the level of stability and displacement of the fracture fragments.

Anatomy

The most prominent portion of the proximal ulna is the olecranon, which is palpated on the dorsal aspect of the elbow. The triceps muscle inserts into the olecranon and provides support that helps prevent subluxation or dislocation. On the anterior aspect of the ulna is the coronoid process. The coronoid process works in concert with the radial head to provide an anterior buttress to the elbow, resisting posterior subluxation. The anterior bundle of the medial collateral ligament attaches to the coronoid process.[4]

Diagnosis and Pathology

Olecranon Fractures

Olecranon fractures typically occur as a result of blunt impact trauma to the posterior elbow. These fractures are classified based on displacement, stability, and comminution. The goals of treatment for olecranon fractures are restoration of joint alignment, motion, and power. Standard anteroposterior and lateral radiographs typically are used to detect olecranon fractures. Multiple surgical approaches for the reduction and fixation are based on the classification of the fracture type. Complications may include ulnar neuropathy, decreased elbow flexion/extension, posttraumatic arthritis, instability, ectopic bone formation, and nonunion.[9]

Coronoid Fractures

Coronoid fractures are referred to as shearing-type injuries because the elbow dislocates by a rotary mechanism. An example is a fall on the outstretched arm while the radial head and proximal ulna supinate away from the humerus. During this action, the trochlea of the humerus shears off part of the coronoid process of the ulna. Radial head fracture also may be evident. Traditionally, coronoid fractures are classified in three types: type I—anterior tip of the bone; type II—up to 50%; and type III—fractures at the base. These fractures typically are detected using standard radiograph lateral views and/or fluoroscopy or computed tomography scans.[10]

Monteggia's Fractures

A proximal ulna fracture with dislocation/fracture of the radial head was first described by Monteggia in 1814 and was classified by Bado into four types according to the direction of the displacement of the radial head.[11] These fractures are seen in children involved in sports or gymnastics or adults following a fall. The mode of injury is described as a direct blow to the proximal ulna or a fall onto the outstretched arm while the forearm is pronated and the elbow is hyperextended. Standard anteroposterior and lateral views of the elbow, forearm, and wrist usually are used to identify this type of ulna fracture. Associated radial nerve injury may occur as a result of direct trauma to the posterior interosseous nerve in the forearm.

Precaution. *Recurrent radial head dislocation may result when proper anatomic alignment of the ulna fracture fragments is compromised.*[10]

Nonoperative Treatment

Olecranon Fractures

Nondisplaced olecranon fractures are referred to as type I fractures. These olecranon fractures can be treated with immobilization for 2 to 3 weeks. Following the immobilization phase, therapy begins with active and active assisted range of motion.

Coronoid Fractures

Because coronoid fractures can occur with associated radial head fractures and/or lateral collateral ligament injuries, operative treatment may be preferred. Treatment depends on the client's age, preinjury health, and functional goals.

Monteggia's Fractures

Because Monteggia's fractures involve injury to the radial head, operative treatment may be preferred. Treatment depends on the client's age, preinjury health, and functional goals.

Operative Treatment

Olecranon Fractures

Internal fixation includes tension band wiring, intramedullary fixation, bicortical screw fixation/plates and dynamic springs. The displaced fractures that are stable are considered type II olecranon fractures. They can be treated with ORIF or olecranon resection. Displaced and unstable olecranon fractures are called type III olecranon fractures and can be treated with internal fixation.[12]

Therapy may begin with early active range of motion at 1 week following the operation if the patient is cleared medically.

Precaution. *Extreme ranges of motion are avoided, especially flexion, until 4 weeks after the operation.*

Strengthening can begin with medical clearance when the union is firm, which is typically about 8 to 10 weeks after the operation.

Coronoid Fractures

Because these fractures typically occur with associated radial head fractures and/or lateral collateral ligament injuries, coronoid fractures may be treated with internal fixation and repair of the associated soft tissue and osseous injuries.

Initial therapy following internal fixation includes finger range of motion and edema management for the first week. Clients are fitted with a long arm splint for support and protection. They can begin protected range of motion with elbow extension limited at 40 to 60 degrees per physician orders while wearing the elbow hinge splint.

Precaution. *Because of associated ligament injuries, be careful to avoid varus and valgus stresses on the elbow.*

The client can increase elbow extension 10 degrees each week starting 4 to 6 weeks postoperatively as permitted by the physician.[10] You usually can initiate forearm active range of motion at 4 weeks postoperatively, based on the level of associated trauma. Coronoid fractures may result in elbow flexion contractures. Static progressive splinting can be initiated at 4 weeks postoperatively (per medical clearance) to prevent or minimize contractures. Passive range and joint mobilizations can start at 6 weeks with medical clearance, and strengthening usually can begin at 8 to 10 weeks. Ligament and fracture stability are key factors in receiving medical clearance to start passive range of motion exercises, strengthening, and joint mobilizations.

Monteggia's Fractures

A low-profile dynamic compression plate may be used to stabilize Monteggia's fracture. Assessment of the radial head dislocation/fracture determines the nonoperative or operative treatment of the radial head. Often, the radial head reduces spontaneously when the ulna fracture is reduced.[11] In some cases the radial head may have an ORIF or excision. See the section on radial head fractures for specific details.

Postoperative immobilization is with the elbow flexed at 90 degrees and the forearm supinated for at least 4 weeks, depending on the rigidity of the fixation. At 4 weeks, active and active-assisted range of motion can be initiated.

Precaution. *Heavy activities should be avoided for 6 months, and passive stretches are to be avoided.*

Questions to Ask the Doctor

- *What is the type of coronoid fracture?*
- *Were there associated radial head and collateral ligament injuries?*
- *What is your protocol for gaining elbow extension?*
- *For Monteggia's fractures, what is the status of the radial head?*
- *Is the fracture stable enough for early active range of motion?*

What to Say to Clients

About the Injury

"This is a diagram of your elbow. The bone you fractured is the proximal ulna. The ulna is a forearm bone that starts at the tip of the elbow and ends on the small finger side of the wrist. The olecranon is the name of the part of the ulna that makes up the 'point' or the back part of the elbow." See the What to Say to Clients section under the discussion of distal humeral fractures for information about splints and exercise.

Evaluation Tips

Evaluation tips for proximal ulna fractures are the same as for distal humeral fractures.

Diagnosis-Specific Information That Affects Clinical Reasoning

- The primary goal for elbow rehabilitation is the restoration of functional active range of motion and reduction of the stress on the collateral ligaments if involved.
- Ulnar fractures occur as a result of axial load and rotation at high force. Associated radial head and collateral ligament damage contributes to loss of motion in forearm rotation and elbow flexion/extension.
- Elbow flexion contractures are common. Begin active range of motion and start early static progressive serial splinting to gain extension at 2 weeks postoperatively if medically permitted.
- Frequently assess the amount of elbow joint swelling because this will affect range of motion recovery. See the section on distal humeral fractures.

Tips from the Field

See the section on distal humeral fractures.

Precautions and Concerns

- *Do not use passive range of motion and dynamic/static progressive splinting until you receive medical clearance.*
- *Early motion for clients with lateral collateral ligament injury should start with the elbow flexed at 90 degrees and the forearm pronated.*
- *Inadequate fixation and early motion can contribute to fracture nonunion.*
- *Aggressive passive range of motion and dynamic splinting/static progressive splinting can lead to ectopic bone formation.*
- *Protect the triceps insertion into the olecranon during early active range of motion by supporting the movement and do not push flexion beyond 90 degrees during the first 4 to 6 weeks.*
  See the section on distal humeral fractures.

RADIAL HEAD FRACTURES

Radial head fractures account for 33% of elbow fractures. One third of radial head fractures have associated trauma. Radial head fractures occur in adults and children; they occur more frequently in the female population. In children, radial head fractures result from falls on the playground, gymnastic stunts, and sports.[13]

Anatomy

The radial head articulates with the capitellum of the distal humerus and the ulna (proximal radial ulnar joint). The radial head is a secondary stabilizer of the elbow joint along with the radial and lateral ulnar collateral ligaments and the annular ligament.[4] The radial head is on the lateral aspect of the proximal forearm/elbow region. The radial head can be palpated with the forearm in full pronation and the elbow flexed to 90 degrees. To palpate, first locate the tip of the lateral epicondyle with your thumb. Then slide your thumb toward the client's wrist approximately ½ inch. The hard feel is the radial head. While holding the thumb on the radial head, have the client rotate the forearm. The radial head will be less prominent in supination.

Diagnosis and Pathology

Radial head fractures typically occur as a result of high-energy impact to the outstretched upper extremity with the elbow partially flexed and the forearm in a pronated position. These fractures are classified based on level of displacement of the fracture fragment. Type I is nondisplaced. Type II is displaced with a single fragment. Type III is comminuted. Type IV is fracture with dislocation. Fractures can be simple and only involve the radial head, or they may be complex and involve other structures. Associated injuries include medial or lateral collateral ligament injury, ulna fracture, triangular fibrocartilage complex (TFCC) tear/interosseous membrane disruption, and/or dislocation (Fig. 11-8).

Radial head fracture plus dislocation of the distal radial ulnar joint and interosseous membrane disruption is called an **Essex Lopresti fracture. Galeazzi's fracture** is a radial shaft fracture and dislocation of the distal radial ulnar joint (DRUJ) with tearing of the TFCC.

Nonoperative Treatment

Radial head fractures typically are treated based on the type of fracture and level of complexity of the associated trauma.

Type I radial head fractures can be treated using a removable immobilization device such as a long arm splint, half cast with Ace wrap, or sling. Clients usually are encouraged to initiate active range of motion and to use the immobilization for comfort.

Type II radial head fractures can be treated nonoperatively with immobilization for 2 to 3 weeks and early motion based on medical clearance. Medical clearance typically depends on the level of displacement with possible delayed excision.[14] Initiate the active range of motion program for flexion and extension of the elbow and rotation of the forearm within the client's pain-free range.

Operative Treatment

Operative treatment for type II radial head fractures includes fracture fragment excision, radial head excision, ORIF, or prosthesis. Postoperative immobilization is typi-

cally in a long arm splint or cast with elbow at 90 degrees and neutral forearm rotation. Start the client on early active range of motion within the first postoperative week based on medical clearance.

Type III radial head fractures can be treated with complete excision of the radial head. Start the client on an early active motion program within the first week postoperatively.

Clients with type IV radial head fractures should have immediate reduction of the dislocation and fracture treatment per type of fracture. In complex fractures, excision or prosthesis may be considered (Fig. 11-9). A hinge

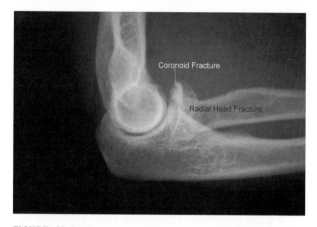

FIGURE 11-8 Lateral radiographic view of the elbow joint showing a small coronoid fracture and radial head fracture.

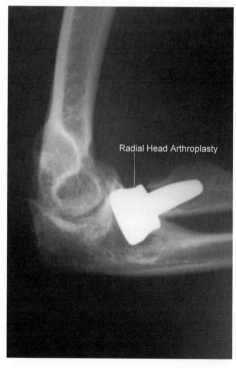

FIGURE 11-9 Lateral radiographic view of the elbow joint highlighting the radial head implant following arthoplasty.

splint typically is used to allow early controlled motion and to protect varus and valgus stresses.[15]

The type of fracture, client factors, and associated trauma can affect postinjury rehabilitation. Ideally, early mobilization starts within the first week to 10 days after injury/surgery. Treatment focus for the first 4 weeks of therapy is restoration of active range of motion within comfort, edema control, and protective splinting. Passive range of motion and strengthening are avoided. Splinting during the first 4 weeks is protective.

During the second phase of rehabilitation, usually at 4 to 5 weeks after injury/surgery, the client may initiate isometric exercises to tolerance if medically cleared and may continue with active range of motion. Splinting for protection is weaned and transitioned to static progressive splinting. Dynamic splints are avoided to prevent the risk of heterotopic calcification.

The third phase focuses on restoration of strength and passive range of motion to improve function.

Questions to Ask the Doctor

- *Are there associated fractures, collateral ligament damage, or wrist problems?*
- *What type of elbow splinting do you prefer?*
- *What are the range of motion parameters?*
- *Are pronation and supination safe based on ligament integrity?*
- *Was there a triangular fibrocartilage complex injury or distal radial ulnar joint disruption?*
- *When will it be safe for passive range of motion exercises?*

What to Say to Clients

About the Injury

"This is a diagram of your elbow, forearm, and wrist. The bone you injured is the radial head. It plays a significant role in bending/straightening the elbow and rotating the forearm. As you can see, the radius is one of the forearm bones that connects to the elbow and wrist. When you fractured the radial head, there is a chance that associated wrist trauma occurred. This may explain some pain you might have on the ulnar side of your wrist. The radius and the ulna connect at the elbow and at the wrist."

About Splints and about Exercise

See the section on distal humeral fractures.

Evaluation Tips

- Measure the elbow active range of motion with the forearm in neutral, supination, and pronation.

- Assess wrist function and pain for possible DRUJ injury.
- Palpate the common extensor tendon at the lateral epicondyle for soreness. You may consider using a volar wrist splint to help minimize lateral epicondylitis pain.

See the evaluation tips in the section on distal humeral fractures.

Diagnosis-Specific Information That Affects Clinical Reasoning

- Acute instability results from radial head excision with unrecognized medial collateral ligament injury.
- Loss of strength in grip and pinch and loss of pronation/supination are possible.

Tips from the Field

Splinting

- Splint for protection during the first 2 to 4 weeks.
- Constant splinting for the first 2 weeks following radial head fractures can lead to flexion contractures.

Exercise

- Perform early active elbow range of motion in pronation to protect the lateral collateral ligaments.
- Supination of the forearm could cause pain because of increased radiocapitellar load.

See the tips from the field under the section on distal humeral fractures.

Precautions and Concerns

- *Wrist pain is associated with radial head excision.*
- *Focus on active and active-assisted range of motion for the first 4 weeks.*
- *Avoid passive range of motion and strengthening until 8 weeks following injury/surgery.*
- *Constant immobilization for more than 2 weeks may cause elbow stiffness.*

See the precautions and concerns under the section on distal humeral fractures.

DISTAL BICEPS TENDON INJURY

Injury of the distal biceps tendon may occur as a complete or partial avulsion of the tendon from the radial tuberosity. Less commonly, injuries to the tendon can occur at the musculotendinous junction.[16] The mechanism of injury consistently is related to contact sports or trying to catch a falling heavy load with an open hand, resulting in forceful extension of the elbow from a flexed and supinated position.[17,18]

Anatomy

The distal biceps tendon passes anterior to the elbow and can be palpated with light resistance to elbow flexion with the forearm in full supination. The biceps muscle originates in the shoulder and inserts as the distal biceps tendon at the radial tuberosity of the radius.

CLINICAL *Pearl*

The primary action of the biceps muscle is supination. The biceps also is a secondary elbow flexor.

The distal tendon feathers as it courses distally to form a tough fibrous connection to the forearm flexors, called the **bicipital aponeurosis.**

Diagnosis and Pathology

Clients who avulse the distal biceps tendon experience a sharp tearing pain in the anterior elbow during lifting. The elbow may demonstrate bruising and discoloration called **ecchymosis.** The muscle mass and contour of the distal biceps will look different compared with the contralateral side. Clients may demonstrate diminished strength in elbow flexion and supination. In partial tears, crepitus might be present. Magnetic resonance imaging may be used to detect biceps tendon ruptures.

The course of treatment depends on the type of rupture. Operative and nonoperative options are available. Results with early repair are favorable. Nonoperative clients can function using the brachialis to flex the elbow and the supinator muscle to supinate the forearm.

Nonoperative Treatment

Nonoperative treatment uses immobilization in a long arm splint or cast with the elbow positioned at 90 of flexion and the forearm neutral for 4 to 6 weeks. While the client is splinted, the client should perform shoulder, wrist, and digital range of motion exercises to minimize stiffness.

Precaution. *Use caution with shoulder range of motion exercises to avoid biceps muscle activation during shoulder flexion. Also, teach your client to limit shoulder extension to 0 degrees.*

Active-assisted shoulder range of motion exercises in the supine position with the splint donned are safer.

When the splint is discontinued, start active and active-assisted elbow and forearm range of motion, avoiding elbow pain. Avoid overexercising, which can irritate tender tissue. Gradually initiate pain-free passive range of motion.

At 8 weeks after injury, begin strengthening with light isometric exercises and gradually upgrade to progressive resistive exercise. Monitor pain and modify the treatment plan as needed for the client to be comfortable.

Operative Fixation and Treatment

Two methods are used for tendon reattachment to the radial tuberosity. The **suture anchor technique** is an anterior approach with one incision and two to three suture anchors to attach the distal biceps tendon to the radial tuberosity. Suture anchors are screw or barb designs. The **two-incision technique** uses an anterior and dorsal incision. A hole is drilled into the tuberosity, and the tendon is pulled through with sutures attached to the distal tendon, which are attached to the tuberosity with the forearm in neutral.[16]

The postoperative treatment begins with protective splinting with the elbow flexed at 90 degrees and the forearm supinated. During these first 2 weeks, initiate edema control and shoulder and wrist/digit range of motion.

At 3 weeks, with medical clearance, initiate elbow and forearm range of motion according to the physician's protocol preference. These initial exercises usually consist of active elbow extension, full passive elbow flexion, active pronation to neutral, and full passive supination. Follow physician-specific limits and precautions for elbow and forearm motions, with gradual increases in extension and adjustments in the position of the elbow splint.

Precaution. *Passive extension range of motion is not safe until 7 to 8 weeks postoperatively and should not be done without medical clearance.*

At approximately 8 weeks, the splint can be discontinued and light strengthening can be initiated if the client is cleared medically. Some physicians do not allow strengthening exercises until 12 weeks postoperatively. If passive range of motion is limited, dynamic or static progressive splinting may be added with medical clearance.

Questions to Ask the Doctor

- *What type of fixation was used?*
- *What protocol do you prefer for splinting and progressing elbow extension motion?*
- *Was there injury to the posterior interosseous nerve?*

What to Say to Clients

About the Injury

"Your biceps muscle is attached to the radius bone of your forearm. The action of the biceps is to turn the palm up to the ceiling when the elbow is bent. The biceps also acts as a secondary elbow bending muscle. You ruptured the tendon from the bone, and your physician reattached it. The initial three weeks of therapy will address your finger, wrist, and shoulder range of motion, swelling, and scar mobility. During the later weeks, we will be able to work on elbow and forearm range of motion according to your physician's postoperative protocols."

About Splinting

"Your physician prescribed a long arm splint with your elbow flexed to ninety degrees and forearm positioned with the palm up to the ceiling. You will be wearing the splint in this position for approximately three weeks or more. As time progresses, the splint will be adjusted to increase your elbow extension."

"If your passive range of motion is limited later on, we can discuss static progressive or dynamic forearm/elbow splinting with your physician. Your physician may recommend that you use a dynamic elbow extension splint to increase your ability to straighten your elbow. This type of splint provides a low-load prolonged stretch to increase range of motion without causing pain. It is important that the force is gentle enough for you to be able to wear the splint for the prescribed time frame."

About Exercise

"Now you are able to start active and passive range of motion exercise to bend the elbow and rotate the forearm. For the next few weeks, straightening the elbow is limited to minimize the stress on the repair. Passive range of motion of elbow extension is not permitted until the doctor authorizes. It is essential that you adhere to these instructions to maximize recovery and minimize potential for rupture or overstretching of the repair."

Evaluation Tips

- Avoid passive range of motion measurements for elbow extension during initial evaluation. Do this only after the protocol allows it.

- Measure active and passive range of motion of the elbow in supine to minimize the effects of gravity.
- Assess motion of the thumb extensors for posterior interosseous nerve function.
- Assess scar adherence.
- Include measurements of the wrist, hand, and shoulder.

Diagnosis-Specific Information That Affects Clinical Reasoning

- Loss of elbow flexion during the first 6 weeks might indicate stretching of the repair. Contact the surgeon immediately if this is suspected.
- Loss of radial nerve function requires resting and dynamic extension assist splinting.

Tips from the Field

Splinting

The initial long arm splint can be a hinge splint with extension blocks. These splints can be custom-molded or prefabricated. Half casts are applied postoperatively and are secured by Ace wraps. This option can cause distal swelling and cumbersome donning/doffing procedures for exercise. Static long arm thermoplastic splints are lighter and easier to don/doff than half casts.

Exercise

Early motion includes active and passive elbow flexion and active elbow extension to 30 degrees. With all phases of exercise, pain must be avoided. If there is pain, reduce the end ranges of motion. Following surgery, active elbow extension is limited intentionally to prevent stretching of the repair. If stretching is suspected, immediately contact the physician. If stretching is confirmed, limit active elbow extension to approximately 60 degrees and adjust the splint to 60 degrees until full active flexion is gained.

Scar Management

Scar mobilization and gentle scar massage help minimize scar adherence. Elastomer, scar gel pads, or light compressive wraps assist with scar softening.

Precautions and Concerns

- *There may be an associated radial nerve palsy.*
- *Early loss of elbow flexion during first 6 weeks postoperatively might indicate stretching of the repair.*
- *Encourage clients to perform digit, wrist, and shoulder motion exercises to minimize associated stiffness and swelling.*

The Role of the Therapy Assistant
In Elbow and Forearm Fractures

- *Edema management*
- *Splint adaptations and modifications per therapist recommendations*
- *Home exercise instruction*
- *Assisting with/instructing in pin care and wound care*
- *Supervision and modification of exercises established by the therapist*
- *Adaptive equipment and activities of daily living training*
- *Reinforcing posture and positioning and precautions*
- *Other possibilities based on the therapy assistant's experience and state licensure regulations*

CASE *Studies*

CASE 11-1: DISTAL HUMERAL FRACTURE

C.W. is a 57-year-old woman who sustained a comminuted supracondylar distal humeral fracture as result of a fall while skiing. She is referred to therapy 5 days after ORIF. Evaluation findings reveal pitting edema at elbow/forearm, significant elbow stiffness in flexion/extension, fair pronation/supination, and no active finger, thumb, or wrist extension because of an associated radial nerve injury. The client's prescription reads, "Evaluation and treatment." The prescription is from a local physician who did not perform the surgery.

The therapist provides supportive elbow splinting, dynamic distal MP extension splinting, and night resting forearm-hand splinting for the radial nerve injury. The therapist contacts the local physician to discuss the fracture stability and other concerns that the operating physician might have communicated.

Initially, this client was diligent in all phases of her care. She wore the splints and performed the exercises consistently. As a result, range of motion improved, edema was minimized, and radial nerve function was showing signs of recovery at 1 month after repair. Elbow active range of motion measured 20 to 120 degrees of extension to flexion and forearm supination/pronation measured 80 to 80 degrees.

This client required a great deal of hands-on therapy to guide range of motion of the elbow, edema management, and stabilization of shoulder actions to focus on isolated forearm and elbow motions. She also received biofeedback to minimize biceps muscle activity during attempts at elbow extension. This was helpful since she was guarding and did not realize that her biceps was firing during elbow active extension.

Unfortunately, C.W. fell in the shower, and the olecranon developed a nonunion. C.W. also developed ulnar nerve neuropathy at the cubital tunnel. She was discharged temporarily from therapy and underwent an iliac bone graft for the olecranon and an ulnar nerve transposition.

CASE 11-2: RADIAL HEAD FRACTURE

D.D. is a 14-year-old right-handed girl who sustained a right type I radial head fracture while attempting a cartwheel. She was diagnosed as having a minimally displaced fracture and was placed in cast for 4 weeks. When the cast was removed, D.D. was apprehensive about flexing or extending the elbow and developed a flexion contracture at 40 degrees. She was referred to hand therapy for range of motion.

During the therapy evaluation, D.D. mentioned ulnar sided wrist pain and weakness in grip. Elbow range of motion was severely limited, with elbow extension to flexion measuring 60 to 95 degrees. Forearm range of motion measured 20 degrees of pronation and 30 degrees of supination. D.D. had functional motion at the shoulder and digits but had significant range of motion loss of wrist ranges. D.D. also had a positive TFCC grind and severe ulnar-sided wrist pain with forearm/wrist motions. The therapist called the physician to discuss the wrist symptoms.

D.D. had further radiographic tests, which revealed a TFCC tear and DRUJ disruption. D.D. was sent back to therapy with revised orders for splinting and range of motion. A sugar tong splint was fabricated and was to be worn for 6 weeks to protect the DRUJ and TFCC (Fig. 11-10). She was started on elbow range of active range of motion in the forearm neutral position during the next 4 weeks. The sugar tong splint was removed for bathing and elbow exercise.

In therapy, D.D. performed elbow flexion/extension exercises in the supine position with the distal humerus supported on a towel and the forearm in the neutral position. D.D. did not perform forearm rotation exercise because these would aggravate the DRUJ and TFCC. With the splint on, she also performed finger and shoulder range of motion exercises to maintain motion. When the splint was discontinued, she began active and active-assisted range of motion for the forearm and wrist. Her elbow range of motion progressed in all planes of forearm positions.

Strengthening exercise began approximately 4 weeks after the splint was discontinued. Her strengthening exercises started with isometric exercises for the elbow, wrist, forearm, and hand. These exercises slowly progressed to progressive resistive exercise as tolerated. D.D. tolerated the progressive strengthening well. She returned to

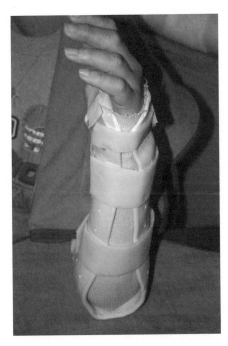

FIGURE 11-10   Sugar tong splint immobilization status after cast removal. This splint is used to support distal radial ulnar joint following open reduction and internal fixation of the distal radius and ulna.

limited gymnastics, avoiding weight-bearing activities. She began elbow and wrist weight bearing on the physioball in therapy but used the sugar tong splint to protect and rest her forearm otherwise. D.D. further progressed to partial weight-bearing gymnastic activities and continued to use the splint periodically. She was discharged from therapy and continued to progress to full floor gymnastics with the supervision of her parents, coach, and trainer.

CASE 11-3: DISTAL BICEPS TENDON RUPTURE

P.J. is a 37-year-old right-hand dominant spa/pool installer who sustained a distal biceps tendon rupture while lowering a spa to the floor. He reported a "pop" followed by pain and immediate loss of elbow motion. He was diagnosed as having an elbow sprain and returned to daily work activities with a compression sleeve for support.

Over the next 2 weeks, P.J. experienced weakness in elbow flexion and ecchymosis over the volar elbow and forearm. Magnetic resonance imaging and clinical exam revealed a distal biceps tendon rupture. P.J. had the tendon repaired with the two-suture anchor approach. He was fitted with a long arm splint with his elbow positioned at 90 degrees and forearm neutral.

At 2 weeks, therapy was initiated for protective range of motion. His therapy program consisted of supine range of motion exercise with the splint removed. The hand therapist provided direction and helped to encourage active and passive flexion to tolerance and active extension to 30 degrees and protected rotation as determined by his surgeon. P.J. wore his splint while performing shoulder active-assisted range of motion. He adhered to precautions during all shoulder motions to protect the elbow. He also performed wrist and digit range of motion. His edema control techniques involved elevation and a compression garment sleeve. P.J. also performed scar massage several times per day.

At 5 weeks, P.J. demonstrated a progressive loss of active elbow flexion. The hand therapist suspected that the repair was starting to have tension or stretching. The therapist immediately contacted the physician, and the splinting protocol was adjusted to 60 degrees of flexion and active elbow extension was blocked at 60 degrees. This adjustment was continued for 2 weeks, and the client was scheduled to follow-up with the surgeon to assess his biceps tendon function.

P.J.'s recovery continued successfully. At 8 weeks, elbow active range of motion was 10 to 130 degrees. Supination was limited to 50 degrees. The hand therapist contacted the physician to discuss possibilities for dynamic or static progressive forearm supination splinting. P.J. was fitted with a static progressive splint to be worn for 30 minutes, 3 times per day, progressing as tolerated in a pain-free way. P.J. slowly regained supination over the course of 6 to 8 weeks and eventually achieved functional pronation and supination.

References

1. Morrey BF, Bernard F: Anatomy of the elbow joint. In Morrey BF, editor: *The elbow and its disorders*, ed 3, Philadelphia, 2000, Saunders.
2. Chinchalkar SJ, Szekeres M: Rehabilitation of elbow trauma, *Hand Clin* 20:363-374, 2004.
3. Morrey BF, An KN: Articular and ligamentous contribution to the stability of the elbow joint, *Am J Sports Med* 11:315, 1983.
4. Magee DJ: *Orthopedic physical assessment*, ed 3, Philadelphia, 1997, Saunders.
5. Jupiter JB, Morrey BF: Fractures of the distal humerus in adults. In Morrey BF, editor: *The elbow and its disorders*, ed 3, Philadelphia, 2000, Saunders.
6. O'Driscoll SW: Supracondylar fractures of the elbow: open reduction, internal fixation, *Hand Clin* 20:465-473, 2004.
7. Ring D, Chin K, Jupiter JB: Radial nerve palsy associated with high-energy humeral shaft fractures, *J Hand Surg* 29A(1):144-147, 2004.
8. Beredjiklian PK: Management of fractures and dislocations of the elbow. In Mackin EJ, Callahan AD, Skirven TM et al, editors: *Rehabilitation of the hand and upper extremity*, ed 5, St Louis, 2002, Mosby.

9. Davila SA: Therapist's management of fractures and dislocations of the elbow. In Mackin EJ, Callahan AD, Skirven TM et al, editors: *Rehabilitation of the hand and upper extremity,* ed 5, St Louis, 2002, Mosby.

10. Cohen MS: Fractures of the coronoid process, *Hand Clin* 20:443-453, 2004.

11. Regan WD, Morrey BF: Coronoid process and Monteggia fractures. In Morrey BF, editor: *The elbow and its disorders,* ed 3, Philadelphia, 2000, Saunders.

12. Cabanela ME, Morrey BF: Fractures of the oleocranon. In Morrey BF, editor: *The elbow and its disorders,* ed 3, Philadelphia, 2000, Saunders.

13. Regan W, Morrey BF: Fractures of the coronoid process of the ulna, *J Bone Joint Surg* 71A:1348-1349, 1989.

14. Morrey BF: Radial head fracture. In Morrey BF, editor: *The elbow and its disorders,* ed 3, Philadelphia, 2000, Saunders.

15. Ring D: Open reduction and internal fixation of fractures of the radial head, *Hand Clin* 20:415-425, 2004.

16. Morrey BF: Injury of the flexors of the elbow: biceps in tendon injury. In Morrey BF, editor: *The elbow and its disorders,* ed 3, Philadelphia, 2000, Saunders.

17. Hamilton W, Ramsey M: Rupture of the distal tendon of the biceps brachii, *Univ Pa Orthop J* 12:21-26, 1999.

18. Ruland RT, Dunbar RP, Bowen JD: The biceps squeeze test for diagnosis of distal biceps tendon ruptures, *Clin Orthop* pp 128-131, Aug 2005.

12

Common Peripheral Nerve Problems

ANNE M.B. MOSCONY

OVERVIEW OF PERIPHERAL NERVE PROBLEMS

Functional recovery from a peripheral **nerve** injury requires the cooperative efforts of the physician, therapist, and client. The potentially grave consequences of these injuries are well known to surgeons and therapists but may not be so obvious to our clients. Diminution or loss of sensation in the hand can result in difficulties performing simple tasks such as safely reaching into one's pocket to retrieve an item or manipulating an object such as a safety pin, especially if vision is occluded. Muscle weakness or paralysis can result in decreased strength and endurance for household and work tasks, with monetary consequences that include lost work time and lost job skills.

Pain is almost always a sequela of a nerve injury, and nerve pain is itself a costly and difficult condition to treat. Inadvertently, clients may damage their nervous system further if they are not educated properly about their injury and relevant precautions and about how full participation in their rehabilitation is essential to optimal recovery.

To understand our client's pathologic peripheral nerve condition, it is vital first to appreciate the normal static and dynamic aspects of the nervous system. We must understand how changes in the peripheral nervous system can lead to changes in the central nervous system These alterations can cause functional disturbances for our clients. A knowledgeable hand therapist is able to anticipate and assist clients in remediation of these functional problems.

Most of us learned about the nervous system as if it has distinct divisions (i.e., the peripheral nervous system and the central nervous system).

CLINICAL *Pearl*

The nervous system is actually one system that crosses multiple joints, moves through multiple muscular and fibrooseous tunnels, and has the same function of continuous electrochemical communication throughout.

Consequently, changes in one part of the nervous system likely will result in changes in other parts of this system, even at those parts of the system that are metrically distant.

The peripheral nerve is composed of many very long cells that originate in the spinal region and that are designed to be conduits for transmitting impulses, no matter how or in what position the body moves. We

know that joints move in a matter of degrees, that muscles contract, and that tendons slide. Nerves also move; they move relative to the tissues that surround them.[1] The nerve cell itself must stretch and slide within its protective tissue coverings, and the nerve trunk must glide relative to the surrounding external tissues while continuing to perform its essential duty: impulse conduction.

The normal nervous system is designed to protect the neurons and their peripheral axons during movement. Movement of the joints is necessary for nerve **homeostasis** (i.e., physiologic balance)[2] and uninterrupted **axoplasmic flow** (flow of cytoplasm or axoplasm within the nerve cell).[2,3] Gliding of the peripheral nerves across the joints and through anatomic tunnels has been speculated to promote axoplasmic flow and to enhance blood circulation to neural tissue. However, certain movements or postures can increase the amount of pressure within the nerve trunk,[2] and if enough pressure is placed on the nerve trunk, temporary anoxia from diminished blood flow to the nerve results. Given the right circumstances, this type of innocuous insult can turn into significant pathologic condition of the nerve.

Impaired axoplasmic flow compromises neural function, with slowed or decreased synaptic activity, and results in **trophic changes** in the tissues served by that nerve.[2,3] Furthermore, an injured nerve can develop an abnormal site of discharge, or an ectopic pacemaker,[3,4] that allows the nerve not only to conduct impulses but also to generate its own impulses without external provocation. That means the peripheral nerve can generate a pain message, even when other local tissue is not damaged!

Changes in a peripheral nerve can have consequences as far away as the cortex of the brain. The adult brain is now known to be more plastic than was once thought; experience with nerve pain, for example, can cause aberrant changes in the somatosensory cortex that can be mapped.[4-6] The central nervous system reorganizes its cortical representations of the hand, following an alteration of skin inputs induced by a peripheral nerve injury. Likewise, neglect of a body part (e.g., following a nerve injury with consequent motor paralysis) can lead to changes in cortical organization.[5,6]

The nervous system is one continuous impulse-conducting system extending from the brain to the toes and fingers. The nervous system is designed for motion, and it needs movement for nervous system homeostasis. Motion is lotion for the nerves. Injuries to a peripheral nerve can have far-reaching consequences, including the development of aberrant cortical changes and the consequent development of a chronic pain state.

Given how much we move and the interesting and varied positions we assume each day, it actually is amazing that the nerves are not traumatized more often. A number of protective mechanisms are inherent in the nervous system. This chapter reviews normal nerve anatomy and looks at factors that can pervert the nerve. The chapter explains how the nerve responds to injury, and how we as clinicians can assist our clients in ameliorating the potentially deleterious affects of commonly seen peripheral nerve injuries of the upper extremity. The chapter concludes with the case studies presented at the beginning of the chapter, using critical reasoning to determine how to treat these clients.

Anatomy

The **neuron** is the basic unit of the nervous system; it consists of a cell body (the **soma**), some **dendrites,** and usually one **axon.** A chain of communicating neurons is called a **pathway.** Within the central nervous system a bundle of pathway axons can be called a tract or a **fasciculus.** Outside the central nervous system a bundle of pathway axons is called a nerve. All peripheral motor nerves have their cell bodies in the anterior horn of the gray matter of the spinal cord, whereas all peripheral sensory nerves have their cell bodies in the dorsal root ganglia, located adjacent to the intervertebral foramen of the vertebral column. The sensory and motor roots join together to form a **spinal nerve** (Fig. 12-1). Sympathetic nerve axons from autonomic ganglia also join the spinal nerve by way of the rami communicantes.

Therefore, spinal and somatic peripheral nerves usually are mixed with sensory, autonomic, and motor axons. Shortly after merging, the spinal nerve splits into dorsal and ventral rami. The ventral rami of all spinal nerves, except for T2 to T12, form networks of nerves called **plexuses.** Of the four main plexuses, the largest are the brachial plexus and lumbar plexus.

The brachial plexus (Fig. 12-2) is formed by the anterior rami of cervical roots C5 to T1. This plexus emerges from the anterior and middle scalene muscles and passes deep to the clavicle before entering the axilla. In the distal axilla the axons from the plexus become the radial, median, ulnar, axillary, and musculocutaneous nerves. The entire upper limb is innervated by branches from this brachial plexus.

Peripheral nerves are ensheathed, protected, and at times constrained by multiple layers of connective tissue coverings: the **endoneurium, perineurium, epineurium,** and **mesoneurium.** The function of these tissue coverings is discussed in more detail later in this chapter. Within these protective tissue coverings, the nerve fibers change position and numbers, frequently entwining and separating as they course in an undulating fashion to their final destination. This meshing serves as a protective mechanism, allowing some play in the overall length

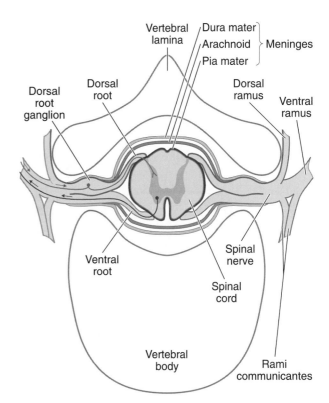

FIGURE 12-1 Schematic of a typical spinal nerve formed from the dorsal and ventral roots of the spinal cord. (From Lundy-Ekman L: *Neuroscience: fundamentals for rehabilitation,* Philadelphia, 1998, WB Saunders.)

of the nerve (Fig. 12-3).[2] Thus peripheral nerve fibers are capable of some degree of stretch, as for example the **ulnar nerve** must do during elbow flexion as it courses behind the medial epicondyle of the humerus.

Diagnosis and Pathology: General Comments about Mechanism of Nerve Injury

Knowing the mechanism of the nerve injury is helpful for estimating prognosis and need for and type of medical and therapeutic intervention. Causes of the injury can include compression or entrapment from internal sources such as a tumor or scar tissue or from an external source such as from crutches or a cast. Nerve injury may occur via traction or stretching to the nerve, by avulsion or laceration, by chemical or electric burns, or by radiation. Nerve injuries may be classified as nerve fibers that are severed or as nerve fibers and their endoneurial tube that remain in continuity despite various degrees of damage to the connective tissue coverings of the nerve and to the nerve fiber itself.

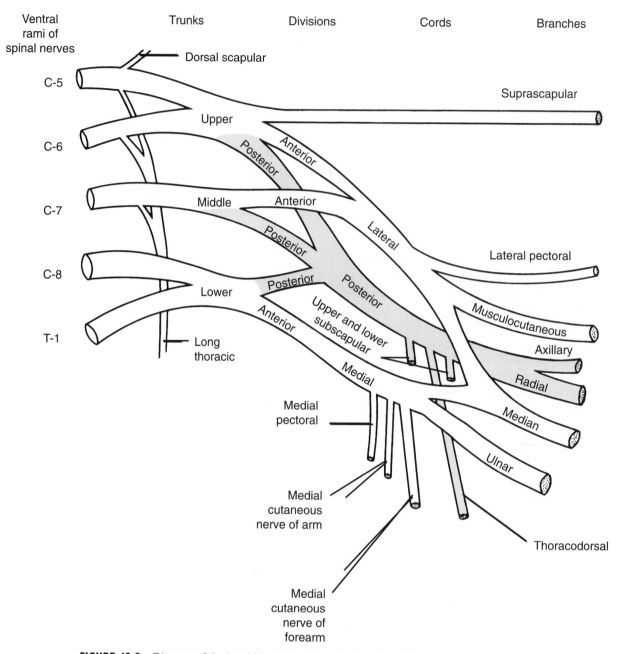

FIGURE 12-2 Diagram of the brachial plexus. (From Jenkins DB: *Hollinshead's functional anatomy of the limb and back,* ed 8, Philadelphia, 2002, Saunders.)

CLINICAL *Pearl*

Nerve injuries where the nerve is severed completely or where the nerve shows serious internal disorganization are considered to have the poorest prognosis for functional recovery,[7] and typically these cases require surgical intervention to allow for some amount of functional recovery.

Incomplete Injuries

Injuries to a nerve in which the external connective tissue coverings remain to some degree intact are known as nerve injuries in which the nerve is in continuity. Also known as incomplete injuries, these injuries have important therapeutic implications. **Mononeuropathy** involves damage to a single nerve. An example would be compression of the median nerve at the carpal tunnel, or **carpal** tunnel syndrome. **Multiple mononeuropathy** is a multifocal asymmetric involvement of multiple nerves.[6] Compression of the right median and ulnar nerves as a complication of occupational stresses that require repetitious elbow and wrist flexion is an example of multiple mononeuropathy.

Metabolic changes can result in neuropathies as well. Typically, one sees **polyneuropathy,** or bilateral damage to more than one peripheral nerve. Peripheral polyneu-

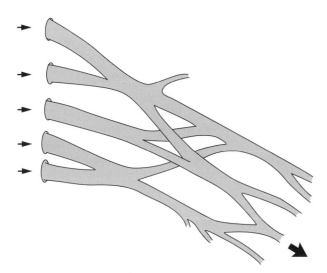

FIGURE 12-3 The peripheral nervous system forms many plexuses and subdivisions, allowing sensory, motor, and autonomic fibers to combine, separate, and recombine. These subdivisions and plexuses are good force distributors. (From Butler DS: *Mobilisation of the nervous system,* Melbourne, 1991, Churchill Livingstone.)

ropathy may involve the feet and the hands, and it occurs most frequently in persons who smoke, who have nutritional deficiencies because of alcoholism, who have autoimmune disease, and who have difficulty controlling their blood sugar levels.[6] Often such nerve damage is in a stocking or glove distribution.[6,8] Neuropathies resulting from pregnancy often resolve gradually as the woman's body returns to its prenatal metabolic state.[8] Other polyneuropathies may be stable with medications, or they may be progressive as the disease advances.

Generally, peripheral nerves are protected from injury by their external protective connective tissue coverings (Fig. 12-4). The outermost covering, the epineurium, functions to surround and cushion nerve fascicles, especially in locations where the peripheral nerve is vulnerable to compression.[2,7] A greater percentage of epineural tissue is present where the nerve is more superficial or located near a joint.[2] For example, the ulnar nerve, as it traverses under the medial epicondyle of the humerus, typically is protected from contusions and compression by the large percentage of epineurial tissue present in that part of the nerve. The deeper layers of epineurium function like packing material to protect the fascicular groups of nerve fibers.[7] Each fascicle is surrounded by a mechanically strong sheath called the perineurium. This connective tissue layer serves as a diffusion barrier, helping to preserve the specialized microenvironment inside the fascicles.[2,7]

The fibers inside the fascicles are embedded in a loose connective tissue called the endoneurium, or basement membrane.[2] Around each nerve fiber, however, the endoneurium becomes closely packed, forming a supporting wall. The endoneurium serves to insulate the axons

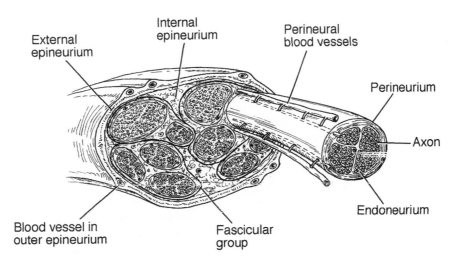

FIGURE 12-4 External protective tissue coverings surrounding a segment of a peripheral nerve. (From Trumble TE, McCallister WV: Physiology and repair of peripheral nerves. In Trumble TE, editor: *Principles of hand surgery and therapy,* Philadelphia, 2000, Saunders.)

electrically from each other. Some of these nerve fibers are myelinated. A longitudinal chain of Schwann cells wraps around the myelinated axon, creating an insulating tube that promotes fast impulse conduction. The **Schwann cell** tissue together with the closely packed endoneurial tissue constitutes the endoneurial tube.[7]

Within the outermost covering, the epineurium, is a well-developed, longitudinally oriented vascular system that feeds the nerve fibers. Peripheral nerves are vulnerable to vascular changes as a result of altered circulation or blood flow within the epineurium of the nerve.[1,2,7] Butler[2] aptly describes nerves as "blood thirsty," with the nervous system consuming 20% of the available oxygen in circulating blood, even though this system consists of only 2% of the body mass.

The vulnerability of axons in the peripheral nervous system to vascular changes is well-documented.[9-11] The effects vary depending on the duration and the magnitude of the trauma. Scarring within the epineurium can occur following prolonged stretch or compression of a peripheral nerve, and this alters blood flow to the nerve fibers, resulting in a mononeuropathy. Prolonged stretch or compression with consequent compromised circulation results in edema within the connective tissue coverings of the nerve once circulation is restored.[2,9-12]

Complete Injuries

An injury in which the peripheral nerve is severed, otherwise known as a complete injury, or in which an entire segment is severely traumatized with consequent serious internal disorganization has serious consequences in terms of motor or sensory loss. Following such an injury, the nerve is divided into two parts: a proximal part attached to the nerve cell body and a distal part that undergoes degeneration. Functional recovery depends on replacement of the lost distal portion by the outgrowth of new axonal processes, growing to reach their corresponding original peripheral targets.[7] These types of injuries require surgical intervention.

Precautions and Concerns

- *If the client has diminished or loss of protective sensation, teach the client to protect the insensate part from temperature extremes (including hot bath water) and from situations in which the insensate part accidentally might get injured because the client is not visually attending to the injured part.*
- *Any client with diminished or loss of protective sensation in the hand or in a part of the upper extremity should be cautioned strictly against exposing this body part to moving machinery because the client could reinjure that body part without immediately realizing it.*

Timelines and Healing

- Nerve compression, or injury in which the nerve remains in continuity, initially results in a loss of proprioception and discriminative touch, followed by a loss of pain and temperature sensation.[13] This loss of proprioception occurs because compression of a nerve affects the large myelinated fibers (that carry information about proprioception and discriminative touch) first.
- If the compression persists or is severe enough, the smaller fibers that carry information about pain and temperature also are lost.
- When the compression resolves, abnormal sensations called paresthesias occur as the blood supply to the nerve resumes. The client may complain of burning, tingling, or pricking sensations.
- Sensation gradually returns in the reverse order in which it was lost: dull, diffuse aching pain; perception of heat; sharp, stinging sensations; cold perception; conscious proprioception; and finally, discriminative touch.[13]

Nerve Response to Injury

In general, nerve cells have limited powers of regeneration (the ability to replicate or repair themselves). Around 6 months after injury, virtually all developing neurons lose their ability to undergo mitosis.[6] This means that when a neuron is damaged or destroyed, it cannot be replicated by daughter cells from other neurons. A destroyed neuron is permanently lost, and only some types of damage, specifically damage to a peripheral nerve, may be repaired. **Neuropathy** is the term frequently used to describe pathologic conditions of the peripheral nerve. Remember that a peripheral nerve is composed of the axons of many nerve cells that are housed in the spinal region of the nervous system.

CLINICAL *Pearl*

A completely severed peripheral nerve presents as loss of sensation, loss of muscle control, and a loss of reflexes in the structures innervated by that specific peripheral nerve.

Stages of Nerve Injury

The stages of nerve injury are well documented and beautifully described by Lundborg.[7] Compression or stretching of a nerve is followed quickly by functional impairment. For example, most of us have experienced our foot "going to sleep" after sitting with our legs crossed for too long. What actually is happening is local compression to the peroneal nerve that runs behind the knee. This results in temporary loss of blood flow to that nerve, then sensory loss, and thankfully, only short-lived motor paralysis. If the pressure on the nerve is of high enough magnitude, a local conduction block could ensue. There may be some damage to the myelin sheaths, which would result in an extended local conduction block. This is called a **neuropraxia,** and this type of nerve compression problem usually resolves within weeks or months. A classic example of this neuropractic lesion (also classified as a Sunderland type 1 nerve injury) is a Saturday night palsy, a radial nerve injury at the humeral level that results from compression from some hard external source.

If the compression was of a severe enough nature, the axons distal to the lesion would degenerate, but the endoneurial tubes of the axons could remain. In this type of nerve injury, called an **axonotmesis** or Sunderland type 2 nerve injury, axonal regeneration would occur, with good recovery of function because the endoneurial tubes would serve as guidelines to the appropriate end-organ of the axon.

In more severe compressions, one would see increasing involvement of the external connective tissue layers of the nerve. A Sunderland type 3 injury, for example, involves destruction of the endoneurial tubes, and a type 4 injury involves destruction of the perineurium. In the latter case, significant internal scarring would occur within the nerve trunk that would impair functional recovery without surgical debridement. Resection of the fibrotic segment of the nerve trunk, followed by nerve repair with a graft, for example, probably would be required.

Laceration of the entire nerve trunk is called a **neurotmesis,** or a Sunderland type 5 injury. These injuries always necessitate surgical repair.

Injured peripheral nerves can achieve complete or partial recovery following injury if certain conditions exist.[14] First, the soma, or nerve cell body, must be viable. Certain severe injures such as nerve root avulsions can kill the motor neurons in the spinal cord and the dorsal root ganglion cells located adjacent to the spinal cord. Damage to the soma results in the death of the entire nerve cell.

Second, physiologic environment in and around the nerve lesion must support axonal sprouting and peripheral growth. Ideally, there is an intact endoneurial tube with undamaged Schwann cells distal to the level of the injury. According to Gutman,[8] Schwann cells produce nerve growth factor, which is key to allowing peripheral nerve damage to resolve. Peripheral growth ceases if the sprouting axons meet scar tissue or bone that blocks access to the empty Schwann sheaths and endoneurial tubes or to the end-organ of the axon.

A third condition for recovery is that the regenerated axon must connect to the appropriate end-organ, and that end-organ still must be viable. The motor nerve fiber must grow to its original motor end plate, and the sensory nerve fiber must connect with its appropriate receptor organ. If a sensory axon is misdirected into a motor distal tubule, the axonal growth will be wasted. Therefore, nerve injuries in which the nerve remains in continuity with intact endoneurial tubes have a better prognosis than neurotmesis, when the whole nerve is disrupted. In the latter case, there are many chances for misguided axons to enter the wrong endoneurial tube. Even if the proper nerve fibers get to the correct sensory end-organ and motor end plate, the receptors and muscle tissue must be viable. Denervated muscle tissue can remain viable for up to 2 years after injury (assuming the muscle tissue does not become fibrotic), whereas sensory end-organs remain viable for only about 6 to 9 months.[13]

A final condition for peripheral nerve recovery is that the central nervous system must perceive and interpret the injured peripheral nervous system signals appropriately. The central nervous system will need to reorganize its cortical representations of the hand, for example, following alteration of skin inputs induced by a peripheral nerve injury. This is an exciting topic in itself, and one that is explored briefly in the section on sensory reeducation.

The classification systems used following nerve injury are summarized in Tables 12-1 and 12-2.

Timelines and Healing When Injured Nerve Is in Continuity

CLINICAL *Pearl*

Although peripheral nerves can be injured in various ways, there are only two possible pathological responses: demyelination and/or axonal loss. Segmental demyelination (or neurapraxia) results in a transient state of disrupted nerve conduction along the injured segment.[17] More severe degrees of injury to a nerve in continuity will always involve some amount of axonal disruption. Those with significant axonal disruption and with concomitant damage to the supporting connective tissue will usually require surgical intervention.[17] Often, an injured peripheral nerve will manifest as a mixed pattern of demyelination and axonal loss. This is because each peripheral nerve is composed of thousands of axons, some of which are more vulnerable at the particular lesion site than others.

If surgery can be avoided, it should. Typically, there is pain after surgery. In addition, postoperative swelling can exacerbate a compression injury. Thus try conservative management first, if at all possible. For example, compression of the median nerve at the wrist (carpal tunnel syndrome) often may be ameliorated with splinting at night, ergonomic interventions, and client education about provocative positions to avoid.

If surgery is necessary, allow the injured nerve time to recover from the trauma of surgery. The amount of time that is necessary for healing depends on a number of factors, including the severity of the nerve injury before surgery and the type of surgery. An endoscopic **carpal tunnel release** is typically less traumatic than the traditional open carpal tunnel release, for example. Other factors may include the presence of systemic diseases such as rheumatoid arthritis or diabetes, which can slow or permanently compromise healing, or the presence of concomitant injuries that may exaggerate the early phases of tissue healing. Gentle active range of motion in the area of the nerve injury typically can begin

when the client has moved beyond the inflammatory stage of healing. The typical timeline for this ranges from 2 to 3 days postoperatively to 2 to 3 weeks postoperatively. Avoid strengthening exercises until the remodeling phase of healing, typically 2 to 5 weeks postoperatively. Knowledge about the phases of wound healing enables the therapist to devise an appropriate postoperative program for each client. Again, the reader is cautioned to address each client as an individual, observing that a person's tissue response to exercise and adjusting each program accordingly.

Timelines and Healing Issues When Nerve Is Severed

- Protect nerve repairs from stress for 3 to 6 weeks afterward.[15]
- Tension at the nerve repair site can compromise results; therefore, position the client's arm or hand to minimize tension on the repair.

Diagnosis-Specific Information That Affects Clinical Reasoning

- Know whether the injured nerve is in continuity. If the nerve was severed, find out whether a nerve repair was done.
- If the nerve was severed, find out if there were other structures that also were injured and repaired.
- Repaired peripheral nerves heal at a rate of about a 1 to 3 mm/day after an initial 3- to 4-week latency

TABLE 12-1

Seddon's Classification

INJURY	RESULT
Neuropraxia	A conduction block; no anatomic disruption; all components intact
Axonotmesis	Disruption of axons and myelin sheaths, but endoneurial tubes are intact
Neurotmesis	Complete severance or serious disorganization; no spontaneous recovery

TABLE 12-2

Sunderland's Classification

DEGREE	DESCRIPTION	MECHANISM OF INJURY	PROGNOSIS
1	All structures remain intact; local conduction block and demyelination	Acute compression (*Seddon's neuropraxia*)	Complete recovery (days/months)
2	Axonal disruption with distal (*Wallerian*) degeneration; however, endoneurial tubes are intact	Mild traction or moderate compression (*Seddon's axonotmesis*)	Typically, complete recovery (months); limiting factor is distance of regeneration required (viable end-organ?)
3	Disruption of axons and endoneurial tubes; mild to moderate functional loss; fascicles remain intact	Moderate to severe traction or crush (*Seddon's neurotmesis*)	Axons may regenerate but in "wrong" endoneurial tube; many result in nerve–target organ mismatch; poor prognosis for proximal injuries
4	Loss of fascicular integrity within the nerve; only epineurium is intact	Severe traction or crush (*Seddon's neurotmesis*)	Moderate to severe functional loss; may be improved by fascicular repair; neuroma in continuity common: regenerating axons lost in scar
5	Complete nerve transection	Severe traction or crush; laceration (*Seddon's neurotmesis*)	Severe functional loss; requires surgery

Revised from 2001, Marilyn Lee, MS, OTR/L, CHT, with permission.

period.[15] Additional delays may occur as the regenerating axon attempts to cross the injury site and reinnervate the end-organ.

- Denervated muscles can remain viable realistically for about 2 years after injury (assuming the muscle tissue does not become fibrotic), whereas sensory end-organs remain viable for about 6 to 9 months.[15]
- Proximal nerve lesions have a worse prognosis for full sensory and motor recovery than distal nerve lesions.
- The presence of scar tissue in and around the healing peripheral nerve can significantly impair the surgical and therapeutic goal of accurate nerve regeneration.
- Nerve regeneration and functional outcomes are age-related. The better functional outcomes in the young may be due to greater cortical plasticity.[5,15]
- Still, cells that fire together will wire together. According to Merzenich and Jenkins[5] and others,[16] practice strengthens and expands the somatosensory cortical representation of the area that is used. Sensory reeducation and cortical retraining may be helpful, even in cases in which the outcome of surgical intervention is poor.

Evaluation Tips

Distinguishing between Central Nervous System, Spinal Segment, and Peripheral Nerve Lesions

- Central nervous system lesions show motor spasticity/flaccidity and whole limb sensory changes, frequently on the side of the body contralateral to the injury site.
- Spinal segment lesions show myotomal and dermatomal changes in the corresponding area. Typically, several adjacent spinal levels must be affected before a dermatomal and myotomal pattern can be appreciated.
- Peripheral nerve lesions show sensory or motor loss specific to the involved nerve and with symptoms and signs at and distal to the site of injury.

Evaluation Protocols for Peripheral Nerve Lesions

Begin with the client interview. Gather information about the client's history and mechanism of injury, medical history, current functional status and current living situation, and the client's goals.

Observation and Palpation

Observe the posture of the involved extremity. Observe how the client uses (or avoids use of) this extremity, for example, while the client is taking off his or her coat or filling out forms. Observe for obvious muscle atrophy, skin lesions, edema, color changes (e.g., areas of erythema, mottled skin, or skin that has a blanched appearance) and trophic changes.

Precaution. *Make note of and caution the client about vulnerability to blisters and other signs of hand injury that may occur with use of a vulnerable insensate hand.*

Palpation of the affected area should be done after informing the client of your intent and asking permission ("Is it okay if I touch your hand?").

Precaution. *Always use universal wound precautions around any lesions and rashes.*

Document areas of edema, **hypersensitivity,** adhesions, and atrophy. Use of a pictorial format in addition to written format may be helpful.

Sensory Function

Refer to Chapter 5 for specific evaluation protocols. The following is meant to serve as a review of the pertinent tests and the procedures used in evaluating clients with nerve injury:

Semmes-Weinstein Pressure Aethesiometer. This is a graded light touch testing instrument consisting of a kit of 20 nylon monofilament probes. The monofilaments are used by the therapist to map light touch sensibility in the hand. An abbreviated kit is also available.

Two-point discrimination testing. According to Moberg (cited by Callahan[13]) (1995), one of the best indicators of eventual function following a peripheral nerve injury is the return of two-point discrimination. Static two-point discrimination[13] and moving Two-Point Discrimination Tests assess the client's ability to discriminate between one point and two points of pressure applied randomly to the fingertip.

Localization of touch. Neither of the aforementioned tests requires the client to identify the location of the stimulus. Localization requires a more integrated level of perception than simple recognition of a stimulus.[13] Localization is appropriate for testing after a nerve repair because difficulty with localization of a stimulus is a common phenomenon following nerve injury. Poor localization can impair function significantly.

The therapist can catalog the client's accuracy in localizing light touch stimuli by using the lowest Semmes-Weinstein monofilament that can be perceived in the area of dysfunction. Ask the client to close the eyes and to indicate verbally if he or she feels the stimulus. Each time the client answers in the affirmative, ask the client to open the eyes and to point to the exact spot touched. The therapist should record the client's results on a gridlike map of the hand, indicating the actual location of stimulation and the sites of referred touch perception. The therapist can draw arrows on the grid to indicate referred perception sites. This test has no formal interpretation or scoring; rather, evidence of poor localization is useful when determining the need for and when planning a sensory reeducation program.

Moberg Pickup Test. This is a useful test for assessing median nerve function. The test may be helpful for testing children or adults who have cognitive involvement or who may have secondary agendas that prevent them from full participation in other sensory tests.

Hoffmann-Tinel sign. Following trauma, gentle percussion along the course of the injured, regenerating nerve produces a temporary tingling sensation in the distribution of the injured nerve up to the site of regeneration. The tingling persists several seconds. Test from distal to proximal for best accuracy. If this sign is absent or is not progressing distally as would be expected with a healing nerve, there is a poor prognosis for continued nerve recovery. Likewise, a progressing **Tinel's sign** is encouraging but does not necessarily predict complete recovery.

Table 12-3 gives a summary of light touch sensibility testing, standardized tests, and techniques for administration and scoring and interpretation of scores.

Sympathetic Function

If sweating (sudomotor function) is still present following a nerve lesion, this suggests that the nerve damage is incomplete, because peripheral autonomic nerve fibers within the nerve are responsible for sweating.[6] Vasomotor homeostasis is likewise a function of the sympathetic

---

TABLE 12-3

Light Touch Sensibility Testing: Standardized Tests and Techniques

TEST/PURPOSE	EQUIPMENT/INSTRUCTIONS TO CLIENT	TESTING PROCEDURE	SCORING	INTERPRETATION OF SCORES*
Semmes-Weinstein Monofilament Aesthesiometer Threshold test for light touch sensibility	*Equipment:* Quiet test area, colored pencils and map or grid of the hand for recording results, kit of 20 nylon monofilament probes, ranging from 1.65 to 6.65. Alternatively, the minikit containing probes: 2.83, 3.61, 4.31, 4.56, and 6.65. *Instructions:* Introduce test and familiarize client with test expectations by demonstrating in proximal area believed to have normal sensibility. Ask subject to say "yes" if stimulus is felt. Ask subject to close eyes during testing. Alternatively, obscure subject's vision with blindfold. Test hand should be stabilized securely on table.	Begin distally and progress proximally along the receptive field of the peripheral nerve. Start with the probe marked 2.83, apply to skin with enough pressure to bow the filament. Apply in $1\frac{1}{2}$ seconds, hold $1\frac{1}{2}$ seconds, and remove in $1\frac{1}{2}$ seconds. Repeat 3 times at each site; progress to next thicker filament if prior one is not perceived. Filaments marked ≥4.31 should be applied only once at each site.	One response out of three is considered affirmative. 2.83 = normal light touch 3.22-3.61 = diminished light touch 3.84-4.31 = diminished protective sensation 4.56-6.65 = loss of protective sensation >6.65 = absence of all sensation	2.83 = normal light touch 3.22-3.61 = stereognosis and pain perception intact, close to normal use of hand 3.84-4.31 = mild to moderate impaired stereognosis and pain perception, difficulty manipulating objects 4.56-6.65 = moderate to significant impaired pain and temperature perception, unable to manipulate objects with vision occluded, marked decrease in spontaneous hand use. Client will need instructions about protective care of impaired area.

TABLE 12-3

Light Touch Sensibility Testing: Standardized Tests and Techniques—cont'd

TEST/PURPOSE	EQUIPMENT/INSTRUCTIONS TO CLIENT	TESTING PROCEDURE	SCORING	INTERPRETATION OF SCORES*
				>6.65 = unable to identify objects or temperature With visual guidance, capable of gross coordination only
Static Two-Point Discrimination Functional Test for determining two-point discrimination and ability to use hand for fine motor tasks	*Equipment:* Handheld Disk-Criminator or Boley gauge *Instructions:* Introduce test and familiarize client with test expectations by demonstrating in proximal area believed to have normal sensibility. Ask subject to say "one" or "two" in response to perception of one point of pressure or two points of pressure. Ask subject to close eyes during testing. Alternatively, obscure subject's vision with blindfold. Test hand should be securely stabilized on table.	Typically, only volar fingertips are tested. Begin testing at 5 mm of distance between two points. Apply one or two points randomly, with the probes held in a longitudinal orientation to avoid crossover from overlapping digital nerves. Force is applied lightly, just until skin blanches. If responses are inaccurate, the distance between the ends is increased by increments of 1-5 mm. Testing is stopped at 15 mm or sooner if digit length is not adequate.	Score is the smallest distance at which client is able accurately to discriminate between two points of pressure and one point of pressure: 7 out of 10 correct responses required. Norms: 3-5 mm = normal, ages 18-70 6-10 mm = fair 11-15 mm = poor One point only perceived = protective sensation only No points perceived = anesthetic	6 mm = normal, needed for winding a watch 6-8 mm = fair, needed for sewing 12 mm = poor, needed for handling precision tools >15 mm = loss of protective sensation to anesthetic; above this, gross tool handling may be possible but only with decreased speed and skill

*Interpretation of scores based on information in Bell-Krotoski J: Correlating sensory morphology and tests of sensibility with function. In Hunter J, Mackin EJ, Schneider L, editors: *Tendon and nerve surgery in the hand: a third decade,* St Louis, 1997, Mosby; Callahan A: Sensibility assessment for nerve lesions in continuity and nerve lacerations. In Mackin EJ, Callahan AD, Skirven TM et al, editors: *Rehabilitation of the hand and upper extremity,* ed 5, St Louis, 2002, Mosby.

nervous system; therefore, abnormal changes in skin temperature and skin color may indicate involvement of these peripheral nerve fibers.

The combination of sympathetic and sensory dysfunction results in characteristic trophic changes in all tissues of the involved area. Specifically, one would expect to see nail changes (blemishes, talonlike appearance), abnormal hair growth (may fall out or become longer and finer), cold intolerance, soft tissue atrophy (most notably in the finger tip pulps), and a slowed rate of tissue healing.[13]

The O'Riain Wrinkle Test (1973) is an objective test that identifies areas of denervation, for denervated skin does not wrinkle when soaked in warm water. The denervated hand is placed in warm water (40° C [104° F]) for 30 minutes, and the presence or absence of finger wrinkling is documented. This test is most useful for children or others who may be unable or unwilling to cooperate with sensibility testing.[13]

Motor Assessment

The following tests are useful for motor assessment:

Goniometric assessment. Evaluation of articular motion and musculotendinous function is performed with a goniometer. Passive range of motion (PROM) is defined as a measurement of the ability of the joint to be moved by an external source through its normal arc of motion. Limitations indicate problems within the joint or capsular structures surrounding the joint. Active range of motion (AROM) is defined as a measurement of the individual's own capability for moving a joint through its normal arc of motion. A limitation in AROM when PROM is full may indicate diminished or loss of muscle power resulting from a nerve lesion. Therefore, assess AROM first, and if limitations exist, then assess PROM.

Manual muscle testing. Muscle paresis or paralysis can result from a peripheral nerve lesion. Careful documentation of muscle strength, using a Manual Muscle Test (MMT), is an important component of the initial evaluation following a nerve injury. If possible, compare strength with the uninvolved side to determine what normal strength is for that client.

Test the muscle or muscle group in the midposition, using a "brake" test. Tell the client to "hold this position, don't let me move you" while exerting a counterdirectional force, attempting to move the client's body part out of the test position. Use a grading system that minimizes the amount of pluses and minuses, for that makes it easier for other health professionals to review the documentation and appreciate what was observed. Table 12-4 gives the recommended grading system.

Strength testing: grip and pinch. Gross grip and pinch strength can be assessed using standardized tools, the Jamar dynamometer and the pinch gauge.

Pain Assessment

Pain is almost always a consequence of a nerve injury; therefore acknowledging this fact and aiming to quantify and qualify this multidimensional experience is important to the therapist and the client. Many pain assessment tools are one-dimensional, attempting to quantify the pain experience numerically. The benefit of such tools is that they are easy and quick to administer and to score, and they produce repeatable, objective results that can be used to assess treatment outcomes. Perform a pain interview at the time of the initial evaluation in addition to these other pain assessments to provide the therapist with a more complete picture of the client's pain experience. This unstructured interview should include questions about topics such as current medication regimen, location and frequency of pain, verbal

TABLE 12-4

Manual Muscle Test Grades and Interpretation

GRADE	INTERPRETATION
5, Normal	Able to move body part full range against gravity, holding position with normal strength
4, Good	Able to move body part full range against gravity, holding position with good strength
3+, Fair plus	Able to move body part full range against gravity, holding position for short time and/or against some resistance
3, Fair	Able to move body part full range against gravity, but unable to hold position against any resistance and/or for any functional length of time
2, Poor	Able to move body part full range in gravity-minimized position
2−, Poor	Able to move body part through partial range in gravity-minimized position minus
1, Trace	Palpable flicker in muscle; no observable movement at joint
0, Zero	No palpable flicker in muscle; no observable movement at joint in gravity-minimized position

description of pain, and what factors exacerbate or decrease pain. Table 12-5 summarizes typical pain assessment tools with a brief synopsis of administration and scoring instructions. This is not an exhaustive list of pain assessments but rather a list of those that can be used efficiently during an initial evaluation of a client with a peripheral nerve injury.[18]

Other Assessments to Consider

Reflexes. Complete severance of the efferent or afferent nerve in a reflex arc abolishes that reflex. However, a reflex can be lost even in partial nerve injuries, so hyporeflexia is not a good guide of injury severity.[6]

Provocative testing. Testing to provoke symptoms frequently is used to clarify the site of injury and to exclude the possibility that other nonneural tissues may be sources of pain. Provocative nerve testing is predicated on the fact that irritated nerve tissue is sensitized or hyperresponsive to any manual stimulus applied along its length. A manual stimulus can be defined as a compressive force to a nerve trunk or a graded force that causes longitudinally directed nerve gliding. In the normal nerve, these forces would not result in an irritated neural response. For example, tapping over a nerve normally would not cause a Tinel's sign unless the nerve was injured. Therefore,

Tinel's testing, or percussion along a nerve that results in an irritated tingling sensation, is considered a positive provocative stress test. Likewise, upper limb tension testing is considered a provocative stress test, for the nerves of the brachial plexus are moved passively and longitudinally. A positive upper limb tension test would present as a pathologic response or symptomatic pain reproduction.[1]

Precautions and concerns with provocative testing include the following:

* Neural provocative testing, especially upper limb tension testing, must be done carefully and by the skilled therapist who understands the testing technique and the interpretations and who can manage symptoms once provoked. Upper extremity provocative tests are not standardized in terms of precise positioning, how long each position is held, or how much force is applied.
* Whenever possible, compare the involved to the uninvolved side to appreciate the client's individual normal response.

Edema measurements. The presence of edema can compromise further the available space for the nerve as it traverses through fibroosseous tunnels and other tightly confined areas, as at the carpal tunnel. Take edema measurements initially or once sutures are

TABLE 12-5

Typical Pain Assessment Tools

NAME	DESCRIPTION/ADMINISTRATION	SCORING/INTERPRETATION*
Numeric pain scale	Subjective rating of pain intensity using a 10-point numeric scale. Client is asked to rate current pain on a 0-10+ scale: 0 = no pain; 10 = worst possible pain imaginable. Client may be asked to rate best and worst pain experienced over the past 30 days or since the onset of pain.	Record the number identified by the client. 0-2 = low level of pain 3-5 = moderate level of pain 6-10+ = high level of pain
Visual analog scale	Subjective quantitative measure of pain intensity using a 10 cm line with descriptors (no pain at all; pain as bad as it could be) at each end. Clients are asked to make a mark through the line to indicate the pain they are presently experiencing.	Measure the distance on the line from the bottom anchor to the client's mark and record in centimeters as the client's pain score. 0-2.9 cm = low level of pain 3-5.9 cm = moderate pain level 6-10.5 cm = high pain level
Pain drawing	Subjective drawing of pain diffusion and localization. Clients are given an outline of the body or body part and are asked to use symbols (that denote different qualities of pain) to reflect the current distribution of symptoms.	No standardized or widely accepted method for scoring. Look for patterns of pain diffusion that may indicate radicular symptoms occurring along a specific dermatone. Widespread or nonanatomic pain drawings may indicate chronic pain or poor psychodynamics.

*Interpretations of these scales are based on information in Galper J, Verno V: Pain. In Palmer ML, Epler ME, editors: *Fundamentals of musculoskeletal assessment techniques,* ed 2, Philadelphia, 1996, Lippincott-Raven.

removed, using a volumeter if there are no wound issues or a tape measure to assess circumference. Establish a baseline before commencement of participation in therapy.

Precaution. *An increase in edema following treatment, along with degradation in sensory status may indicate that your treatment program was too aggressive.*

Canadian Occupational Performance Measure (COPM). The COPM is a client-centered assessment tool for use by occupational therapists. The COPM is designed to assess a client's self-perceived change in occupational performance problems over time.[19] The COPM is intended for use as an outcome measure. The test is designed to assist the client and the therapist in identifying problem areas of occupational performance and in setting treatment goals. Instructions for administration are indicated clearly in the manual.[20] In a semistructured interview, the problem areas are identified and then rated in terms of importance to the client. The five most important problems are then the focus of intervention. These problems are rated by the client to determine the client's perception of ability to perform the identified task/activity and the client's

satisfaction with that performance. After a period of time, the COPM form is revisited, and possible changes in the client's perceptions are recorded. The difference between the initial and subsequent scores gives the measure of outcome, with a two point difference in either direction indicating significant change.

Although this at first may appear to be a time-consuming assessment tool, the semistructured interview can be adapted by the therapist to streamline the problem identification portion. For example, most clients easily can identify five things that are important to them that they can no longer do as well or at all. I incorporate these into initial goal setting and treatment planning. After these goals are achieved, I will ask clients whether there are any other activities that they cannot do at all or as well as they could before this injury, and I incorporate these into the new goals.

Clinical Reasoning: When to Use Which Tests

Table 12-6 contains a list of recommendations for determining which assessment tools to use when evaluating a nerve injury in continuity versus a nerve injury not in continuity.

TABLE 12-6

Recommendations for Therapist's Evaluation Battery

NERVE LESIONS IN CONTINUITY: NONOPERATIVE	NERVE LACERATIONS: POSTOPERATIVE
Client history	Client history
Observation/palpation of involved tissues	Observation/palpation of involved tissues, with special attention to trophic, sudomotor, and vasomotor changes (possible sympathetic dysfunction?)
Tinel's test at suspected compression site	Tinel's test to determine distal progression of regenerating axons
Semmes-Weinstein monofilament test	Semmes-Weinstein monofilament testing followed by localization (determine light touch sensibility, need for sensory protection techniques and/or sensory reeducation)
	Two-point discrimination testing if client is able to perceive ≤4.31 monofilament (predicts functional status, need for sensory reeducation)
Pain assessments (including pain interview)	Pain assessments (Is there a need for desensitization program?)
Provocative stress testing, if client reports intermittent symptoms aggravated by certain positions/activities	
Moberg Pickup Test (for functional assessment with a median nerve injury)	
AROM, followed by PROM if limitations are present with active movement	AROM, followed by PROM (if needed) of involved extremity as permitted by postoperative protocol
Strength test: MMT to isolate muscle involvement, grip and pinch testing to assess functional grasp and pinch strength.	
Modified COPM for goal setting	Modified COPM for goal setting

AROM, Active range of motion; *PROM*, passive range of motion; *MMT*, Manual Muscle Test; *COPM*, Canadian Occupational Performance Measure.

Questions to Ask the Doctor

Following Nerve Injury Not Requiring Surgical Intervention

- *What nerve was injured?*
- *What was the mechanism of injury? Was it a clean injury or a crush injury?*
- *Were an electromyelogram and nerve conduction study done? What were the results?*
- *Is surgical decompression indicated at this time?*

Following Nerve Injury with Surgical Intervention

- *What was the date of the repair?*
- *Was the nerve repair under tension? Was there need for a nerve graft?*
- *Was there a delay from the time of injury to the time of the nerve repair?*
- *Are there other structures that were injured and repaired?*
- *Do you have a particular postoperative therapy protocol you would like to be followed? How long do you want the nerve repair to be protected by immobilization?*
- *Can we begin range of motion of the parts distal and proximal to the repair site to maintain joint suppleness and tissue length and gliding?*

RADIAL NERVE

Anatomy

Table 12-7 gives a summary of radial nerve anatomy, common lesion sites, and typical deficits/deformities associated with radial nerve lesions.

The radial nerve is the largest branch of the brachial plexus, arising from the posterior cord (C6 to T1; Fig. 12-5).[21] Many of the fibers that innervate the triceps muscle arise high in the axilla. This nerve runs distally in the arm by winding around the posterior aspect of the humerus from medial to lateral under the cover of the triceps. The radial nerve sends a branch to the medial head of the triceps that continues downward to innervate the anconeus. Cutaneous branches supply the posterior region of the arm and the lower lateral arm. A small cutaneous branch also emerges posterolaterally in the lower third of the arm to supply the posterior skin of the forearm. The main trunk continues distally, emerging on the lateral side of the humerus between the triceps and the brachialis. The main trunk passes anterior to the extensor forearm group, lying between the brachioradialis and brachialis before passing into the forearm. In the forearm the radial nerve gives off motor branches to the brachioradialis and the radial wrist extensors. At the level of the radial head, the radial nerve divides into

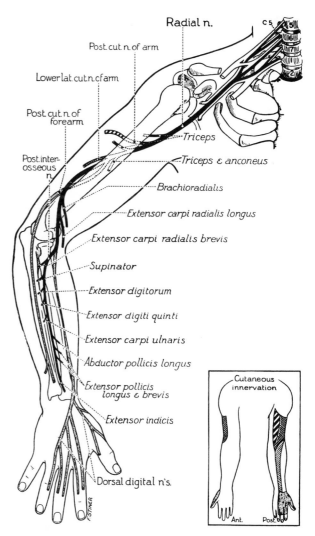

FIGURE 12-5 Schematic of the radial nerve. (From Haymaker W, Woodhall B: *Peripheral nerve injuries: principles of diagnosis,* Philadelphia, 1953, WB Saunders.)

two terminal branches: the anterior superficial sensory branch, which runs into the forearm under the brachioradialis, and a posterior motor branch, the posterior interosseous nerve, which penetrates the supinator muscle by passing under its fibrous origin called the arcade of Frohse. This posterior motor branch winds around the neck of the radius for a short distance and then emerges from the supinator muscle in the posterior-lateral compartment of the forearm. The posterior branch gives off branches to the extensor carpi ulnaris and to all the extensors of the digits.

The superficial cutaneous branch is the smaller of the two terminal branches. At the wrist, the cutaneous branch divides into digital branches that supply the lateral two thirds of the dorsum of the hand, the dorsal

TABLE 12-7

Summary of Radial Nerve Anatomy, Lesion Sites, and Typical Deficits/Deformities

Sensation	*Brachial cutaneous branches* supply the posterior region of the arm and lower lateral arm. An *antebrachial branch* supplies the posterior skin of the forearm. The *superficial sensory branch* of the forearm supplies the lateral two thirds of the dorsum of the hand, the dorsal thumb, and the proximal portion of the dorsal index, and long digits and radial half of the proximal ring.
Motor	*Innervations, proximal to distal:* triceps (long head), triceps (medial head), branch to anconeus, triceps (lateral head), brachioradialis, extensor carpi radialis longus, extensor carpi radialis brevis, supinator, extensor digitorum communis, extensor digiti minimi, extensor carpi ulnaris, abductor pollicis longus, extensor pollicis longus, extensor pollicis brevis, extensor indicis proprius
Function	An intact radial nerve allows for elbow extension and is *essential to the tenodesis action that is fundamental to the grasp-release pattern of normal hand function.* The radial nerve powers all wrist extension, all metacarpophalangeal joint extension, and thumb extension and radial abduction.
Common sites of entrapment/injury	*Crutch palsy* (axilla level, motor and sensory involvement) *Saturday night palsy/high radial nerve palsy* (midhumeral compression or shaft fractures—triceps spared, motor and sensory involvement) *Posterior interosseous nerve palsy* (fracture/dislocations of elbow joint, tendinous edge of extensor carpi radialis brevis, between two heads of supinator—radial wrist extensors spared); primarily motor involvement *Radial tunnel syndrome* (compression between radial head and supinator muscle); primarily a pain syndrome *Superficial radial sensory nerve palsy* (compression between extensor carpi radialis longus and brachioradialis tendons or at wrist from tight cast/splint—sensory involvement only)
Results of lesion	*Motor palsy* has significant functional consequences. A lesion to this nerve as it passes medially to laterally across the posterior shaft of the humerus results in *"wrist drop,"* with a loss of all active wrist, digit, and thumb extension. Supination of the forearm remains functional because the intact biceps brachii is a powerful supinator of the forearm. Likewise, the triceps is spared because it receives its innervation more proximally. Only high lesions to the radial nerve (as in the axilla) result in loss of all active elbow extension and the aforementioned problems. Lesions to the *posterior interosseous nerve branch* in the forearm spares the brachioradialis and radial wrist extensors, but thumb, digit, and ulnar wrist extension are lost. A *lesion to the superficial radial sensory nerve* results in some loss of sensation on the dorsal lateral hand. This typically does not present a debilitating problem for clients. Following radial nerve palsy, clients report an inability to use the hand for grasp or release. The loss of stability at the wrist results in an inability to use the long flexors to make a fist. Clients cannot move their thumb away from their hand to grab hold of a cup or utensil, for example, or skillfully to let go of an object once placed in their hand.

thumb, and the proximal portion of the dorsal lateral digits.

High (Proximal) Radial Nerve Palsy and Posterior Interosseous Nerve Palsy (Low Motor Radial Nerve Palsy)

Diagnosis and Pathology

The radial nerve is the most commonly injured of the three major peripheral nerves in the upper extremity.[22] The radial nerve is particularly vulnerable about mid-humeral level as it traverses around the spiral groove of the humerus, moving medially to laterally. Injury at this level is called a high radial nerve palsy. The triceps muscle is spared, for nerve fibers innervating this three-headed muscle branch off the main trunk at or just distal to the axilla. Thus elbow extension is intact. The supinator and brachioradialis muscles are paralyzed; however, elbow flexion and forearm supination remain because the musculocutaneous-innervated biceps brachii muscle is the primary elbow flexor and forearm supinator. Paralysis of all wrist extensors, loss of finger extension at the metacarpophalangeal joints, and an inability to extend and radially abduct the thumb result. This injury is called wrist drop deformity[15,22] (Fig. 12-6), named for its classic dropped or flexed wrist posture.

The most common cause of radial nerve palsy is direct trauma to the nerve, often resulting fractures of

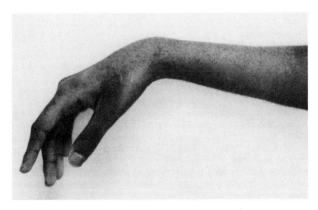

FIGURE 12-6 Wrist drop deformity resulting from radial nerve palsy. (From Stanley BG, Tribuzi SM, editors: *Concepts in hand rehabilitation*, Philadelphia, 1992, FA Davis.)

the humerus, elbow dislocations, and Monteggia's fracture-dislocations.[21] According to Barton (cited in Colditz[22]), about 1 in 10 humeral shaft fractures is complicated by a high radial nerve palsy. External compression, as from a crutch in the axilla or along the midhumeral level where the nerve runs superficially between the triceps muscle and the humeral shaft, also can result in neuropathy of the radial nerve. The latter case frequently is referred to as Saturday night or drunkard's palsy.[21] Depending on the level of injury, triceps paresis may exist, as well as some posterior arm sensory loss. One sees paralysis of all the wrist and finger extensors and sensory loss along the dorsal lateral aspect of the forearm and hand.

In the forearm, about the level of the radial head, the radial nerve divides into a superficial sensory branch and a motor branch, the posterior interosseous nerve. An injury to this motor branch spares the radial wrist extensors, which receive their innervation above the level of the elbow joint. The clinical picture of this low radial nerve palsy (or posterior interosseous nerve palsy)[15,23] is one of radially directed wrist extension but absent finger metacarpophalangeal joint extension, thumb extension, and thumb radial abduction. Injuries to the nerve at this level can occur following compression of the nerve between the humeral and ulnar heads of the supinator muscle (called the arcade of Froshe), from radial head fracture-dislocations, from tumors, or from a history of repetitive and strenuous pronation and supination. In the latter cases, men are affected twice as often as women, and the dominant arm is involved twice as often as the nondominant arm.[21]

Timelines and Healing

Typically, radial nerve palsies that result from closed injuries represent a neuropraxia that resolves spontaneously over a period of a few days to 3 to 4 months. Clients

who fail to show clinical improvement after 3 months of conservative management should be considered for surgery.[21]

Evaluation Tips

- Begin with a thorough interview to ascertain the history of the injury and the medical care received to date.
- Posterior interosseous nerve palsy is distinguished from high radial nerve palsy by the preservation of radial wrist extensors, brachioradialis function, and superficial radial nerve sensibility. Check for intact sensibility using the Semmes-Weinstein monofilaments at the first dorsal web space. Assess radial wrist extension via an MMT with the forearm positioned in pronation and the elbow flexed.
- For preoperative and nonoperative cases, perform a comprehensive MMT to document the level of impairment and to have a baseline for assessing recovery. Assess muscle function moving from the most distally innervated muscle and progressing proximally. (Table 12-7 lists the anatomic progression of innervation.) Because most radial nerve motions can be achieved by substitutions, or "tricks,"[15] the examiner should look for the classic drop wrist posture when the elbow is flexed and pronated. Muscle wasting over the dorsal arm (or brachial) area would indicate a high radial nerve lesion, with triceps involvement.
- If the client requires a splint, evaluate and document cutaneous sensory involvement using the Semmes-Weinstein monofilament test before splint fitting. This will provide the information needed to protect insensate skin adequately from hot splinting material and to educate the client about visually monitoring skin for breakdown.

Nonoperative Treatment

- A number of different splint designs are compatible with radial nerve motor palsy with wrist drop. In 1987, Colditz[22] reviewed popular splint options and presented her design for a custom-made dorsal forearm-based dynamic splint that "harnesses" the normal tenodesis pattern of the hand while awaiting motor return (Fig. 12-7). She argues that this splint remains the recommended choice whether the injury is a high radial nerve palsy or a posterior interosseous palsy because her splint design does not preclude use of active wrist extension and does assist with finger extension with slight wrist flexion. Colditz's low profile splint is an ideal daytime choice for clients with dominant arm injuries. During the night, the client may use a simple prefabricated, wrist cock-up

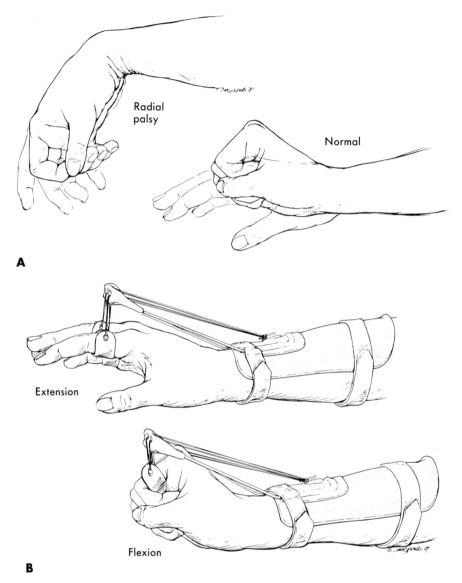

FIGURE 12-7 A, Radial nerve palsy results in a loss of normal tenodesis action. **B,** Colditz radial nerve palsy splint. (From Colditz J: *J Hand Ther* 1:19-21, 1987.)

splint to support the wrist, preventing the denervated wrist extensors from overstretching. If the injury is on the nondominant side, many clients prefer to use the prefabricated wrist cock-up splint only for activities such as dressing in long-sleeved clothing becomes a challenge with even a low-profile splint. The therapist must be vigilant to prevent joint contractures from developing, particularly at the metacarpophalangeal joints of the digits, if the client insists on using only a static wrist splint.

- Instruct the client in passive and active-assisted range of motion exercises in the clinic, and have the client continue these daily at home. (I recommend 3 to 5 sets/day, 10 repetitions each set to start, and adjust-

ment according to the client's response.) The goal is to prevent joint contractures and to promote general joint health by encouraging frequent movement through the normal available arc of motion.
- Educate the client about the need to protect the joints and denervated muscles from overstretching by using proper positioning techniques such as splinting.
- As muscle strength returns and the client is able to demonstrate full movement in the gravity minimized plane (MMTs are 2/5 strength), begin place-and-hold exercises (or isometric contractions) in the against-gravity plane. Initially, these exercise sessions will be brief because the muscle fibers will fatigue quickly.

- Isotonic strengthening exercises to correct proximal weakness and muscle imbalance should begin once there is adequate muscle strength to hold the body part against gravity for a functional period (MMT is 3+/5). As noted before, these initial isotonic strengthening sessions should be short but frequent.
- Muscle retraining should begin as soon as possible. Encourage the client to use the involved extremity as normally as possible during the day whether the client needs a splint to assist or not. Use of the involved extremity can become part of the client's daily home exercise regimen. It is important that the client does not develop a habit of performing daily activities with the uninvolved arm only because the brain will forget how to incorporate the impaired extremity, even when motor power returns.

Radial Tunnel Syndrome: Conservative Management

Diagnosis and Pathology
Radial tunnel syndrome[21,23] is a condition caused by compression of the radial nerve in the proximal forearm. The clinical picture is one of dull aching or burning pain along the lateral forearm musculature rather than one of frank muscle weakness or sensory loss.

CLINICAL *Pearl*

The cause of radial tunnel syndrome is most often compression of the nerve at the fibrous edge of the supinator muscle from an external source such as a counterforce brace used to treat epicondylitis, if applied too tightly, or from repetitive forceful supination with concurrent wrist extension.

Evaluation Tips: Differential Diagnosis
Symptoms may be confused with lateral epicondylitis, but the two conditions can co-exist.[23] Lateral epicondylitis is an inflammatory and degenerative process that primarily involves the tendinous origin of the extensor carpi radialis brevis. With lateral epicondylitis, there is pain localized over or just distal to the lateral epicondyle. This pain is provoked by palpation over the lateral epicondyle area and by resisting wrist extension. With radial tunnel syndrome, placing the wrist in flexion and resisting long finger extension provokes symptoms of dull pain or aching and burning in the lateral forearm. Symptoms also may be reproduced when forearm supination is resisted while the elbow is extended.

Nonoperative Treatment
- *Splinting:* Conservative management of radial tunnel syndrome during the acute phase of treatment involves reducing pain and inflammation by resting the involved extremity in a long arm splint with the elbow flexed, the forearm in supination, and the wrist in neutral.[23,24] Advise the client to wear this splint as much as possible, removing it for hygiene and AROM exercises only. The splint is used until the client reports a significant decrease in pain with rest and with activities (typically about 4 to 6 weeks).
- *Pain management:* Besides resting of the inflamed tissue, pain can be addressed through the use of over-the-counter oral pain medications as prescribed by the physician and with various therapeutic modalities and massage.[24,25]
- *Massage:* Massage techniques designed to increase blood flow and reduce pain are also helpful.
- *Therapeutic exercises:* Clients should perform pain-free active, active-assisted, and passive range of motion exercises daily at home. Instruct clients to remove their splint 3 to 5 times per day to perform these exercises to avoid joint stiffness from immobilization. Composite compartmental stretching, (i.e., stretching of the extensor-supinator compartment of the forearm) may be included once the client's nerve irritability decreases. When the client's symptoms have quieted down significantly (typically about 4 to 6 weeks), strengthening exercises can commence. Isometric exercises are easiest on the soft tissues and joints, so they are a good choice for these initial strengthening sessions. Progressive resistive exercises that target muscle groups rather than individual muscles and that are designed to address endurance rather than power may be added as necessary to help the client to attain functional goals.

Precaution. *Repetitive forceful wrist extension and supination should be avoided at all times.*

- *Nerve gliding:* (See the section on nerve glides at the end of this chapter.) For the radial nerve glide[24] (Fig. 12-8), tell the client to look at the hand (palm surface) and then move the hand back and away from the body (shoulder extension, abduction, internal rotation; elbow extension; forearm pronation and wrist flexion), as if the client were a waiter, inauspiciously asking for a tip. Nerve glides should be performed slowly with attention to any change in symptoms.

Precaution. *Nerve glides should never be painful!*

- *Activity modification:* Modifications of a task or a tool may be necessary so that the client avoids the provocative activity of forceful, repetitive wrist

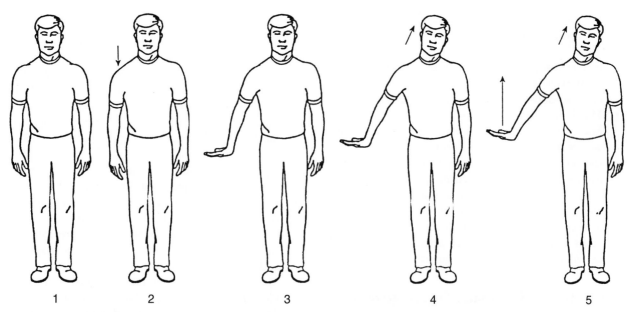

1   2   3   4   5

FIGURE 12-8 Traditional radial nerve glide exercises. (From Alba CD: Therapist's management of radial tunnel syndrome. [Redrawn from a Spectrum Health Rehabilitation and Sports Medicine Services home program form.] In Mackin E, Callahan AD, Skirven TM et al, editors: *Rehabilitation of the hand and upper extremity*, ed 5, St Louis, 2002, Mosby.)

extension and supination. An ergonomic evaluation of the work site may be necessary to identify those tasks that aggravate radial tunnel symptoms. When possible, tool grips should be built up to lessen the adverse effects of a tight power grasp. Use of long lever arms on tools also can decrease the force and range of motion needed to complete a task successfully.

Operative Treatment
If conservative management is not effective in relieving pain, surgical release of the compressive structures (e.g., the arcade of Frohse) may be done.[21]

Timelines and Healing
Consider the following guidelines[23,24,26]:

- A long arm splint to support the elbow, forearm, and wrist is used for the first 2 weeks postoperatively; a wrist cock-up splint may be used intermittently during weeks 2 to 4.
- Begin passive and active pronation and supination within the first postoperative week.
- Hand strengthening, as with putty, may begin around 3 weeks postoperatively.
- Progressive resistive exercises for the elbow, forearm, and wrist can begin around week 6 postoperatively.
- Functional recovery of strength may take 3 to 4 months, whereas relief of muscular aching can take several months to a year.

Tips from the Field

CLINICAL *Pearl*

Client education and behavior modification are critical to successful therapeutic intervention.

Because radial nerve palsy is dynamic, reoccurrence is likely. The client must learn to manage the disorder by understanding and using various methods of prevention or by recognizing early symptoms so they can be addressed before a flare-up occurs. A wrist cock-up splint may reduce some of the load on the forearm and wrist muscles during provocative activities. Teach the client slow, sustained stretching of the forearm and wrist (simultaneous wrist flexion and forearm pronation). Instruct the client to perform these stretches daily: after rest to address stiffness and before engaging in any activity that may be provoking.

What to Say to Clients

- "This is a syndrome that is likely to reoccur, so a good understanding of the causes and symptoms and techniques for managing a flare-up is important for future self-management. Think of me as your coach or teacher. I can answer questions and concerns and help you recognize a possible flare-up in order to manage symptoms early on."

- "Try to avoid provocative postures such as forearm rotation and wrist extension or straightening unless you are performing your controlled stretches. Avoid repetitive activities that put the injured arm in these provocative positions. Alternate arms whenever possible. Minimizing the accumulation of stress on your injured forearm tissues is a key component of prevention. When one of these positions is necessary, try to limit the time you spend in this posture. Try to alternate activities that require forearm rotation and wrist extension with ones that rest the forearm and wrist to allow the soft tissue time to recover from these stressful postures. Use your wrist splint to decrease some of the stress on the wrist and forearm muscles when you plan to participate in an activity that requires simultaneous wrist straightening and repetitive forearm rotation (like using a screwdriver)."

- "Slow, sustained stretching of the forearm and wrist should be done daily and before any activity that puts load or resistance on the forearm and wrist. Think of an injured athlete. Would you expect the athlete to engage in a sports activity without stretching first? You are the injured athlete; you also must stretch from now on before engaging in anything that could stress your vulnerable tissue."

- "A heating pad or warm soaks may be helpful in reducing early morning muscle stiffness; ice packs may be helpful in reducing muscle spasms after activity."

Superficial Radial Sensory Nerve Lesions

Diagnosis and Pathology

Precaution. *Superficial radial sensory nerve lesions can occur because of an ill-fitting wrist cast or a splint that is tight or chafes the radial styloid.*[21]

Superficial radial sensory nerve lesions can result from external trauma, such as tight handcuffs or a snug watchband. The condition can occur because of proximity of the nerve to pinning or external fixation following a wrist fracture. Chronic localized edema or scar tissue that develops after surgery or repeated injections in this area (as with de Quervain's tenosynovitis) also can cause a radial sensory nerve irritation. Occasionally, entrapment of this superficial branch of the radial nerve can occur between the extensor carpi radialis longus and extensor carpi radialis brevis tendons. Clients typically complain of numbness, tenderness, and burning pain along the dorsal, lateral aspect of the hand.

Evaluation Tips

This condition can be misdiagnosed as de Quervain's tenosynovitis[21] because of an overlap of signs and symptoms. Both conditions present as pain and tenderness along the dorsal, lateral aspect of the hand. Both conditions can be provoked by a posture of wrist hyperflexion and ulnar deviation. A diagnosis of superficial radial sensory nerve irritation is likely if there is first dorsal web diminished sensibility in addition to the aforementioned symptoms. De Quervain's tendonitis is the likely diagnosis if there is pain with forced flexion and adduction of the thumb in addition to the aforementioned symptoms. Both diagnoses can co-exist.

Nonoperative Treatment

Conservative management involves identifying the source of compression and, when possible, removing it.

Precaution. *The poorly fitted splint or cast should be remolded so as to relieve pressure over the radial styloid, where the superficial radial nerve is particularly vulnerable to external compression.*

Treatment protocols[26] incorporating thumb spica splints, modalities to address pain and edema, antiinflammatory medications, and **desensitization** programs appear to be most helpful. Also helpful is to modify activities of daily living and to instruct the client in biomechanics to avoid those provocative motions that stretch and further irritate the nerve.

Operative Treatment for Radial Nerve Palsy

Compression resulting in motor weakness that does not improve with several months of splinting, antiinflammatory medications, and activity modification usually is treated with surgical decompression. Results after radial nerve decompression are not as favorable as those following carpal tunnel release or cubital tunnel release.[21]

When it is clear that the muscles are not going to be reinnervated, tendon transfers frequently are performed.[15] The tendonous insertion of an innervated muscle is rerouted or transferred to a different site to compensate for the paralyzed muscle. For example, the insertion of the pronator teres, a frequent donor choice to provide wrist extension, is surgically cut, repositioned, and anchored to allow for active radial wrist extension. The goal of this procedure is to redistribute the available motor power in an attempt to improve function.

Timelines and Healing Issues
Following Radial Nerve Repair above the Elbow, Below the Axilla
Consider the following guidelines[23,26]:

- Fit a static elbow splint, positioning the elbow in 90 to 100 degrees of flexion and the forearm in neutral.

In addition, fit a radial nerve palsy splint to the client.

- At 4 weeks, extend the elbow to 60 degrees of extension.
- At 5 weeks, extend the elbow to 30 degrees of extension.
- At 6 weeks, discontinue use of the splint altogether to allow full elbow extension. Initiate AROM and PROM exercises to the elbow, forearm, wrist, and hand.
- Have the client continue the radial nerve palsy splint until adequate motor return occurs or tendon transfers are done.

Following Radial Nerve Repair at the Elbow or Forearm

Consider the following guidelines[23,24,26]:

- Within the first or second postoperative week, fabricate a static wrist extension splint, positioning the wrist in 30 degrees of extension, to protect the nerve repair juncture. Dynamic extension outriggers for the digit metacarpophalangeal joints and for thumb extension can be fabricated. Initiate AROM exercises for the digits.
- At 4 weeks postoperatively, adjust the wrist immobilization splint to 10 to 20 degrees of extension.
- In the fifth week postoperatively, have the client begin active and active-assisted range of motion exercises. The wrist should continue to be splinted between exercise sessions until there is adequate wrist extensor muscle strength to maintain the wrist in extension against gravity.

Following Tendon Transfers

Consider the following guidelines[15]:

- Clients undergoing tendon transfers typically are immobilized for 3 to 6 weeks in a protected cast or splint that minimizes tension on the repair.
- Begin brief sessions of active muscle contractions and place-and-hold exercises by week 5 or 6. Clients will need muscle reeducation to help them learn how contracting the donor muscle results in a new movement. Biofeedback and electric stimulation of the donor muscle can be used to help increase the client's awareness and isolated control. Splinting is continued in between exercise sessions so as not to overload the healing tendon.
- Resistive exercises can begin by week 7 or 8, and the daytime protective splint can be discontinued at this time. Typically, by week 12, the client may resume all prior activities without restrictions.

MEDIAN NERVE

Anatomy

Table 12-8 provides a summary of median nerve anatomy, common lesion sites, and typical deficits/deformities associated with median nerve lesions.[27-29]

The median nerve (Fig. 12-9) arises from the lateral and medial cords of the brachial plexus. The median nerve runs distally in the anteromedial compartment of the arm. In the cubital fossa of the anterior elbow and in the forearm, the median nerve lies medial to the brachial artery. Just distal to the elbow joint, the median nerve passes below the bicipital aponeurosis and between the two heads of the pronator teres. The median nerve gives off a purely motor branch, the anterior interosseous nerve, to the flexor pollicis longus, to the flexor digitorum profundus tendon to the index finger, and to the pronator quadratus.

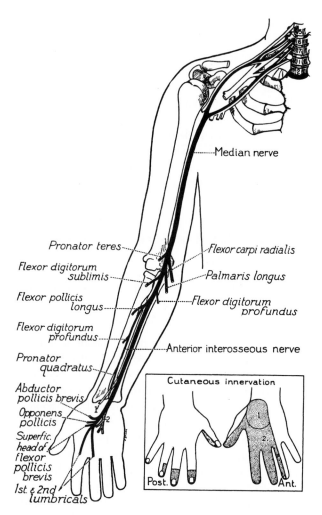

FIGURE 12-9 Schematic of median nerve. (From Haymaker W, Woodhall B: *Peripheral nerve injuries: principles of diagnosis,* Philadelphia, 1953, WB Saunders.)

TABLE 12-8

Summary of Median Nerve Anatomy, Lesion Sites, and Typical Deficits/Deformities

Sensation, includes the palmar cutaneous branch	Volar hand: thumb, index, long, radial aspect of ring, volar radial palm, dorsal 20%-35% of terminal dorsal thumb, index, long, and radial ring rays
Motor	Innervations proximal to distal in this order: pronator teres, flexor carpi radialis, palmaris longus, flexor digitorum superficialis (FDS), radial two flexor digitorum profundus (FDP), flexor pollicis longus (FPL), pronator quadratus, abductor pollicis brevis, flexor pollicis brevis (superficial head), opponens pollicis, index lumbrical muscle, middle digit lumbrical muscle
Function	The median nerve allows for forearm pronation; thumb, index, and long digit flexion; and thenar palmar abduction and opposition. These movements combine to position the hand for grasping (as a piece of candy off the table, for example) and allow for precision pinch. The sensory contribution of the median nerve is huge: without intact sensation along the radial volar aspect of the hand, fine motor coordination is not possible.
Common sites of entrapment/injury	*Pronator syndrome:* compression at ligament of Struthers, lacertus fibrosis, hypertrophy of pronator teres or at arch of FDS; pain syndrome, sometimes sensory involvement *Anterior interosseous syndrome:* compression of deep motor branch, paralysis of FPL and FDP to index, sensory symptoms absent, forearm pain present *Carpal tunnel syndrome:* compression at carpal tunnel resulting from provocative positioning, anatomic anomalies, metabolic conditions, trauma to wrist, or space occupying lesions; nocturnal pain and dysesthesias and thenar weakness
Results of lesion	Loss of median nerve integrity at the elbow *(high-level lesion)* results in *ape hand deformity*, with loss of precision pinch, loss of thenar opposition, paralysis of FDS and radial two FDP muscles. Forearm pronation is significantly compromised following paralysis of both pronator muscles. Pronation can occur only by abduction of the shoulder and the assistance of gravity. A *lesion to the anterior interosseous nerve* results in paralysis of the FPL and index and (sometimes) long digit FDP, making it difficult to make an "O" when attempting to pinch *(Ballentine's sign)*. A more distal *(low-level) lesion* of the nerve, as at the *carpal tunnel*, results in loss of thenar opposition, with frequently observable thenar muscle wasting. The thumb lies to the side of the radial palm, and a web space contracture may develop because of the unopposed pull of the thumb adductor. The *loss or diminution of sensation* in the tips of the thumb, index, and long digits results in significant functional deficits with regard to all fine motor tasks such as writing, winding a watch, tying a shoe, or picking up a small object, particularly if vision is occluded. Clients complain about nocturnal dysesthesias, dropping objects, diminished fine motor coordination, and debilitating numbness.

The main trunk of the median nerve continues on under the fibrous origin of the flexor digitorum superficialis. The nerve emerges to become a more superficial structure in the distal forearm. Just proximal to the wrist, the palmar cutaneous (or sensory) branch arises and runs superficial to the flexor retinaculum to innervate the midpalm. The terminal portion of this nerve, along with the nine extrinsic digit flexor tendons, runs under the flexor retinaculum, then through the carpal tunnel and under its roof, the volar carpal ligament.

Precaution. *In the shallow carpal tunnel, the nerve sits superficially in relation to these tendons, making it particularly vulnerable to compression in this area because it is sandwiched between these tendons and the volar carpal ligament.*

The distal thenar motor branch of the median nerve innervates the thenar intrinsic muscles; the common digital branches innervate the first two lumbrical muscles to the index and long digits. The nerve continues through the palm as sensory branches that primarily provide sensation to the volar thumb, index, long, and medial half of the ring digits.

High (Proximal) Median Nerve Palsy: Anterior Interosseous Nerve Palsy and Pronator Syndrome

Diagnosis and Pathology

Compressive neuropathies of the median nerve in the proximal forearm are unusual lesions.[27] The two major compression neuropathies of the proximal median nerve occur with similar symptoms. Both syndromes involve entrapment of the nerve in the proximal forearm, and both are associated with pain in the proximal (volar) forearm that typically increases with activity.

The more proximal entrapment is called **pronator syndrome.** Diffuse pain in the medial forearm or distal volar arm along with dysesthesias in the radial three and one-half digits of the hand are hallmarks of this syndrome. Symptoms may be provoked by resisted elbow flexion, often with concurrent resisted forearm pronation. Provocation of symptoms with flexion of the proximal interphalangeal (PIP) joint of the long finger also may indicate pronator syndrome with the site of compression likely to be at the arch of the flexor digitorum superficialis.[27]

Four possible sites of nerve entrapment are associated with pronator syndrome. The first is at the distal third of the humerus, between the ligament of Struthers and the humeral supracondyloid process. The second site is at the elbow joint as the nerve courses under the lacertus fibrosis. A third potential site of compression is within the pronator teres, especially if that muscle is hypertrophied. The final site occurs at the arch of the flexor digitorum superficialis as the median nerve passes deep to it.[27]

Anterior interosseous syndrome is an entrapment neuropathy of the motor branch of the median nerve. This syndrome presents as nonspecific, deep aching pain in the proximal forearm that increases with activity. Usually there are no sensory symptoms. Paralysis of the flexor pollicis longus to the thumb and index and long finger flexor digitorum profundus results in collapsed distal interphalangeal joints when attempting to pinch (called **Ballentine's sign;** Fig. 12-10, A). Although paresis of the pronator quadratus may be present, it is difficult to appreciate, given the overlapping action of the stronger pronator teres. Potential sites and sources of compression are the same as with pronator syndrome and include local edema, hypertrophy of the pronator teres, or prolonged and excessive elbow flexion (120 degrees or greater).[27]

Evaluation Tips

- Pronator syndrome typically occur with diffuse forearm pain aggravated by resisted elbow flexion and forearm pronation and sensory changes along the volar, radial three and one-half digits of the hand.
- Anterior interosseous syndrome typically occurs with diffuse forearm pain, a positive Ballentine's sign with tip pinch, and no sensory changes.

Timelines and Healing

Many clients have vague symptoms for months or even years before a definitive diagnosis is made. This is frustrating for the client and may require serial clinical examinations and repeat electrodiagnostic studies to confirm anterior interosseous syndrome or pronator syndrome. Prolonged compression of the median nerve indicates a poor prognosis for full recovery, even following surgical decompression.[27]

Ideally, clients with proximal median nerve entrapment neuropathies are evaluated and are given a home exercise program and a short course of in-clinic pain management, followed by interim therapy visits every 2 to 4 weeks until resolution of symptoms occurs. Insurance and financial constraints may necessitate altering this timeline.

Nonoperative Treatment

- *Splinting:* Fabricate a splint to rest the irritated tissues, and give it to the client with instructions to use it as much as possible over the initial 3 to 4 weeks, removing it for hygiene. If the suspected site of entrapment is at the ligament of Struthers, at the lacertus fibrosis, or at the pronator teres, fabricate a long arm splint or a sugar tong splint. Place the elbow at 90 to 100

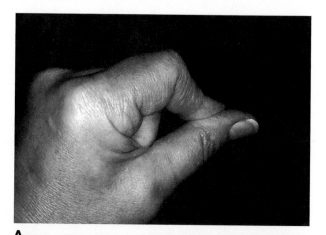

A

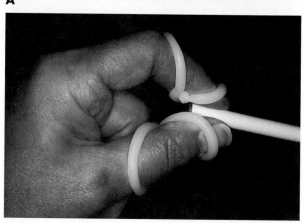

B

FIGURE 12-10   A, Anterior interosseous palsy. **B,** Tip splinting for anterior interosseous palsy. (From Colditz JC: Splinting the hand with a peripheral nerve injury. In Mackin E, Callahan AD, Skirven TM et al, editors: *Rehabilitation of the hand and upper extremity,* ed 5, St Louis, 2002, Mosby.)

degrees of flexion, and position the forearm in neutral rotation. If the suspected site of entrapment is along the flexor digitorum sublimus arch, include the wrist in the splint and immobilize it in a neutral position.

- Because the anterior interosseous syndrome makes tip pinch difficult (resulting from paresis of the flexor pollicis longus and the flexor digitorum profundus to the index finger), static tip splints blocking full extension at the distal interphalageal joints of the thumb and index finger may assist the client in activities such a holding a pen and writing (Fig. 12-10).
- *Pain management:* Pain can be addressed through the use of physician-prescribed over-the-counter oral pain medications and various therapeutic modalities and massage.
- *Therapeutic exercise:* Once symptoms have diminished at rest and with self-care activities, the client can be weaned from the splint. Encourage clients to incorporate a regular, lifetime stretching program designed to condition the forearm soft tissue before using the arm. Show clients how to perform gentle, prolonged stretching with the elbow in extension, forearm in full supination, and the wrist and digits in full extension. If necessary, address proximal muscle weakness with an appropriate exercise program that minimizes the irritating positions of full elbow flexion and full forearm pronation.
- *Activity modification:* The therapist should assist the client in identifying inciting activities and postures. Performing repetitive forearm rotation against resistance at work or maintaining prolonged elbow flexion, such as when sleeping prone in the fetal position, are two common examples of positions the client should avoid. When possible, activities should be modified to decrease load and repetition and to limit elbow extremes of flexion. Suggest using a padded soft elbow sleeve on the symptomatic arm when sleeping, but reverse it so that the padded portion is located on the volar surface. This will make it difficult for the client fully to flex the elbow when sleeping. Sometimes I will have a client fill this soft elbow pad with old (clean) socks to add bulk to this makeshift splint and to limit elbow flexion further during sleep.

Precautions and Concerns

- *With pronator syndrome, there may be sensory changes along the volar, radial three and one-half digits; therefore, performing a light touch sensory threshold exam to identify sensory status is imperative.*
- *Be careful when splinting a body part that is insensate or that has diminished sensation.*

- *Use extra layers of stockinette to protect the skin from burns from hot plastic splinting material.*
- *Educate the client in ways to protect the insensate hand or the hand with diminished sensation.*

Decompression of the Median Nerve
Operative Treatment
Surgical exploration and release is done if there is no spontaneous recovery in 8 to 12 weeks of conservative management.[27]

Timelines and Healing Following Decompression Surgery
Consider the following guidelines[26,27]:

- Use a removable half cast or splint that supports the elbow and forearm to protect and rest the newly decompressed tissue. Support for the wrist usually is included.
- Encourage early AROM exercises of all joints, unless the pronator teres was released completely from its insertion into the radius. In this case, forearm AROM is limited to a protective arc of 45 degrees of pronation to full pronation for several weeks postoperatively.
- Muscle strengthening can begin 7 to 10 days postoperatively if the pronator teres was not released, or after 3 to 4 weeks if the pronator teres was released and reattached.
- Full AROM should be achieved by 8 weeks after surgery, and normal strength should return by 6 months postoperatively.

Median Nerve Not in Continuity, Elbow to Wrist Level
Diagnosis and Pathology
Severance of the median nerve in the forearm or wrist typically occurs from knife or glass lacerations. Clinical presentation is one of sensory and motor involvement, with specific deficits depending on the site of injury. Loss of median nerve integrity at the elbow or proximal forearm (high-level lesion) results in **ape hand deformity,**[15] with loss of precision pinch, loss of thenar opposition, paralysis of the flexor digitorum superficialis and radial two flexor digitorum profundus muscles and their corresponding two lumbrical muscles. The thenar eminence is atrophied, with the thumb lying to the side of the palm. Loss of ability to oppose and palmarly abduct the thumb occurs. Index finger metacarpal and PIP joint flexion is lost, as is thumb interphalangeal flexion. Forearm pronation is significantly compromised because of paralysis of the pronator teres and the pronator quadratus. Some forearm pronation can occur, however, with the assistance of gravity when the shoulder is abducted

slightly.[27] Sensory loss typically includes the radial three and one-half digits and the radial, volar palm.

Low-level lesions[15] (occurring at the wrist) also occur with thenar eminence flattening and with loss of thumb opposition and thumb palmar abduction because of paralysis of the median-innervated intrinsic muscles (Fig. 12-11). As with a high-level lesion, a thenar web space

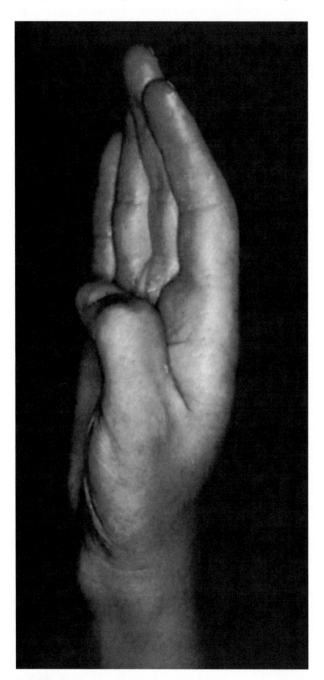

FIGURE 12-11   Ape hand deformity resulting from median nerve palsy. (From Colditz JC: Splinting the hand with a peripheral nerve injury. In Mackin E, Callahan AD, Skirven TM et al, editors: *Rehabilitation of the hand and upper extremity*, ed 5, St Louis, 2002, Mosby.)

contracture can develop because of the unopposed pull of the thumb adductor muscle. Sensory loss to the radial three and one-half digits is also present.

Timelines and Healing Following Surgical Repair

Consider the following guidelines[26]:

- Remove the bulky compressive dressing and apply a light compressive dressing for edema control.
- Fabricate a custom-made dorsal wrist blocking splint with the wrist in approximately 30 degrees of palmar flexion but not more than 45 degrees of palmar flexion. The amount of wrist flexion is predicated upon the amount of tension at the nerve repair site. Replicate the wrist position of the postoperative cast if the surgeon is not immediately available to give you guidelines.
- *Have the client wear the splint continuously for 4 to 6 weeks except for protective skin care. Hygiene should occur with the splint on.*
- Begin AROM and PROM of the digits and thumb, 10 repetitions every waking hour within the splint. Instruct the client in active tendon glide exercises so that the extrinsic flexor tendons glide separately and do not become adherent at the area of surgical repair. Fig. 12-12 depicts tendon glide exercises.
- Scar massage and scar mobilization techniques may begin 24 to 48 hours after sutures are removed but should be gentle initially.
- At 4 weeks postoperatively, adjust the dorsal wrist blocking splint to 20 degrees of palmar flexion.
- At 5 weeks postoperatively, adjust the dorsal wrist blocking splint to 0 to 10 degrees of palmar flexion.
- By 6 weeks postoperatively, discontinue use of the dorsal wrist blocking splint and initiate progressive strengthening for the hand and wrist. Begin by having the client incorporate the postoperative hand into daily activity use. Strengthening can be as simple as setting a table or tying a shoe or writing a grocery list.
- By 8 weeks postoperatively, the client can begin a work rehab program designed to address residual strength and coordination deficits that adversely affect return to work.

Clinical Reasoning

In the adult client with a high median or ulnar nerve injury, return of normal motor and sensory function is rare.[23] Therefore, splinting to maintain PROM may be necessary in preparation for tendon transfers.

Precaution. *With a median nerve injury, adduction contractures of the thumb are the most common and preventable deformity that should be addressed by proactive splinting.*

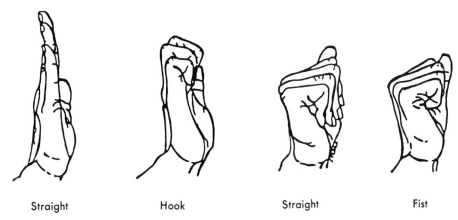

Straight   Hook   Straight   Fist

FIGURE 12-12 Tendon glide exercises. (From Hayes EP et al: Carpal tunnel syndrome. In Mackin E, Callahan AD, Skirven TM et al, editors: *Rehabilitation of the hand and upper extremity,* ed 5, St Louis, 2002, Mosby.)

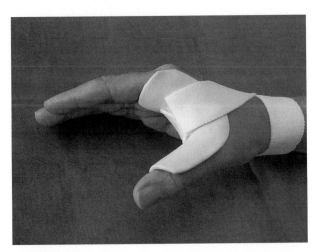

FIGURE 12-13 Static thenar web spacer splint to prevent adduction contracture following median nerve palsy. (From Skirven TM, Callahan AD: Therapist's management of peripheral-nerve injuries. In Mackin E, Callahan AD, Skirven TM et al, editors: *Rehabilitation of the hand and upper extremity,* ed 5, St Louis, 2002, Mosby.)

Fabricate a static hand-based night splint (Fig. 12-13) that holds the thumb in full abduction, and provide the client with instructions about wear and care, with a clear explanation as to the purpose of the splint. A small daytime splint made of neoprene or leather can be used to hold the thumb in a stable and opposed, if not fully abducted, position. This splint can be fabricated or purchased from one of the commercial splint catalogs. The advantage to this type of splint is that it does not block the index finger metacarpophalangeal joint from flexion, thereby diminishing the possibility of an extension contracture developing at that joint.

Precautions and Concerns

- *Watch for thenar web space and index finger metacarpophalangeal joint contracture associated with this injury. Incorporate proactive splinting and PROM exercises in the treatment program until muscle function returns or until tendon transfers are done.*
- *Client education is critical regarding sensory impairment. Teach the client protective sensation techniques, including visually monitoring all activities performed with the insensate hand until there is adequate protective sensory return.*
- *An isolated median nerve laceration at the forearm or wrist is rare. More commonly, concurrent flexor tendon injuries occur. Also address postoperative protocols for flexor tendon repairs and nerve repairs.*

Low Median Nerve Palsy: Carpal Tunnel Syndrome

Diagnosis and Pathology

CLINICAL *Pearl*

Median nerve compression at the carpal tunnel of the wrist is the most common nerve compression syndrome of the upper extremity.[28]

Classic symptoms of carpal tunnel syndrome (CTS), as this low median nerve entrapment is called, include nocturnal pain and dysesthesias, diminished fine motor coordination, intermittent daytime numbness and tingling, and in advanced cases, thenar weakness with significantly decreased pinch strength.[28] CTS is seen more often in women than men, and the symptoms are often bilateral.[28,29] About 50% of the cases occur in persons between 40 to 60 years of age.[28]

The carpal tunnel is a narrow channel. The median nerve and the nine extrinsic flexor tendons to the digits and thumb pass through this tunnel. At this level, each of the nine flexor tendons is encased by a synovial fluid-filled sheath. (Think of the sheath as a type of bursa, or fluid-filled sac, that protects and nourishes the tendon it surrounds.) The dorsal floor and sides of the carpal tunnel are formed by a concave arch of carpal bones. The volar roof of the canal is formed by the transverse carpal ligament. The median nerve sits superficially, just below this ligament and on top of all nine synovial ensheathed tendons.

Median nerve compression occurs in the carpal tunnel because there is too little space or too much tissue within the tunnel.[28] In either case, the result is ischemia, or decreased blood flow to the nerve. Persistent vascular insufficiency results in anoxia and edema within the epineurium, or outer connective tissue covering of the nerve. Prolonged congestion within the nerve results in (initially) intermittent disturbances in nerve conduction that ultimately, if not treated, results in permanent damage to the nerve.

Any condition or circumstance that can result in diminished space within the carpal tunnel can cause CTS. A common condition that can lead to CTS is nonspecific tenosynovitis, or inflammation of the synovium within the sheaths that surround the tendons within the carpal canal. This scenario is associated with otherwise healthy individuals who perform repetitive forceful tasks with their wrists flexed or with significant loading of their digital flexors. Tenosynovitis within the carpal canal can lead to constriction of the median nerve and hence diminished blood flow to this nerve. Other causes of CTS include fluid retention from systemic states, such as pregnancy or endocrine disorders; space-occupying lesions such as ganglions or tumors; systemic medical conditions such as rheumatoid arthritis or diabetes; or trauma to the wrist, such as from a severe wrist fracture or lunate dislocation.[28,29]

Evaluation Tips

- Early diagnosis is important to ensure accurate, appropriate conservative treatment and to minimize potential for disability.

Precaution. *Clients complaining of hand pain and referred to hand therapy by a non–hand specialist may be diagnosed incorrectly with CTS.*

An evaluation should always include light touch threshold testing, grip and pinch testing, fine motor coordination testing (I recommend the Nine-Hole Peg Test because of ease and speed of administration), and a pain interview.

- Clients may be able to compensate for median nerve sensory loss during fine motor testing by visually attending to the task. In situations in which the client's verbal reporting is suspect or unreliable, a nonstandardized Moberg Pickup Test can provide insight about the functional status of the involved hand. Observe and time the client picking up a number of small objects and placing them in a cup or container, first with eyes open and then with eyes closed. Test the involved and uninvolved hands. Observe and record changes in prehension patterns associated with occluded vision. Clients tend to avoid using the part of the hand that has poor sensibility when locating and picking up objects with vision occluded.

- Suspect CTS if the client complains of the hand feeling "fat" or "swollen"; if the client reports weakness or clumsiness and dropping of small objects; and if the client reports nocturnal paresthesias that wake him or her from sleep and improve by shaking or massaging the hand. The nocturnal symptoms are likely the result of venous stasis, aggravated by wrist postures of hyperflexion or extension sustained when sleeping.

- Observe for thenar eminence atrophy. In advanced cases, an adductor contracture of the thumb can occur as a result of the unopposed pull of the adductor pollicis.

- **Phalen's Test,**[30] also called the Wrist Flexion Test, involves placing the wrist in a position of full flexion for 1 minute and asking the client to describe any changes in sensation during or after this posture. A positive Phalen's Test response, indicative of CTS, involves reports of numbness and tingling in the median-nerve distribution of the hand. A review of the literature[31] reveals a wide range of sensitivity for identifying CTS with this provocative test.

CLINICAL *Pearl*

When performing a Phalen's Test, try to prevent simultaneous elbow flexion because this is a separate provocative test for the ulnar nerve at the elbow and could confound your findings.

Nonoperative Treatment

- *Splinting:* Use of a wrist splint to rest the inflamed tissues and to minimize intratunnel pressures on the median nerve is well documented.[15,23,29,32] The proper position for wrist splinting is neutral, with the wrist at 0 to 2 degrees of flexion and about 3 degrees of ulnar deviation.[32] Prefabricated wrist cock-up splints are readily available in pharmacies.

Precaution. *Unless these splints are adjusted correctly to position the wrist in neutral, they may elevate carpal tunnel pressure significantly, thereby aggravating carpal tunnel symptoms.*[32]

Often, the metal insert of the prefabricated splint can be replaced with a custom-molded thermoplastic insert that provides proper wrist positioning. The splint should be used at night for 6 to 8 weeks and may be used selectively during the day to assist with wrist positioning during provoking activities such as computer use.

- *Nerve gliding:* The use of nerve and tendon gliding exercises in a conservative management program for CTS was shown significantly to decrease the number of clients undergoing surgery at an average of 23 months' follow-up.[33] You can teach traditional median nerve glides to the client. However, incorporating the movements of the nerve glide into a functional activity makes them easier to remember. For the median nerve glide, I instruct my clients to begin by making a closed fist and bringing that fist up, thumb side, close to their face. I then instruct the client to open the hand and extend the elbow and wrist slowly (with a supinated forearm), pretending to be playing with a yo-yo. The client returns to the start position and repeats this 5 to 10 times. The goal of these glides is to slide the nerve gently through its available range to promote axoplasmic flow and general nerve health. Fig. 12-14 outlines traditional median nerve gliding exercises.

- *Tendon gliding* (Refer to Fig. 12-12).

- *Pain management:* Over-the-counter or prescription nonsteroidal antiinflammatory medications are often

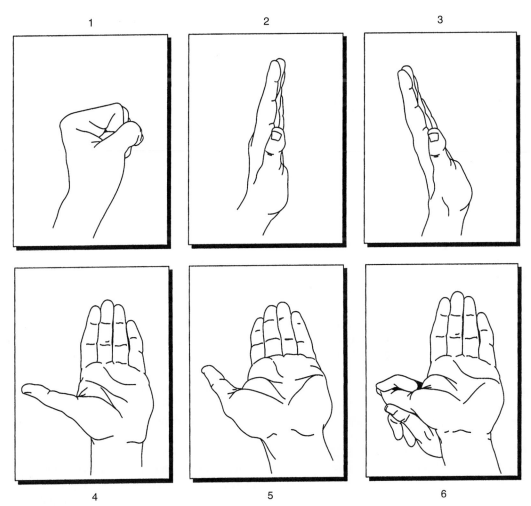

FIGURE 12-14 Traditional median nerve glide exercises. (Redrawn from Totten PA, Hunter JM: *Hand Clin* 7(3):505-520, 1991. In Mackin E, Callahan AD, Skirven TM et al, editors: *Rehabilitation of the hand and upper extremity,* ed 5, St Louis, 2002, Mosby.)

part of the conservative treatment program for clients with CTS, although oral medications have not been shown to be effective in reducing clinically measurable symptoms. Likewise, ultrasound has not been shown to be effective in conservative treatment of CTS.[29]

- *Activity modification:* Whether a client's CTS is related to work tasks, avocational pursuits, pregnancy, or other causes, it is important to discuss how certain postures and tasks can contribute to typical CTS symptoms. Reducing the duration, frequency, and intensity of forceful, repetitive work and reducing extreme wrist postures and vibration can decrease the severity of carpal tunnel symptoms.[32] Antivibration gloves, or bicycle gloves that contain volar gel pads over the wrist crease, can be purchased to help dampen the adverse effect of vibration experienced with a lawn mower, for example. An ergonomic evaluation of the work site and of household tasks and leisure tasks that may contribute to the CTS symptoms can be helpful. For example, the person who works on a computer in the office all day may need educating about how work place postures and home avocational computer pursuits may be aggravating the symptoms. Educate the client about which wrist and finger postures to avoid and which ones to assume.

Precaution. *Caution clients against tight fisting activities or repetitive, resistive finger flexion.*

Recommend rest breaks and rotation of tasks at work and home that require provocative postures or repetitive movements.

- *Exercise:* Proximal conditioning exercises and postural training may be helpful, especially for the deconditioned client with poor postures (such as forward rounded shoulders and flexed cervical spine). Altered axoplasmic flow that results from compression of the nerve at the carpal tunnel can cause the entire nerve to become sick and to become vulnerable to multiple sites of irritation along its axon.[2-4]

CLINICAL *Pearl*

Poor posture can contribute to further median nerve problems as the already distally irritated nerve is exposed to proximal compression when good body mechanics are not used consistently.

Repetition, cueing, and client motivation are absolute prerequisites to abolishing bad habits.

What to Say to Clients

- "Try to keep your wrist in a neutral position when performing daily activities."
- "Avoid sustained pinch or gripping, particularly prolonged pinching when your wrist is in a flexed or bent posture."
- "Avoid positioning your wrist in a bent or flexed posture (the fetal position) when sleeping. Use your splint at night to help keep your wrist in the safe, neutral position."
- "Think of your median nerve as the cord that attaches the vacuum to the wall outlet. If you bend that cord too often or if you bend it with enough force, you might damage the cord, and the vacuum won't work as well. That is how your nerve is: if you bend it too often or with too much force at your wrist, the nerve can get damaged and it won't work as well or it won't work at all. Be proactive and try to prevent further damage by limiting the extremes of wrist motion at work and at home and when you sleep."
- "Whenever possible, use tools in the kitchen, the workplace, and the garden that have larger grips that are contoured to the arches of your hand. Your hand should close easily around the handle. You don't want one that is too big or too small for your hand. The grip handle can be adjusted with dense foam to increase the diameter (if necessary) and to pad the surface somewhat so that it is easier on the structures, like your nerve, that lie underneath the skin of your hand."
- "Look at a work station design handout to figure out how to set up your home office or your work office. These ergonomic work station designs are available at no charge on the Internet."

Operative Treatment

If there is a lack of symptomatic relief with conservative management or if there is electrodiagnostic evidence of denervation of the median nerve, transection of the transverse carpal ligament (called a carpal tunnel release, or CTR) is performed.[28] CTR is estimated to be among the 10 most commonly performed operations in the United States.[33] A traditional open CTR surgery or a less invasive endoscopic release may be performed. The latter technique has the advantage of less postoperative pain, a quicker recovery of strength, and faster return-to-work time. However, endoscopic release also is associated with increased complications, including accidental severance of or injury to the ulnar nerve, the palmar cutaneous branch of the median nerve, the ulnar artery, and the flexor tendons. Incomplete release of the transverse carpal ligament with consequent reoccurrence of CTS following surgery is another complication of this surgical method.[29]

The traditional open CTR is always performed if the surgeon suspects that a flexor tenosynovectomy or a neurolysis may need to be done and for a better result. The goal of the tenosynovectomy is to remove the diseased synovial tissue so that there will be better gliding between the tendons and the nerve and to decompress the nerve further within the hand. A neurolysis may be done to resect constricting scar tissue that is affecting the circulation within the nerve adversely. In either of these cases, the therapist will see a larger scar postoperatively.

Postoperative therapy is guided by wound healing principles, the procedures performed, and tissue response to stress. For the uncomplicated client, little or no follow-up therapy may be necessary. For the complicated client, such as the client with a premorbid health condition of diabetes or for those clients with worker's compensation insurance, a course of therapy following CTR most likely will be necessary to maximize functional return.[32]

Follow-up therapy consists of the following:

- *Wound and scar care:* Begin wound and scar care as soon as the client is referred and evaluated. Scar pain is common after a CTR, and the client's occupational performance may be affected such that the client avoids using the postsurgical hand. Apply an appropriate compressive dressing that minimizes edema and subsequent scar formation after surgery. I use an elastic stockinette for edema control initially and add a silicone gel insert over the scar to improve scar cosmesis once the sutures are removed. This silicone gel pad insert has the added benefit of acting as a shock absorber when the client attempts to use that hand. Evans[32] recommends the use of Micropore paper tape in place of a gel pad or silicone insert for improved scar cosmesis.
- *Pain management:* Pain can be addressed through the use of over-the-counter, oral pain medications and various therapeutic modalities and massage. See Tips from the Field about Pain Management for further discussion of this topic.
- *Splinting:* The use of a supportive splint that maintains the wrist in neutral or slight extension traditionally has been advocated for 2 to 3 weeks postoperatively. The thought process was that splinting would prevent potential complications associated with wound dehiscence (or the wound not healing) and anterior displacement of the median nerve and flexor tendons after the transverse carpal ligament is excised. Recent studies suggest that the incidence of either of these is minimal, and therefore a splint is probably not necessary.[32] A short course of postoperative splinting is appropriate for the client who

complains of nocturnal pain associated with flexed postures of the wrist when asleep and for those clients who are likely to overdo it when they return to their occupational roles.

- *Mobilization:* Begin active exercises of the wrist, thumb, and digits within the first 24 to 48 hours to ensure adequate glide of the median nerve and flexor tendons. Tendon glide exercises are a good choice for encouraging full glide of the digit flexor tendons. Introduce median nerve glides and progress according to the client's tolerance.
- *Strengthening:* Gentle strengthening exercises can begin in the third postoperative week if significant pain and edema are not present. Advise the client that he or she can begin to resume household tasks such as laundry and light house cleaning at this time. If the client has inadequate strength to perform work, household, or avocational tasks, initiate progressive strengthening for the wrist and hand between weeks 3 and 6 after surgery, depending on the client's tissue tolerances. A work rehab program, if necessary, can begin about 5 to 6 weeks after surgery to address residual strength and endurance issues and specific critical job demands that may present difficulties on return to work.

Tips from the Field

- **Pillar pain,** or pain on either side of the CTR incision, is a normal postoperative occurrence. This pain can be debilitating, making it difficult to grip or perform palmar weight-bearing activities. Return to work often is delayed because of pillar pain.[29] The exact cause of pillar pain is unknown; the various theories suggest that it is ligamentous or muscular in origin or a result of an alteration of the carpal arch. Typically, this pain decreases over the first year after surgery. Intervention strategies are discussed infrequently in the literature. Gel pads that cross the irritated sites may ameliorate the soreness experienced with weight bearing. Educating the client about the nature of this pain and that this pain eventually will dissipate is also helpful.
- If possible, instruct the client to perform a home strengthening program using activities that she wants and needs to do during the course of her day, rather than using putty and hand weights. Although this type of individualized strengthening program is more difficult for the therapist to design, it has more meaning for the client, and client follow-through will be better. Use of the COPM, if appropriate to the therapist's scope of practice, will assist the therapist in identifying meaningful tasks that can be graded appropriately for an alternative strengthening program.

Precautions and Concerns

Be cautious about introducing putty, hand grippers, or repetitive gripping tasks such as the Baltimore Therapeutic Equipment (BTE) work simulator in the clinic following a CTR. The development of trigger finger (stenosing tenosynovitis) that was not present before the CTR can complicate the postoperative course.[32] Repetitive hand gripping and pinching exercises may contribute to this inflammatory condition following a CTR. Some experts advocate delaying resistive grip exercises until 6 weeks after CTR.

ULNAR NERVE

Anatomy

Table 12-9 gives a summary of ulnar nerve anatomy, common lesion sites, and typical deficits/deformities associated with ulnar nerve lesions.

The ulnar nerve (Fig. 12-15) arises from medial cord of the brachial plexus (C7 to T1 roots). The nerve runs medial to the humeral artery, travels through the medial intermuscular septum, and passes superficially between

TABLE 12-9

Summary of Ulnar Nerve Anatomy, Lesion Sites, and Typical Deficits/Deformities

Sensation: dorsal cutaneous branch and superficial sensory branch	Ulnar/medial side of palm (volar and dorsal); entire fifth digit and ulnar aspect of fourth digit (volar and dorsal)
Motor	Innervations, proximal to distal: flexor carpi ulnaris, flexor digitorum profundus to digits 4 and 5, abductor digiti minimi, flexor digiti minimi, opponens digiti minimi, fourth and third lumbrical muscles, three palmar interossei muscles and four dorsal interossei muscles, deep head of the flexor pollicis brevis, and adductor pollicis
Function	The ulnar nerve allows for simultaneous strong wrist flexion and ulnar deviation, as well as power grip via full flexion of the ulnar two digits. This is necessary for tasks such as swinging a golf club or a hammer. Ulnar nerve integrity is also necessary to allow for powerful tip and lateral or key pinch, for the adductor pollicis and first dorsal interossei assist in stabilizing the thumb and index during pinching. The hypothenar muscles and the interossei muscles allow the hand powerfully to cup an object, such as a doorknob or a basketball.
Common sites of entrapment/injury	*Cubital tunnel syndrome:* causes include direct compressive trauma, repetitive or sustained elbow flexion, cubitus valgus deformities, second-degree supracondylar fractures, disease processes; symptoms include pain, dysesthesias, motor weakness
	Guyon's canal compression: causes include pisiform or hook of hamate fractures, arthritis, thrombus, and mass/ganglion; symptoms include pain, dysesthesias, and/or motor weakness
Results of lesion	Motor ulnar palsy has significant functional consequences. The balance between extrinsic and intrinsic muscles is lost, following paresis of most of the intrinsic muscles of the hand. This results in a flattening of the normal arches of the hand. Low-level lesions, as at the wrist, produce the *classic claw deformity* of the digits, with hyperextension of the metacarpophalangeal joints and flexion of the interphalangeal joints. (This posture is less noticeable in the index and long digits because the lateral two lumbrical muscles, which serve to flex the metacarpophalangeal joints, remain innervated by the median nerve.) There is wasting of the interosseous muscles, of the thenar adductor, and of the hypothenar eminence. Paralysis of the thenar adductor causes *significant loss of pinch strength.* If the client attempts to pinch, the distal phalanx typically assumes a position of flexion *(Froment's sign)*, and the proximal phalanx may hyperextend *(Jeanne's sign)* as the unimpaired flexor pollicis longus and the extensor pollicis brevis attempt to stabilize the thumb. High-level lesions, such as lesions to the nerve proximal to the innervation of the flexor carpi ulnaris, result in all of the aforementioned deficits and loss of simultaneous wrist flexion and ulnar deviation.
	Typically a client complains about significant loss of grip strength (i.e., for swinging a golf club or a hammer), difficulty with gross grasp (i.e., unable effectively to grasp a doorknob), and loss of ability to perform in-hand manipulation tasks such as shaking dice or moving coins into position to place into a slot. The client may report difficulty with lateral pinch (i.e., unable to turn a key in the ignition) and difficulty abducting and adducting the digits to don gloves or type (resulting from paresis of the interossei). Sensory loss, although problematic, is not as severely disabling as with the median nerve. Clients tend to complain of difficulty gauging the force needed to hold an object (such as a glass).

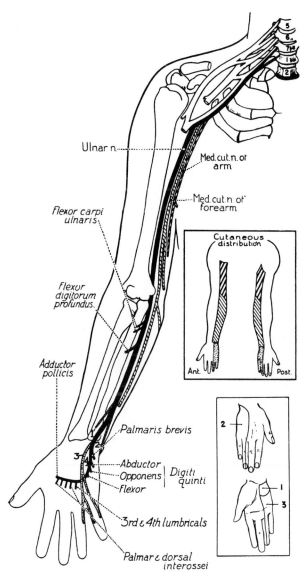

FIGURE 12-15 Schematic of the ulnar nerve. (From Haymaker W, Woodhall B: *Peripheral nerve injuries: principles of diagnosis,* Philadelphia, 1953, WB Saunders.)

the medial epicondyle of the humerus and the olecranon at the elbow joint. The ulnar nerve enters the forearm between the two heads of the flexor carpi ulnaris and descends within the anteriomedial forearm under the cover of the flexor carpi ulnaris. In the lower third of the forearm the ulnar nerve gives off a dorsal cutaneous branch, which supplies the skin of the ulnar half of the dorsum of the hand. At the wrist the ulnar nerve sits medially to the ulnar artery and runs with this artery in the osseofibrous carpal canal called **Guyon's canal,** a superficial passageway between the pisiform and hamate bones of the carpus. Just distal to the pisiform the ulnar nerve divides into two terminal branches: the superficial

(palmar) cutaneous branch and the deep motor branch. The motor branch winds around the hook of the hamate and innervates the three intrinsic hypothenar muscles, the ulnar two lumbrical muscles, and the three palmar adductors and four dorsal abductors. The ulnar nerve terminates at the adductor pollicis and the deep head of the flexor pollicis brevis. The sensory branch supplies the skin of the ulnar half of the volar hand and the fifth digit and the medial half of the fourth digits.[34-36]

Proximal Ulnar Nerve Compression: Cubital Tunnel Syndrome (High Level of Injury)

Diagnosis and Pathology

> **CLINICAL** *Pearl*
>
> Ulnar nerve compression at the cubital tunnel of the elbow is the second most common site of nerve entrapment in the upper extremity.[35]

This condition can occur in older persons with elbow arthritis or in younger individuals as a result of repetitive elbow motion.[35] The cubital tunnel is a fibrosseous space bound by the medial epicondyle anteriorly, the ulnohumeral ligament laterally, and the fibrous arcade of the two heads of the flexor carpi ulnaris posteromedially. A fibrous band extending from the olecranon to the medial epicondyle of the humerus forms the roof of this tunnel. The ulnar nerve can be palpated easily within this superficial tunnel.

The elbow has five potential sites for nerve entrapment.[35] They are under the arcade of Struthers, at the medial intramuscular septum, at the medial epicondyle, within the cubital tunnel itself, and beneath the deep aponeurosis of the flexor carpi ulnaris.

A variety of causes for ulnar nerve compression occur at the elbow.[34,35] Systemic disease such as diabetes or chronic alcoholism may predispose one to compression neuropathies. External sources of compression can include tourniquets or pressure from a hard surface on which the elbow was leaning. Compression can be induced by occupational activities such as in assembly line work that requires repetitive or sustained elbow flexion. Fractures and dislocations of the medial epicondyle and supracondylar area of the humerus may lead to acute or chronic nerve compression. Elbow deformities, congenital or as a result of a posttraumatic cubitus valgus deformity (essentially, too much lateral angulation of the forearm), can result in nerve compression.

The clinical picture depends on the severity and duration of the compression. Typically, pain occurs along the medial aspect of the elbow and tenderness over the cubital tunnel. Paresthesias in the ring and little finger are present. Motor weakness and wasting of the ulnar-innervated intrinsic muscles are present in more severe cases. This muscle involvement results in decreased power grip and decreased pinch strength. In advanced cases, one sees clawing of the ring and small fingers, resulting paralysis of the ulnar-innervated interossei and lumbrical muscles.

Evaluation Tips

- **Froment's sign**[30]: When the client attempts powerful lateral pinch, one sees flexion of the interphalangeal joint of the thumb as the flexor pollicis longus attempts to compensate for the paralyzed or weak adductor pollicis and flexor pollicis brevis.
- **Wartenberg's sign**[34] is present if the fifth finger is postured or held in an abducted position from the fourth finger. This indicates interosseous muscle weakness (specifically paresis of the palmar adductor interossei).
- **Elbow Flexion Test**[30,34]: This provocative maneuver is designed to reproduce the symptoms of ulnar nerve compression. The elbow is flexed fully and the wrist is held in neutral for up to 5 minutes. A positive test is a reproduction of symptoms.
- The muscle strength of the flexor digitorum profundus can be an important diagnostic tool to help determine the level of compression along the ulnar nerve. Normal muscle strength would indicate a distal or low-level entrapment, most likely at Guyon's canal.

Nonoperative Treatment
- *Splint*
  - Fabricate a static long arm resting splint for the client in order to rest the irritated tissues. The purpose of the splint is to limit elbow flexion and thus prevent further stress on the ulnar nerve as it passes through the cubital tunnel. The cubital tunnel is at its narrowest in full flexion, which contributes to nerve compression. The splint should position the elbow in 45 to 60 degrees of elbow flexion and the forearm and wrist at neutral, and the digits should be free to move. The splint can be fabricated anteriorly or posteriorly, though if a posterior splint is used, the elbow must be well padded so as not to cause increased surface pressure at the cubital tunnel. Generally, instruct the client to wear the splint at night for at least 3 weeks. If the symptoms do not improve, instruct the client to wear the splint as much as possible, removing it only for hygiene.[26,34]

- If clawing is evident (Fig. 12-16), a hand-based static splint that blocks the metacarpophalangeal joints from extension allows the extensor digitorum communis tendon to shunt its terminal force to the distal interphalangeal joint, thus allowing interphalangeal joint extension[15,23] (Fig. 12-17).
- Provide an *elbow pad* to protect the vulnerable cubital tunnel area whenever the client is unable to wear the long arm splint or for when the client discontinues the use of the long arm splint. This soft elbow pad cushions the elbow when it is resting on a hard surface. The pad also can be used at night to prevent or discourage the client from sleeping in a fetal position with the elbows in a fully flexed posture. I rec-

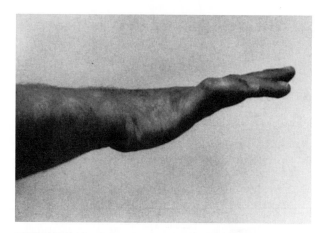

FIGURE 12-16 Claw hand deformity resulting from ulnar nerve palsy. (From Stanley BG, Tribuzi SM, editors: *Concepts in hand rehabilitation,* Philadelphia, 1992, FA Davis.)

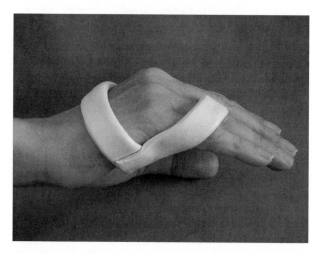

FIGURE 12-17 Hand-based splint designed to prevent clawing caused by ulnar nerve palsy. (From Skirven TM, Callahan AD: Therapist's management of peripheral-nerve injuries. In Mackin E, Callahan AD, Skirven TM et al, editors: *Rehabilitation of the hand and upper extremity,* ed 5, St Louis, 2002, Mosby.)

ommend that the client don the elbow pad backward so that the padding is sitting on the volar aspect of the elbow joint. The client can place a wadded up (clean) sock or stocking inside the elbow pad to provide further bulk. This bulk acts as a barrier to full elbow flexion, thus serving as a gentle reminder to the sleeping brain to avoid this position.

- *Pain management:* Prescription medication, splinting/rest, and activity modification are most helpful in dampening the client's pain.
- *Activity/work modification:* Educate clients about their syndrome and about modifications needed for sleep and work habits. An ergonomic assessment of the work place may be helpful in identifying those tasks that contribute to perpetuation of symptoms. In general, tell clients to avoid repetitive elbow flexion/extension and sustained elbow flexion postures. Educate clients about ways to minimize pressure on their ulnar nerve by using the elbow pad under clothing during the day and by resting the elbow on padded surfaces or pillows rather than on hard surfaces.

What to Say to Clients

"You have an injury to your nerve at your elbow. You know when you hit your funny bone? It doesn't feel funny, does it? That's because you're actually hitting your nerve, which is like a live wire close to the surface. You need to be careful and protective of that nerve, especially right now, when it's so sensitive. One way to protect the nerve is to avoid what I call the 'telephone position.' That's the elbow position you assume when you're holding the phone receiver up to your ear. That's a provocative position for your nerve; it doesn't like that position. If you have to use the phone a lot, you should consider getting a headset, so you can avoid that position. Also, you'll need to avoid that bent elbow position when you sleep."

Demonstrate elbow pads to clients. If the clinic does not have elbow pads, small pillows lightly Ace-wrapped to the volar elbow may substitute.

Timelines and Healing
According to Blackmore,[34] successful conservative management should demonstrate a reduction in symptoms within 3 weeks and should be apparent to the client and the therapist.

Operative Treatment
Cubital Tunnel Release
A simple cubital tunnel release consists of releasing or opening up the cubital tunnel of the elbow. All restricting fibrous bands are excised. This eliminates the restriction and pressure that has occurred along the ulnar nerve at the elbow. This procedure is done if the symptoms do not respond to conservative management and if the ulnar nerve does not dislocate around the medial epicondyle groove of the humerus.[26,35]

Anterior Transposition of the Ulnar Nerve: Subcutaneous versus Submuscular
A number of surgical options are available to address persistent **cubital tunnel syndrome** that may be aggravated further by painful subluxation of the ulnar nerve. Typically, the nerve is exposed, elevated from its bed, and transferred anterior to the medial epicondyle. In a **submuscular ulnar nerve transposition,** the nerve is placed in a well-vascularized muscular bed. To do this, the flexor-pronator muscle origin must be separated and then reattached to its origin on the medial epicondyle. With a **subcutaneous ulnar nerve transposition,** the nerve is transferred anteriorly and positioned below the subcutaneous fascia of the anterior forearm, medial to the median nerve.[26,35]

Precautions and Concerns

- *If the flexor-pronator muscle origin was reflected and reattached in surgery, the initiation of gentle AROM of the elbow, forearm, and wrist typically is delayed for about 3 weeks to allow the reattachment to heal enough to withstand motion.*
- *If the flexor-pronator muscle origin was reattached, passive forearm supination with wrist and finger extension is contraindicated because this will stress the repair site.*
- *Premature stretching and strengthening activities can result in avulsion of the flexor/pronator origin. Regarding initiation of strengthening, it is always best to err on the cautious side with clients who have had a submuscular transposition.*
- *Following any of these procedures, strong gripping and lifting are contraindicated for 3 to 8 weeks, depending on the procedure and the client's individual response to the trauma of surgery.*

Timelines and Healing
According to Blackmore,[34] postoperative rehabilitation for any type of cubital tunnel decompression should be divided into three progressive phases: protection, active motion, and strengthening. The stages vary in length based on the surgical procedure and consequent precautions, wound healing principles, and the individual's response to surgery and therapy.

- Protection phase (day 1 to 3 weeks)
  - *Splinting:* The amount of rigid protection the client needs varies according to the procedure, client comfort, and the surgeon-therapist protocol. Traditionally, a long arm splint placing the elbow in 70 to 90 degrees of flexion and the

forearm and wrist in neutral is fabricated and provided.[26,34] Other options include a bulky dressing and a sling. Following a submuscular transposition, the long arm splint may need to position the forearm in slight pronation.[34]

Precaution. *When fabricating a splint without clear positioning orders, it is always best to simulate the position in which the client was casted.*

- *Treatment:* At this stage the therapist should focus on wound care, edema control, pain management, improving AROM of uninvolved joints, and addressing activities of daily living issues/one-handed techniques. If the flexor-pronator origin *has not* been repaired, gentle active elbow, forearm, and wrist can begin outside the splint within the first few days postoperatively. If a repair was done, gentle AROM of these joints can begin by week 3. (See the following for parameters for an early mobilization program.) Whether or not motion is allowed for all joints in the first 3 weeks, do not emphasize end-range elbow motion.[34]
- Active motion (day 1 to weeks 3 to 5 or 6)
  - *Splinting:* Protective long arm splints usually are discontinued between 2 and 3 weeks postoperatively, depending on the surgery.[26] If necessary, the client may continue to use the long arm splint to rest from overuse or for protection as when traveling or sleeping. If the scar site remains tender, the client can use an elbow pad. Provide a hand-based anticlaw splint to correct claw deformity to improve function (Fig. 12-17). If a fixed joint deformity or soft tissues contracture is present because of prior muscle paresis, address additional splinting at this point.
  - *Treatment:* Scar management begins as soon as the wound is healed. Edema and pain control should continue. AROM of all joints should continue with the goal of achieving normal functional range that is within the limits of the client's discomfort. Desensitization techniques may need to be introduced now, for clients often experience hypersensitivity following this surgery. Ulnar nerve gliding also may begin, with the client cautioned about proceeding slowly and stopping at any point in the sequence if numbness, discomfort, or pain increases. Advise the client that nerve gliding can increase symptoms and nerve irritability if not done carefully and correctly. Incorporating the movements of the nerve glide into a functional activity makes them easier to remember.
  - *Early mobilization following submuscular transposition (beginning 1 to 2 weeks postoperatively):* Start

active elbow motion with forearm first in pronation and then gradually progress to elbow motion with forearm supination. Start wrist motion with elbow first in flexion and then progress to wrist motion with the elbow extended.[26,34]

- Strengthening (weeks 5 to 7; continue as needed)
  - *Splinting:* Padding of the elbow area may continue if there is persistent hypersensitivity. Splints to address muscle imbalance resulting from the initial ulnar neuropathy should continue until this problem is resolved with return of muscle strength or until tendon transfers are done.
  - *Treatment:* If distal muscle weakness is present, the therapist may need to do an MMT to develop a baseline. Assess grip and pinch strength, and address residual strength issues at this point. A strengthening program should always begin with a good warm-up or gentle stretching program. If individual muscle weakness was identified by the MMT, isolated strengthening should begin with isometric exercises. A general conditioning program may be necessary if the injury has been long-standing. If the injury is work related, a work rehab program can address back-to-work issues.

Tips from the Field

- Expect tenderness over the medial aspect of the elbow after any of these surgeries, and pad any splints appropriately.
- Clients with subcutaneous ulnar nerve transfers will have a shorter course of rehab than those with a submuscular transposition. However, their nerve will be less protected from environmental elements, such as compression or irritation from some external source (e.g., a purse strap worn routinely on the supinated forearm).
- Achieving full elbow AROM following a submuscular transposition is often difficult. Focus on functional elbow range rather than physiologic range. Assist return of elbow extension by allowing the arm to hang at the side while holding a light weight (e.g., a shopping bag or briefcase with a few ounces to a pound or so in it). Monitor for any increase in paresthesias when stretching the elbow joint.

Distal Ulnar Nerve Compression: Ulnar Tunnel Syndrome or Entrapment at Guyon's Canal (Low Level of Injury)

Diagnosis and Pathology

The ulnar tunnel at the wrist, called Guyon's canal, contains the ulnar nerve and artery and fatty tissue. The canal is bounded by the pisiform and tendinous insertion of the flexor carpi ulnaris ulnarly and the hook of the hamate radially. The roof of the canal is the flexor retinaculum.[35,36]

After giving off the dorsal cutaneous branch about 5 to 6 cm proximal to the wrist, the ulnar nerve enters Guyon's canal medial to the artery. Within the canal, the ulnar nerve divides into two branches: the superficial sensory branch and the deep motor branch.[36]

The most common cause of ulnar nerve compression at the wrist is a ganglion, followed by occupational neuritis. Other causes include a pisiform or hook of hamate fracture, pisotriquetral arthritis, thrombus, or vessel anomalies.[36] Smoking or the use of a pneumatic drill can predispose the client to ulnar artery thrombosis.[36]

The clinical picture is one of sensory loss and motor paresis affecting the intrinsic ulnar-innervated muscles, including the interossei, and the adductor pollicis. Occasionally, the hypothenar opponens, abductor, and flexor digiti minimi muscles are spared.[36] The sensory deficit involves the palmar ulnar aspect of the hand, both sides of the little finger, and the ulnar border of the ring finger. The dorsal, ulnar aspect of the hand is spared because it is supplied by the more proximal dorsal cutaneous branch.[36]

Motor ulnar palsy has significant functional consequences. The balance between extrinsic and intrinsic muscles is lost, resulting from paresis of most of the intrinsic muscles of the hand. This results in a flattening of the normal arches of the hand. Low lesions produce the classic **claw hand deformity,** with hyperextension of the metacarpophalangeal joints and flexion of the interphalangeal joints[15] (Fig. 12-18). (This posture is less

noticeable in the index and long digits because the lateral two lumbrical muscles, which serve to flex the metacarpophalangeal joints, remain innervated by the median nerve.) Wasting of the interosseous muscles, of the thenar adductor, and of the hypothenar eminence occurs. Paralysis of the thenar adductor causes significant loss of pinch strength, especially lateral or key pinch. If the client attempts to perform this type of pinch, the distal phalanx typically assumes a position of flexion (Froment's sign) and the proximal phalanx may hyperextend (*Jeanne's sign*) as the unimpaired flexor pollicis longus and the extensor pollicis brevis attempt to stabilize the thumb.

Evaluation Tips

- A detailed sensory exam (Semmes-Weinstein monofilament testing) of the volar and dorsal hand assists the clinician in detecting the site of compression.

CLINICAL *Pearl*

Sensory loss on the dorsal and volar hand would indicate a lesion proximal to Guyon's canal, whereas intact dorsal hand sensation with diminished volar hand and little digit and ulnar half of the ring digit would indicate compression within or just distal to Guyon's canal.

- Froment's sign[30] is seen when the client attempts powerful lateral pinch. One sees flexion of the interphalangeal joint of the thumb as the flexor pollicis longus attempts to compensate for the paralyzed or weak adductor pollicis and flexor pollicis brevis.
- Wartenberg's sign[34] is present if the fifth finger is postured or held abducted from the fourth. This indicates interosseous muscle weakness.

Nonoperative Treatment for Low Ulnar Nerve Palsy or Ulnar Tunnel Syndrome

Consider the following treatment options[15,23,26]:

- *Splinting*
  - Design an ulnar nerve palsy splint, also called an anticlaw splint, to prevent overstretching of the denervated lumbrical muscles and interossei of the ring and small fingers (see the tips from the field for more information on this). Instruct the client to remove the splint for hygiene only. Continue use of the splint until the muscle imbalance resolves or until tendon transfers are performed. If PIP flexion contractures of the involved digits have developed, a dynamic PIP extension splint is needed to address joint contractures before

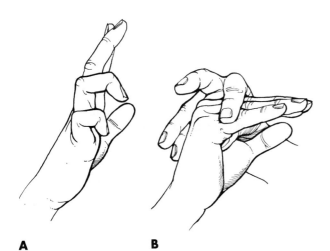

A   **B**

FIGURE 12-18 Drawing of clawing of the fourth and fifth digits following loss of intrinsic flexion and unopposed pull of the extensor digitorum communis. (From Fess EE, Gettle KS, Philips CA et al, editors: *Hand and upper extremity splinting*, ed 3, St Louis, 2005, Mosby.)

using the static anticlaw splint. I have found commercially available spring coil splints effective for mild contractures (about 30 degrees).

- A padded antivibration glove, a bicycle glove that has a gel pad that crosses the wrist crease, or a custom-made padded glove can be used to protect Guyon's canal from further external irritation during activities such as riding a mountain bike, maneuvering a lawn mower, or using traditional hand bike brakes.

- *Activity modification:* Ergonomic tools that are designed to minimize or eliminate stress on the ulnar wrist are good choices for clients with **ulnar tunnel syndrome.** An ergonomic hammer, for example, has a shaft that is designed to conform to the arches of the hand and has the tool head angled so that hammering can occur with the wrist in neutral. Educate the client about provocative postures and activities. Tell the client to avoid prolonged positions of simultaneous ulnar deviation and wrist flexion, for example. For the biking enthusiast, suggest foot brakes or having the hand brakes repositioned so as to avoid this posture. Have the client avoid vibratory input as much as possible, or at least to use dampening splints such as gel pads or padding on the handles of the equipment (lawn mower, vacuum, motorcycle).

Tips from the Field

- Intrinsic function does not commonly return in adults. Tendon transfers are typically necessary to correct the muscle balance that results from an ulnar nerve palsy.[15,26]

- When making an anticlaw splint for a low ulnar nerve palsy, take care to fabricate the splint so that the metacarpal phalangeal joints do not buckle or pop out of the splint inadvertently when the client attempts digit extension. Make sure that the palmar bar is form-fitting and wide enough to cover the entire metacarpophalangeal joint. Also, make sure the carefully molded dorsal hood of the splint extends all the way to the PIP joints, ending at the axis for PIP joint movement. At the same time, the splint should allow full finger flexion of all digits (Fig. 12-19). Construction of this splint can be tricky.

Operative Treatment

Low Ulnar Nerve Palsy or Ulnar Tunnel Syndrome

According to Moneim,[36] surgical exploration and decompression is recommended with ulnar tunnel syndrome because of the high incidence of space-occupying lesions. Postoperative therapy involves splinting as described before, wound/scar management as appropriate, and activity modification as described before. A postsurgical wrist immobilization splint typically is not needed fol-

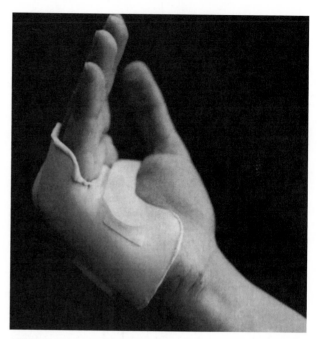

FIGURE 12-19 Hand-based ulnar nerve anticlaw splint with good volar support. (From Stanley BG, Tribuzi SM, editors: *Concepts in hand rehabilitation,* Philadelphia, 1992, FA Davis.)

lowing decompression; rather a bulky dressing serves the purpose of resting the tissues for the first 3 to 10 days postoperatively.

Repair of Ulnar Nerve Not in Continuity, Elbow to Wrist Level

Lacerations to the ulnar nerve can occur following injuries from a knife or glass. Typically, these injuries occur with concurrent flexor tendon injuries or ulnar artery injuries. Postoperative protocols need to consider all injured structures.

Timelines and Healing

Consider the following guidelines[15,26]:

- *Splint:* Fabricate a dorsal blocking splint with the wrist in 20 to 30 degrees of flexion, depending on the amount of tension at the nerve repair junction. If in doubt, position the wrist in the same amount of flexion as in the postoperative cast. Incorporate into the splint a metacarpophalangeal dorsal block that limits metacarpophalangeal joint extension to −45 degrees. This further minimizes tension on the nerve repair by limiting nerve excursion during digit extension and simultaneously blocks clawing or hyperextension at the metacarpophalangeal joints of the ring and little digits.

- *Wound care/scar mobilization:* Wound care should reflect wound healing timelines and can commence as soon as the client is referred and evaluated. Begin by assessing the incision site and documenting your findings. Immediately report the presence of clinical signs of infection (such as foul-smelling exudate or pus present at the incision site) to the physician. Once the sutures are removed, gentle scar massage may begin. The goal of scar management is to facilitate optimal scar formation that can withstand external friction stresses—that is, not hypersensitive to nonnoxious cutaneous stimuli—and that does not impede the normal gliding of underlying structures, such as tendons or the neurovascular bundle.

- *Desensitization* for hypersensitive scar tissue may begin after sutures are removed and wounds are healed.
- *Between weeks 3 and 5 to 6 postoperatively*, gradually adjust the dorsal blocking splint at the wrist, bringing it closer to neutral or 0 degrees extension. Progression is dictated by the surgeon, surgical procedure, and the client's relevant medical history.
- By *week 6* the dorsal blocking splint is discharged. A hand-based anticlaw splint may be needed until intrinsic muscle function returns.
- AROM of the wrist and hand can begin by week 6. Progressive strengthening exercises and resumption of self-care activities can occur over the next 2 weeks.
- By *week 8*, address residual strength issues that limit return to work in a work-conditioning program.

Tips from the Field
Sensory reeducation should begin once protective sensibility has returned. Typically, this is about 10 to 12 weeks following the repair.[26]

DOUBLE CRUSH SYNDROME

Diagnosis and Pathology

Normal axoplasmic flow is necessary for nerve maintenance and impulse conduction. Axoplasmic flow requires a constant energy source, which it gets from the blood. A complex vascular system exists that allows for an uninterrupted supply of blood to the nerve. If the vascular system of the nerve becomes compromised, the flow of its axoplasm is impaired. The consequences of altered axoplasmic flow include an alteration in the quality and quantity of synaptic transmissions and damage to the nerve cell body and to the axon itself. The nerve does not need to receive a specific injury, such as a crush or a stretch injury. Rather, over time, altered axoplasmic flow in a nerve that results from diminished blood flow to the nerve can cause the entire nerve to become sick and thus to become vulnerable to one or more sites of irritation along its axon.[2-4]

CLINICAL *Pearl*

Mononeuropathy caused by entrapment or compression of a peripheral nerve also may predispose the rest of the nerve trunk to general irritability and thus secondary neuropathies.

Because the peripheral nerve is one long, continuous cell, injury in one part of the cell almost certainly has consequences in other areas of the cell. Locations of increased susceptibility for a secondary impingement lesion may develop in areas where the nerve must traverse through spaces of increased friction (e.g., fibroosseous tunnels).[2-4] At that point the nerve cell would be most likely to demonstrate some amount of vascular impairment and thus slowed axoplasmic flow.[2,3] Conditions are thus ripe for gradual development of a pathologic condition. When a nerve has serial impingements or dual sites of pathologic manifestations that developed without a history of acute trauma, it is called **double crush syndrome.** Dellon[3] suggests that the sick nerve could have more than two sites of compression, each being insufficient in itself to cause clinical symptoms, but with the effects of each summating to create symptomatology. These clients with multiple crush syndrome would have diffuse upper extremity complaints and multiple sites of minor peripheral nerve irritation or entrapment.

Usually, electrodiagnostic testing, such as an electromyography, objectively demonstrates and quantifies abnormal peripheral nerve function. According to Butler,[2] with multiple crush syndrome, minor changes in the nerve fibers may not register as abnormal on electrodiagnostic tests, or these tests may not be specific enough to identify the presence of multiple sites of nerve irritation. Therefore the clinician may need to use the nonstandardized exams, such as nerve tension testing, to assess the presence of and the exact locations of multiple-site nerve irritation. Typically, clients complain of an intermittent diffuse upper extremity pain of varying intensity with a spread of symptoms from one area to another (e.g., from the wrist to the elbow).[3] Pain and paresthesias may be induced with specific postures of the arm that place the involved neural structures on tension.[2,3] As the nerve irritation progresses, the client may assume a protective posture of the involved extremity that minimizes tension on the irritated nerve or nerves or may develop a disuse atrophy as a means of coping with a chronic pain that seems to "have a mind all of its own."[1,2,4]

The most commonly studied double crush syndrome is the carpal tunnel syndrome–cervical spine injury,[2,3] followed by cubital tunnel syndrome and associated thoracic outlet syndrome. Metabolic conditions such as alcoholism, diabetes, and thyroid dysfunction may predispose the peripheral nervous system to double or multiple crush syndromes.[3]

Nonoperative Treatment and Operative Treatment

Not much has been written about the nonoperative and postoperative treatment of double crush syndrome. As with any peripheral nerve irritation, the therapist must follow protocols for tissue tolerances and wound care. Dellon[3] notes that the surgical release of one compression site may relieve the client's symptoms so that there is no further need to release other/all sites.

If surgical decompression is performed, the postoperative protocols should follow those specific for that surgery. For example, if a CTR is done, follow the postoperative protocols for this surgery, and augment therapy with interventions aimed at addressing the other more proximal "crush" sites. If multiple sites of entrapment are decompressed, then the timeline for healing is lengthened. Following Dellon's suggestions for managing the client with double or multiple crush syndrome,[3] I have listed some additional tips to assist the clinician in designing an appropriate and successful intervention program. Refer to Chapter 11 for further information and suggestions.

Treatment suggestions are as follows:

- *Early compression stage:* Clients in this stage have intermittent and position-dependent symptoms with only slight provocation of symptoms on physical examination. There may be a hypersensitive response to vibratory stimuli. Surgery is not recommended unless the symptoms fail to improve after at least 3 months of conservative management. Use appropriate splinting and instruct clients to decrease those activities that cause repetitive compression of the nerve.
- *Moderate compression stage:* Clients in this stage have symptoms that are intermittent but are more pronounced than in the earlier stage. For example, motor weakness is evident and measurable. Sensory threshold testing indicates changes from normal sensibility perception. Symptoms may interfere with daily activity performance and occupational roles. Surgery still is not indicated until a 3 month conservative management program has been tried and deemed unsuccessful. Dellon[3] suggests that steroid injections at the site of compression may be temporarily helpful.
- *Severe compression stage:* Clients in this stage have persistent symptoms with muscle wasting, finger numbness, abnormal two-point discrimination, and significant limitations in role performance because of pain. Surgery is recommended, for these clients will not improve without surgical intervention. Following surgery, it is important that the decompressed nerve not be immobilized for more than 1 week. Introduce range of motion exercises at the joint crossed by the released nerve and nerve gliding exercises early. The postoperative client may not become symptom-free when performing certain repetitive activities or using vibratory or pneumatic impact tools.[3]

Tips from the Field

- *Client education and cooperation are keys to successful management.* Educate the client about the underlying pathologic condition and about conditions that can aggravate further the already irritable nervous system. Encourage the client to find a safe and comfortable imaginary zone in which to move the arms without pain or increased symptoms. Have the client practice "staying within the box" (see Chapter 11) when performing self-care and work tasks. Reinforce concepts by reviewing the client's responses to staying within the box. Later, as the nerve irritation diminishes, the boundaries of the box can be increased.
- *Ergonomics can help lessen the external stresses on the irritable nerve.* Avoid repetitive upper extremity movements in the ranges and postures that aggravate the nerve. For example, instead of reaching overhead to put dishes away, use a sturdy step stool and keep the shoulder close to the body. Instead of bending the elbow to hold the telephone receiver to the ear, use a headset. Avoid using vibratory or pneumatic impact tools. If these are necessary, use an antivibration glove with a palmar gel pad to absorb some of the vibratory shock.

Precaution. *Nerve gliding should never be painful; find a way to encourage movement without irritating the nerve further.*

- Even a little bit of movement at a joint where the nerve crosses is better than none. If, for example, the client is unable to perform the entire brachial plexus glide without pain, adapt the glide so that the proximal joints remain still, minimizing some of the tension on the nerve, while the distal joints move, creating nerve gliding in the distal extremity. Then hold the distal joints still, in a position that minimizes tension on that nerve, as the proximal joints move to create proximal nerve gliding.
- Exercises for scapular stabilization, posture, and core trunk strengthening are important for treating distal

peripheral nerve entrapments and for minimizing the risk of developing double or multiple crush syndrome. Too often clients work at home and at the work site with a forward head posture, rounded shoulders, and a slumped back, and exercises to address these bad habits can facilitate nerve recovery and prevent future problems.

- Sometimes incomplete symptom resolution is the best that it gets. Not all clients recover completely from double or multiple crush syndrome. In fact, many do not. Help the client make the psychological adjustment necessary to living with a chronic and painful condition by teaching the client pain management strategies and by allowing the client to verbalize grief about this. Listen, acknowledge the client's grief, and when necessary, refer the client to a psychologist or psychiatrist.

Questions to Ask the Doctor

- *Does nerve testing (electromyogram/nerve conduction study) support the diagnosis of double crush syndrome?*
- *Where are the proximal and distal sites of entrapment?*
- *Is the client a candidate for carpal tunnel release (or some other decompression surgery)? What is the likely outcome of surgical intervention (e.g., incomplete symptom resolution)?*

DIGITAL NERVE INJURY AND REPAIR

Sources of entrapment include Dupuytren's disease or scar tissue following surgery to the hand. Direct pressure from a ring or a bowling ball can cause compression to a digital nerve as well. Symptoms include pain and dysesthesias. Digital nerves can be lacerated from glass or knife injuries; typically there are concurrent vascular and often tendon injuries. Digital nerve injuries respond best to exploratory surgery, decompression, and surgical repair.[37]

Postoperative Treatment

Postoperative treatment consists of the following[26]:

- *Splinting:* A dorsal blocking gutter splint is fitted in 30 degrees of PIP joint flexion for continuous wear for the first 3 to 6 weeks, depending on the surgeon's protocol and surgical procedure. If the splint is continued for the full 6 weeks, the therapist can begin to adjust the dorsal blocking splint into lesser degrees of PIP flexion beginning 4 weeks postoperatively. After 6 weeks of protective splinting, a slight PIP contracture may have developed. A static extension gutter splint may be fabricated to wear at night and

for brief periods (two to three sessions of 45 minutes during the day.
- *Edema control:* Edema control is initiated within the first postoperative week. Use 1 inch Coban or a similar compressive dressing, instructing the client gently to wrap the digit from the fingertip to the base of the finger.

Precaution. *Be sure any dressing to control edema is not tight because this compresses the repair.*

The very tip of the finger should be left free for visual inspection. The client may do the exercises with the wrap on. The wrap should be removed regularly for hygiene and to monitor skin integrity.
- *Desensitization* can begin within 24 to 48 hours following suture removal.
- *Range of motion exercises:* Within the splint, range of motion exercises are initiated to the digit. Active extension is limited by the splint for the first 3 to 6 weeks.
- *Strengthening* can be initiated 6 weeks postoperatively, if needed. Strengthening exercises should address residual weakness for specific functional tasks.
- *Sensory reeducation* can begin once signs of sensory return are noted. Typically, this is about 10 to 12 weeks after repair. In the interim, teach the client protective sensory techniques.

Precautions

- Always instruct the client how to use Coban or a similar elastic wrap correctly. Have the client apply the Coban starting at the distal part and progressing proximally. Do not leave sections in the middle of the finger uncovered because that is where the edema will accumulate.
- Application should not be under tension, for any elastic wrap can constrict the vascular system further, causing additional damage to the injured nerve and its corresponding blood vessels. The client should be able to bend the finger within the wrap. Treat any diminution of sensation or warmth in the finger following application immediately by removing the constricting wrap.
- Instruct the client to call the physician immediately if finger temperature or sensation does not return to its prewrapped status shortly after removal of the constricting wrap.

Tips from the Field

Therapeutic intervention for any nerve injury likely will incorporate techniques to address pain, hypersensitivity, nerve gliding, client education, and possibly, sensory reeducation. The following tips may be useful when considering such interventions.

About Nerve Gliding

Normally, longitudinal gliding of the peripheral nerve in relation to adjacent tissues occurs with extremity motion. If the nerve is constrained by adhesions or a compressive anatomic structure, these normal movements create stress and strain at and proximal to the site along the nerve where it is stuck. Decompression is an early medical goal for these nerves, either by surgery or by rest and medication or modalities designed to ameliorate swollen tissues that constrain the nerve. Once the nerve is decompressed, introduce therapeutic exercises as soon as possible to restore and maintain the normal longitudinal excursion of the nerve.[1,4,38]

Nerve gliding should be done slowly, moving the extremity as if one were a dancer. Advise the client to pay attention to how these exercises feel and to stop at any point in the sequence if numbness, discomfort, or pain increases.

Precaution. *Instruct the client that nerve gliding can increase symptoms and nerve irritability if not done carefully and correctly. Creating nerve tension by pulling on both ends of a nerve to complete an exercise surely will increase symptoms.*

The idea of a glide is to place tension on one area of the nerve while releasing tension at another area.[38] The concept of nerve glides as a treatment technique may be visualized as sliding a piece of floss through teeth. While one end (of the floss) is pulled, the other end is relaxed or free from tension. Likewise, as the peripheral nerve is pulled across a joint, or through a tunnel, tension must be eased proximal or distal to this site so as not to create or increase adverse neural tension. Changing the position of an adjacent joint or joints can ease the length-tension requirements of the nerve. For example, moving the elbow and wrist from neutral position (the anatomic position) to a position of full flexion would put the ulnar nerve on some tension; this tension could be dampened by moving only one joint at a time while the other was maintained in neutral. Clearly, the therapist must know his or her anatomy before designing an appropriate nerve gliding program for a client.

Incorporating the movements of the nerve glide into a functional activity makes them easier to remember. Remember that the goal of these glides is gently to slide the nerve through its available range to promote axoplasmic flow and general nerve health.[4]

CLINICAL *Pearl*

Positive changes from nerve gliding exercises may take months to become noticeable.

Help the client recognize improvements in abilities in everyday activities and celebrate this.

About Sensory Reeducation

An important part of rehab for clients with sensory loss associated with peripheral nerve damage is sensory reeducation. Peripheral nerve lesions can result in a shuffling of skin "addresses" or end-organ sites with respect to central nervous system addresses. In other words, individual regenerating axons may not end up reinnervating the exact same end-organs after the injury. This results in an altered, and likely diminished, pattern of input coming from this area of the periphery to the somatosensory cortex. The cortex will reorganize in response to this altered pattern or picture.[5]

The goal of sensory reeducation is to improve the client's perception of sensory information arising from receptors in the hand so that the client can interpret correctly the (altered) pattern of incoming sensory signals. Assuming that the higher cortical somatosensory pathways for object recognition are intact, once a client has achieved sufficient return of protective sensation, sensory reeducation can begin.

Various sensory reeducation programs are found in the literature.[39,40] Similarities between these programs include incorporation of localization tasks, graded stimulus tasks, and recognition tasks.[40] A popular choice among upper extremity rehab specialists is Callahan's program, which divides sensory reeducation into two types: protective and discriminative.[39]

Protective Sensory Reeducation

The goal of protective sensory reeducation is to educate the client in techniques of compensation for loss of sensory protection. These clients are unable to discriminate protective sensation; they are unable to evaluate the potential harmfulness of hot and cold or of sharp objects.

Precaution. *These clients are at significant risk for unknowingly injuring their insensate hand, especially when vision is occluded.*

Education about the injury, the potential risks for reinjury, and about compensation strategies typically can be done in one to two sessions. Tell the client to avoid working around machinery or anything with moving parts and to avoid situations in which the environmental temperature is below 60° F. Advise the client to use vision to compensate for sensory loss. Reaching into a pocket becomes a potentially harmful situation for a client without protective sensation.

Discriminative Sensory Reeducation

The goal of discriminative sensory reeducation is the recovery of discriminative sensibility. Following nerve injury, there is a predictable pattern of sensory recovery, beginning with pain perception and progressing to vibration of 30 cps, moving touch, and constant touch. The return proceeds from proximal to distal. Callahan's proposed discriminative program follows Dellon's sensory reeducation program, with graded training tasks involving localization and graded discrimination of textures, shapes, and objects. A visual-tactile matching process is used, where the client attempts to identify correctly the stimulus location or modality type, first with eyes closed. If the client is wrong, then the stimulation is repeated with eyes open, and the client concentrates on matching what he or she feels with what he or she sees.

Protective and discriminative sensory reeducation should begin as soon as possible after a nerve injury in order to encourage the client to use the affected extremity before abnormal use patterns can develop.[5] To minimize compensatory use of the uninvolved arm and resultant neglect of the involved extremity, integrate the involved arm into normal functional use as early as possible. This is more difficult if the deficit is on the non-dominant side.

A prerequisite for successful carryover of newly developed discriminative sensory skills is that the client has enough motor skills for object manipulation. A potential barrier to functional recovery is that the client ultimately must be able to hold onto and manipulate an object for a short time without the object slipping through the fingers, even with vision occluded.

The treatment for sensory deficits and retraining for fine motor skills requires functional use of the involved hand and a high degree of motivation and commitment from the client. Repetition and motivation are key concepts; therefore, task completion must be meaningful to the client and must have just enough degree of difficulty, yet possibility of success, for the therapy to be successful.[5,39] Research indicates that without a sensory reeducation program, the prognosis for recovery of discriminative sensibility following a proximal (or high-level) peripheral nerve injury is poor for adults, though better for children.[5,7,39]

About Desensitization

Immediately after injury to tissue, the local neural tissue lowers its sensory stimulus threshold in response to the sensitizing effects of inflammation.[1] In other words, it is easier for the nerve to achieve an action potential. Sensory input that is nonnoxious, such as palpation or percussion along the nerve, may be perceived as irritating or painful.

CLINICAL *Pearl*

Prolonged irritation to the neural tissue can result in a state of hyperalgesia, or hypersensitivity, with local sensitivity changes that eventually reflects changes in the way the central somatosensory system processes sensory inputs.

Clients with **hyperalgesia** may complain of extreme discomfort or irritability with tactile stimulation to their involved body part. For example, hypersensitivity of the skin around the radial styloid and proximal thumb is a fairly common phenomenon occurring with radial sensory nerve irritation. Interestingly, even when the source of irritation such as a tight cast or splint is removed, the hypersensitivity may remain. This can result in significant functional problems for clients. For example, they may find wearing a watch unbearable. They may even develop an intolerance to the touch of a sleeve or a shirt or coat on the injured area.

Desensitization is the systematic process of applying nonnoxious stimuli to peripheral tissues to reeducate and retrain the nervous system. As with sensory reeducation, the ideal client is encouraged to participate in a home program. For desensitization to be successful, frequent sessions with various tactile stimulations must occur throughout the day. The more the client does, the quicker the results. Initially, clients may need to apply the stimulus around the irritated tissues, rather than directly on these tissues. The client applies the stimulus, so the client controls the amount of pressure that is applied.

What to Say to Clients *about Hypersensitivity and Desensitization*

"Your nerve is irritable at this time, and that's why things that shouldn't be painful feel painful. This pain does not indicate that there is something medically wrong with the nerve; it's just mixed up. To get yourself better, you will need to reeducate your nerve. Right now, that nerve is firing too soon. To help it go back to how things were before, you will need to touch the irritated skin regularly. Try short sessions at first, about five to ten minutes each. Try to touch the irritated skin every waking hour or every other hour. Make sure you are relaxed when you do this. You can put on nice music or watch a favorite television show or go into a quiet room. Try touching or tapping your skin with a towel or a piece of cotton; or massaging the area with cream. Any type of cream is fine. The key to getting better is to do this treatment often and every day. If you don't do this, your brain will learn that this pain is normal, and the pain message will become permanently fixed, like a memory."

Tips from the Field about Pain Management

According to Paul Brand,[41] pain can be diminished if the client understands the cause of pain and loses fear associated with unknown variables such as healing expectations and timelines. This is an opportunity for therapists to be powerful pain relievers. The following also may be helpful in mitigating the client's pain experience:

- *Modalities:* The subsequent list is not meant to be an exhaustive accounting of available modalities nor of the parameters for using these modalities. The therapist is encouraged to seek out and follow guidelines for modality use as listed by the appropriate state regulating agency for his or her profession (registered occupational therapist, physical therapist, occupational therapy assistant, or physical therapy assistant). Ongoing courses in modality use keep the practitioner up to date on current research and practice issues.[24,25]
  - *Continuous wave ultrasound,* a deep heat modality, has been shown to increase tissue extensibility, to improve blood flow and tissue permeability, and to increase the pain thresholds. Ultrasound can reach tissue depths of 5 cm or more; therefore this is a good modality choice for addressing pain emanating from structures deep to the skin. Pulsed ultrasound can facilitate the resolution of the inflammatory phase of healing; therefore this is a good choice in the acute phase of tissue healing.
  - *Iontophoresis,* the use of direct current to introduce topically applied ions to underlying tissue, may alter pain perception and reduce edema.
  - *Transcutaneous electrical nerve stimulation* (TENS) can be an effective modality for addressing acute and chronic pain. I think of TENS as providing white noise or a safe distraction that can dampen those unhelpful pain messages that interfere with function. Various theories exist about how TENS is effective in controlling pain. The **gate theory,** proposed by Melzack and Wall in the mid-1960s,[25] is perhaps the most widely recited. Recent research has led to modifications of this theory. Gating off

pain by using TENS is predicated upon the fact that a message of pain is brought to the spinal cord by small-diameter, slow-conduction nociceptive nerve fibers with little or no myelin (type A-delta or C fibers). Large-diameter, myelinated, A-beta sensory fibers can inhibit the activity of these nociceptive nerve fibers in the spinal cord by activating local interneurons in the substantia geltinosa (of the dorsal horn of the spinal column). These interneurons depress the transmission of nociceptive signals to the brain by releasing a neurotransmitter that dampens the nociceptor nerve cell activity.[6,8] Activation of the cutaneous mechanoreceptors by light touch/massage, percussion, vibration, or stretch stimulates A-beta nerve fibers. TENS that provides a low-level cutaneous stimulation therefore may provide temporary pain relief—at least until the client acclimates to that TENS setting. (Eventually, human beings acclimate to any nonnoxious cutaneous stimulation.) Use of large electrode pads may help recruit a more optimum number of A-beta nerve fibers than one would get with small pads.
  - *The application of superficial heat,* such as a heat pack, before range of motion exercises or stretching can diminish stiffness and muscle spasms.
  - *Fluidotherapy,* a type of superficial convection heat, is a dry whirlpool that has the added advantage of desensitizing irritable scar tissue while simultaneously heating this tissue before stretch and exercise.
  - A *paraffin bath,* another type of superficial heat modality, is advantageous because the client can be taught how to use this pain relief modality appropriately at home. Paraffin baths are relatively inexpensive and readily available at many department stores and pharmacies.
  - *Cryotherapy,* or cold therapy is a modality frequently used for pain that results from muscle spasms. Post exercise pain and edema can be managed effectively by cold packs or ice massage.
- *Massage:* Massage techniques designed to increase blood flow and reduce pain are also helpful. Therapeutic touch can be augmented by discussions about stress management, relaxation, visualization, and activity pacing. Incorporating these cognitive-behavioral techniques with manual therapies, in my experience, facilitates pain reduction by acknowledging the presence of pain and by gently and supportively instructing the client in pain management strategies. Discussion of soft tissue mobilization and myofascial release techniques are beyond the scope of this chapter. The reader is encouraged to seek out

courses in these areas to develop appropriate knowledge and skills before applying these techniques.

- *Brushing:* When TENS is not accessible to a client, it may be possible to get a similar (temporary) analgesic response by using anything that stimulates the A-beta sensory fibers. Vibration, massage, or brushing may do this. Have the client use a soft baby's hair brush and brush the irritated limb, moving along the entire peripheral nerve. Initially, have the client move from proximal to distal, using large firm but gentle sweeping motions to recruit as many large A-fibers as possible. Later, a more random pattern of brushing, using circular motions for example, may be used so that it is more difficult for the client to acclimate to the brushing sensation.

- *Occupation-based interventions:* Research supports the concept that pain management is most effective when it is client-centered, when the therapy program allows the client to be actively engaged in goal setting and intervention planning.[42] Interventions should be meaningful and motivating for each individual client. Using the COPM (as appropriate to one's role or discipline) to elucidate areas of performance difficulty and dissatisfaction assists in developing an appropriate collaborative intervention program.

Typical Concerns and What to Say to Clients

Clients are often fearful about their injury, about life changes that have occurred or may yet occur following their injury, about reinjury, and about expectations for recovery. These fears frequently present as pain and pain behaviors in and outside of the clinic. Therapists are in the best position to address many of these concerns simply because we spend more time with the client than the physician can. Therefore client education is an integral part of any treatment program. Therapists should anticipate some of these concerns and fears and be prepared to address them.

Why is my hand/wrist/forearm/elbow still swollen?

Typical answer: "Swelling is a normal part of healing. Your body is producing the cells that are needed for healing. Following an injury or surgery to a nerve, you can see swelling for up to a year afterward."

Will my scar open up if I massage over it?

Typical answer (once sutures are out and the wound is showing adequate tensile strength): "No, your wound won't break open if you apply cream and massage your scar. You can begin gently, using any kind of lotion. I prefer something with an oily feel, because while the nerve is healing, it can't maintain the normal healthy elasticity of the skin.

Why do I have pain? Or, Why do I still have pain? Should I keep going if I have pain?

Typical answer: "Pain is the normal mechanism of your body for telling you that something is wrong. It's actually one of our senses, like smell or taste. Usually that's a good thing, letting you know that you're doing too much or that something is amiss. Sometimes this warning mechanism continues to alert you, even when you've taken care of the initial problem. Your brain comes to expect pain, even when what you're doing should not be painful. When that happens, you need to learn how to self-manage your symptoms. Knowing the difference between pain that is a 'good' warning pain and pain that needs to be self-managed is difficult. I can help you with this. You should always ask me if you have pain with anything I give you in therapy, and I will tell you if it's okay to continue that exercise or activity. I also can share some ideas with you about coping with pain, if you do experience pain with the exercises or activities that you need to do."

The Role of Therapy Assistants

Depending on state regulations and the competence level of the therapy assistant, any or all of the following may be appropriate duties for the therapy assistant:

- *Splint modifications and refurbishing*
- *Instruction in home program, splint application, splint wear and care schedule, and splint precautions including skin care*
- *Assistance in skin inspection and wound care*
- *Scar massage*
- *Edema management*
- *In-clinic supervision of desensitization and/or sensory re-education program, as identified and designed by the therapist*
- *In-clinic supervision of tendon glide exercises, nerve glides, and strengthening program as identified and designed by the therapist*
- *Activities of daily living modifications and adaptations*

CASE *Studies*

CASE 12-1

P.R. is a 32-year-old, right-hand dominant female executive who sustained puncture injuries to her right third and fourth digits, volar surface, from her cat's claws. She was seen by her family physician, who prescribed antibiotic medication for her to prevent infection. She continued to complain of pain, numbness, stiffness, and swelling at her follow-up appointment. P.R.'s physician referred her for a course of hand therapy to address her complaints.

At her initial visit, which was approximately 1 month after injury, P.R. had significantly swollen and stiff long, ring, and fifth digits, per circumference measures. The volar puncture wounds had healed with minimal observable scar tissue, although P.R. reported some hypersensitivity with gentle palpation to these areas. AROM measurements were taken; isolated joint motion indicated that all extrinsic flexor tendons were intact. Active flexion to the distal-palmar-crease ranged from −2.2 cm (fifth digit) to −4.5 cm (long digit). Semmes-Weinstein monofilament testing indicated normal light touch (2.83) at the tip of the fifth digit, tip of the index finger, and along the ulnar aspect of the fourth digit. The radial aspect of the ring finger responded with diminished light touch (3.61) at the base of the digit to diminished protective sensation (3.84) at the tip. The ulnar aspect of the long finger responded with diminished protective sensation (3.84 to 4.31). The radial aspect of the long finger responded with diminished light touch (3.22 to 3.61). P.R. reported tingling radiating to the tips of her ring and long fingers with percussion to the digital nerves about 1 cm distal to the puncture sites. P.R. reported that her finger "numbness" had not improved since the date of injury. P.R. reported concerns about the integrity of her nerves and voiced concern that she might need surgery to "fix them." The sensory findings were reviewed with P.R., and she was told that these were consistent with the physician's diagnosis of a nerve injury in continuity. Persistent sensory symptoms likely were aggravated by venous stasis.

A modified COPM was performed to establish client goals. It became clear that P.R. was avoiding normal use of her right hand during work and at home because "it hurts." She was typing one-handed and was using her left hand to cook and clean whenever possible. She was observed to hesitate to grip her briefcase with a hook fist, preferring to use a modified pinch grasp (between the index finger and thumb) to secure the handle.

P.R. was instructed in tendon glide exercises and blocking exercises for the digits to encourage better pull through and gliding of the extrinsic flexor tendons. She also was instructed in edema control measures, including use of 1 inch Coban, retrograde massage, and active fisting to assist the overwhelmed venous system. She was instructed in the likely repercussions of continuing to avoid use of her right hand, and she was encouraged to begin to incorporate her hand in activities such as holding onto the toothbrush while brushing her teeth. Cylindric foam was provided, and P.R. was instructed in how to apply the foam to her tooth brush, her eating utensils, and even her brief case handle so that she could grip these items comfortably and securely during use. Finally, P.R. was instructed in how nerves respond to trauma and was given a timeline and guidelines for what she could expect as the nerves continued to heal. Protective sensory education strategies were discussed, and appropriate cautions (such as not reaching into a suds-filled basin for a knife) were reviewed.

P.R. returned to therapy 1 week later. Although she did not have a complete fist, she now was able to touch her palm with each finger tip after a few warm-up exercises. Her swelling was less noticeable, and she demonstrated correct application of the Coban wrap. She requested another roll, indicating consistent use of it. She continued to complain of some scar hypersensitivity and of intermittent "zinging" up to the tips of her involved fingers. She was assured that this was a normal response as the nerves healed and was told to continue with scar massage and normal hand usage. She also reported some cold intolerance, with marked change in the ability of the fingers to tolerate the office air conditioner blowing on them. This would appear to indicate a concomitant digital vascular injury. She was instructed to continue her tendon glide exercises even after full digit motion was achieved to encourage nerve gliding (and promote nerve homeostasis) within the digits.

P.R. was seen once a week for short sessions over the next 3 weeks. She was now approximately 9 weeks from her injury. Digit motion was full. P.R. reported that she had resumed all preinjury work and home activities using her right hand as she had before this injury. Sensory testing showed moderate improvements in light touch sensibility, with the ring and long neurologically impaired areas responding with diminished light touch (3.61). Because it was likely that the digital nerves would continue to heal at a rate of about 1 mm/day and because PR had returned successfully to all preinjury activities and had achieved the goals she had set for herself (via the COPM), a final but optional visit was offered (1 month later) to document continued nerve healing. P.R. reported that she would call if she had further issues; she was satisfied that her hand would continue to heal as she had been instructed.

CASE 12-2

L.E. was an 11-year-old right-hand dominant boy at the time of his injury. He was playing with his brother when he fell into a plate glass door. He suffered numerous lacerations and punctures, including a severe puncture to his right axilla. Almost immediately, he was covered in blood. His mother's cousin, an emergency room nurse, happened to be visiting that day, and she was able to pinch off the impaired artery until the trauma team arrived. L.E. was transported by helicopter to the nearest trauma center, where he underwent several hours of surgery. Because of the severe blood loss, his parents were told he might not survive.

L.E. arrived at the outpatient clinic with his parents and an health maintenance organizaton (HMO) referral 6 weeks after surgery. The HMO referral stated, "Evaluate and treat, splint fabrication." L.E. was wearing a long arm half cast that had been removed to date "only by the surgery team." The prescription from the hand surgeon, requesting a long arm splint and bearing a diagnosis of right axillary artery laceration and repair, eventually was produced from mother's purse. A telephone call to the surgeon to clarify orders and surgical procedures further was not successful; the surgeon was in surgery. The half cast therefore was removed carefully with attention paid to minimizing movement at the shoulder. L.E.'s arm and forearm showed significant atrophy of the triceps (posterior compartment of the arm) and of the lateral-posterior compartment of the forearm. His unsupported wrist and digits fell into the classic wrist drop posture. Muscle strength of the triceps (elbow extension) was 0/5. Sensory loss included the posterior lateral aspect of the distal arm and the dorsal radial hand. Skin appeared dry and inelastic. Surgical incisions, while closed and suture free, presented as raised and red-purple, with evidence of early hypertrophy.

A long arm splint replicating the position of the half cast was fabricated and provided with wear and care instructions. The family was instructed to begin a regimen of scar massage and mobilization. A follow-up appointment was made for several days later. Aggressive telephone calling was necessary to reach the busy surgeon before L.E.'s next visit. Concerns about a high radial nerve palsy were addressed. The surgeon reported that he was one of a team of surgeons who worked on L.E. and that the brachial plexus had been visualized and appeared to be intact at the time of this surgery. It was possible that the posterior cord of the plexus was now acutely compressed from edema or from scar tissue. The surgeon instructed the therapist to monitor the radial nerve palsy with appropriate testing and to proceed with appropriate splinting and therapy.

At L.E.'s next therapy visit, a dynamic extension assist splint was fabricated. L.E. was allowed to come out of his long arm splint for initial short exercise sessions. During these sessions, the dynamic splint was to be worn to prevent overstretching of the paralyzed muscles and to encourage L.E. to use the right dominant arm with light activities. Already L.E. had (competently) switched to his left hand to complete many tasks; he was at risk for developing a disuse atrophy of the right upper extremity. Therapy sessions focused on age-appropriate play activi-

ties, such as playing a board game (where the right hand had to move the pieces).

L.E. was weaned from the long arm splint over the first 3 weeks of therapy. A nighttime static volar splint was fabricated to hold his wrist and metacarpophalangeal joints in extension, and the dynamic splint was to be used during the day. L.E. preferred the static short arm splint because the outrigger of the dynamic splint got in his way with dressing. Therapy continued to focus on incorporating the right arm into daily life activities; still, the loss of stability at the elbow and wrist (resulting from muscle paresis) was a strong hindrance. At this time, L.E. was actively able to flex his elbow and to use gravity to extend his elbow; however, he had no control over how fast his elbow straightened. MMTs continued to show no palpable muscle fiber contractions in the triceps or in any of the radial wrist extensors. L.E.'s scar, while mobile, was hypertrophic, despite use of scar compression gel pads.

Because of the extraordinary nature of the injury, L.E.'s parents were able to get an HMO extension beyond the typical 2 months of therapy. At the 3 months after injury, electrodiagnostic testing was conducted. No activity was seen in the radial nerve. Surgery options were discussed; however, the family and the vascular surgeon felt the risks of an exploratory neurolysis of the radial nerve outweighed the benefits. Therefore, approximately 5 months from the initial injury, L.E. underwent tendon transfers to correct his wrist drop. At this point, it was clear that switching dominance made sense because the left unimpaired arm had better strength overall and good elbow stability in particular. Postoperative rehab therefore included change of dominance training and was uneventful. Again, therapy focused on age-appropriate activities, including playing with a yo-yo, a paddle ball, and eventually bouncing a basketball to facilitate strength and motor reeducation of the transferred muscles.

Postscript: Two years after the injury, L.E. did undergo an exploratory neurolysis. The radial nerve was found to be bound down in scar tissue and adhered to the brachial artery. Repair was attempted in hopes that L.E. would gain some functional triceps muscle return. L.E. went through another course of therapy, but no return of strength to the triceps muscle was seen.

CASE 12-3

T.B. is a 52-year-old left-hand dominant machine shop worker with bilateral CTS. He underwent a CTR for his right hand; then 6 weeks later had his left carpal tunnel released. His medical history includes insulin-dependent diabetes, cardiac issues, sleep apnea, and obesity. T.B. lives with his sickly wife, on whom he clearly dotes, and with his mother-in-law, whom he describes as demanding and lazy. Because of his wife's illness and his mother-in-law's presence, he is solely responsible for cooking, cleaning, shopping, and household maintenance. His grown son lives in the area and has been in some recent legal trouble. Recently, this son had his driver's license temporarily revoked. T.B. is on call to drive the young man to and from work. T.B. is helping his son fix the motor on his car, so that once the driving restrictions are lifted, the son can drive himself in his own car. T.B. is also the self-appointed guardian of his neighborhood. Because of his size (and he is indeed a large, imposing man), neighbors call on him to deal with errant teenage children. He has been known to take a disrespectful teenager on a tour of the local prison. Leisure interests include hunting with a bow and arrow. He wants to return to work and to hunting yesterday!

T.B. arrives late at the clinic for his initial evaluation; he got lost. He becomes agitated and is vocal with the receptionist. He is taken back quickly to the evaluation room, where he immediately complains of serious left hand pain, swelling, and weakness. He insists that he had no trouble when recovering from surgery with his right (nondominant) hand. A couple of discrete questions allow the therapist to glean the aforementioned personal, social, and community demands upon T.B. while also allowing him time to calm down.

T.B. is now 12 days past a left CTR. Sutures are still in place, and he is wearing a beaten-up, prefabricated wrist splint that does not quite close around his swollen hand and wrist. Both hands are large and clean but with calluses. Some yellow exudate is oozing from the incision site on the left hand, indicating infection. The old splint is thrown out. The incision area is cleaned and dressed with a sterile, nonadherent dressing. The physician is called and notified that there is concern that the incision may be infected. The physician instructs the therapist to fabricate a new wrist splint that the client is to wear full time until his next doctor's appointment. A prescription antibiotic is called in to the client's pharmacy by the client's physician.

The new splint is fabricated and provided with wear and care instructions reviewed verbally and in written format. Activity restrictions are outlined clearly with repercussions emphasized should T.B. not follow through. T.B. is told that his right hand most likely healed better because he was not using it as much. (Remember, he is left-hand dominant). He is told that he will need to give his left hand similar time off if he wants it to heal. The real carrot for T.B., though, is when he is told that he will not be able to engage in hunting in the next 2 or 3 months, given his present response to surgery and postoperative recovery. T.B. has a hunting trip scheduled for early fall, and he desperately wants to go. Rigid adherence

to the activity restrictions provided by the surgeon and therapist will be a necessary prerequisite; though at this point, no promises are made.

T.B. is seen 3 days later. The wounds are clean, and the splint shows signs that T.B. has been using it regularly. The evaluation is completed. T.B. has limited finger flexion to the distal palmar crease and is unable to oppose his thumb past his long finger. A sensory evaluation indicates diminished light touch to diminished protective sensation in all fingertips. This is not an uncommon finding for someone with diabetes; it is likely T.B. has polyneuropathy. There appears to be significant edema in the hand, but the sutures preclude volumetric measurements. Wrist range of motion is not assessed per the physician's orders. T.B. is instructed in tendon glide exercises and thumb opposition exercises. Activity restrictions are again reviewed. Time is spent instructing T.B. about tissue tolerances, wound healing timetables, and the need to balance rest with the stimulation of AROM exercises.

T.B. is seen 3 times a week for the next 3 months. He continues periodically to overdo his home program and to overdo his activities at home. He has significant scar hypersensitivity and pillar pain in the left hand, probably exacerbated by his postoperative infection. Modalities for pain relief are tried, including iontophoresis. However, the iontophoresis played havoc with his blood sugar, and he reported a bad headache after the first trial session; therefore, this modality was not used again.

T.B.'s job is considered a medium physical demand level, meaning he must be able to perform a maximum lift of 50 lb. Strength issues and general body mechanics are addressed in preparation for return to work. T.B. reports that he may be required to hammer between 8 and 288 nails into a board that is approximately 2 inches thick, though he can pace himself. Ergonomic leather gloves with the palmar surface padded and the fingertips free are procured for use at work. T.B. demonstrates good tolerance for hammering with the gloves on.

As the date of the hunting trip looms closer, T.B. anxiously explores his options. Apparently, shooting a bow and arrow requires considerable bilateral hand strength and endurance, which T.B. does not yet have. A particular bow design, called a crossbow, would allow him to participate in hunting with less stress to his hands. He will need special medical approval to get a permit to use this design. His physician is contacted, the prescription is written, and T.B. successfully attends his hunting trip, with his new crossbow. (Unfortunately, because of the weather that year, there were no deer to be had.)

T.B. did return to work successfully. He pops up at the clinic about every 4 to 6 months, requesting new work gloves. Because his gloves take such a beating at work, they regularly wear out.

CASE 12-4

F.L. is a 17-year-old right-hand dominant girl who has been seen at an outpatient hand therapy clinic by colleagues for about 1 month for postoperative treatment of a subcutaneous ulnar nerve transposition. F.L. has HMO insurance that capitates her visits to 60 consecutive days. Because she is a high school senior, she can attend therapy only in the later afternoons or early evenings. She was being seen by a therapist to address the protective and active motion phases of healing. F.L. is now ready for strengthening, but the primary treating therapist is out sick. Therapy notes indicate that F.L. is quiet, with a flat affect and downward gaze. Hypersensitivity at the scar site is a continuing issue. Recent strengthening exercises prescribed by the colleague included free weights, putty, and a BTE program.

F.L. arrives on time and speaks quietly in response to the new therapist's questions. She sits in a slouched posture, with forward rounded shoulders and her hair covering her face. She reports a very high level of pain today, rating her symptoms as an 8/10. She reports suffering a bad night last evening with pain severe enough that she was unable to sleep; she reports frequently crying about her pain. Upon further questioning, it becomes clear that her pain is in multiple joints, not just in the right postoperative elbow. A quick assessment reveals hypermobile joints and low muscle tone throughout the upper extremity. Her scapulae appear to "clunk" as they move during shoulder abduction; this is associated with increased pain perception in the shoulder region.

A good rule of thumb is that too much movement at a joint results in too little stability and thus a loss of strength at that joint. In F.L.'s case, her joints are very mobile, and her muscle strength is inadequate to compensate for the potential instability at these joints. Her activity level had decreased significantly following onset of her ulnar nerve symptoms (about 1 year prior) and the consequent surgery on her right elbow. She is clearly deconditioned. The exercises prescribed by the primary treating therapist did not engage F.L.'s interests; therefore she participated in strengthening only when she attended therapy.

Using a modified COPM, mutually acceptable goals are identified and a treatment program is established that incorporates her interests in reading, gymnastics, dance, and swimming. Nerve gliding is introduced as part of a balletlike dance move, with F.L. cautioned to stop if her symptoms increase. F.L. reports that she has an exercise ball at home that she can use. Using a large exercise ball in the gym, F.L. is shown postural exercises to do at home, such as moving from a slumped position to sitting up straight. Exercise balls are fun for all ages; it is hard not to smile when sitting or bouncing on one of these. She is encouraged to replace her desk chair with the exercise ball, for she will need to maintain a good posture sitting on this while doing homework or she will fall off the ball. She is encouraged to read books while lying on her belly and with the books propped up on a binder to encourage the prone extension posture. Simply holding this position against gravity for periods of time can strengthen the back muscles.

Future sessions include time in a heated pool walking and performing ballet arm (AROM) exercises against the resistance of the water. F.L.'s family belongs to a YMCA; therefore she is encouraged to continue these exercises after therapy ends to address proximal strength issues and to encourage gentle nerve gliding simply by moving the joints safely and slowly. During these aqua therapy sessions, client education is provided about the need to engage in a regular daily strengthening program to prevent future joint and nerve problems. This becomes a good time also to talk about activities and positions to avoid, such as avoiding sustained elbow flexion while holding a phone and talking to a girlfriend. She is encouraged to participate in exercises such as tai chi and yoga rather than high-impact aerobics that might lead to joint dislocations/subluxations and other nerve compression syndromes.

F.L.'s flat affect and detachment from therapy and the therapeutic relationship shifts in response to the redesign of the therapy program so that it now incorporates her interests and age-appropriate activities. Her pain reports decrease to a 4/10 or 5/10, and she is able to identify ways that she can continue to address her strengthening issues once formal outpatient therapy ends.

References

1. Elvey RL: Physical evaluation of the peripheral nervous system in disorders of pain and dysfunction, *J Hand Ther* 10:122-129, 1997.
2. Butler DS: *Mobilisation of the nervous system,* Melbourne, 1991, Churchill Livingstone.
3. Dellon AL: Client evaluation and management considerations in nerve compression. In Rayan GM, editor: *Hand clinics: nerve compression syndromes,* Philadelphia, 1992, WB Saunders.
4. Butler DS: *The sensitive nervous system,* Adelaide, Australia, 2000, Noigroup Publications.
5. Merzenich MM, Jenkins WM: Reorganization of cortical representations of the hand following alterations of skin inputs induced by nerve injury, skin island transfers, and experience, *J Hand Ther* 6(2):89-104, 1993.
6. Lundy-Ekman E: *Neuroscience: fundamentals for rehabilitation,* Philadelphia, 1998, WB Saunders.

7. Lundborg G: Peripheral nerve injuries: pathophysiology and strategies for treatment, *J Hand Ther* 6(3): 179-188, 1993.

8. Gutman S: *Quick reference neuroscience for rehabilitation professionals*, Thorofare, NJ, 2001, SLACK.

9. Lundborg G, Dahlin L: The pathophysiology of nerve compression. In Rayan GM, editor: *Hand clinics: nerve compression syndromes*, Philadelphia, 1992, WB Saunders.

10. Rydevik B et al: Effects of graded compression on intraneural blood flow, *J Hand Surgery* 6:3-12, 1981.

11. Gelberman RH et al: Tissue pressure threshold for peripheral nerve viability, *Clin Orthop* 178:285-291, 1983.

12. Lundborg G, Rydevik B: Effects of stretching the tibial nerve of the rabbit: a preliminary study of the intraneural circulation and the barrier function of the perineurium, *J Bone Joint Surg* 55B:390-401, 1973.

13. Callahan AD: Sensibility assessment for nerve lesions in continuity and nerve lacerations. In Mackin EJ, Callahan AD, Skirven TM et al, editors: *Rehabilitation of the hand and upper extremity*, ed 5, St Louis, 2002, Mosby.

14. Frykman G: The quest for better recovery from peripheral nerve injury, *J Hand Ther* 6(2):83-88, 1993.

15. Skirven TM, Callahan AD: Therapist's management of peripheral-nerve injuries. In Mackin EJ, Callahan AD, Skirven TM et al, editors: *Rehabilitation of the hand and upper extremity*, ed 5, St Louis, 2002, Mosby.

16. Dannenbaum RM, Jones LA: The assessment and treatment of clients who have sensory loss following cortical lesions, *J Hand Ther* 6(2):130-138, 1993.

17. Holland N: Traumatic peripheral nerve lesions. Retrieved March 12, 2005 from http://www.emedicine.com/neuro/topic382.htm

18. Galper J, Verno V: Pain. In Palmer ML, Epler ME, editors: *Fundamentals of musculoskeletal assessment techniques*, ed 2, Philadelphia, 1998, Lippincott-Raven.

19. Law M et al: The Canadian Occupational Performance Measure: an outcome measurement protocol for occupational therapy, *Can J Occup Ther* 57:82-87, 1990.

20. Law M et al: *Canadian Occupational Performance Measure manual*, Toronto, 1991, CAOT Publications ACE.

21. Eaton CJ, Lister GD: Radial nerve compression. In Rayan GM, editor: *Hand clinics: nerve compression syndromes*, Philadelphia, 1992, WB Saunders.

22. Colditz JC: Splinting for radial nerve palsy, *J Hand Ther* 1:18-23, 1987.

23. Colditz JC: Splinting the hand with a peripheral nerve injury. In Mackin EJ, Callahan AD, Skirven TM et al, editors: *Rehabilitation of the hand and upper extremity*, ed 5, St Louis, 2002, Mosby.

24. Alba CD: Therapist's management of radial tunnel syndrome. In Mackin EJ, Callahan AD, Skirven TM et al, editors: *Rehabilitation of the hand and upper extremity*, ed 5, St Louis, 2002, Mosby.

25. Bracciano A: *Physical agent modalities: theory and application for the occupational therapist*, Thorofare, NJ, 2000, SLACK.

26. Cannon N, editor: *Diagnosis and treatment manual for physicians and therapists*, ed 4, Indianapolis, 2001, Hand Rehabilitation Center of Indiana.

27. Eversmann E: Proximal median nerve compression. In Rayan GM, editor: *Hand clinics: nerve compression syndromes*, Philadelphia, 1992, WB Saunders.

28. Omer GE: Median nerve compression at the wrist. In Rayan GM, editor: *Hand clinics: nerve compression syndromes*, Philadelphia, 1992, WB Saunders.

29. Hayes EP et al: Carpal tunnel syndrome. In Mackin EJ, Callahan AD, Skirven TM et al, editors: *Rehabilitation of the hand and upper extremity*, ed 5, St Louis, 2002, Mosby.

30. *The hand: examination and diagnosis*, ed 2, Edinburgh, 1983, Churchill Livingstone.

31. MacDermid J: Accuracy of clinical tests used in the detection of carpal tunnel syndrome: a literature review, *J Hand Ther* 4(4):169-176, 1991.

32. Evans RB: Therapist's management of carpal tunnel syndrome. In Mackin EJ, Callahan AD, Skirven TM et al, editors: *Rehabilitation of the hand and upper extremity*, ed 5, St Louis, 2002, Mosby.

33. Rozmaryn LM et al: Nerve and tendon gliding exercises and the conservative management of carpal tunnel syndrome, *J Hand Ther* 11:171-178, 1998.

34. Blackmore SM: Therapist's management of ulnar nerve neuropathy at the elbow. In Mackin EJ, Callahan AD, Skirven TM et al, editors: *Rehabilitation of the hand and upper extremity*, ed 5, St Louis, 2002, Mosby.

35. Rayan GM: Proximal ulnar nerve compression: cubital tunnel syndrome. In Rayan GM, editor: *Hand clinics: nerve compression syndromes*, Philadelphia, 1992, WB Saunders.

36. Moneim MS: Ulnar nerve compression at the wrist: ulnar tunnel syndrome. In Rayan GM, editor: *Hand clinics: nerve compression syndromes*, Philadelphia, 1992, WB Saunders.

37. Dobyns JH: Digital nerve compression. In Rayan GM, editor: *Hand clinics: nerve compression syndromes*, Philadelphia, 1992, WB Saunders.

38. Walsh MT: Rationale and indications for the use of nerve mobilization and nerve gliding as a treatment approach. In Mackin EJ, Callahan AD, Skirven TM et al, editors: *Rehabilitation of the hand and upper extremity*, ed 5, St Louis, 2002, Mosby.

39. Fess EE: Sensory reeducation. In Mackin EJ, Callahan AD, Skirven TM et al, editors: *Rehabilitation of the hand and upper extremity*, ed 5, St Louis, 2002, Mosby.

40. Dellon AL: *Somatosensory testing and rehabilitation*, Bethesda, Md, 1997, American Occupational Therapy Association.

41. Brand P: Pain—it's all in your head: a philosophical essay, *J Hand Ther* 10(2):59-63, 1997.

42. Carpenter L et al: The use of the Canadian Occupational Performance Measure as an outcome of a pain management program, *Can J Occup Ther* 68(1):16-22, 2001.

13

Common Wrist and Hand Fractures

ANNE M.B. MOSCONY

"Thank goodness it's only a fracture. I thought it might be broken."

Client quote, with thanks, from Paul LaStayo, Kerri Winters, and Maureen Hardy[1]

KEY TERMS

Anatomic snuff box

Articular cartilage

Base

Bennett's fracture-dislocation

Biaxial ellipsoid joint

Bony mallet injury

Boutonniere deformity

Boxer's fracture

Colles' fracture

Complex regional pain syndrome (CRPS or RSD)

Diaphysis

Distal radioulnar joint (DRUJ)

Distal transverse arch

Epiphyses

External fixator

Fall on outstretched hand (FOOSH) injury

Fracture

Head

Inflammatory phase

Kienböck's disease

Longitudinal arch

Neck

Negative ulnar variance

Periosteum

Positive ulnar variance

Primary healing

Proximal transverse arch

Purulence

Radiocarpal joint

Reduction

Remodeling phase

Repair phase

Secondary healing

Shaft

Smith's fracture

Triangulofibrocartilage complex (TFCC)

Tuft

Ulnocarpal abutment syndrome

Uniaxial pivot joint

Unstable fractures

Watson's test

Wrist

Bone fractures are common injuries. The American Academy of Orthopedic Surgeons estimates that on average, each person will experience two bone fractures over the course of a lifetime.[2] A **fracture** results in impairment of the skeleton's mechanical integrity, which typically leads to functional deficits and pain, especially when the hand is involved. Bone stability is a prerequisite for initiation of hand therapy after a fracture, therefore hand therapists must understand the biologic process of bone healing and the various methods used to surgically enhance bone stability (and thus healing).

GENERAL TIMELINES AND HEALING

The goal of fracture healing is to regenerate mineralized tissue in the fracture area and restore mechanical strength to the bone. Ultimately, all fractures must heal with new bone, not scar tissue.[1]

After a fracture occurs, the body initiates a three-stage, organized, and predictable process of bone healing that is similar to the process seen with a soft tissue injury. The first stage is the **inflammatory phase,** in which the immediate cellular and vascular responses to the injury promote the formation of a hematoma, which provides some early fracture stabilization. The second stage is the **repair phase,** in which the damaged cells, including the hematoma, are removed and replaced with callus bone. The callus is gradually converted to bone tissue by a process of mineralization called **enchondral ossification.** The third stage is a **remodeling phase,** in which the repaired tissue is replaced and reorganized, over months to years, to provide the bone with its preinjury strength and structure. This ordered process of bone tissue repair and reorganization is called **secondary healing** (also *callus healing* or *indirect healing.*)

Healing of a bone fracture requires stability at the injury site; without stability, healing may be delayed or nonunion of the fracture fragments may result. Some fractures, such as the nondisplaced type (i.e., fractures in which the bone fragments remain correctly aligned) do not require medical intervention to restore normal bony configuration. Other fractures require some type of manipulation by the physician to obtain normal or near normal alignment; this is called **reduction.** Physicians use various techniques to realign the fracture ends.

Once a fracture has been appropriately realigned, it must be kept stable by external or internal support to ensure healing. **Unstable fractures** are fractures that displace spontaneously or with motion; they require some type of fixation method to ensure that healing occurs without malunion, angulation, or rotation of the bone. The medical goal of maintaining anatomic reduction of the fracture ends is achieved by various internal or external means (or both), such as plates, screws, pins, casts, or splints. If traction across the fracture site is required, an **external fixator** typically is used. Various types of external fixators are commercially available. These devices consist of pins, wires, or screws that attach the appropriately aligned and stabilized injured bone to an external, low-profile scaffold. The tension provided by the device can be adjusted relatively easily by the physician. Reduction by means of an external fixator allows the therapist access to the hand and wrist for hygiene and edema control and may make it easier for the client to perform active range of motion (AROM) of uninvolved adjacent joints because a bulky cast does not block motion.

If the physician can secure the bone fragments through an open surgical procedure using stiff metal (plates and/or screws) with enough integrity to ensure essentially no movement and if vascularity at the fracture site is good, fracture healing bypasses the typical three phases and occurs without the secondary process of callus conversion to bone. This is called **primary healing.** Primary healing permits direct regrowth of bone across the fracture line, because it provides for adequate compression across the fracture (i.e., all interfragmentary gaps are eliminated) and adequate stability (i.e., no motion occurs between the fracture fragments). The internal rigid stability offered by a plate and/or screws serves as a substitute external callus, ensuring the absence of motion required for bone healing.

The advantages of rigid fixation of a fracture and consequent primary healing include avoidance of callus formation (and possible local tissue adherence), immediate access by the therapist to the hand for wound care, edema control, and early initiation of motion (immediately after surgery). Rigid fixation also has a number of disadvantages. These include a greater risk of soft tissue scarring and the possible development of adhesions and infection after surgical positioning of the plate and/or screws. Also, plates or screws, particularly those placed dorsally, can cause long-term discomfort for the client and problems with tendon gliding. In these cases, a second surgery may be needed to remove the hardware. Finally, the use of rigid fixation does not accelerate the development of tensile strength in the new bone after primary healing.[1]

Precaution. *Strengthening exercises cannot be introduced any sooner with primary fracture healing than with secondary fracture healing.*

Fracture healing timelines, soft tissue tolerances, and the client's personal interests, life-style, health, and functional goals dictate the progression of therapy and the choice of therapeutic activity or exercise.

CLINICAL *Pearl*

If the physician uses rigid internal fixation to secure the fracture, AROM can and should begin immediately after surgery.

Secondary fracture healing requires an average of 7 weeks or longer, depending on the location and type of fracture.[3] Initiation of AROM with these fractures depends on the adequacy of fixation and the client's health and life-style. Controlled AROM often can begin sometime between the third and sixth weeks after immobilization (i.e., before x-ray evidence of bone healing can be seen).[1,3] Stability at the fracture site must be sufficient to maintain reduction so that the fracture does not displace either spontaneously or with controlled motion. Reduced fractures still require intermittent protection, which usually is accomplished by an interim removable splint.[1] About 2 weeks after AROM is allowed at a previously immobilized joint, passive motion and dynamic splinting can be initiated, if needed, to address joint limitations.[1] By 8 to 10 weeks after immobilization, most clients can begin progressive resistive exercises or more forceful work, leisure, or homemaking tasks using the involved extremity. For resistive exercises, the healing bone must be structurally capable of tolerating high muscle forces across it.[1,3] For this reason, the introduction of resistance into the therapy plan first must be approved by the physician.

Precaution. *Early resumption of resistive or repetitive work, homemaking or avocational tasks, and/or premature introduction of progressive resistive exercises likely will cause pain and increased swelling and may compromise the integrity of the healing bone.*

Instead, the client should be encouraged to use the involved hand early on for pain-free, light activities of daily living (ADL), work, or leisure interests. Clients may need help identifying and grading these tasks appropriately so that they don't overdo use of the injured extremity.

ASSOCIATED SOFT TISSUE INJURIES AFTER BONE FRACTURE

Fractures of the radius, ulna, and phalanges are diagnosed radiographically in the emergency department with little difficulty; however, associated soft tissue trauma may not be so easily recognized. Given the forces required to break a bone, concomitant soft tissue injuries can be expected. In some cases these injuries heal adequately during the fracture immobilization period, but in other cases they require further rest, support, and protection.

Soft tissue injuries commonly associated with fractures may include injury of the triangulofibrocartilage complex, peripheral nerve injury, joint collateral ligament injury, and aggravation of pre-existing osteoarthritis. Early detection of these conditions allows the therapist to explain associated symptoms to their clients, aids the therapist in determining appropriate modifications in the plan of care, and leads to more successful treatment outcomes. It is important to communicate these findings and reported symptoms to the client's referring physician through telephone and/or written reports.

Distal Radial Fractures

ANATOMY

The **wrist** is the common term used to describe the multiple articulations between the distal radius, the ulna, and the eight carpal bones (Fig. 13-1). The distal radius articulates with the scaphoid and lunate; this articulation is called the **radiocarpal joint.** It is a **biaxial ellipsoid joint,** which means that it has two axes of motion: (wrist)

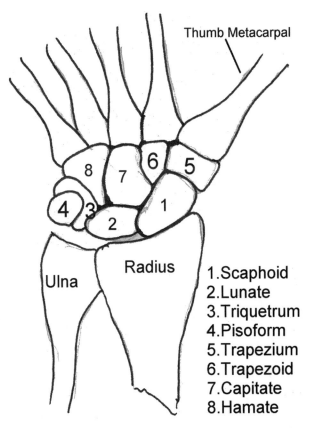

FIGURE 13-1   Schematic of the bones and multiple articulations of the wrist.

flexion/extension and radial/ulnar deviation. A normal radiocarpal joint has a slight palmar tilt or angulation of about 10 to 15 degrees when viewed laterally on x-ray films.[4,5] Preservation of this palmar tilt after a radial fracture has been linked to a good functional outcome, including the return of pain-free, normal range of motion (ROM).[5]

The ulna does not directly articulate with the proximal carpal row (Fig. 13-2). Instead, the **triangulofibrocartilage complex (TFCC),** a hammock-like structure composed of cartilage and ligaments, suspends the ulnar carpus and acts as both a force distributor between the ulnar head and triquetrum and a primary stabilizer for the distal radioulnar joint. The central portion of the TFCC, an articular disk that provides a smooth gliding surface for the ulnar carpus, has no blood supply and therefore does not heal if torn.[6] The peripheral portions are ligamentous and capable of bearing tensile loads generated during gripping or weight bearing on the wrist. These portions have a fair to excellent blood supply and thus a fair to good capacity for healing after injury. With weight bearing on the wrist or with gripping, about 80% of the load traveling through the carpal bones is transferred to the radius and 20% is transferred to the ulna by way of the TFCC.[6,7] Therefore injury of this soft tissue structure has significant functional repercussions, including loss of grip strength and also pain with loading of the wrist or distal forearm or both.

The distal radius articulates with the distal ulna to form the **distal radioulnar joint (DRUJ)** (see Fig. 13-2). This is an important joint because it is a major site

of persistent symptoms and residual disability after fracture of the distal radius.[7] The DRUJ is a **uniaxial pivot joint,** which allows rotatory motions called *supination* and *pronation*. In forearm rotation, the radius pivots around a relatively stable ulna, although the ulna is not completely stationary. During pronation, a proximal-to-distal translation of the ulna occurs with regard to the radius.[6] In fact, the ulna slides distally up to 2 mm in relation to the radius.[6] This subtle movement is important, because a fracture of the radius or ulna can result in changes in the relationship between the length of the radius and ulna and/or how much the ulna translates, or moves, during pronation.

> **CLINICAL** *Pearl*
>
> A change in the proportion of force distributed to the radius or ulna during gripping or loading of the wrist often produces a pathologic effect and pain.

For example, if the ulna heals shorter than its original length, a **negative ulnar variance** exists, which can cause the radius to impinge on the proximal carpal row during forearm rotation. This leads to dorsal and radial wrist pain and increases the likelihood of DRUJ arthrosis. If the radius heals short of its preinjury length and, as a result, the ulna is longer, a **positive ulnar variance** is present. In this case, the ulna impinges on the TFCC, particularly during forearm rotation. This kinematic alteration can cause a wear-and-tear injury of the TFCC, thus compromising ulnar wrist stability (Fig. 13-3). Restoration of the length relationship between the radius and the ulna therefore is an important goal in fracture treatment, because it is necessary for preservation of normal, pain-free motion at the wrist joint.

DIAGNOSIS AND PATHOLOGY

Distal forearm or wrist fractures typically result from an impact on the outstretched hand and wrist during a fall; this type of injury is called a **fall on outstretched hand (FOOSH) injury.** Colles' fracture and Smith's fracture are common distal radial fractures. **Colles' fracture** is the most common type of wrist fracture and among the most common fractures seen in the human body.[5,8,9] It is a complete fracture of the distal radius with dorsal displacement of the distal fragment and radial shortening (Fig. 13-4). Traditionally, it has been described as extraarticular, minimally displaced, and stable, which means the fracture will stay reduced when the extremity is placed in a cast or fracture brace.[5] Most of these fractures occur in postmenopausal women with osteoporotic bone.[10]

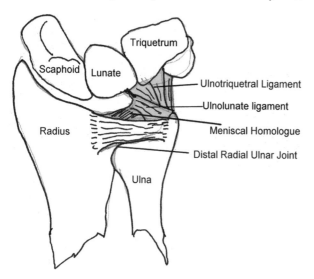

FIGURE 13-2 Anatomy of the wrist, showing the triangulofibrocartilage complex (TFCC) and distal radioulnar joint (DRUJ). Note that the ulna does not directly articulate with the proximal carpus. (Copyright the Mayo Foundation. From Cooney WP: *The wrist: diagnosis and operative treatment,* St Louis, 1998, Mosby.)

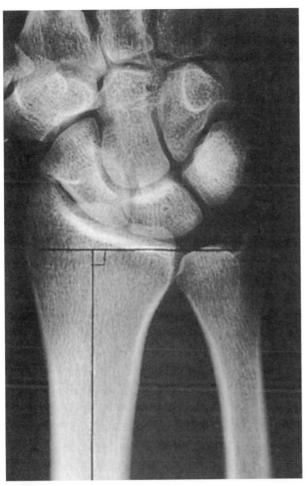

FIGURE 13-3 Standard posteroanterior (PA) x-ray view showing positive ulnar variance. Ulnar variance is considered neutral when the PA x-ray taken in neutral forearm rotation shows the head of the distal ulna to be even with the distal end of the radius. In negative ulnar variance, the ulna is shorter than the radius. In positive ulnar variance, the ulna extends beyond the distal radius. This x-ray film shows a 1 mm positive ulnar variance. (From Jaffe R, Chidgey L, LaStayo P: *J Am Acad Othop Surg* 3:95-109, 1995.)

CLINICAL *Pearl*

Therapists should be aware that the label "Colles' fracture" frequently is applied to more complex types of dorsally displaced fractures that may require more than reduction with casting to restore anatomic alignment.[5]

Smith's fracture is a complete fracture of the distal radius with palmar displacement of the distal fragment (Fig. 13-5). This is the second most common distal radial fracture. A Smith's fracture frequently is unstable and requires some type of internal fixation to hold the displaced distal fragment in correct alignment for healing.

TIMELINES AND HEALING

- Extraarticular, stable fractures usually are treated with closed reduction and casting for 3 to 8 weeks.[5] The position of immobilization is one of moderate wrist flexion and ulnar deviation, because this position uses the surrounding intact soft tissue to help maintain the fracture reduction.

Precaution. *This position can cause or aggravate carpal tunnel symptoms, because prolonged moderate wrist flexion increases carpal tunnel pressures to dangerous levels.*[5]

The client's sensory complaints must be monitored during the period of cast immobilization, when possible, and changes must be reported promptly to the physician. Some clients with this type of uncomplicated fracture need little or no therapy after removal of the cast.

- Unstable distal radial fractures may be treated with percutaneous pinning alone or in conjunction with casting, external fixation, or arthroscopic reduction. Frequently an external fixator is used to maintain reduction of comminuted or severely displaced fractures (Fig. 13-6).[9] Immobilization averages about 8 weeks,[5] and the complication rate with these difficult fractures is high. Complications include median neuropathies, irritation of the dorsal sensory branch of the radial nerve, damage to finger or wrist tendons (or both), finger stiffness and, most commonly, pin tract infections.

- For a particularly complex distal radial fracture, such as a volar-displaced fracture-dislocation of the distal radius (i.e., a Barton's fracture), or when a concomitant open wound with soft tissue damage is present, the surgeon may perform open reduction and internal fixation (ORIF) of the fracture using a metal plate. In these cases, stability should be adequate to allow early active motion of the wrist, starting within the first 2 weeks after surgery. Edema control, wound care, scar management, pain management, and restoration of digit motion are priorities, along with return of wrist and forearm motion during the first 2 months of therapy. Close communication between the therapist and the physician is necessary for at least 8 to 10 weeks after surgery.[5]

- Maximum functional improvement may take months to years after a distal radial fracture; it can take 6 months for uncomplicated fractures and 1 to 2 years for complicated fractures. However, with the current emphasis on managed care and capitation for treatment, therapists and clients may be required to com-

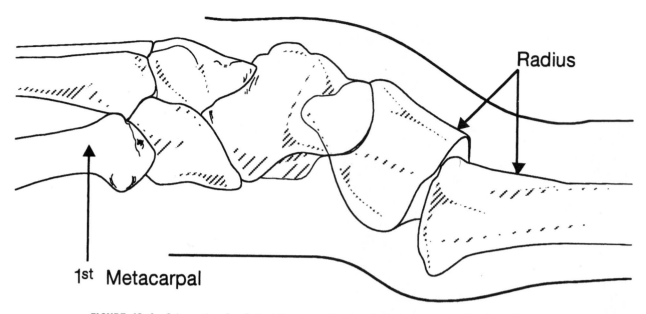

FIGURE 13-4 Schematic of a Colles' fracture with dorsal displacement of the distal fragment. (From Stanley BG, Tribuzi SM, editors: *Concepts in hand rehabilitation,* Philadelphia, 1992, FA Davis.)

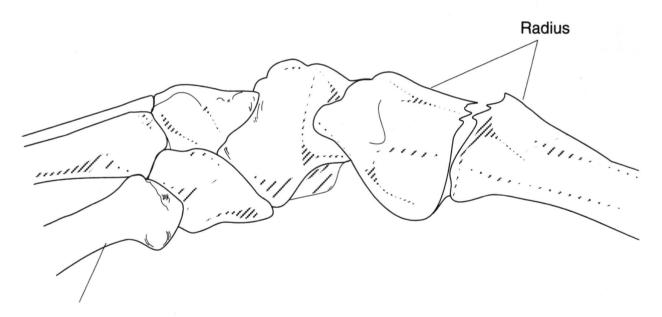

FIGURE 13-5 Schematic of a Smith's fracture with palmar displacement of the distal fragment. (From Stanley BG, Tribuzi SM, editors: *Concepts in hand rehabilitation,* Philadelphia, 1992, FA Davis.)

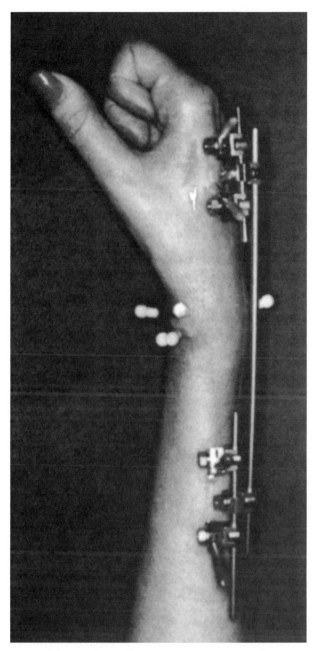

FIGURE 13-6 Distal radial fracture stabilized with an external fixator and percutaneous pins. (From Stanley BG, Tribuzi SM, editors: *Concepts in hand rehabilitation,* Philadelphia, 1992, FA Davis.)

plete rehabilitation within a time frame that is not compatible with anatomic healing and functional recovery.

NONOPERATIVE TREATMENT

The goal of therapy for any distal radial fracture is restoration of preinjury function. This is achieved by facilitating the return of strength and of maximum

pain-free ROM of the joints of the involved extremity, including the shoulder if it was adversely affected by the period of immobilization. Return of preinjury strength and motion depends on resolution of the bone and concomitant soft tissue impairment. In other words, a good outcome, as defined by the client, may not be possible if, for example, radial shortening has occurred.[9] A review of the literature suggests that therapeutic management of distal radius fractures can follow a number of courses and that treatment planning depends on the therapist's clinical decision making.[5,8,9,11] The therapist must take into consideration the type and severity of the impairment, associated injuries, and individual client factors, including the client's occupation and interests, overall health, cognition, access to therapy, hand dominance, which wrist is injured, and finances. The following interventions are recommended strategies.

THERAPEUTIC RECOMMENDATIONS

- **Splinting**
  - After the cast has been removed, a removable, forearm-based wrist splint can be used for intermittent, continued protection of the fracture site and of the local soft tissue during the first 2 weeks of controlled active motion. If the physician has not prescribed a splint, consider requesting one for the client to use for 1 to 2 weeks to address the day's-end pain and fatigue that are typical for clients with newly healed wrist fractures.
  - With an external fixator, the client's comfort can be improved with a removable, forearm-based ulnar wrist splint that supports the ulnar wrist and the mobile transverse arch of the hand (Fig. 13-7).[5]
- **Pin care:** Clients with percutaneous pins or an external fixator need careful monitoring for proper pin care, because the pins provide bacteria with direct access to the subcutaneous tissues and healing bone. Physicians have different preferences for pin sites and wound care, therefore the therapist must make sure to ask the referring physician about the proper protocol and must reinforce it with the client.

CLINICAL *Pearl*

When sterile cotton swabs are used to clean the pins, make sure the client uses only one swab per pin per application. The client should never use the same swab on more than one pin.

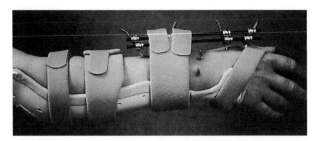

FIGURE 13-7   Ulnar gutter support splint, elbow included, for use with an external fixator. This splint supports the transverse arch of the hand and allows full motion of the thumb and fingers but limits forearm rotation. The length of the splint can vary, from short arm to above the elbow, depending on the need to limit forearm rotation. (From Laseter G, Carter P: *J Hand Ther* 9:122, 1996.)

This carefulness minimizes the risk of infection. Be sure to teach the client the signs and symptoms of infection: a foul smell, increased pain, heat and redness at the pin site, and **purulence** (viscous, yellowish-white pus oozing from the pin site). Make sure clients know they should contact the physician if they think a pin site has become infected.

- **Edema control**
  - The affected extremity should be elevated above the heart. Positioning devices such as pillows can be used when the client is relaxing at home.

Precaution. *Avoid using slings whenever possible. They encourage the protected posture clients often assume after injuring the upper extremity (i.e., internal rotation and adduction of the shoulder and flexion of the elbow).*

The protected posture promotes shoulder and elbow stiffness and hand edema and discourages functional use of the involved extremity. Furthermore, the weight of the arm in a sling is born by the contralateral neck, sometimes compromising that vulnerable site where the brachial plexus exits the scalenes.

  - AROM exercises should be performed to increase venous and lymphatic outflow. As muscles contract and relax, they help move edema; if the exercises are done with the arm elevated above heart level, gravity can assist the muscles in transporting the fluid proximally.
  - Retrograde massage, or "milking the fluid," can be performed by massaging the fingers, wrist, and forearm, moving distal to proximal. This moves the lymph through the superficial lymphatics in the skin and subcutaneous tissues toward normal areas of drainage (i.e., the sweat glands in the

axilla).[5] First perform proximal AROM exercises, and then take care to use very light pressure with this massage to avoid collapsing the lymphatics (see Chapter 3).

  - Compressive dressings or elastic gloves or finger sleeves can temporarily help the overwhelmed venous and lymphatic systems of the dorsal hand move fluids from the interstitial subcutaneous tissue spaces in the hand toward normal areas of drainage. These aids should not be tight.

- **Scar management and desensitization:** Assess the scars that form at pin sites and surgical sites (if ORIF was performed) to determine whether the underlying tissues are adherent and restricting normal tendon gliding. Adhesions that form beneath cutaneous scars should be addressed with scar massage and tendon gliding exercises. Topical scar compression dressings designed to improve scar cosmesis can be introduced within 24 to 48 hours of suture removal or when all scabs (eschar) are gone. Scar hypersensitivity can be addressed with a desensitization program that encourages the client to touch and massage the affected area regularly, providing various nonnoxious stimuli throughout the day.

- **AROM:** Remember to instruct the client in exercises for all joints of the injured arm, and introduce wrist and forearm active exercises as soon as the physician allows. Have the client hold the end-range position for a sustained 5 second stretch. Begin with three or four sets a day of 10 repetitions of each exercise; the number of repetitions and sets should be adjusted according to the client's response. For example, if the client develops shoulder stiffness during the fracture healing phase, the number of sets of shoulder exercises should be increased. As the client resumes functional activities using the injured extremity, the number of sets and/or repetitions of AROM exercises of nonstiff joints can be reduced, or the exercises can be discontinued.

  - Weakness of the radial wrist extensors allows the wrist flexors to overpower them during attempted grasp. This flexed wrist position further limits finger flexion and weakens grip. In addition, unless cautioned otherwise, clients often substitute with the digital extensors to initiate wrist extension (Fig. 13-8).

CLINICAL *Pearl*

It is important to isolate the radial wrist extensors during early controlled AROM and to add target strengthening exercises when appropriate.

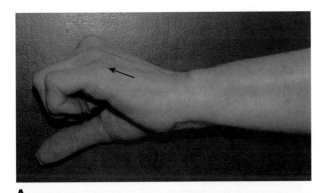

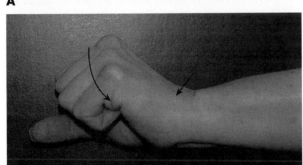

FIGURE 13-8 A, Many distal radius fracture patients have a well-established substitution pattern of using the digital extensors—particularly those in the ring and small fingers—to extend the wrist. **B,** Independent wrist extension is critical to developing the ability to make a fist and in regaining power grip after a distal radius fracture. (From Laseter G: External and internal fixation of unstable distal radius fractures. In Burke S, Higgins J, McClinton M et al, editors: *Hand and upper extremity rehabilitation: a practical guide,* ed 3, St. Louis, 2005, Churchill Livingstone.)

Instruct the client in active wrist extension exercises by having the client make a gentle fist when performing wrist extension. Encourage tenodesis, with simultaneous wrist extension and finger flexion, followed by simultaneous wrist flexion and finger extension.

- Instruct the client in individual tendon gliding exercises for the flexor digitorum superficialis and flexor digitorum profundus tendons. The hook fist position isolates the metacarpophalangeal (MCP) extensor and the extensor digitorum communis (EDC); it also addresses interphalangeal (IP) flexion while stretching the intrinsic muscles of the digits.
- **Strengthening**

Precaution. *Resistive exercises should not be introduced without the specific consent of the treating physician, who must determine whether the healing fracture is capable of withstanding high muscle forces across the fracture site.*

- Many therapists use a hammer as a weight to stretch the DRUJ joint and strengthen the forearm muscles. This exercise can be graded by having the client grasp the shaft of the hammer either closer to or farther from the head, thus increasing or decreasing the lever arm and hence the force generated during forearm rotation. If this exercise causes ulnar-sided wrist pain, the client should perform it while wearing a wrist splint and should rotate the hammer only in the midrange (between clock positions 10 and 2). The splint will protect the vulnerable ulnar carpus, and strengthening in the midrange is just as effective for muscle rehabilitation and less stressful to the ligaments and joint capsule of the ulnar wrist (Fig. 13-9). As an alternative to the splint, the client can support the DRUJ with the other hand while performing pronation and supination stretching exercises designed to increase forearm AROM.
- **Resumption of functional activities and ADL:** Light functional activities that are familiar to the client should be reintroduced as soon as possible to discourage "disuse atrophy." Clients may need help in appropriately adapting and grading (and upgrading) activities and tasks. For example, give the client some cylindric tubing, along with instructions on how to put it on a toothbrush. Enlarging the handle of a toothbrush, pen, hairbrush, safety razor, or spoon makes it much easier to grasp, which limits the force required to complete a task such as brushing the teeth or signing a check. Most clients relish the return to independence in self-care tasks; encourage them and cheer their successes!
- **Passive range of motion (PROM) and dynamic splinting**
  - The index MCP joint typically is stiffer than its neighbors after immobilization with an external fixator. Early in therapy, PROM should target digit MCP joint flexion, IP joint extension, and the thumb web space.

Precaution. *Passive stretching of the joints should never be painful.*

- If ROM of the wrist or distal forearm (or both) plateaus before the client has achieved functional ranges, dynamic and/or static progressive splinting should be considered. Dynamic splinting applies a low-load, prolonged stretch to tight, adaptively shortened tissues or adhesions to encourage the tissue to grow longer. Typically supination is more impaired than pronation,[9] and loss of functional wrist extension is more a concern than loss of wrist flexion. A number of

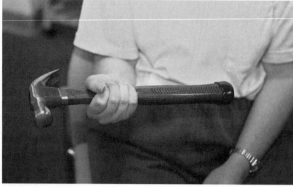

A

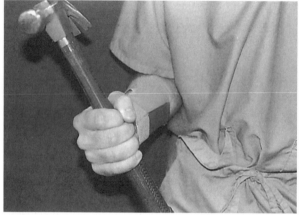

B

FIGURE 13-9   A, A hammer can be used to passively stretch the forearm and/or to strengthen the muscles of forearm rotation. The torque force can be adjusted by changing the point where the client grasps the handle (thereby increasing or decreasing the lever arm). **B,** Exercising the forearm with a hammer may require the use of a wrist splint to protect the vulnerable ulnar carpus. (**A** from LaStayo PC: Ulnar wrist pain and impairment: a therapist's approach to the triangular fibrocartilage complex. In Mackin EJ, Callahan AD, Skirven TM et al, editors: *Rehabilitation of the hand and upper extremity,* ed 5, St Louis, 2002, Mosby; **B** from Jaffe R, Chidgey L, LaStayo P: *J Hand Ther* 9:136, 1996.)

commercially available dynamic splints can be used to address wrist tightness and decreased forearm rotation (Fig. 13-10).

• **Complications: Complex regional pain syndrome (CRPS),** also known as **reflex sympathetic dystrophy (RSD)** is a primary complication of distal radial fracture. Be alert for signs of increased sympathetic activity and vasomotor instability. Look for discoloration of the skin (especially over the dorsal digital joints); shiny, waxlike skin; increased warmth in the injured hand compared with the uninjured hand; brawny edema (swelling that is firm to the touch); increased sweating (hyperhidrosis); and persistent, unrelenting stiffness. Pain often is out of proportion to the injury. Inform the physician of your findings

and concerns. Early treatment of these symptoms increases the chances of resolving them and of preventing the well-known dysfunctional consequences of CRPS (see Chapter 18).[5]

Questions to Ask the Physician

• *Is disruption of radial length, inclination, or tilt involved?*
• *Is the TFCC injured?*
• *Are AROM parameters restricted in any way?*
• *What is the preferred protocol for pin care?*
• *When does the physician plan to remove the hardware (if at all)?*
• *Are there any other soft tissue considerations?*
• *Does the client have pre-existing thumb or wrist arthritis that would affect rehabilitation?*

What to Say to Clients

About Exercises

"Reducing swelling and improving movement are important goals during the initial phase of hand therapy. We will focus on motion for the thumb, fingers, wrist, forearm, and elbow. I would like you to start by doing three to five sets of your exercises each day. I will adjust the number of repetitions and sets based on how you respond to these exercises. It is very important to exercise the fingers often during the day to minimize swelling in the hand and promote normal hand motion. It also is very important to learn how to isolate your wrist muscles from your finger muscles. We will practice the exercises together now, and I will give you a handout with pictures of the exercises so that you can remind yourself how to do them correctly. Please remember that you should not have any pain with these exercises, although you may have some discomfort related to moving joints that haven't moved in a while. Always do your exercises slowly and hold the end position so that you get a little stretch."

About Swelling

"Swelling is a normal bodily response to injury or surgery. It means your body is doing what it needs to do to bring the cells necessary for healing, assisting the injured tissue in the repair process, and providing a way to remove the debris and waste products that accumulate as the body heals. If you had no swelling, you couldn't heal, so thank goodness for swelling! It can last for a long time after an injury, especially if a lot of soft tissue trauma was involved. Swelling typically resolves gradually over weeks or months as your body's tissues return to a state of homeostasis. I'm telling you this so that you won't be overly concerned about the presence of swelling and morning stiffness and so you won't go out and get your rings resized or your watchband enlarged until you've waited about a year after the injury date."

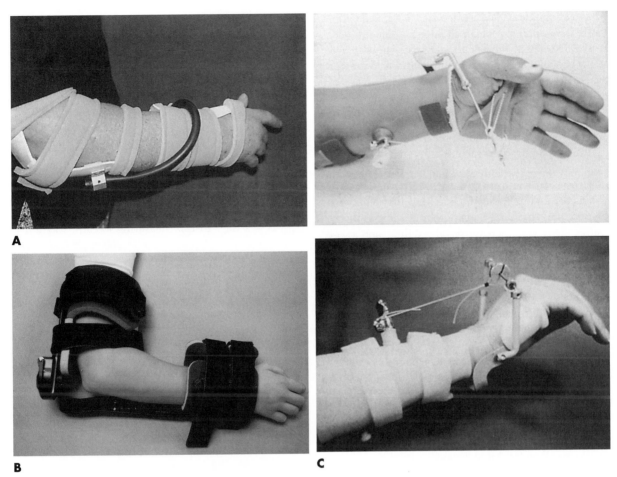

FIGURE 13-10 Dynamic splints used to address forearm and wrist ROM limitations after a distal radial fracture. **A,** A dynamic forearm rotation splint using components made of Rolyan. **B,** A dynamic forearm supination splint. **C,** A static progressive wrist flexion and extension splint using the Phoenix wrist hinge and the maximum end range (i) time (MERiT) component. (**A** from Jaffe R, Chidgey L, LaStayo P: *J Hand Ther* 9:136, 1996; **B** from Fess EE, Gettle KS, Philips CA et al: *Hand and upper extremity splinting: principles and methods,* ed 3, St Louis, 2005, Mosby; **C** from King JW: *J Hand Ther* 5:36-37, 1992.)

"Now, even though swelling is a healthy, normal response to injury, we don't want the fluid to accumulate and sit 'stagnant' in your hand. If this happens, you'll find it hard to move your fingers, and you could develop contractures or limitations in movement. That's why I want you to address this swelling, assisting your body in the regular exchange of fluids by exercising as I've shown you and also by massaging or lightly milking the fluid out of your fingers. Try to limit the amount of time you allow your injured arm to hang by your side. Instead, keep your hand above your elbow when possible, maybe by using a pillow or a pocket to position it. This allows gravity to help get rid of the fluid that accumulates in your hand. If the swelling becomes problematic and exercise, positioning, and massage don't seem to control it, we may use some elastic gloves or sleeves or a compressive bandage to help your body move the fluid, with its waste products, out toward your armpit, where your body will naturally get rid of it.

These elastic sleeves or bandages work like the support hose people sometimes wear to assist leg circulation."

EVALUATION TIPS

Client-rated outcome measurement tools are an important component of the evaluation, because they facilitate identification of the client's interests and concerns. This information is collected and evaluated in a standardized format and used to develop goals and to demonstrate positive functional outcomes after therapy. The disabilities of the arm, shoulder, and hand (DASH index) (see Reference 54, Chapter 6) is an easy to administer, client friendly outcome tool with excellent validity and reliability measures. It identifies client-specific disabilities that either proximal or distal arm impairments can cause, and it allows the therapist easily to evaluate the effectiveness of a single (or more than one) treatment session in mitigating these disabilities. The Patient-Rated Wrist Evaluation (PRWE)[12] is a similar popular, client-rated outcome tool. Like the DASH, it is quick to administer and easy to score, with low scores indicating little or no upper extremity debility (see Chapter 6).

Other evaluation measures also are important.

- Check for shoulder AROM and pain. Identify and address secondary shoulder problems immediately to prevent complications such as a frozen shoulder.
- Observe the client's arm and hand posture. Some clients keep the arm in a sling with the shoulder adducted and internally rotated, the elbow and wrist flexed, and the hand hanging out of the end of the sling. This can increase distal swelling and cause elbow and shoulder stiffness.
- Poor finger motion can be caused by limited tendon gliding at the wrist and by swelling. Check this and document it.
- Take composite measurements, such as digit flexion to the distal palmar crease and digit extension off the table with the wrist held in a steady neutral position. This indicates whether extrinsic flexor and/or extensor tendon tightness has developed.
- Passively flex the MCPs gently to assess capsular tightness that may have developed secondary to cast immobilization, especially when the distal volar portion of the cast extends too far distally or is too bulky to allow full MCP flexion.
- The extensor pollicis longus (EPL) tendon changes direction as it wraps around the dorsal bony tubercle on the distal radius (Lister's tubercle). Sometimes, just by virtue of its location, the EPL can become attenuated or can rupture with a distal radial fracture. To assess the function of the EPL, have the client position the involved hand with the palm flat on the table and then instruct the client to raise the thumb to the ceiling (Fig. 13-11). Report pain or

problems with extending the IP joint of the thumb to the physician.

- When measuring forearm rotation at the DRUJ, have the client sit with the elbow flexed at 90 degrees and the arm close to the side of the body. Maintaining this arm position is important to preventing substitution movements at the shoulder. Align the goniometer's stability arm parallel to the humerus. For supination, align the mobility arm parallel to the proximal volar wrist crease. The axis is just medial to the ulnar styloid. For pronation, the stability arm remains the same; the mobility arm is placed on the dorsum of the wrist at the level of the styloid processes (Fig. 13-12). Measuring forearm rotation this

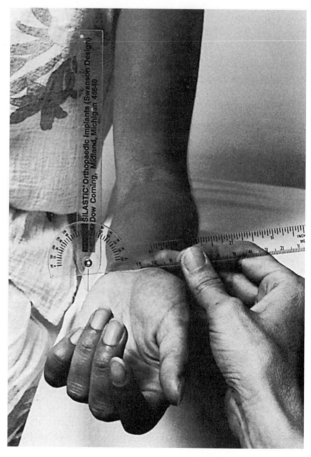

FIGURE 13-12   To assess forearm supination (and pronation) correctly, position the client with the test arm in adduction and the elbow flexed to 90 degrees. The axis of the goniometer is just medial to the ulnar styloid. The movable arm is placed across the volar aspect of the wrist for supination, at the level of the ulnar styloid. The stationary arm is aligned with the humerus. (From Cambridge-Keeling CA: Range-of-motion measurement of the hand. In Mackin EJ, Callahan AD, Skirven TM et al, editors: *Rehabilitation of the hand and upper extremity*, ed 5, St Louis, 2002, Mosby.)

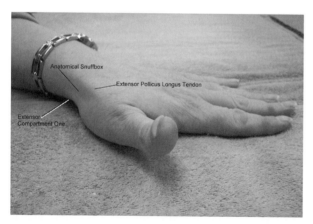

FIGURE 13-11   Test to determine EPL patency.

way allows the therapist to appreciate true forearm rotation as opposed to rotation at the carpus.

- Check the ulnar side of the wrist for swelling and palpate it for pain. Ask the client whether pain is felt during forearm rotation. Document your findings and report them to the physician.
- Perform sensory testing as appropriate, using Semmes-Weinstein monofilaments to identify or rule out sensory nerve problems. Report your findings immediately to the physician and discuss guidelines for any required treatment modifications.

DIAGNOSIS-SPECIFIC INFORMATION THAT AFFECTS CLINICAL REASONING

If possible, the therapist should determine whether the fracture is extraarticular or intraarticular, because an intraarticular fracture involves at least some disruption of the articular cartilage, which puts the joint at risk for traumatic arthritis. If the fracture is the intraarticular type, knowing whether the DRUJ or the radiocarpal joint (or both) is involved can also be helpful. Although a fracture of the distal tip of the ulnar styloid typically creates no long-term problems,[11] it is helpful to be aware of its presence or absence in explaining early-on versus later-developing ulnar-sided wrist pain.

Other diagnostic-specific information also may be important.

- More than half of fractures of the ulnar styloid occur in conjunction with distal radial fractures; however, these ulnar styloid fractures do not typically require formal medical intervention.[6,11] They generally do not impede function or cause lasting discomfort, even though many result in a nonunion.[6] When clients know they have an ulnar styloid fracture, reassure them that these fractures typically are treated with benign neglect and that early ulnar-sided wrist pain may indicate nothing more than the body's attempt to heal this fracture. A wrist splint that stabilizes the ulnar side of the wrist may be helpful for managing pain associated with these fractures. Keep in mind that prolonged pain in the distal ulnar wrist area that is aggravated by motion or appropriately introduced strengthening exercises may be a sign of injury to soft tissue structures rather than to the bone itself.
- A fracture of the proximal or middle one third of the ulnar styloid may involve the TFCC and possibly the insertion of the extensor carpi ulnaris tendon. If the fracture is not displaced, a long arm cast is worn for 3 to 4 weeks to prevent wrist and forearm motion until the fracture has healed. If the fracture is displaced, ORIF is necessary, followed by immobilization in a long arm cast for about 3 to 4 weeks.[11]

- Distal ulnar shaft fractures can also disrupt the DRUJ. These fractures may require either open or closed reduction and some type of fixation for 4 to 6 weeks to achieve stability.[6]
- Distal radial fractures that heal with an incongruity (incompatibility) of the articular surfaces between the distal radius and the proximal carpus and/or between the distal radius and the distal ulna at the DRUJ often develop a painful degenerative condition or posttraumatic arthritis. Radiocarpal arthrosis manifests as pain with wrist flexion and extension. DRUJ arthrosis is characterized by pain with forearm rotation.[6]
- If a distal radial fracture heals with significant dorsal angulation (rather than normal volar angulation) of the distal radius, DRUJ problems are likely. If the radius heals in a shortened position relative to the ulna, more force will be transmitted to the TFCC, the ulnar carpus, and the ulnar styloid. This can lead to TFCC degeneration and **ulnocarpal abutment syndrome,** with the development of pain and traumatic arthritis of the ulnar wrist, restricted ulnar deviation of the wrist, and diminished grip strength.[6]

TIPS FROM THE FIELD

Pain

Therapists are not required to be the expert in determining the exact cause of ulnar-sided wrist pain that develops after a distal radial fracture. Instead, carefully document your findings, indicating conditions in which the pain is exacerbated, and report them to the physician. Remember that sometimes even the best therapy cannot ameliorate pain and dysfunction that occur secondary to bony alignment issues.

Normal versus Functional Range of Motion

In some cases the return of "normal," pain-free wrist ROM cannot be achieved after a distal radial fracture. The therapist may need to help such clients refocus, so that their goal becomes gaining pain-free ROM within a functional range. Studies disagree on what constitutes *functional* wrist motion, with reports ranging from 35 to 80 degrees of total wrist flexion/extension as a prerequisite for functional activities.[5] Typically, if the injured hand is the dominant hand, greater ROM is necessary for return of function. To determine how much functional ROM the client needs, the therapist should help the client identify the specific activities the person wants or needs to do with the involved hand. Therapy sessions should include practicing these specific activities, which can be graded in terms of repetition, load, or both.

Splinting

A custom-molded or prefabricated wrist splint can be very helpful for minimizing pain and swelling after the cast or external fixator is removed and the client resumes light activities and exercises with the involved hand. As mentioned previously, if the physician has not written orders for a splint, the therapist may want to ask whether short-term use of a splint would be beneficial for the fatigue and pain these clients typically have at the end of the day.

Sometimes a wrist splint is prescribed because it offers needed additional support for the healing fracture. Some clients get very attached to the splint and eventually use it too much. Use of the splint beyond the therapeutic interval delays the recovery of motion and functional hand use. These clients may need gentle encouragement to wean themselves from the splint.

The therapist should identify signs of extrinsic flexor tightness and use a night platform extension splint, which can be serially adjusted, with the fingers and wrist positioned in extension. The client should feel only a light stretch to the finger flexors when the splint is adjusted in the clinic. Clients do not tolerate aggressive stretching from a splint while trying to fall asleep, and a stretch that feels mild when the client is awake and alert will feel intolerable in the quiet of the night. Also, remember that a slow, sustained stretch allows the tissues to remodel to become longer without causing pain, tearing, or other tissue deformation.

Client Compliance

Some clients may fear that they will rebreak the wrist when performing exercises or activities at home. If the client is not following the prescribed program, consider first reassuring the person that the bone is well-enough healed to tolerate the exercises, which will further strengthen the newly healed bone. If fear or pain is not the limiting factor, the therapist must reconsider the program.

CLINICAL *Pearl*

If the exercises are not meaningful to the client or if it is not clear how the exercises will allow resumption of an important activity, the client may not be invested in the program and may refuse to comply.

The true art of therapy involves engaging the client and incorporating the person's interests into treatment planning.

Precautions and Concerns

Pin Care

- *Inspect the skin around the pin sites and check for purulence (yellowish-white pus oozing from the wounds). Wound odor may also be a sign of infection. Notify the physician if any discharge at the pin sites is malodorous (has a pungent smell) or purulent.*

Splinting and Joint Mobilization to Regain Forearm Motion

- *Remember that the carpus is composed of eight small, mobile bones and that after a distal radial fracture, the ligaments that restrain and support these bones may be compromised. The job of a ligament is to provide stability at a joint. Aggressive stretching, exercising, or splinting of the forearm and wrist that does not protect the vulnerable ulnar carpal ligaments can result in ligamentous laxity that will give the appearance of greater supination. Encouraging supination at the carpus (rather than the DRUJ) is detrimental in the long run because stability and strength at the wrist are lost in exchange for more motion. Be careful to support the ulnar carpus with a splint when trying to stretch the forearm with joint mobilization or resistive exercises (see Fig. 13-9).*

COMPLICATIONS

Complications are common after a distal radial fracture. Some require medical management and some can be ameliorated therapeutically. DRUJ dysfunction is a common complication requiring medical intervention; it also is one of the problems that most often limit the potential for therapy gains. Clients complain of persistent pain and limited forearm rotation. Other complications include carpal tunnel syndrome, malunion, radiocarpal arthritis, and rupture of the EPL tendon.[9]

Complications that can be addressed in the therapy clinic include stiffness in uninvolved joints, contracture of intrinsic muscles as a result of prolonged edema, and CRPS. Many of these problems can be prevented or mitigated by an excellent therapy program that incorporates early exercise, edema control, and instructions about the timing of activity resumption. However, CRPS may require more intensive intervention by both the physician and the therapist to remedy this devastating complication (see Chapter 18).

CARPAL FRACTURES

The eight small carpal bones are highly mobile and largely covered by articular cartilage. They can be divided into two rows: a proximal row, consisting of the scaphoid, lunate, triquetrum, and pisiform, and a distal row, consisting of the trapezium, trapezoid, capitate, and hamate (Fig. 13-13).[13]

Precaution. *The blood supply to the carpals is tenuous. After injury, avascular necrosis can develop even in the best of circumstances.*[14]

Most carpal fractures occur when a force is applied with the wrist in extension.[9] The incidence of carpal fractures is one tenth that of distal radial fractures, and the scaphoid bone accounts for 60% to 70% of carpal fractures.[10,15]

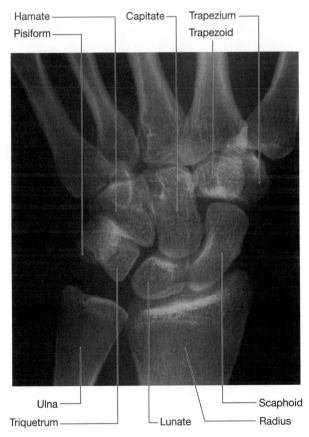

FIGURE 13-13 Posteroanterior (PA) x-ray film of a normal wrist with the carpal bones identified. (From Drake RL, Vogl W, Mitchell AWM: *Gray's anatomy for students,* Philadelphia, 2005, Churchill Livingstone.)

SCAPHOID FRACTURE

Anatomy

The scaphoid, the second largest carpal bone, is shaped somewhat like a kidney bean. It has a proximal pole, a distal pole (or tubercle), and a waist, which separates the two poles.[4] Although the scaphoid is considered part of the proximal carpal row,[13] it actually spans the midcarpal joint. Proximally, it sits in a shallow facet at the distal end of the radius, where, along with the lunate bone, it makes up the radiocarpal joint. The blood supply enters at the dorsal, distal pole; therefore, if a fracture disrupts the blood supply to the proximal pole, the result may be a delay in bone union, avascular necrosis (AVN) of the bone fragment, or nonunion.[15,16]

Diagnosis and Pathology

The mechanism of injury for a scaphoid fracture usually is a fall on an outstretched hand with the wrist extended and radially deviated, resulting in compression of the waist of the scaphoid against the radial styloid. The typical client is a young adult, most often male. It is not unusual for this type of injury to go unreported for a time, because clients often consider it "just a sprain." Acute fractures may not be evident on initial x-ray films. If the client has a history of a FOOSH incident and pain over the scaphoid, x-ray films are repeated until the pain resolves or the fracture line appears.[16]

Clients with a scaphoid fracture have tenderness and pain over the scaphoid that are aggravated by palpation of the **anatomic snuff box** (the dorsal wrist distal to the radial styloid process). ROM, particularly wrist extension, is restricted, and grip strength is reduced by more than 50%.[15]

Timelines and Healing

Nondisplaced scaphoid fractures can be treated adequately with cast immobilization. Many physicians use a long arm thumb spica cast for the first 6 weeks of immobilization and then a short arm thumb spica cast until the fracture is healed.[11,16] Herbert[15] recommends using a short arm cast, leaving the thumb completely free, because excluding the carpometacarpal (CMC) and MCP joints of the thumb does not seem to have any adverse effects. Typically, a distal pole fracture heals in 6 to 8 weeks, a waist fracture heals in 8 to 12 weeks, and a fracture of the proximal pole (where vascularity is poor) heals in 12 to 24 weeks.[11,16] About 70% of scaphoid fractures occur at the waist.[11]

Displaced fractures, comminuted fractures, or fractures with associated injuries frequently are treated with surgical fixation, most often a bone screw.[16] Immobilization after surgery depends on the location of the fracture, whether a bone graft was used, the method of internal fixation. and the stability of the fracture. The immobilization period can range from 2 to 16 weeks.[11,14]

Nonoperative Treatment

Hand therapy may begin while the client is still casted. During these sessions, the therapist should address edema control of the digits and active ROM of the uninvolved joints. (See edema control suggestions in the section on treatment of distal radial fractures.)

After removal of the cast, the client typically is fitted with a forearm-based thumb spica splint to use between prescribed exercise sessions for the next 2 weeks. This splint provides interim protection for the scaphoid and local soft tissue, especially if the client engages in strenuous activities with the involved hand. The client is instructed in a home exercise program of active ROM of the wrist and thumb. Because stiffness often is a problem after the long period of immobilization needed for scaphoid healing, frequent exercise sessions (i.e., hourly or every other hour) are recommended. The client is encouraged to use the hand to perform familiar functional tasks, gradually resuming self-care and light household maintenance over the first month after immobilization. The therapist can slowly introduce specific strengthening exercises, monitoring swelling and any reports of pain or discomfort with these added activities. The client should be able to return to full activity by 10 to 12 weeks after cast removal.[16]

Clients who undergo ORIF with screw fixation for a scaphoid fracture often are referred to therapy after a short period in a cast (about 10 to 14 days) for soft tissue healing.[14] A flexible wrist splint (Fig. 13-14) can be used for the next 2 to 4 weeks to allow controlled active wrist flexion and extension during light ADL. The proposed advantages of early controlled motion in this splint include decreased bone osteopenia, maintenance of articular cartilage health, and promotion of bone mineralization of the fracture site.[17] Clients who engage in contact sports or who work in physically demanding environments may require another month of some type of rigid splint protection until bone union is confirmed by an x-ray film.[15]

Significant joint stiffness and, frequently, pain are hallmark complaints from clients who have undergone lengthy immobilization before a fracture is deemed unstable and from clients in whom a fracture has developed into a nonunion. Treatment of delayed union or nonunion of a scaphoid fracture usually requires either ORIF or a vascularized bone graft, followed by prolonged immobilization. After this period, clients often need

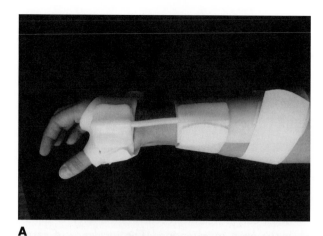

A

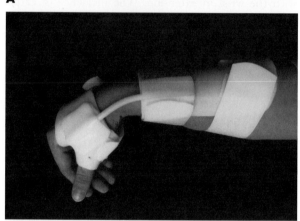

B

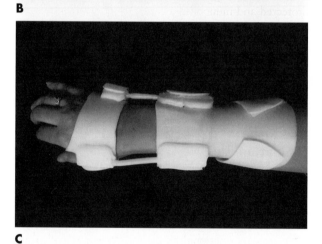

C

FIGURE 13-14 A removable, flexible wrist splint that allows some wrist flexion and extension yet restricts deviation. The splint was designed in 1989 by Terri Skirven, OTR/L, CHT, for use as an interim fracture brace that allows some protected, safe active motion while the client performs light activities of daily living (ADL). The splint is introduced after a period of rigid immobilization for a scaphoid fracture. Use of this splint has been shown to reduce bone osteopenia, reduce the severe stiffness seen after prolonged casting, promote bone mineralization at the fracture site, and maintain articular cartilage health. (Courtesy Terri Skirven, OTR, CHT, King of Prussia, PA.)

dynamic or static progressive splinting, beginning at 6 weeks after surgery,[15] to regain mobility. A work rehabilitation program may be required if the client is returning to a job that requires heavy lifting or manual labor.

Questions to Ask the Physician

- *In what area of the scaphoid is the fracture site located?*
- *Do you want the thumb included in the postcast splint?*
- *How acute is the fracture?*
- *If surgical repair was required: What type of fixation was used? Was a vascular bone graft used?*
- *What is the splinting protocol after cast removal for clients who have had surgery?*
- *What exercise precautions should be observed?*

What to Say to Clients

"You fractured the scaphoid bone. This bone is located on the thumb side of the wrist and is positioned between the thumb and your wrist joint. The scaphoid is a bone with a limited blood supply, and its ability to heal is not predictable. To promote healing, it is important for you to assess your pain symptoms accurately and to avoid overusing or straining the hand or wrist."

"It is also important that your wrist and thumb be protected and immobilized while the fracture is healing. Your physician will closely assess the fracture at regular intervals. During this immobilization period, make sure you move your shoulder normally and maintain the range of motion in the fingers and elbow to speed up your recovery and to prevent further complications when the cast is removed."

Evaluation Tips

- Take goniometric measurements of wrist flexion and extension and ulnar and radial deviation; expect initial limitations in all directions, especially wrist extension.
- Consider functional measurements when evaluating the thumb, specifically thumb radial abduction, palmar abduction, and opposition. Good abduction is needed for cylindric grasp, and thumb movement can be compromised by prolonged splinting.
- Once strengthening exercises are allowed, volumetric measures taken before and after exercise sessions can help establish safe guidelines for exercise and tissue loading. A study by McGough and Surwasky[18] examined the effect of exercise on the asymptomatic hand. Although the study involved only a small sample of uninjured hands, its results provide some guidelines

for assessing normal (and abnormal) response to exercise. The study showed that females demonstrate a 3.6% increase in volumetrics after exercise, and males demonstrate a 5.2% increase in volume.[18] Volume changes that exceed these values, especially when accompanied by symptom complaints, would seem to indicate that the level of resistance or the number of repetitions (or both) during exercise exceed the healing tissues' tolerance. Subsequent treatment sessions should take this information into account. Further research is needed on postexercise edema in injured extremities.

Diagnosis-Specific Information That Affects Clinical Reasoning

Radial wrist pain can be caused or aggravated by a number of factors, including dorsal radial sensory neuritis, acute scaphoid fracture, thumb basal joint arthritis, scaphoid nonunion, and de Quervain's tenosynovitis. If the client's injury involved a high-energy impact, yet repeated x-ray films show no evidence of a scaphoid or distal radial fracture, the scapholunate (S-L) ligament may be damaged. The physician makes this diagnosis partly on the basis of a positive result on **Watson's test,** also known as the scaphoid shift test. (For the specifics of this test, see Skirven's article on the clinical examination of the wrist.[19])

Tips from the Field

Clients who have pain and tenderness over the scaphoid despite the absence of radiographic evidence of fracture should wear a forearm-based thumb spica splint until the pain has resolved or until further testing identifies the cause of the symptoms. Ideally, these clients are reevaluated weekly for pain and tenderness and the findings are reported to the physician.

Sometimes such clients are sent to hand therapy with a diagnosis of "wrist sprain/strain." In these circumstances a careful evaluation must be performed, including documentation of the history of the injury and a good biomechanical evaluation of the tissue. Active motion, pain, volumetrics, and grip strength should be noted. A primary responsibility of hand therapists is to use clinical reasoning to help monitor progress or lack of progress. Volumetrics taken before and after exercise can provide information about tissue tolerances for exercise. Remember to take volumetric measures of both the involved and uninvolved hand so that you can compare the client's individual response to activity. Light activities should not significantly increase swelling and pain if the involved hand has healed enough to tolerate such loads.

Precaution. *If light exercise or activity consistently aggravates the involved extremity, stop loading the injured hand and wrist and notify the referring physician.*

Compression of the dorsal radial sensory nerve can develop secondary to the prolonged immobilization required for scaphoid healing or as a result of irritation caused by the thumb spica cast or splint. The condition manifests as pain, numbness, tingling, and/or burning over the dorsal radial wrist. These symptoms are aggravated by percussion of the area and by wrist flexion and ulnar deviation and thumb flexion, because these postures stretch the radial sensory nerve. Instruct the client to perform radial nerve gliding exercises gently five times a day (see Chapter 12).

Precautions and Concerns

- *The primary goal of therapy for scaphoid fractures is to restore function after the fracture has healed. At the start of therapy, it is important to restore movement and strength within the client's pain tolerance. Aggressive therapy results in persistent wrist symptoms, including pain. Remember that scaphoid fractures and their associated soft tissue trauma require a great deal of care and time to heal. Avoid any painful exercises.*

OTHER CARPAL FRACTURES

Fractures of the other carpal bones occur less often than scaphoid fractures and are treated in the same manner.[15] As many as 90% of these other types of fractures occur as a result of a force applied when the wrist is in extension.[10]

Diagnosis and Pathology

The trapezium is a component of the distal carpal row. It articulates proximally with the scaphoid and distally with the thumb metacarpal, with which it forms a highly movable saddle joint. Trapezium fractures account for 1% to 5% of all carpal fractures.[15] Fractures of this bone occur most often with a fall on a hyperextended and radially deviated wrist with the thumb in abduction. Clinically, point tenderness is noted at the base of the thumb. Resisted wrist flexion typically aggravates the pain, and carpal tunnel syndrome may be associated with the injury.[15]

The trapezoid, one of the smallest carpal bones, is interposed between the trapezium and the capitate. Trapezoid fractures are rare, accounting for less than 1% of carpal fractures. This type of injury usually occurs when a high-velocity force pushes the index metacarpal into

the trapezoid, causing either a fracture or dislocation of the trapezoid.

Capitate fractures also are rare (1% to 2% of carpal fractures).

CLINICAL *Pearl*

The capitate is the largest carpal bone; it is considered the keystone of the carpus. As with the scaphoid, the blood supply to the proximal portion of the capitate is tenuous, therefore avascular necrosis can develop here.

Eighty percent of the force generated with hand use is transmitted across the capitate onto the lunate and proximal third of the scaphoid and subsequently onto the radius.[14] Isolated fractures of the capitate are uncommon; more typically, capitate fractures are seen with other wrist injuries.[14,15]

The hamate, one of the larger carpal bones, forms the ulnar border of the distal carpal row. It has a volar protrusion, called the *hook of the hamate.* Fractures of the hamate account for 2% to 4% of carpal fractures, and fractures of the hook are more common than fractures of the body. Hook fractures may occur with a fall on an extended wrist or in association with a forceful swing of a golf club or bat.[14,15] Clinically, these fractures are marked by pain when the person holds a racket or club, acute tenderness over the hook of hamate, and discomfort with resisted abduction or adduction of the little finger.[14,15] Ulnar nerve neuropathy may accompany these fractures because a branch of the ulnar nerve passes into the hand between the pisiform and the hook of the hamate. Fractures of the hook frequently are overlooked,[14] and the result is symptomatic nonunion.

The pisiform is a sesamoid bone that resembles a pea. It is situated in the proximal ulnar carpal row and serves as the attachment for the flexor carpi ulnaris tendon. Pisiform fractures account for 1% to 3% of carpal injures. The cause of these fractures typically is direct trauma to the volar aspect of the wrist or a chip avulsion caused by the pull of the flexor carpi ulnaris against strong resistance. These fractures are characterized by acute tenderness over the pisiform.

The triquetrum is a small, irregularly shaped bone adjacent to the lunate in the proximal ulnar carpal row. Triquetral fractures usually occur with lunate dislocations or other associated carpal injuries; they account for 3% to 4% of all carpal fractures.

The lunate, named for its lunar (moon) shape, is wedged between the scaphoid and the triquetrum in the proximal carpal row. Like the scaphoid bone, the lunate has a tenuous blood supply, and its vascular viability depends on the ligamentous attachments.[4] Isolated lunate fractures account for 2% to 7% of carpal fractures. Fractures of the lunate are more likely to be caused by repeated compression or stress than by a single force.[10]

CLINICAL *Pearl*

Lunate fractures are strongly associated with the development of avascular necrosis, or Kienböck's disease.

AVN is common in the wrist, where the blood supply to many of the carpal bones is tenuous. AVN of the lunate (**Kienböck's disease**) typically is the result of repetitive microtrauma that compromises the blood flow to the bone. It also is associated with negative ulnar variance.[14]

Timelines and Healing

Most carpal fractures are treated with cast immobilization and heal within 6 to 8 weeks if they are nondisplaced and have a good blood supply. Pisiform and stable triquetrum fractures are the exception; they typically require protection in a splint or cast for approximately 3 weeks. If the carpal fracture is unstable, ORIF may be necessary. If AVN develops, the injury is treated with prolonged casting and may require a salvage procedure such as bone grafting or arthroplasty or some type of partial or total wrist fusion.[10,14-16]

Nonoperative Treatment

During the acute phase of healing, instruct the client in AROM exercises of all the uninvolved joints of the injured arm to minimize stiffness and reduce swelling. After the cast is removed and when the fracture is stable enough to permit controlled active motion, the client should wear a removable thermoplastic splint for continued intermittent protection between exercise sessions. Light self-care and ADL activities can be introduced during this time to encourage motion and resumption of normal hand use.

When the physician confirms that the fracture has fully healed, PROM and dynamic splinting can be used, if needed, to help restore wrist and/or thumb motion. Grip strengthening also can be introduced.

Precautions and Concerns

- *Be aware that pain often is a continuing problem, and the possibility of refracture always exists with the carpal*

bones.[10] *Therefore exercises and activities to regain ROM and strength should be within the client's pain tolerance. Never use aggressive therapy.*

METACARPAL FRACTURES

Metacarpal fractures account for 30% to 50% of all hand fractures.[20] They are most prevalent in males age 10 to 29.[21] These fractures typically are caused by a motor vehicle or bike accident, although injuries resulting from a fistfight are also quite common.[21]

ANATOMY

The five metacarpal bones are considered miniature long bones.[20] Each has a central **shaft,** or **diaphysis,** which is composed of cortical bone, and proximal and distal ends, which are composed primarily of cancellous bone. In general, healing is more efficient (i.e., occurs faster) in cancellous bone than in cortical bone.

The distal end of the metacarpal is called the **head** and the proximal end is called the **base.** The **neck** is proximal to the head, at the junction of the head and shaft. These bones have a rich blood supply, which enables them to heal well after a fracture. The metacarpals vary in length; the index metacarpal is the longest, and the thumb metacarpal is the shortest. An interesting relationship exists between the length of the metacarpal and how much mobility each has at its CMC joint. The index and long metacarpals (i.e., the second and third digits) have a rigidly interlocking joint anatomy at the corresponding CMC joints; this contributes to the stability of these digits and creates the **longitudinal arch,** or *fixed unit,* of the hand.[13] The shorter ring and small finger metacarpals have greater joint mobility at the CMC joints; this allows for some flexion at these joints and contributes to the palmar cupping appearance of the hand at rest. This palmar concavity is enhanced by the **proximal transverse arch** of the hand, which is created by the interlocking carpal bones. Just distal to this arch, at the metacarpal heads, lie deep ligaments that support the **distal transverse arch** of the hand (Fig. 13-15). The intrinsic and extrinsic muscles provide added support to this skeletal arch system.

CLINICAL *Pearl*

Interruption of the longitudinal, proximal transverse, and/or distal transverse arch system, as can occur with a metacarpal fracture, allows the muscles of the hand to exert potentially deforming forces, creating a disruption of the bony scaffold and leading to significant loss of hand function.[20]

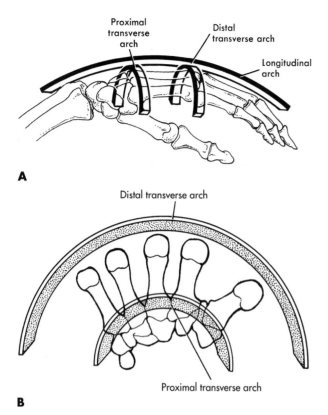

FIGURE 13-15 **A,** Skeletal arches of the hand. **B,** Proximal and distal transverse arches of the hand. (From Fess EE, Gettle KS, Philips CA et al: *Hand and upper extremity splinting: principles and methods,* ed 3, St Louis, 2005, Mosby.)

DIAGNOSIS AND PATHOLOGY

Metacarpal fractures most often involve the first and fifth digits, because they are highly mobile border digits and therefore more susceptible to injury. These digits can also be more difficult to treat.[10] Metacarpal fractures frequently occur in conjunction with open injuries. They may be *intraarticular fractures*, or fractures that occur at the joint and include some involvement of the joint's articular cartilage.[20] Late developing traumatic arthritis is an unavoidable and common consequence of an intraarticular fracture.[20]

Fractures of the base of the metacarpal usually are the result of a direct blow or a crush injury, in which case several metacarpals may be involved. Fractures of the shaft typically are caused by torsion, direct impact, or longitudinal compression. They can be categorized as comminuted, transverse, or oblique, depending on the number of fragments or the line of the fracture, or both. An oblique fracture can result in bone shortening and malrotation. A transverse fracture may manifest with dorsal angulation as a result of the deforming forces of the interossei and long flexor muscles.

CLINICAL *Pearl*

Fractures of the neck of the metacarpal are most commonly seen, because this is the weakest area of the bone.

Fractures of the base of the metacarpal typically result from a compression force, such as a direct blow with a closed fist. Often the impact causes comminution of the distal shaft of the bone and volar displacement of the metacarpal head. This type of extraarticular fracture, called a **boxer's fracture,** occurs most often in the fourth and fifth metacarpals. Open injuries on the dorsal aspect of the hand are often seen with these fractures, and these "fight bites" must be monitored for signs of infection and treated with antibiotics before operative repair of the fracture.[20]

Fractures of the thumb metacarpal, which typically occur at or near the base of the bone, are classified as extraarticular or intraarticular. **Bennett's fracture-dislocation** is a common intraarticular fracture. The mechanism of injury is an axial blow against a partly flexed metacarpal, such as occurs during a fistfight. These are unstable, two-fragment fractures of the base of the thumb metacarpal; because of the competing forces of the adductor pollicus and abductor pollicus longus tendons, they result in dislocation or subluxation of the thumb's CMC joint.[20]

Because injuries to the metacarpal bones can compromise the basic structural support of the hand, medical management must include maintenance or restoration (or both) of the natural arches.

The thumb, which has the shortest and most mobile metacarpal, also demonstrates the interesting relationship between metacarpal length and mobility.[20] The thumb's CMC joint is particularly mobile, allowing for three classes of movement: flexion/extension, abduction/adduction, and anteposition (opposition)/retroposition. Strong ligaments contribute to the stability of the thumb CMC joint. Any interruption of this stability results in a loss of thumb strength.

The digital extensor tendons are particularly sensitive to any change in the length of the metacarpal bones; bone shortening of 3 mm or more can result in an extensor lag in the corresponding digit.[21] Extensor adhesions at the metacarpal level lead to loss of composite finger flexion.

TIMELINES AND HEALING

Fractures of metacarpals two through five tend to be stable because of the numerous muscles and ligaments that attach to these bones. These fractures heal within 3 to 7 weeks, depending on the location of the fracture (i.e., head, neck, shaft, or base).[10] However, under certain conditions the same muscles and ligaments that help stabilize the associated joints and arches of the hand can produce a deforming force, causing dorsal angulation at the fracture site[10] and interrupting the normal arch system. Bennett's fracture-dislocations are unstable and require some type of internal or external fixation for reduction and repair.

- **Base fractures:** Base fractures of the second or third metacarpal are uncommon and usually are stable. Base fractures of the fourth or fifth ray may demonstrate a small amount of rotation at the base, which is magnified many times at the flexed fingertip.[10]

CLINICAL *Pearl*

Rotational malunion can cause scissoring or overlapping of the fingers when they attempt to flex, functionally limiting grasp and impeding grip strength.

- **Shaft fractures:** An impacted comminuted fracture usually is stable and can withstand controlled active motion in 12 to 14 days.[10] An unstable shaft fracture requires ORIF or percutaneous pinning. Transverse fractures usually are stable, and protected active motion often can be started in 3 weeks.[10] Oblique fractures that shorten and malrotate require open reduction or percutaneous pinning.
- **Neck fractures:** Various surgical and nonsurgical options for treatment of metacarpal neck fractures have been discussed in the literature.[10,19,21] Clients treated with nonsurgical closed reduction are immobilized for 3 to 4 weeks in a safe position ulnar or radial gutter splint. This splint maintains MCP joint flexion and allows protected but full active IP flexion and extension (Fig. 13-16).[20]
- **Head fractures:** If joint involvement is less than 20%, these fractures are treated with closed reduction and internal fixation. The involved digit is immobilized in a protective radial or ulnar gutter splint (see Fig. 13-16) or a cast for 3 weeks with the wrist in 0 to 20 degrees of extension, the MCPs in 90 degrees of flexion, and the IP joints in 0 degrees of extension.[20] An adjacent finger is included for comfort and to increase stability. ORIF is indicated if more than 20% of the articular surface is involved. Because

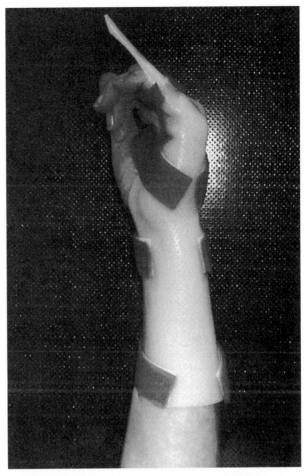

FIGURE 13-16 A safe position ulnar or radial gutter splint for metacarpal neck fractures. This splint maintains MCP joint flexion and allows protected but full active IP flexion and extension within the splint. (From McNemar T, Howell J, Chang E: *J Hand Ther* 16:148, 2003.)

access to the injured joint may require a longitudinal incision in the extensor tendon, it is very important to start motion almost immediately after surgery to prevent tendon and capsular adhesions and to ensure full AROM of the MCP joint.

- **Bennett's fracture-dislocation of the thumb metacarpal:** Closed reduction with percutaneous pinning frequently is the treatment of choice for these injuries.[20] Clients are immobilized for 6 weeks in a short arm thumb spica cast or splint with the thumb IP joint included. After 2 to 3 weeks, the surgeon may allow controlled AROM of the thumb IP joint, but resistance is deferred until there is evidence of stable fracture healing. If the thumb metacarpal is treated with rigid internal fixation, controlled assisted ROM of the thumb and wrist usually is allowed after only 1 week of immobilization, but again resistance is avoided until there is evidence of stable fracture healing.

NONOPERATIVE TREATMENT

Early therapeutic management of most types of metacarpal fractures is similar regardless of the fracture's location. Immobilization with a splint or cast is necessary to allow healing, and the risk of joint contractures can be minimized by using a position of 70 to 90 degrees of MCP flexion, 0 degrees of IP extension, and 20 degrees of wrist extension. When the thumb is splinted for a first metacarpal fracture, it is important to preserve the thumb-index web space and to include the IP joint of the thumb initially, until the physician indicates that enough healing has occurred at the fracture site to allow controlled active IP joint motion. All splints should be carefully molded to incorporate and maintain the longitudinal and transverse arches of the hand.

During this early phase of healing, the client should be instructed in AROM of all uninvolved joints that are not splinted or casted. Dorsal hand edema usually is pronounced with these fractures, and interventions such as manual edema mobilization (MEM), gentle retrograde massage, elevation, and active finger exercises should be instituted as soon as possible. If percutaneous pinning is used, the client must be instructed in pin care (see pin care instructions in the section on distal radial fractures).

- **Closed reduction:** Controlled AROM of the wrist and MCP joints can begin when the physician determines that stability at the fracture site is adequate (typically between 3 and 5 weeks after injury). Intermittent splinting with a removable hand-based protective splint to protect the healing metacarpal should continue between exercise sessions for approximately 2 more weeks. Gentle PROM can be added gradually with the goal of regaining MCP joint ROM, but forceful resistance exercises are withheld until the physician determines that adequate healing has occurred at the fracture site (typically 6 to 8 weeks after injury).[11,20,21]

  Dorsal edema often is a continuing problem for clients with a metacarpal fracture. After the cast or full-time splint is removed, a compressive glove or sleeve can be used to manage chronic edema. Although tendon adherence to the metacarpal is an unusual complication,[21] all tissues can adhere to each other given the right environment (e.g., prolonged and chronic swelling). Clients should be encouraged to exercise hourly, performing isolated extensor digitorum exercises (e.g., "make a claw") and composite flexion, tendon gliding, and independent MCP joint flexion exercises (e.g., "tabletop" or "duck bill" position). Splinting the hand at night in a safe intrinsic plus position may prevent the development of "claw posture," which is seen with shortening of the collateral ligaments and intrinsic muscles of the MCP joint. If a contracture of the thenar web space develops after a thumb metacarpal fracture, a night web stretcher splint may be helpful.

- **ORIF:** Metacarpal fractures that are rigidly stabilized can be remobilized at 24 to 72 hours after surgery. Initial considerations are edema control and AROM and PROM exercises. The exercise program after rigid fixation of a digit metacarpal should include isolated extensor digitorum exercises ("make a claw") and composite flexion, tendon gliding, and independent MCP joint flexion exercises ("tabletop" or "duck bill" position). An exercise program after rigid fixation of the thumb metacarpal should include AROM and PROM exercises to regain wrist and thumb motion. Instruct the client in composite thumb flexion and extension exercises, opposition, and thumb palmar and radial abduction exercises to stretch the thenar web space. A hand-based opponens splint can be used to provide additional intermittent support during the final phase of healing and until functional thumb muscle strength returns.

  If dorsal scarring presents a problem, a silicone elastomer insert may be applied within a splint and scar mobilization techniques can be initiated by 2 weeks after surgery (i.e., once the sutures have been removed and healing is complete).

Questions to Ask the Physician

- *Where is the fracture located (i.e., base, shaft, neck, head)?*
- *What type of fracture is it (i.e., comminuted, displaced or nondisplaced, intraarticular or extraarticular, transverse, oblique)?*
- *How stable is the fracture fragment (or fragments)?*
- *With surgical stabilization: Did a tendon or ligament injury (or injuries) occur that needs to be considered in the therapy program?*
- *Did other associated soft tissue injuries occur?*
- *When can controlled AROM of the MCP joints begin? Are there any restrictions on the initiation of AROM of the IP joints?*
- *When can strengthening exercises begin?*

What to Say to Clients

About the Injury

"Here is a diagram of the bones of the hand and fingers. You fractured this bone. As a result, your physician chose

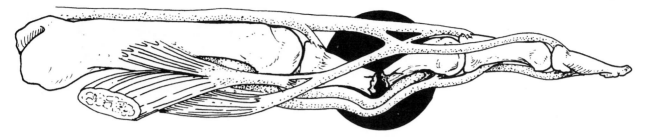

FIGURE 13-17 Fractures of the proximal phalangeal shaft typically have an apex palmar angulation, with the fracture gap appearing wider when viewed volarly and seeming compressed when viewed dorsally. This appearance is produced by the deforming forces of the intrinsic muscles. (From Purdy BA, Wilson RL: Management of nonarticular fractures of the hand. In Mackin EJ, Callahan AD, Skirven TM et al, editors: *Rehabilitation of the hand and upper extremity,* ed 5, St Louis, 2002, Mosby.)

the injured bone forms callus. Oblique fractures can cause digital rotation or scissoring, such that the injured digit overlaps with adjacent fingers when flexing. For these reasons and others, P-1 fractures are considered difficult to treat.[10]

Timelines and Healing

- Most closed, nondisplaced P-1 shaft fractures are stable, and buddy-taping or splinting the digit to an adjacent uninvolved digit for 4 weeks is sufficient treatment.[24]
- If the fracture is nondisplaced but unstable, treatment usually involves a hand-based static splint with the MCP joints in 50 to 70 degrees of flexion and the PIP and DIP joints in 0 degrees of flexion to minimize contracture.[24]
- Minimally displaced fractures are often treated with manual reduction and Kirschner wire (K-wire) stabilization for 3 to 4 weeks.
- If a fracture requires internal fixation (e.g., because of associated soft tissue damage that must be surgically repaired, fracture comminution, bone loss, or rotational deformity), rigid fixation is needed to allow early controlled AROM and successful rehabilitation.

Nonoperative Treatment

- Simple, nondisplaced, stable P-1 fractures treated with buddy taping are allowed immediate, gentle progressive AROM exercises. Edema control measures should be initiated during the first therapy session.
- Simple phalangeal fractures treated nonoperatively with a static splint usually are healed enough to allow gentle (pain free) progressive AROM exercises by 4

weeks after injury or sooner.[24] Fracture callus calcification should be apparent on x-ray films (as determined by the physician) before strengthening exercises are introduced.

- With P-1 fractures treated with K-wire fixation, AROM exercises are begun about 3 to 4 weeks after reduction. The exercises are performed six to eight times a day in short sessions. Emphasis is placed on composite flexion and extension of the digits, isolated blocking of the FDS and FDP, and gentle passive positioning of the MCP joint of the involved digit in flexion with active extension of the PIP joint. A hand-based safe position splint that includes the involved digit and an adjacent digit is fitted for wear between exercise sessions and at night. Edema control measures should be instituted using appropriate massage and compression wraps (e.g., 1-inch Coban). Scar massage should address subcutaneous adhesions that may have developed at the pin sites. When the fracture has clinically healed, as determined by the physician, PROM and dynamic splinting may begin, typically about 6 to 7 weeks after reduction. Strengthening exercises must wait until the physician determines that the fracture is well healed; this often has occurred by approximately 8 weeks after reduction.[11]
- With P-1 fractures treated with open reduction and rigid fixation, introduction of active and gentle passive ROM exercises should be possible by 24 to 72 hours after surgery.[11] Exercises can be done hourly and should focus on composite active and active assistive flexion and extension of the digits, isolated blocking of the PIP and DIP joints, and positioning of the MCP joint in flexion while attempting IP joint extension. Edema control should be initiated using a light compressive dressing (e.g., Coban). A hand-based splint that holds the MCP joints in 70 degrees

of flexion and the IP joints in 0 degrees of flexion should be worn between exercise sessions and at night for about 8 weeks after surgery.[11] If more than one digit is involved, a forearm-based splint that incorporates the above positions should be provided. Within 24 to 48 hours after suture removal, scar massage can begin and a topical scar compression dressing can be introduced to address scar cosmesis. The introduction of dynamic splinting to address residual joint contractures and the initiation of strengthening exercises are determined by the physician.

Tips from the Field

CLINICAL *Pearl*

Two major causes account for most cases of PIP joint extensor lag after a proximal phalanx fracture: (1) soft tissue adhesions between the extensor mechanism and the fracture site and (2) persistent skeletal deformity, such as shortening of the bone with consequent redundancy of the extensor mechanism.[24]

The therapist can address soft tissue adhesions with a program of blocked PIP extension exercises (see previous discussion), scar massage, and treatments such as ultrasound. Ultrasound can be used as a thermal agent to increase the tissue temperature of tendons, ligaments, joint capsules, and scar tissue. Once heated, these structures demonstrate increased tissue extensibility. Redundancy of the extensor mechanism secondary to shortening of the proximal phalanx after a fracture results in an extensor lag that is not amenable to therapeutic intervention.

• The recovery of digital motion is perhaps the most important determinant of final functional outcome in all hand fractures. Waiting as long as 4 weeks to begin AROM can make this goal more difficult to achieve. For fractures requiring more than buddy strap support, Freeland and colleagues[24] recommend using a functional positional splint (Fig. 13-18) rather than a circumferential cast or splint for all but displaced P-1 fractures that remain unstable after closed reduction. This splint has the advantage of allowing early controlled motion starting 6 to 7 days after immobilization. (The initial immobilization period is needed to allow the acute inflammatory response to resolve and to permit the injured site to develop a modicum of fibroblastic activity, which is necessary for developing wound strength). The splint places the

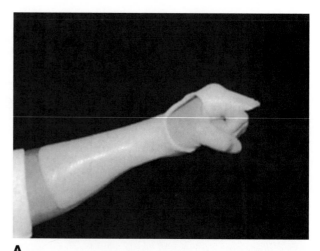

A

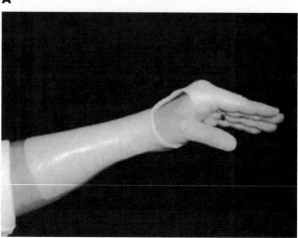

B

FIGURE 13-18   Short arm functional position splint for closed-reduced, stable proximal phalangeal fractures that require more than buddy taping. The metacarpal is blocked in flexion to maximize active extension of the PIP joint. A volar component can be added at night to maintain IP joint extension when the client is resting. (From Freeland A, Hardy M, Singletary S: *J Hand Ther* 16:137, 2003.)

wrist in slight flexion to increase tension in the extensor mechanism and simultaneously relax the tension engendered by the flexor tendons. The splint is a forearm-based model initially and then is reduced to a hand-based splint after about 3 weeks. The MCP joint is placed in flexion, and a dorsal block keeps the extensor tendon tension focused at the PIP joint while preventing hyperextension at the MCP joint during extensor tendon gliding exercises. A volar component can be added for night use to maintain IP joint extension and to reduce the risk of a PIP flexion contracture. As with any new protocol, the referring physician must approve its use and must write a prescription stating this.

- Dynamic splinting and serial casting may be used when active exercises are insufficient for recovering joint motion. A flexion loop splint composed of a loop of pajama elastic works well for regaining passive IP flexion. Clients should be advised to wear this loop no longer than 5 to 10 minutes at a time and to use a gentle tension, because the amount of force exerted can damage the IP joints if left on too long. Serial casting works best for PIP joint flexion contractures with a hard end-feel (Fig. 13-19). A few finger-based, dynamic PIP splints are commercially available that work well for PIP joint flexion contractures of 30 degrees or less (Fig. 13-20).

MIDDLE PHALANGEAL (P-2) FRACTURES

Diagnosis and Pathology

Nonarticular middle phalangeal fractures are rare, occurring most often in sports-related injuries and machinery accidents.[22] These bones are broader, shorter, and there-

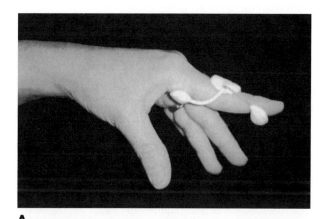

A

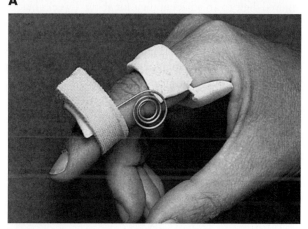

B

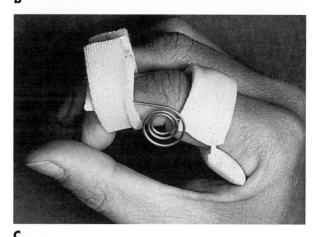

C

FIGURE 13-20 Commercially available dynamic PIP extension splints that can be used for PIP flexion contractures. **A,** A finger-based, prefabricated splint that allows PIP joint flexion. **B,** A Capener splint, which permits active flexion while providing a dynamic extension force. (**A** from Freeland A, Hardy M, Singletary S: *J Hand Ther* 16:138, 2003; **B** from Campbell PJ, Wilson RL: Management of joint injuries and intraarticular fractures. In Mackin EJ, Callahan AD, Skirven TM et al, editors: *Rehabilitation of the hand and upper extremity*, ed 5, St Louis, 2002, Mosby.)

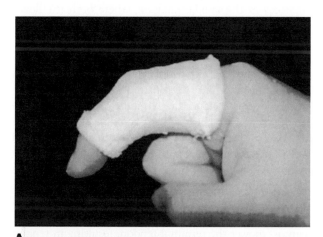

A

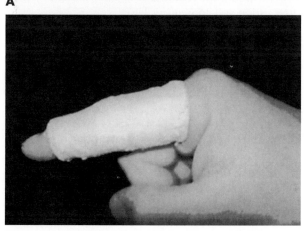

B

FIGURE 13-19 Serial casting for PIP flexion contractures with a hard end-feel. (From Freeland A, Hardy M, Singletary S: *J Hand Ther* 16:138, 2003.)

fore stronger than their neighbors, the proximal phalanges and metacarpals. Concomitant soft tissue injury at the PIP joint is common with these fractures. Typically, the more vulnerable PIP joint capsule or its ligaments (or both) deform or fail before the bone fractures.[22] Fractures of the middle phalanx may deform or angulate in response to the pull of the FDS insertion, the pull of the central slip insertion, or to both of these working in concert.

Timelines and Healing

Nondisplaced and closed reduced middle phalangeal fractures are stable and require only buddy taping of the injured digit to an adjacent digit for about 3 weeks before unrestricted motion can be resumed.[22] These fractures require little, if any, hand therapy.

Displaced fractures that can be reduced and stabilized without internal fixation typically are immobilized for 3 to 4 weeks to allow fracture consolidation before AROM exercises are permitted. An unstable middle phalangeal fracture may require either percutaneous fixation after reduction or ORIF. Some of these fractures remain unstable even with some type of fixation, and the physician may decide that early AROM is not possible without risking malunion or nonunion at the fracture site.[22] These unstable fractures are immobilized for 3 to 6 weeks, depending on the location of the fracture (i.e., the shaft versus the neck of the bone).

Nonoperative Treatment

A displaced fracture that can be reduced and stabilized without internal fixation is immobilized in a cast or splint with the wrist in slight extension (20 degrees), the MCP joints at 70 to 90 degrees of flexion, and the PIP and DIP joints in full extension. Some physicians may request a hand-based splint that leaves the wrist free and incorporates an adjacent digit into the splint for comfort and additional protection of the fracture. Although the IP joints may show early stiffness once active ROM is allowed, splinting these joints in extension early on minimizes the risk of a more difficult problem, namely, an extensor lag or a PIP joint contracture.

Once AROM of the MCP and IP joints is allowed (about 3 to 4 weeks after injury), the emphasis in therapy should be on restoring composite finger flexion. Blocking exercises can be introduced gradually to encourage flexor tendon pull-through at the IP joints. A hand-based protective splint often is worn between exercise sessions for about 2 weeks. The client can use this splint at night to address a residual extensor lag by resting the joint and the terminal tendon in extension. PROM and dynamic splinting (if necessary) usually can be introduced by 6 weeks after injury, depending on fracture healing.[11,22]

Unstable fractures that require ORIF with K-wire fixation may need to be immobilized for 3 to 6 weeks to allow healing. These fractures present a challenge to the therapist once AROM is allowed. The soft tissue structures along the middle phalanx become adherent to the bone, adversely affecting flexor tendon gliding and terminal extensor tendon gliding. Exercises should focus on isolating the extensor and flexor tendons. To isolate the terminal extensor tendon, instruct the client to flex or bend the MCP joint while trying to straighten the IP joints. Using a finger from the uninvolved hand, the client can provide gentle resistance over the dorsal PIP joint to shunt the force of the extensor mechanism to the DIP joint, thus isolating the terminal extensor tendon. Blocked DIP flexion exercises isolate the FDP tendon.

Tips from the Field

To achieve an excellent outcome for middle phalangeal fractures, therapists must understand the complex anatomy at the middle phalanx, where both the flexor and extensor tendons share an intimate relationship with this bone. Complications include limited tendon gliding, decreased joint mobility, and the development of an imbalance in the extensor mechanism, resulting in a swan neck deformity (hyperextension of the PIP joint and an extensor lag at the DIP joint).[22]

If an extensor lag at the DIP joint develops, try using a night DIP joint extension splint to rest the tendon and the joint capsule in extension. Remember that the terminal tendon is paper thin at this level and may require intermittent splinting to prevent overstretching by the stronger FDP. Resistive DIP exercises, such as with putty, should not be used because the resistance of the putty can overpower the terminal tendon, resulting in tendon attenuation and consequent lag.

If DIP flexion is not full, work on gentle passive flexion of the joint by using dynamic splinting or Coban. If the joint is passively supple, active DIP flexion exercises can be emphasized, using blocking motions and putty. Full, active DIP flexion is necessary for grip strength.

DISTAL PHALANGEAL (P-3) FRACTURES
Diagnosis and Pathology

Distal phalangeal fractures occur more often than other hand fractures because the fingertips are exposed to more trauma than other parts of the hand.[10] The long finger is the most frequently involved digit, followed by the thumb.[10,22] Intraarticular fractures typically involve the dorsal lip of the base of the bone and, if associated with avulsion of the terminal insertion of the extensor tendon, result in a **bony mallet injury.** Common mechanisms of injury for distal phalangeal fractures include jamming of the finger and crush injuries. In young children, getting a finger caught between two objects (e.g., in a door) is the most common cause of injury; in children over 9 years of age, sports-related injuries are the typical cause; in adults, industrial accidents and crush injuries are the most common causes.[22] Concurrent soft tissue injuries often seen with this fracture include nail bed injuries, dorsal skin lacerations, and hematomas.[10] Complications include nail bed deformities and prolonged pain and hypersensitivity secondary to irritation of the nerve endings in the finger pulp.

Timelines and Healing

A bony mallet injury requires ORIF if subluxation of the distal phalanx palmarly has occurred, if the bony fragment has displaced proximally to a significant degree, or if more than one third of the joint surface is involved.[13] Comminuted fractures may be treated with percutaneous K-wire stabilization, placed across the DIP joint to immobilize it.

Nonoperative Treatment

Fractures of the tuft of the distal phalanx that are uncomplicated by nail bed injuries and that do not require internal fixation typically heal without residual problems. Provision of a protective cap splint and instructions in edema control and desensitization often are adequate. Hypersensitivity related to crush injuries and resultant distal phalangeal fracture may continue for 3 to 4 months after injury.[11]

With internal fixation of a distal phalangeal fracture, the goals of therapy during the first 6 postoperative weeks are as follows:

- Edema control with Coban
- AROM and gentle PROM for the uninvolved joints
- If pins were used: pin care per the physician's preferences to prevent a pin tract infection
- Use of a protective tip splint, fitted for continual wear

When the fracture has consolidated (about 3 weeks after surgery) or, with terminal extensor tendon involvement, once the tendon has healed adequately (about 6 weeks after surgery), the pin is removed and treatment progresses as follows:

- AROM exercises and gentle blocking exercises for the DIP joint
- Desensitization to address persistent fingertip pain

- Continued use of the tip protector splint for protection and pain management as needed

Typically, PROM and grip strengthening, if needed, can begin 1 to 2 weeks after AROM is initiated. The tip protector splint is discontinued about 4 to 6 weeks after surgery if there was no tendon involvement and about 10 to 12 weeks after surgery if tendon involvement was a factor. The tip protector splint can be gradually discontinued when no more than 10 degrees of extensor lag is present at the DIP joint following use of the involved hand with the client's normal activities.

Tips from the Field

- **Protective splinting of the distal phalanx and DIP joint:** Various custom-made splint designs immobilize the DIP joint and protect the distal phalanx during fracture healing. The keys to splinting this area successfully are (1) to make sure the splint does not inadvertently slide off during PIP joint flexion or during sleep and (2) to minimize splint pressure over the dorsal DIP joint. Securing the splint with Coban or paper tape may solve the first problem. A sugar tong splint design or a circumferential splint design (with access on the lateral aspect of the splint) ensures that the surface pressure from the splint is distributed equally across the dorsal aspect of this bone. Instruct the client to perform daily skin inspection and to inform the therapist immediately of any reddened or ulcerated areas. A $^3/_{32}$-inch, perforated splint material is a good choice because it allows the skin to breathe and typically is dense enough to protect the healing fracture.
- **Bony mallet injury**
  - An extensor lag of less than 10 degrees is the goal of therapy. The DIP joint often is stiff when the protective splint is removed and AROM is initiated.

Precaution. *It is important to increase active DIP flexion gradually, because overzealous efforts tend to result in a significant extensor lag.*

Remember that the FDP is stronger than the terminal portion of the extensor tendon and that the FDP typically can and does overcome its weaker counterpart, given time. Strengthening exercises for grip should be performed only if grip strength has been compromised. Do not attempt isotonic strengthening exercises for the terminal extensor tendon; isometric exercises should be adequate. Instruct the client to block the MCP and PIP joints in flexion and to attempt extension of the DIP joint, holding for an 8 second count. Short sessions of this exercise repeated hourly are most beneficial for regaining terminal extensor tendon strength. Inform the physician if an extensor lag greater than 10 degrees develops after initiation of AROM and discontinuation of the protective tip splint. It may be helpful to try having the client resume wearing the protective splint at night when sleeping and, if necessary, for short periods during the day. Slowly wean the client from this splint over 2 to 3 weeks.

- Watch for hyperextensible PIP joints, which may indicate an imbalance of the extensor mechanism and a propensity for developing a swan neck deformity. Inform the physician of your concern. If the physician agrees, you might fabricate a finger-based splint that immobilizes the DIP joint in 0 degrees of extension, blocks the PIP joint from hyperextension with a dorsal hood, and allows full PIP joint flexion.

PROXIMAL INTERPHALANGEAL JOINT FRACTURES AND DISLOCATIONS

Diagnosis and Pathology

PIP joint injuries range from mild sprains to unstable, irreducible fracture-dislocations. Fracture-dislocations are caused by axial compression on a semiflexed or hyperextended digit[26]; this typically results in dorsal dislocation of the middle phalanx in relation to the proximal phalanx. Less often, volar dislocation occurs, with the middle phalanx moving volarly in relation to the proximal phalanx. These injuries manifest clinically as a **boutonniere deformity,** with interruption of the central slip of the digital extensor tendon, flexion of the PIP joint, and hyperextension of the DIP joint.[26]

Timelines and Healing

If less than 30% of the articular surface is involved, the fracture is considered stable and managed with closed reduction techniques.[26] If more than 30% of the articular surface is damaged, the fracture usually is unstable and requires management with some type of ORIF technique.

Nonoperative Treatment

Treatment of nondisplaced fractures requires splint immobilization (with the PIP joint in full extension) for 2 to 3 weeks,[27] followed by a program of controlled AROM. The finger-based extension splint is worn between exercise sessions for several more weeks. PROM typically is not initiated until 6 weeks after the injury.

Stable hyperextension and dorsal dislocation injuries of the PIP joint are treated with a dorsal block splint or cast, sometimes with the injured digit buddy taped within the splint to an adjacent digit for 3 to 6 weeks.[10,25] The PIP joint should be allowed full flexion and arrested at −20 to −45 degrees of full extension, depending on the relative stability of the joint.[10,25,27] Edema control measures should be introduced during the first therapy session. Hourly ROM exercises within the dorsal block splint should be performed. Motion at the PIP joint encourages gliding of the joint capsule and excursion of the extensor mechanism and promotes joint homeostasis. Instruct the client in active DIP joint blocking exercises to encourage the FDP to glide past the location of injury rather than become tethered at this site. When the acute risk of redislocation has resolved, the injured digit may be given additional protection, either by buddy-taping the digit to an adjacent digit for several more weeks or by adjusting the dorsal block splint gradually into full extension over 3 weeks. At the point when the physician determines that the PIP joint has healed enough to allow unrestrained extension and the splint has been discontinued, a PIP joint flexion contraction often is seen. Static progressive or serial static splinting of the joint should be considered to address this problem.[25]

Open reduction and ligament repair are indicated if the joint is unstable. Surgical intervention involves stabilizing the joint and preventing redislocation, often by advancing the volar plate ligament into the articular surface of the middle phalanx. A pull-out wire secured to a button on the dorsum of the middle phalanx may be used to stabilize the newly repaired joint surgically, maintaining it in 30 degrees or more of flexion during the early healing phase.[10,25] These clients often wear a bulky cast or dressing for 3 weeks. After the wire and button are removed, the client is placed in a dorsal blocking splint for the next 2 weeks. Hourly AROM and PROM exercises of the PIP joint within the splint are encouraged, and edema management techniques are introduced. At 5 weeks after surgery, most clients can move to an interim extension gutter splint, which can be serially adjusted as PIP joint extension improves. During the fifth through eighth weeks after surgery, therapy should focus on regaining full PIP motion. Dynamic extension splinting often can be initiated by the sixth to eighth week, as determined by the physician. Gentle progressive strengthening frequently can be initiated by the eighth postoperative week.[10] What to Ask the Physician: what to Say to Clients, Evaluation Tips, Diagnosis-Specific Information That Affects Clinical Reasoning; Tips from the Field; and Precautions and Concerns.

Tips from the Field

With any joint injury, the focus of rehabilitation is to begin ROM as soon as possible. Remember, motion is lotion to the joint. Also, the articular cartilage is avascular and has no nerve supply, therefore it depends on motion for health. For these reasons, regular communication between the physician and therapist on a client-by-client basis is a must!

• Clients often have pain that limits functional grasp after a fracture or fracture-dislocation of the PIP joint. Encourage functional grasp by enlarging the handle of the client's toothbrush, hairbrush, razor, fork, and spoon with rubber tubing whenever possible. Encourage hourly exercises, avoiding pain. Paraffin is a great means of easing joint pain and is readily available to the public.

• If the joint can be reduced and remains stable, a finger-based, figure 8 splint (Fig. 13-21) usually is adequate for blocking PIP joint extension while allowing full flexion.

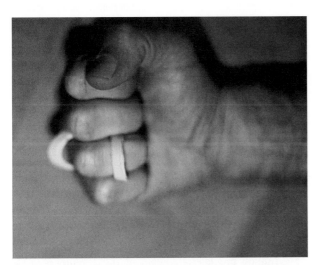

A

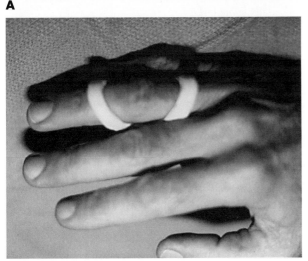

B

FIGURE 13-21 Figure 8 splint used to block full PIP extension but allow full flexion. (From Campbell PJ, Wilson RL: Management of joint injuries and intraarticular fractures. In Mackin EJ, Callahan AD, Skirven TM et al, editors: *Rehabilitation of the hand and upper extremity*, ed 5, St Louis, 2002, Mosby.)

• A residual flexion contracture is a common complication after a PIP joint dorsal fracture-dislocation. Don't confuse this with a boutonniere deformity. The extensor tendon has not been injured, and the DIP joint remains flexible. For flexion contractures with a hard end-feel, serial casting of the PIP joint tends to correct this issue more efficiently than static progressive or dynamic splinting.

DIAGNOSIS-SPECIFIC INFORMATION THAT AFFECTS CLINICAL REASONING

• Base and head/neck fractures permit AROM and subsequently PROM earlier than midshaft fractures, because fractures in cancellous bone heal faster than fractures in cortical bone. Generally, midshaft fractures heal in 6 to 8 weeks, and base and head/neck fractures heal in 3 to 4 weeks.[11] Controlled active motion often can start before clinical healing is evident. Determining when the fracture is clinically healed to the point of tolerating passive stress or resistance is always a decision made by the physician.

• Helpful information for the therapist includes the location of the fracture and whether the joint is involved.

CLINICAL *Pearl*

If the fracture occurs at the base of the phalanx, greater effort will probably be needed to regain motion at the joint just proximal to the fracture. If the fracture occurs at the head or neck, the joint just distal to the fracture will require more intensive therapy.

• Fractures of the digit typically result in significant swelling. Edema can produce predictable patterns of deformity, such as a swollen, moderately flexed PIP joint with an extended DIP joint. Early edema control measures (e.g., joint positioning using protective splinting, elastic bandaging) can mitigate pain associated with a distended joint and prevent the development of a fixed, contracted joint.

Precautions and Concerns

• *Do not attempt isotonic strengthening exercises (as with putty) for the terminal extensor tendon. Isometric exercises should be adequate.*

- *To prevent pin tract infection, the client should clean each percutaneous pin daily with a separate cotton-tip applicator, according to the physician's preferences.*
- *If the fracture is stabilized with one or more percutaneous pins that are not flush with the skin, advise the client to be careful not to inadvertently pull out the pin by getting it caught in a towel or blanket.*
- *It is important not to sacrifice PIP extension to gain full PIP flexion. An extensor lag greater than 25 to 30 degrees presents a functional limitation for most clients.[11] An extension assist splint (see Fig. 13-20) is a good choice for addressing PIP joint stiffness, because the client can flex the PIP joint while it is in the splint, and the splint holds the joint in extension when at rest.*
- *The development of an extensor lag at the DIP joint is a common complication of either a bony mallet injury or a middle phalangeal fracture, especially as passive tension is introduced to the terminal tendon and the oblique retinacular ligament.[22] To help minimize the development of a lag, avoid isolated passive flexion of the DIP while the PIP joint is extended. Instead, once passive ROM exercises are initiated, emphasize composite flexion and extension of the digit.*

Questions to Ask the Physician

- *What type of fracture is it and where is it located?*
- *What method of fracture reduction was used?*
- *Was internal fixation used to maintain the fracture reduction? If so, what type was used and does it cross a joint?*
- *How stable is the fracture? Could motion cause the fracture fragments to displace?*
- *What soft tissue structures are involved or compromised?*
- *When can AROM of the joints immobilized by the splint or cast begin?*
- *With bony mallet injuries and PIP joint fracture-dislocations: Should a specific protocol be followed in beginning mobilization of the involved joint?*
- *When can passive stress at or near the fracture site begin? When can strengthening exercises begin?*

EVALUATION TIPS

- Ask the client about the history of the injury, including when and how it happened, and about any previous treatment. The goal is to recognize all the injured structures, whether bony or soft tissue.
- Inspect the involved digit for swelling and document the amount (using a circumference gauge) and location. Remember to document the circumference of the contralateral digit at the same time for comparison.

- Gently palpate the digit and note areas of tenderness.
- Note whether any lateral instability is evident at the PIP or DIP joint during active flexion and extension of the finger. Also note any scissoring of the digit.
- Check for and document any hypermobility or lateral laxity of other uninvolved digits.
- Check and document composite flexion of the uninvolved digits and the involved digit.
- Document isolated active and passive joint digit extension, then active extension potential at the IP joints when you block the MCP joint in flexion and ask the client to actively extend the IP joints.

What to Say to Clients

See the sections earlier in the chapter on metacarpal fractures.

The Roles of the Therapy Assistant

- *Edema management*
- *Splinting (fabrication based on experience level), instructions on application and wear and care guidelines, and modifications as necessary*
- *Home exercise instruction*
- *Assisting with pin care and/or wound care*
- *Supervising and modifying exercises as established by the therapist*
- *Training in adaptive equipment and activities of daily living (ADL)*
- *Reinforcing precautions as determined by the therapist*

CASE *Studies*

CASE 13-1

N.D. is a 37-year-old, right-hand dominant (RHD) female who sustained significant injuries when her motor scooter crashed while she was on vacation in Bermuda. She was flown back to the United States so that her internal injuries could be addressed. Once her condition stabilized, she underwent surgery to rebreak and correctly set a left distal radial fracture. An external fixator was applied to keep the fracture correctly aligned and reduced. She was seen at an outpatient hand therapy clinic once a week for the first 6 weeks, until the external fixator was removed, for treatment of edema; ROM of the digits, thumb, elbow, and shoulder; and pain management. Gentle active forearm rotation also was allowed at this time. Early in her therapy, an ulnar wrist splint was fabricated to support the ulnar carpus and to provide some pain relief. N.D. was instructed in pin care, light retrograde massage, tendon gliding exercises, composite fisting, and thumb opposition within her comfort range during this time.

After the external fixator was removed, N.D. was seen two or three times a week for 12 weeks to address ROM limitations, edema control, scar management, pain management, and strength and endurance issues related to her goals of returning to work as a waitress and returning to playing weekend golf with her husband.

At her first visit after removal of the external fixator, N.D. initially was tearful, reporting a fear of "hospitals and doctors" and stating that she believed she would "never be able to play golf again!" She rated her pain over the past week as 5/10 at its lowest level and 7/10 at its worst. The pain was worst at the end of the day and at night when she was trying to sleep. She had decreased AROM of the wrist (flexion = 25 degrees, extension = 30 degrees) and the forearm (pronation = 35 degrees, supination = 10 degrees). Her PRWE score was 92. (The worst possible score on the PRWE is 100). She reported some hypersensitivity in the area of the pin sites. Light touch sensibility testing showed diminished light touch (3.22 to 3.61) along the dorsal radial sensory nerve distribution but normal sensation otherwise. N.D. reported episodic "hand numbness," especially at night. When questioned closely, she reported that the numbness was worse in her thumb and index finger.

Initial therapy sessions addressed pain and scar hypersensitivity with treatments such as fluidotherapy. Soft tissue massage addressed scar adhesions and sensitivity and the persistent edema so often seen after this type of fracture. N.D. was instructed to continue tendon glide exercises and composite fisting and thumb opposition exercises. Additional active exercises included wrist AROM and specific exercises to address forearm rotation. Because N.D. was RHD and the injury was to the left side, the therapist gave her specific functional tasks to try at home, including folding the laundry and using a built-up fork to stabilize her meat while she cut it with her right hand. She was also given median nerve gliding exercises to do, along with specific cautions to pay attention to her body's response to these nerve exercises.

By 4½ weeks after removal of the external fixator, N.D. demonstrated increased functional use of her left hand, reporting that she used it to wash her hair and to button her clothing. However, she noted continued difficulties with forceful gripping, reporting trouble pulling up her jeans and carrying a grocery bag in that arm. Grip

strength on the dynamometer (position 2, right/left) was 45 lb/4 lb. Three-jaw pinch strength (right/left) was 13 lb/2.5 lb. She reported supination as the motion most functionally limiting, because she could not turn her palm up enough to receive money, a task she would need to perform once she returned to work as a waitress. (Active supination had increased from 10 to 20 degrees, pronation had increased from 35 to 45 degrees). The therapist contacted the physician, requesting orders to begin strengthening and for a dynamic supination splint.

When the orders were received, N.D. was fitted with a prefabricated dynamic supination splint to use at home. She was told to build up her wearing tolerance gradually to several hours at a time; once this level was reached, she could use the splint while sleeping. She was started on a light upper extremity strengthening program in the clinic, using free weights, the BTE machine, and Nautilus equipment. She brought in a golf club and practiced chipping using plastic golf balls. Within a week, she began complaining of increasing left thumb pain. Palpation over the dorsal wrist at Lister's tubercle provoked her symptoms, as did active and resisted thumb IP motion. All resistive exercises were stopped, and the physician was informed of this development. The physician agreed that N.D. had developed EPL tendonitis and that she should use an interim neoprene thumb spica splint with a removable metal or plastic stay. Also, strengthening exercises were halted until the symptoms resolved. N.D. was allowed to continue with the dynamic supination splint and AROM exercises.

N.D. was discouraged by this setback. Discussions in the clinic made it clear that N.D. had been "going to town" with her strengthening exercises and her determination to resume all preinjury activities. The therapist coached N.D. on soft tissue tolerances and on the likely repercussions of pushing through or ignoring pain. During this time N.D. appeared depressed and missed a number of her scheduled appointments. She admitted to not sleeping well and reported anxiety about returning to work and about the "mountain of bills we've accumulated."

N.D.'s pain subsided within 2 weeks, and she was able to resume a light strengthening program. A week and a half later, she returned to work on modified duty, working fewer shifts per week than she normally would and taking the less busy shifts. At the therapist's encouragement, she made sure she had a busboy available to clear her tables. Her successful return to even this modified schedule alleviated much of N.D.'s anxiety about her future capabilities. Eight weeks after removal of the external fixator, N.D.'s AROM was as follows: pronation, −45 degrees; supination, −55 degrees; wrist flexion, 37 degrees; and wrist extension, 60 degrees. Her PRWE score was 45. Although supination was significantly improved, N.D.

reported difficulty and radial wrist pain when she attempted to supinate her forearm while carrying a weight (e.g., a plate or tray) in her left hand. Left hand grip strength was 15 lb on the Jaymar dynamometer. The left hand weakness was most evident after N.D. worked a shift, because she reported an inability to use that hand for much at home afterward. She reported generalized left arm fatigue, and she feared reinjuring her hand if she tried playing golf. Left thumb pain returned periodically, and this concerned her. She was encouraged to use the neoprene splint at work to provide some light thumb and wrist protection when lifting the heavy plates. She was reminded not to do strengthening exercises on the same days she worked a busy shift.

N.D. continued her supervised therapy for another month. On the last day of scheduled therapy, N.D. reported, "I did a double shift yesterday; I feel ready to be discharged from therapy." At this point her AROM was as follows: supination, −65 degrees; pronation, 50 degrees; wrist flexion, 55 degrees; extension, 75 degrees. Her PRWE score was 16, and she reported minimal episodes of pain and stiffness, which she associated with "overdoing it." She had been gradually weaning from the dynamic supination splint and had not lost supination motion. She had not resumed playing golf; she reported that she would wait until next summer to do this.

N.D. returned to visit the clinic a little over a year after she started therapy. She proudly showed off her first-place golf trophy, stating, "I never thought I'd play again, and look at this!"

CASE 13-2

E.O. is a 76-year-old, right-hand dominant male who fractured the proximal phalanx of his right small finger in a fall. Two percutaneous pins were placed. He has a history of osteoarthritis and has had a previous stroke, although he has no residual upper extremity (UE) problems related to the stroke. He mentioned at the initial evaluation that he was "forgetful." He was sent to hand therapy when the pins were removed.

E.O.'s goal for therapy was to be able to make a better fist so that he could drive again. E.O. initially had moderate edema of the right hand, particularly the small finger. He had limited composite active flexion of all digits and lacked 2 to 3 cm to the distal palmar crease for the index, long, and ring fingers actively. He had marked stiffness of the small finger. His AROM values were MP, 0-35; PIP, 0-0; DIP 0-10. Gentle assessment of PROM revealed MP, 0-50; PIP 0-10; and DIP 0-15.

E.O. was started on edema control with proximal AROM and Coban wrap. AROM was begun, including tendon gliding and gentle blocking exercises of all digits, as well as functional and coordination activities that promoted fisting and opposition to all fingers. A small finger cylinder was made to isolate MP flexion and extension AROM. A DIP cap also was made to promote isolated PIP flexion AROM. Gentle place and hold fisting exercises were performed. An MP block was provided to promote isolated PIP AROM, and this was used for functional activity as much as possible.

E.O. made good progress in recovering full flexion of the index through ring fingers over the first 2 weeks of therapy. However, he remained very stiff at the small finger PIP joint. The therapist contacted the physician and asked whether any bony block or articular restrictions might be limiting PIP motion. The physician stated that there were no articular limitations and agreed to the therapist's request to initiate low-load, long-duration dynamic splinting for small finger PIP flexion.

E.O. gained active MP and DIP flexion of the small finger and passive PIP flexion (as a result of the use of the dynamic splint). His tendon pull-through was limited, and this was the cause of his PIP flexion limitations. He had a tendency to forget to exercise or to use the dynamic splint only some of the time, as the therapist had specified. All home instructions were simplified, written down, and reviewed with E.O. at each visit.

Despite gaining passive PIP flexion, E.O. still had active limitations because of tendon adherence, a common and challenging problem after proximal phalangeal fractures. Six weeks after starting therapy, E.O.'s small finger AROM was MP, 0-70; PIP, 0-35; and DIP, 5-40. Passive PIP ROM was 0-55. At the time of discharge, E.O. stated that he had returned to preinjury function, including driving. He was using buddy straps to help position his small finger more effectively for gripping, and he continued with home exercises. He was hopeful that he would continue to make further progress over time.

References

1. LaStayo P, Winters K, Hardy M: Fracture healing: bone healing, fracture management and current concepts related to the hand, *J Hand Ther* 16:81-93, 2003.
2. American Academy of Orthopedic Surgeons. Available at www.aaos.org
3. Smith K: Wound healing. In Stanley B, Tribuzi S, editors: *Concepts in hand rehabilitation*, Philadelphia, 1992, FA Davis.
4. Berger R: The anatomy and basic biomechanics of the wrist joint, *J Hand Ther* 9:84-93, 1996.
5. Laseter G: Therapist's management of distal radius fractures. In Mackin EJ, Callahan AD, Skirven TM et al, editors: *Rehabilitation of the hand and upper extremity*, ed 5, St Louis, 2002, Mosby.
6. Frykman G, Watkins B: The distal radioulnar joint. In Mackin EJ, Callahan AD, Skirven TM et al, editors:

Rehabilitation of the hand and upper extremity, ed 5, St Louis, 2002, Mosby.

7. Wang J, Jupiter J: Introduction to distal radius fractures. In Mackin EJ, Callahan AD, Skirven TM et al, editors: *Rehabilitation of the hand and upper extremity,* ed 5, St Louis, 2002, Mosby.

8. Laseter G, Carter P: Management of distal radius fractures, *J Hand Ther* 9:114-128, 1996.

9. MacDermid J, Richards R, Roth J: Distal radius fracture: a prospective outcome study of 275 patients, *J Hand Ther* 14:154-169, 2001.

10. Mannarino S: Skeletal injuries. In Stanley B, Tribuzi S, editors: *Concepts in hand rehabilitation,* Philadelphia, 1992, FA Davis.

11. Cannon N, editor: *Diagnosis and treatment manual,* ed 4, Indianapolis, 2001, The Hand Rehabilitation Center of Indiana.

12. Beaton D, Katz J, Fossel A et al: Measuring the whole or the parts? Validity, reliability and responsiveness of the disabilities of the arm, shoulder and hand outcome measure in different regions of the upper extremity, *J Hand Ther* 14:128-141, 2001.

13. *The hand: examination and diagnosis,* ed 2, Edinburgh, 1983, Churchill Livingstone.

14. Dell P, Dell R: Management of carpal fractures and dislocations. In Mackin EJ, Callahan AD, Skirven TM et al, editors: *Rehabilitation of the hand and upper extremity,* ed 5, St Louis, 2002, Mosby.

15. Prosser R, Herbert T: The management of carpal fractures and dislocations, J Hand Ther 9:139-147, 1996.

16. Brach P, Goitz R: An update on the management of carpal fractures, *J Hand Ther* 16:152-160, 2003.

17. Wright T, Michlovitz S: Management of carpal instability. In Mackin EJ, Callahan AD, Skirven TM et al, editors: *Rehabilitation of the hand and upper extremity,* ed 5, St Louis, 2002, Mosby.

18. McGough C, Surwasky M: Effect of exercise on volumetric and sensory status of the asymptomatic hand, *J Hand Ther* 4:177-182, 1991.

19. Skirven T: Clinical examination of the wrist, *J Hand Ther* 9:96-107, 1996.

20. McNemar T, Howell JW, Chang E: Management of metacarpal fractures, *J Hand Ther* 16:143-151, 2003.

21. Purdy B, Wilson R: Management of nonarticular fractures of the hand. In Mackin EJ, Callahan AD, Skirven TM et al, editors: *Rehabilitation of the hand and upper extremity,* ed 5, St Louis, 2002, Mosby.

22. Cannon N: Rehabilitation approaches for distal and middle phalanx fractures of the hand, *J Hand Ther* 16:105-116, 2003.

23. Hritcko G: Finger fracture rehabilitation. In Clark G, Wilgis E, Aiello B et al, editors: *Hand rehabilitation: a practical guide,* New York, 1993, Churchill Livingstone.

24. Freeland A, Hardy M, Singletary S: Rehabilitation for proximal phalangeal fractures, *J Hand Ther* 16:129-142, 2003.

25. Chinchalkar S, Siang Gan B: Management of proximal interphalangeal joint fractures and dislocations, *J Hand Ther* 16:117-127, 2003.

26. Brown AP: Proximal interphalangeal joint fracture dislocation. In Clark G, Wilgis E, Aiello B et al, editors: *Hand rehabilitation: a practical guide,* New York, 1993, Churchill Livingstone.

27. Campbell P, Wilson RL: Management of joint injuries and intraarticular fractures. In Mackin EJ, Callahan AD, Skirven TM et al, editors: *Rehabilitation of the hand and upper extremity,* ed 5, St Louis, 2002, Mosby.

14

Common Forms of Tendinitis/Tendinosis

CYNTHIA COOPER AND HOPE A. MARTIN

Clients with tendinitis/tendinosis experience pain that can significantly limit their daily activities. Simply picking up a coffee cup may be a task that is too painful. Stirring food, putting away groceries, or using a computer keyboard may provoke pain, and exercise routines can be interrupted. These clients may put off going to the physician, hoping that the symptoms will pass. Unfortunately, those who wait may develop chronic changes, which can be more difficult to treat.

Symptoms associated with tendinitis/tendinosis include pain with active range of motion (AROM), resistance, or passive stretching of the involved structures. It is very important to identify the activities contributing to the problem and to make as many ergonomic changes as possible. These often can be accomplished with clever improvising and do not necessarily require expensive purchases. For example, simply placing large pillows in the lap to provide forearm and wrist support while reading or knitting can be very helpful. Many clients recover well by improving their posture and upper extremity (UE) biomechanics and by participating in an ongoing exercise program.

GENERAL ANATOMY

Tendons are viscoelastic structures with unique mechanical properties. They are composed of connective tissues made of collagen, and they are poorly vascularized. Relatively speaking, cells play a small role in the makeup of the tendons; fibroblasts account for approximately 20% of the tissue volume. The extracellular matrix of tendons accounts for approximately 80% of the tissue volume. Of this matrix, 70% is water and 30% is composed of solids, mostly collagen.[1]

The strength of a muscle depends on its cross-sectional area. A larger cross-sectional area provides greater contraction force, with transmission of greater tensile loads through the tendon. Tendons with a larger cross-sectional area also are able to bear higher loads.[1]

The factors that most affect tendons' biomechanical properties are aging, pregnancy, mobilization (or immobilization), and use of nonsteroidal antiinflammatory drugs (NSAIDs). Up to the age of 20, the collagen cross-links in tendons increase in number and improve in quality, which equates with increased tensile strength. With aging, tensile strength decreases.[1]

CLINICAL *Pearl*

Tendons remodel in response to the stresses or mechanical demands imposed on them. They become stronger by being exposed to increased stress (e.g., movement). They become weaker when stress is reduced or eliminated (e.g., immobilization, such as splinting).[1]

GENERAL PATHOLOGY

Tendinitis is defined as an acute inflammatory response to injury of a tendon that produces the classical signs of heat, swelling, and pain.[2] Physicians and therapists historically have treated tendinitis as a phenomenon of tendon inflammation. However, recent, compelling histologic evidence has resulted in a change of terminology. The term **angiofibroblastic hyperplasia** or **angiofibroblastic tendinosis** (hereafter referred to as **tendinosis**) describes the pathologic alterations seen in the tissue of clients diagnosed as having tendonitis. A visible change occurs in the gross appearance of the tissue. Microscopically, normal tendon fibers are arranged in an orderly fashion. With tendinosis, the tendon fibers are invaded by fibroblasts and atypical vascular granulation tissue, and the adjacent tissue becomes degenerative, hypercellular, and microfragmented. Typically, only a few, if any, inflammatory cells are seen histologically. Tendinosis now is thought to be a degenerative pathologic condition, not an inflammatory one. Experts currently believe that true tendinitis is rare and that the condition hand therapists see in clients is tendinosis.

This histologic evidence has some intriguing implications for therapists: (1) we should question traditional approaches to the treatment of tendonitis as an inflammatory condition, and (2) we should alter our hand therapy treatments to fit the evidence of a tendinosis pathology.[2,3]

Individuals most likely to have tendinosis (1) are over age 35; (2) engage in a high-intensity occupational or sports activity three or more times a week for at least 30 minutes per session; (3) use a demanding technique for the activity; and (4) have an inadequate level of physical fitness. Symptoms occur when the tissue is worked beyond its tolerance (i.e., overused).[3]

GENERAL TIMELINES AND HEALING

The key to promoting healing is to help your clients avoid pain. Timelines and healing vary. Symptoms may persist or recur over years but do not always do so; some clients recover completely. In therapy, some clients may be able to start pain-free isometric or AROM exercises immediately, whereas others may find this too painful initially. Generally speaking, if your client is following therapy guidelines but has not made progress after a few weeks, suggest a return visit to the physician.

GENERAL TREATMENT SUGGESTIONS

General treatment suggestions are presented in the following sections. Lateral epicondylitis, medial epicondylitis, de Quervain's tenosynovitis, and digital stenosing tenosynovitis are addressed individually because they are common tendinitis/tendinosis diagnoses. The chapter ends with a table designed to promote structure-specific clinical reasoning and treatment for these and other diagnoses of UE tendinitis/tendinosis.

Posture and Conditioning

Always promote good posture, regardless of which UE structures are diagnosed with the tendinitis/tendinosis. Likewise, proximal UE AROM and tolerable aerobic exercises are valuable for stimulating lymphatic flow and promoting circulation to the distal structures.

Biomechanics and Symptom Management

Instruct clients in biomechanical guidelines promoting physiologic UE motions that are not strenuous. Teach them to keep their elbows at their sides with the forearms and wrists in neutral positions and to use softer force for pinch and grip activities. Encourage the use of padded and enlarged handles on tools. Explain that two-handed activities done frontally put much less strain on distal UE structures than one-handed activities done far away from the body, overhead, or with trunk twisting.

Ergonomic modifications and life-style changes, including pacing, can be very beneficial, but convincing clients of this sometimes can be difficult. An even more difficult task is persuading some clients to take better care of their bodies and to delegate more chores or tasks at home if possible. It is essential to learn your client's priorities and goals so that contributory life-style issues can be addressed appropriately and effectively. Adjustments as simple as moving closer to the telephone and using a headset can be quite helpful.

Progression of Treatment

Rest may be necessary initially, depending on the severity of symptoms. Splints or soft straps may be helpful for pain, and treatments that relieve pain (e.g., application of superficial heat) should be used. The goal is to bring these clients to the point where they are ready for pain-free isometric and short arc AROM of the involved structures. If exercising the involved structure is too painful, be sure to exercise proximally. Always incorporate aerobic exercise and proximal AROM if possible.

Begin short arc AROM of the involved structures as soon as this can be done without causing pain. If necessary for pain control, eliminate gravity and keep the arc of motion small. Try isometrics with a gentle contraction in a position of comfort and upgrade with varying positions.

Progress to AROM of the involved structures in greater arcs of motion against gravity when this can be done without pain. Gradually add resistance. In most cases, performing more repetitions with a lighter load is better than performing few repetitions with a higher load. Eccentric exercises stimulate the production of collagen and are particularly important for clients who want to return to sporting activities that require eccentric contractions (e.g., tennis). Monitor the client's responses to this upgrade.

As hand therapists, we are taught to believe that we should perform passive stretching of the involved structures. However, this poses a dilemma, because passive stretching can injure tissue. Clients find it difficult to truly relax for passive self-stretching, partly because of an appropriate anticipation of pain. Some experts have found that clients recover full passive stretching capability when pain-free, upgraded exercises are used instead of therapist-assisted passive stretching. This point deserves further research. In the meantime, if you perform passive stretching of involved structures, be very careful to avoid pain and monitor the client's pain after the stretching session.

Precaution. *Always avoid pain with exercise; pain is a sign of injury.*

(See Chapter 4 for more information on tissue-specific exercises.)

LATERAL EPICONDYLITIS (TENNIS ELBOW)

ANATOMY

The lateral epicondyle of the humerus is the origin of the symptomatic muscle-tendon units in lateral epicondylitis, commonly known as tennis elbow (Fig. 14-1). The extensor carpi radialis brevis (ECRB) is most often involved, followed by the extensor digitorum communis (EDC).

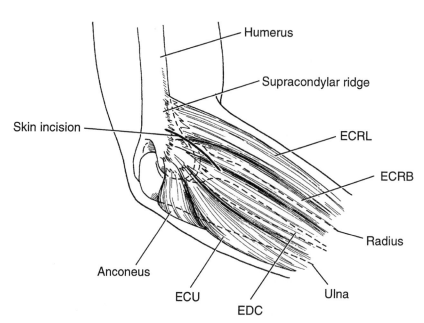

FIGURE 14-1 Muscles that attach at the lateral epicondyle of the distal humerus. (From Trumble TE: Tendinitis and epicondylitis. In Trumble TE, editor: *Principles of hand surgery,* Philadelphia, 2000, WB Saunders.)

DIAGNOSIS AND PATHOLOGY

Clients usually have point tenderness at the lateral epicondyle, possibly anterior or distal to it. Point tenderness at the supracondylar ridge may indicate involvement of the extensor carpi radialis longus (ECRL). Clients with lateral epicondylitis complain of nighttime aching and morning stiffness of the elbow. Gripping provokes pain, as does resisted wrist extension, supination, digital extension, and wrist radial deviation. Grip strength is reduced when the elbow is extended, and pain may be worse with this position (e.g., when carrying a briefcase). Tightness of the extrinsic extensors is common, and stretching of these muscles causes pain (Fig. 14-2).

The test for tennis elbow is called **Cozen's test** (Fig. 14-3). The examiner's thumb stabilizes the client's elbow at the lateral epicondyle. With the forearm pronated, the client makes a fist and then actively extends and radially deviates the wrist with the examiner resisting the motion. Severe, sudden pain in the area of the lateral epicondyle is a positive test result.[4]

Mill's tennis elbow test originally was described as a manipulation maneuver, but it can be used as a clinical test. The client's shoulder is in neutral. The examiner palpates the tenderest area at or near the lateral epicondyle, then pronates the forearm and fully flexes the wrist while moving the elbow from flexion to extension. Pain at the lateral epicondyle is a positive test result. (For more information on this topic and other provocative tests, see Fedorczyk's work.[4])

Differential diagnoses include cervical radiculopathy, proximal neurovascular entrapment, and radial tunnel syndrome. X-ray films can rule out osseous or articular conditions such as calcification or arthritis. When the triceps is most symptomatic, the condition is called *posterior tennis elbow*.

Radial tunnel syndrome differs from lateral epicondylitis in that the pain is more diffuse and occurs within the muscle mass of the extensor wad rather than at the lateral epicondyle (Fig. 14-4). The middle finger test can be used to detect radial tunnel syndrome (Fig. 14-5). Another test for this syndrome is to tap (percuss) over the superficial radial nerve in a distal to proximal direction. The test result is positive if paresthesias are elicited.[5,6]

NONOPERATIVE TREATMENT

Treatment can be divided into two phases, acute and restorative. In the acute phase, the client reports pain at rest that is worsened by daily functional use of the

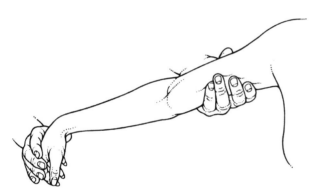

FIGURE 14-2 Stretching of extrinsic extensors. (From Wadsworth TG: Elbow tendinitis. In Mackin EJ, Callahan AD, Skirven TM et al, editors: *Rehabilitation of the hand and upper extremity*, ed 5, St Louis, 2002, Mosby.)

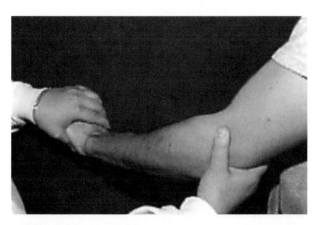

FIGURE 14-3 Cozen's test. (From Fedorczyk JM: Therapist's management of elbow tendinitis. In Mackin EJ, Callahan AD, Skirven TM et al, editors: *Rehabilitation of the hand and upper extremity*, ed 5, St Louis, 2002, Mosby.)

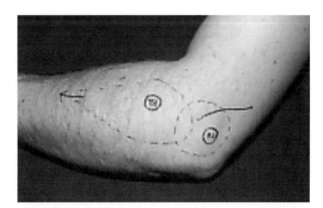

FIGURE 14-4 Radial tunnel syndrome differs from lateral epicondylitis in that the pain is more diffuse and occurs within the muscle mass of the extensor wad rather than at the lateral epicondyle. (From Fedorczyk JM: Therapist's management of elbow tendinitis. In Mackin EJ, Callahan AD, Skirven TM et al, editors: *Rehabilitation of the hand and upper extremity*, ed 5, St Louis, 2002, Mosby.)

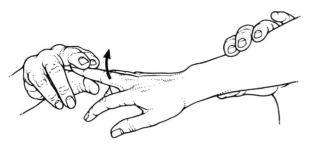

FIGURE 14-5 Middle finger test for radial tunnel syndrome. (From Wadsworth TG: Elbow tendinitis. In Mackin EJ, Callahan AD, Skirven TM et al, editors: *Rehabilitation of the hand and upper extremity*, ed 5, St Louis, 2002, Mosby.)

extremity or by range of motion (ROM). The emphasis in this phase is on reducing pain and promoting healing.

CLINICAL *Pearl*

> Because lateral epicondylitis is not an inflammatory condition, the traditional use of treatments intended to reduce inflammation (e.g., iontophoresis, phonophoresis, corticosteroid injections, nonsteroidal antiinflammatory drugs) should be questioned.

The application of superficial heat may be beneficial for managing pain and improving tissue extensibility.

Precaution. *Do not use heat if the injury site is inflamed or swollen.*

Ice also may be used for pain relief. The vasoconstrictive effect of ice may help normalize the neovascularization associated with the condition.[7] Continuous-wave ultrasound and high-voltage pulse current (HVPC) have been reported to reduce pain.[3,4] Although friction massage has been recommended for healing and pain relief, many clients find this technique too painful to tolerate. Fedorczyk[4] notes that more research is needed on the use of soft tissue mobilization to treat tendinosis.

Splinting is provided in the acute phase to support the wrist extensors. Either a prefabricated or a custom-made volar wrist cock-up splint can be used. The wrist should be positioned in 35 degrees of extension. A counterforce brace is worn over the extensor muscle mass, but this should not be used until the client is able to tolerate it comfortably. Most experts suggest removing it at night to avoid nerve compression problems. The counterforce brace is thought to disperse forces and to promote rest of the involved tendon.

Precaution. *Be very careful not to apply a counterforce brace tightly, because this can cause nerve compression. If the client develops sensory symptoms of the superficial radial nerve distribution (dorsal forearm and hand), discontinue use of the counterforce brace.*

In the acute phase, AROM should be within pain-free ranges. Gentle **isometric exercises** (muscle contraction with no movement) in varying positions are done at the elbow, forearm, and wrist. *Make sure that these exercises can be performed without pain.* Isolated AROM of the ECRB can begin in short arcs of motion, with gravity eliminated if necessary, to stimulate and nourish tissue in a pain-free manner. Be sure the client gently contracts the ECRB with a soft fist, to prevent substitution with the EDC. Also make sure the client relaxes the contraction as the motion is released (wrist flexion with digital extension) so that an eccentric ECRB exercise does not occur at this stage, because it most likely would be painful. Proximal ROM and light strengthening of periscapular and hand intrinsic muscles may begin. Functional activities should be included wherever possible, with attention given to posture and pacing.

In the restorative phase, the client's pain has improved. AROM and light functional activity are no longer painful. The emphasis in this phase is on helping the extensor mass recover flexibility, strength, and endurance. Periscapular and hand strengthening exercises should be continued, and graded conditioning exercises for the common extensors should be added. Assess ergonomic needs and sports participation with biomechanical modifications as needed.

Isometric exercises are advanced with the use of stronger contractions. As muscle contracts more, the tendon is subjected to greater stress. Progressive resistive exercises with **isotonic contraction** (contraction with muscle shortening) are started with low weight. Gradually, **eccentric contraction** (contraction with muscle lengthening) may be added.

Precaution. *Eccentric exercises should be performed with caution because they are more forceful.*

Eccentric exercise helps restore tissue tolerance of the eccentric loads associated with sports and other functional activities.[4] Eccentric exercise is believed to stimulate collagen production, which is considered the key to recovery from tendinosis.[7]

OPERATIVE TREATMENT

Various surgical procedures can be performed for lateral epicondylitis.[3,8] Splinting may be ordered after surgery to support the wrist or elbow or both. ROM guidelines and upgrades for strengthening are determined by the surgeon.

Questions to Ask the Physician

- *Has the client had any corticosteroid injections?*
- *Would any x-ray findings affect the progression of therapy?*

What to Say to Clients

About Tendinitis/Tendinosis

"Consider this a wake-up call. Your body is telling you that certain structures are overworked and need to recover. Often a few small changes in your body mechanics or improved awareness of posture can make a huge difference in resolving the symptoms. Also, this may be a signal that you should take better care of yourself, get more rest, pamper yourself a little more, exercise more regularly, and delegate more tasks to others if possible. You know yourself and your body the best, but sometimes clients need to feel permitted to take better care of themselves. So I am instructing you to do so, if possible, because it will help you recover more quickly."

About Splinting

"The purpose of your splint is to rest your muscles so that your pain resolves. Then you will be able to begin gentle, pain-free exercises. However, when tissue is immobilized, it does not get the same blood flow, oxygen, or stimulation; therefore it is important not to use the splint more than necessary. As a general guideline, remove the splint for any activity you can perform without pain; use the splint for any activity that otherwise would be painful."

About Exercises

"You will recover the quickest by avoiding pain. Pain is a sign of reinjury. The best way to heal your tissues is to provide controlled stimulation with exercises that cause no pain. If you cannot tolerate light stimulation, such as a gentle isometric exercise, therapy will focus on resolving the pain so that you become ready to tolerate this stimulation. Thereafter your exercises will be upgraded gradually. If any new exercises cause pain, it is very important to discontinue them."

About Activities of Daily Living

"Your arms and hands work harder when your upper extremity is away from your body. As much as possible, try to keep your elbows at your side when you are using your arms. Use two hands for activities you normally would do with one hand. Do as many of your daily activities as possible in front of you rather than to the side. Avoid reaching whenever possible by moving in closer.

Try to use the gentlest force possible when gripping and pinching items such as a pen or the steering wheel. These modifications will promote faster recovery and help reduce your pain."

EVALUATION TIPS

- Clarify whether the onset of symptoms was due to trauma or was atraumatic.
- Do not cause unnecessary pain with your evaluation.
- Use the Patient-Rated Forearm Evaluation Questionnaire (PRFEQ) (see Chapter 6).
- Find out what activities of daily living (ADL) and recreational activities provoke pain and incorporate this information into your treatment plan.
- Check the client's posture and proximal scapular muscle strength.

DIAGNOSIS-SPECIFIC INFORMATION THAT AFFECTS CLINICAL REASONING

The smaller, more delicate structures of the upper extremity work harder when the upper arm is unsupported. Biomechanical guidelines for neutral arm position, bilateral frontal UE activity, and softer force with grip and pinch are very helpful.

TIPS FROM THE FIELD

- Built-up and padded handles reduce the forces on joints and tendons. Recommend a sheepskin or padded steering wheel cover, pens with a larger girth, cylindric tubes for toothbrushes, and adapted kitchen implements with larger, padded handles.
- Manual edema mobilization (MEM) techniques promote UE pain relief and can facilitate proximal ROM (see Chapter 3). Light compressive garments may also give comfort. If the lateral epicondyle is quite tender, positioning a chip bag over that area at night may provide relief. The bag usually can be kept in place with a cotton stockinette sleeve.
- The soft, four-finger buddy strap can be helpful for clients with lateral epicondylitis who also have EDC symptoms (see Chapter 1 for more information). This strap helps support the EDC, and clients report that it improves pain-free arcs of motion for digital flexion and extension. The strap can be used in conjunction with a volar wrist splint or a counterforce brace. Kinesio Tape has been used successfully for various types of tendinitis/tendinosis. Courses providing instruction in proper techniques are available.

- Help clients determine which of their daily activities may be provoking pain and suggest changes that promote less strenuous UE biomechanics. Some clients may not realize that they are making progress. Whenever possible, give feedback about objective findings to reassure the client. For example, the arc of pain-free AROM may be greater, the positions of isometric exercises may be upgraded, or the number of exercise repetitions may be increased. A more important point is that clients may now be brushing their teeth with the involved extremity but may not realize that this is a sign of improvement.

Precautions and Concerns

- *Make sure the counterforce brace is not too tight.*
- *Do not encourage any painful exercises.*

MEDIAL EPICONDYLITIS (GOLFER'S ELBOW)

With medial epicondylitis, or golfer's elbow, the medial epicondyle of the humerus is the origin of the symptomatic muscle-tendon units. The pronator teres (PT), flexor carpi radialis (FCR), and palmaris longus (PL) are most often involved, although the flexor carpi ulnaris (FCU) and flexor digitorum superficialis (FDS) also may be implicated.[3]

Medial epicondylitis is less common than lateral epicondylitis. These clients have point tenderness of the medial epicondyle at the common flexor origin. Pain occurs with resisted elbow extension when the forearm is supinated and the wrist is extended. Repetitive or forceful pronation and resisted wrist flexion also cause pain.[4]

Differential diagnoses include cervical radiculopathy, proximal neurovascular compression, and referred pain caused by a shoulder or wrist problem. Ulnar neuropathy or neuritis and ulnar collateral ligament problems are possible associated conditions.[4]

The treatment of medial epicondylitis follows the same guidelines as those for lateral epicondylitis, but the emphasis is on supporting the symptomatic flexor structures rather than the extensors. With medial epicondylitis, the volar wrist splint positions the wrist in neutral (Fig. 14-6). Some recommend splinting the wrist in slight flexion, but caution should be used because this position may produce or aggravate symptoms of carpal tunnel syndrome. A counterforce brace is used on the flexor muscle wad. Some clients find the soft, four-finger buddy strap helpful for pain and gripping function, possibly because it supports the extrinsic flexors.

DE QUERVAIN'S TENOSYNOVITIS

ANATOMY

The abductor pollicis longus (APL) and the extensor pollicis brevis (EPB) tendons make up the first dorsal compartment of the wrist, where they share a common tendon sheath (Fig. 14-7).

DIAGNOSIS AND PATHOLOGY

De Quervain's disease is also called *stenosing tenovaginitis* or *stenosing tenosynovitis*. This condition causes pain over the radial styloid process, and the pain can radiate

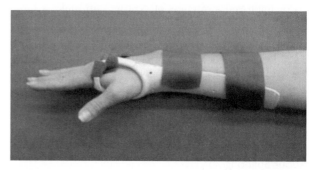

FIGURE 14-6 Volar wrist splint with wrist in neutral position.

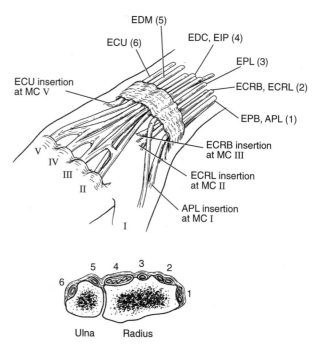

FIGURE 14-7 The six dorsal compartments of the extensor tendons. (From Trumble TE: Tendinitis and epicondylitis. In Trumble TE, editor: *Principles of hand surgery*, Philadelphia, 2000, WB Saunders.)

proximally or distally. Pain also occurs with resisted thumb extension or abduction, and Finkelstein's test (Fig. 14-8) frequently has a positive result. Thickening or swelling often is palpable over the symptomatic area. Histologically, clients with de Quervain's disease show fibrotic, thickened tissue with hypervascular changes and tendon degeneration.[2]

The anatomy of the first dorsal compartment varies greatly. The EPB may be absent in 5% to 7% of the population. When present, the EPB may have its own compartment.[9] The APL often has multiple tendinous slips, and these may insert in varying locations.

Forceful, repetitive, or sustained thumb abduction with ulnar deviation of the wrist may contribute to the development of this condition. Activities that may provoke pain include wringing out washrags, opening or closing jars, using scissors, typing on a computer keyboard, playing piano, knitting, racquet sports, or doing needlepoint. Some experts feel that radial deviation of the wrist with pinch is most likely to provoke pain because of the angulation of the involved tendons in this position.[9]

Women are four times more likely than men to have de Quervain's disease. The onset occurs most often between 35 and 55 years of age, but pregnant women in the third trimester and mothers of young children also are at risk.[9] Differential diagnoses include thumb carpometacarpal (CMC) osteoarthritis, scaphoid fracture, wrist arthritis, intersection syndrome, and radial nerve neuritis.

NONOPERATIVE TREATMENT

A forearm-based, thumb spica splint that leaves the interphalangeal (IP) joints free is used to prevent painful motions. Some recommend positioning the wrist in neutral and the thumb in radial abduction. Others recommend slight wrist extension of about 20 degrees with the thumb in extension. A radial or volar splint may be used. The radial gutter spica splint seems to allow more

UE function but should not be used unless the client can wear this splint without pain. Studies suggest greater clinical success with this condition when splinting is combined with corticosteroid injection, compared with splinting alone.[9] As pain resolves, the client may progress to a soft or semirigid splint.

Treatments and graded exercises have the same role in de Quervain's disease as in lateral epicondylitis. Isometric exercise of the APL and EPB, short arc AROM of these structures, isolated wrist flexion and extension, and isolated thumb IP flexion and extension should be included.

CLINICAL *Pearl*

Symptom-provoking motions of radial and ulnar deviation and thumb composite flexion and extension should be avoided until the client can perform them without pain.

Strengthening exercises for the APL and EPB can be added gradually when pain has resolved. Eccentric exercises have been described,[2] but caution is warranted to avoid causing pain or injury.

OPERATIVE TREATMENT

Surgical release of the first dorsal compartment is an option for clients in whom conservative treatment has failed. High success rates have been reported for this procedure.[9] After surgery, the surgeon indicates the type of splint to be used and the precautions to be observed. Generally, the splint is weaned over a few weeks, with isolated AROM progressing to composite motions of the APL and EPB. Strengthening exercises are begun when they have been approved by the surgeon, usually after a few weeks. Scar management and desensitization are important aspects of therapy.

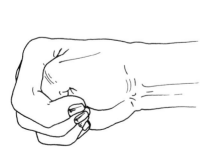
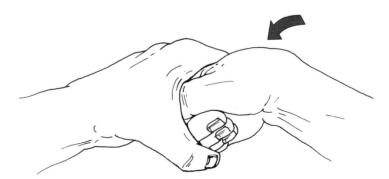

FIGURE 14-8 Finkelstein's test. (From Magee DJ: *Orthopedic physical assessment*, Philadelphia, 2002, WB Saunders.)

Questions to Ask the Physician

- *Has the client had any corticosteroid injections?*
- *Would any x-ray findings affect the progression of therapy?*

What to Say to Clients

About Tendinitis/Tendinosis

"Consider this a wake-up call. Your body is telling you that certain structures are overworked and need to recover. Often a few small changes in your body mechanics or improved awareness of posture can make a huge difference in resolving the symptoms. Also, this may be a signal that you should take better care of yourself, get more rest, pamper yourself a little more, exercise more regularly, and delegate more tasks to others if possible. You know yourself and your body the best, but sometimes clients need to feel permitted to take better care of themselves. So I am instructing you to do so, if possible, because it will help you recover more quickly."

About Splinting

"The purpose of your splint is to rest your muscles so that your pain resolves. Then you will be able to begin gentle, pain-free exercises. However, when tissue is immobilized, it does not get the same blood flow, oxygen, or stimulation, therefore it is important not to use the splint more than necessary. As a general guideline, remove the splint for any activity you can perform without pain, but use the splint for any activity that otherwise would be painful."

About Exercises

"You will recover quickest by avoiding pain. Pain is a sign of reinjury. The best way to heal your tissues is to provide controlled stimulation with exercises that cause no pain. If you cannot tolerate light stimulation, such as a gentle isometric exercise, therapy will focus on resolving the pain so that you become ready to tolerate this stimulation. Thereafter your exercises will be upgraded gradually. If any new exercises cause pain, it is very important to discontinue them."

About Activities of Daily Living

"Moving your wrist from side to side [demonstrate radial and ulnar deviation] with your thumb held either straight or bent is likely to cause pain. Try to keep your wrist straight so that the long finger is in line with the middle of your forearm. From this position you may be able to perform light pinch and grip activities without pain."

Computer Ergonomics

"Try not to deviate your wrist [demonstrate radial and ulnar deviation] when working at the computer keyboard. Instead, keep your elbows at your side and pivot from the elbow, not at the wrist. You may want to investigate computer keyboard designs that make it easier to maintain this neutral position."

EVALUATION TIPS

- Irritation of the superficial radial nerve may be present (Fig. 14-9). Note this in your evaluation findings.
- Note whether the client wears a watchband or tight bracelet; if so, suggest that it be worn more loosely on the contralateral side.
- Clients often test their symptoms by performing a Finkelstein's stretch on themselves to see whether this motion is still painful. I ask them not to do this for at least 1 week. Thereafter, if they must do it, I recommend that they try it once only, as gently as possible. The presence of more pain-free passive stretch than in the previous week is a favorable sign.

DIAGNOSIS-SPECIFIC INFORMATION THAT AFFECTS CLINICAL REASONING

Most ADL require combined wrist and thumb motions, which makes de Quervain's disease very challenging to treat. Providing more than one splinting option often is helpful.

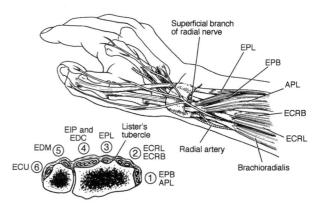

FIGURE 14-9 Proximity of superficial radial nerve and first dorsal compartment. (From Trumble TE: Tendinitis and epicondylitis. In Trumble TE, editor: *Principles of hand surgery,* Philadelphia, 2000, WB Saunders.)

TIPS FROM THE FIELD

- Pad the dorsal radial wrist area before splinting, because the superficial radial nerve may be irritated or may become irritated. If the client has had surgery, scar sensitivity and hypersensitivity may be noted at this site. Splint the client in the position of maximum comfort and function, if both are possible, but be sure the position is pain free.

- Provide materials for built-up pens and cylindric cushions for toothbrushes or kitchen implements. Instruct the client to use the softest force necessary when pinching. The more quickly the client can begin pain-free functional use, the better. Remind the client that pain-free motion most nourishes and stimulates the production of collagen.

Precautions and Concerns

- *Monitor for signs of superficial radial nerve irritation; if these appear, modify the splints immediately.*

DIGITAL STENOSING TENOSYNOVITIS (TRIGGER FINGER)

ANATOMY

With **digital stenosing tenosynovitis,** or trigger finger, a discrepancy exists between the volume of the flexor tendon and the size of the pulley lumen. The site of the problem typically is the first annular pulley (A1), which lies volar to the metacarpophalangeal (MCP) joint in the area of the distal palmar crease (Fig. 14-10).[9] The area between the A1 and A2 pulleys is described as a hypovascular watershed, which predisposes the tissue to problems of attrition due to lack of nourishment.[10]

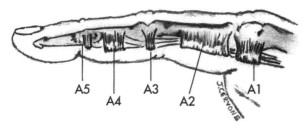

FIGURE 14-10 Finger annular pulleys. (From Falkenstein N, Weiss-Lessard S: *Hand rehabilitation: A quick reference guide and review,* St. Louis, 1999, Mosby.)

DIAGNOSIS AND PATHOLOGY

The characteristic symptom of trigger finger is an inability to perform smooth digital flexion or extension. The ring finger and thumb most often are involved, followed by the long, index, and small fingers. Trigger finger can occur in several digits. Most clients describe a painful snapping as they make a fist and an inability to actively extend the affected digit. Palpation in the area of the A1 pulley elicits pain, and crepitus often is heard with active composite digital flexion. When symptoms are more severe, the digit locks in flexion.[11]

The inflammatory pathology of trigger finger is classified as either nodular or diffuse, based on palpation of the tendon sheath. With nodular inflammation, the swelling is contained and a distinct nodule can be palpated as the digit triggers. With diffuse inflammation, the swelling is less defined. Nodular trigger fingers respond more successfully to conservative treatment. Symptoms that last longer than 6 months are less likely to respond to nonoperative treatment.[11]

Women develop trigger finger more often than men. Differential diagnoses include flexor tendon masses, such as tumors, ganglia, or lipomas. Associated diagnoses include diabetes, rheumatoid arthritis, gout, carpal tunnel syndrome, and Dupuytren's contracture.[11] Children also can have trigger finger, typically at the thumb. This usually is caused by nodules on the flexor pollicis longus (FPL) and is corrected with surgery.

NONOPERATIVE TREATMENT

Evans and colleagues[10] described a comprehensive program for conservative management of trigger finger in clients who did not have rheumatoid arthritis. Clients must refrain from all activities that aggravate the symptoms (i.e., gripping activities). A hand-based, volar splint is fabricated to support the involved MCP joint or joints at 0 degrees (neutral position). The splint must allow full IP flexion (Fig. 14-11). The client is taught to perform a hook fist (complete flexion and extension of IPs with MCP neutral) with the splint on, 20 repetitions every 2 hours while awake. After hook exercise, the splint is removed for gentle place and hold, full fist motions. The client is instructed to massage the flexor tendon sheath and palm area. If a flexion contracture is present, a night gutter splint is used to correct the contracture.

The client follows this program for 3 weeks and then is re-evaluated. If no improvement is seen, the physician decides whether corticosteroid injection or surgery should be done. If improvement is noted, the program is continued for a total of 6 weeks. It is extremely important that

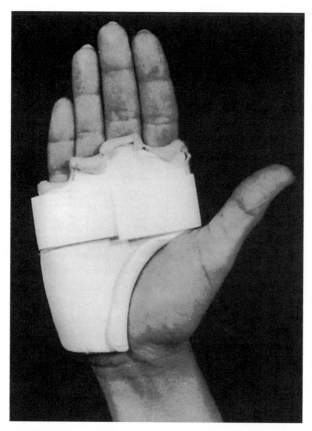

FIGURE 14-11 Hand-based volar splint for treatment of trigger finger. (From Evans RB, Hunter JM, Burkhalter WE: Conservative management of the trigger finger: a new approach, *J Hand Ther* 1:60, 1988.)

clients avoid all possibility of triggering throughout the program.

OPERATIVE TREATMENT

Operative treatment involves surgical release of the A1 pulley. Surgical and percutaneous techniques can be used for this purpose. After surgery, clients may be sent to hand therapy for edema control, scar management, ROM, or splinting if needed. Most clients do not need postoperative therapy.

Question to Ask the Physician

• *Has the client had any corticosteroid injections?*

What to Say to Clients

About Splinting and Exercise

"Your splint prevents your finger from triggering. Along with the proper exercises, this will better nourish the tendon and help it to heal. It is very important to perform the exercises gently and to accomplish full motions in bending and straightening to recover flexibility and function of the tendon."

About Activities of Daily Living

"Please think about any activities you are doing that may apply repeated pressure to your palm at the painful area. For example, using the palm of your hand like a hammer or repeated use of a staple gun can contribute to trigger finger symptoms. Sometimes scissors rub the area inside the affected thumb. Gardening may contribute to the symptoms if you grip the tools tightly for a long period. It will help to change these activities, to frequently change hand and upper extremity positions, to take a break regularly to stretch and reposition yourself, and to try padded gloves. We want you to be able to do the activities you enjoy, but initially some changes must be made so that the symptoms can improve."

EVALUATION TIPS

• Assess for flexion contractures and treat accordingly.
• Distinguish between possible extrinsic flexor tightness and joint contracture.
• Document pain at the A1 pulley.
• Document crepitus with composite active digital flexion.
• Monitor edema.
• Check that the symptom occurs at the A1 pulley (symptoms sometimes can occur at a different pulley).

DIAGNOSIS-SPECIFIC INFORMATION THAT AFFECTS CLINICAL REASONING

Composite digital flexion is very difficult to avoid in daily life, and certain tasks are difficult to perform with the MCP splint. In some cases an alternative splint can be helpful for maximizing function while preventing triggering. For example, a small proximal interphalangeal (PIP) volar gutter splint can be used as long as it prevents triggering. The splint must prevent composite digital flexion, and this is achieved by splinting one of the digital joints. Use of a PIP volar gutter splint may enhance clients' ability to perform some of their daily activities. It also may minimize the risk of maceration by varying the areas of splint contact and coverage.

TIPS FROM THE FIELD

• Trigger splints should be worn at night to prevent locking. For the thumb, splinting can limit either MCP or IP motion. A volar IP gutter splint is very easy to use and can be taped in place if necessary. The distal volar end should be trimmed to allow volar thumb pad exposure for sensory input and improved function. The hand-based MCP splint can be similar to that used for thumb CMC osteoarthritis (see Chapter 17).

- As with the other diagnoses, teach your clients not to test their symptoms, because this can interfere with their recovery. Sometimes treating the edema is the most important step in resolving trigger finger symptoms.

Precautions and Concerns

- *Warn the client to avoid any activities that could result in triggering for 6 weeks.*
- *Modify place and hold exercises so that no triggering occurs; this may mean limiting these exercises to less than full composite digital flexion initially.*
- *Watch for and manage skin maceration related to splint use.*

OTHER FORMS OF TENDINITIS/TENDINOSIS

Table 14-1 presents a summary of the involved structures, provocative tests, differential diagnoses, and splinting considerations for the common forms of tendinitis/tendinosis described in this chapter. It also provides an overview of other UE diagnoses seen by hand therapists.

The Role of Therapy Assistants

- *Splinting based on individual experience and competencies*
- *Instruction of client in symptom management, body mechanics, and home exercise program, as determined by supervising therapist*
- *Edema control*
- *Provision of adaptive devices, built-up handles, and other ADL modifications*
- *Instruction of client in pacing and work simplification*

CASE *Studies*

CASE 14-1

D.L., a 30-year-old, left-dominant male, was referred to hand therapy with a diagnosis of left wrist pain. He reported that he was unemployed, was receiving disabil-ity payments, and that he was taking medication for obsessive-compulsive disorder. He had a history of sub-stance abuse. The client had left ulnar wrist pain that worsened with wrist ulnar deviation and flexion. He had swelling at the ulnar wrist and pain over the pisiform. The therapist asked him if he had been doing any activities recently that might have aggravated his symptoms. He stated that his favorite pastime was to twirl scarves and that he was working on a scarf-twirling routine that he hoped would become an entertainment skit for future employment. He was twirling scarves with repetitive extreme wrist flexion/ulnar deviation motions for 6 hours daily. He rarely took rest breaks. He stated that he liked the repetition of the activity, that it helped pass the time, and that he found it comforting to do.

D.L. was fitted with a custom forearm ulnar gutter splint and was instructed to wear it for pain relief. He was started on proximal and postural exercises. Heat and ultrasound were used for pain relief (he had tried ice but did not like it). Gentle AROM for wrist flexion and exten-sion, differential flexor tendon gliding, and light digital strengthening were started when his pain had subsided. These routines were presented as a temporary replace-ment for twirling with the explanation that they would help his tissue condition improve so that he could resume twirling. D.L. was eager to resume twirling scarves and found it difficult to refrain from performing this activity. In the clinic he practiced modified scarf twirling with short arcs of wrist motion that did not cause pain. This activity was incorporated into his exercise program; he was cautioned not to exceed 5 minutes per hour initially. D.L. followed this guideline carefully and gradually was able to increase the twirling time and to wean off the wrist splint. He learned that if he monitored his posture, performed home exercises, and took frequent, brief rest breaks, he could perform longer sessions of scarf twirling once again.

CASE 14-2

A 45-year-old veterinarian was referred to hand therapy with trigger thumb. She had considerable pain in the area of the A1 pulley of the thumb, which was locking in flexion at night. She would awaken with pain when this occurred. She was seen for fabrication of a hand-based thumb splint that supported the MCP joint, which was to be used at night, and a very thin ($1/16$ inch) thumb IP volar gutter splint, to be used during the day. Care was taken to ensure that the day splint would fit inside her sterile gloves for animal surgery. In discussing her biome-chanics and contributing activities, she realized that she used surgical tools that often pressed against the thumb A1 pulley, provoking symptoms. Simulation in the therapy clinic led to alternative tool positions that protected the

TABLE 14-1

Overview of Tendinitis/Tendinosis of the Upper Extremity

DIAGNOSIS	STRUCTURES MOST INVOLVED	PROVOCATIVE TESTS	DIFFERENTIAL DIAGNOSES	SPLINTING CONSIDERATIONS
Lateral epicondylitis	ECRB, EDC	• Cozen's test • Mill's test • Palpation of lateral epicondyle • Resisted wrist extension • Gripping with elbow extended	• Cervical radiculopathy • Proximal neurovascular entrapment • Radial tunnel syndrome	• Volar wrist cock-up splint at 35 degrees wrist extension • Counterforce brace on extensor wad • Soft four-finger buddy strap
Radial tunnel syndrome	Superficial radial nerve	• Middle finger test • Percussion of superficial radial nerve (distal to proximal)	• Lateral epicondylitis	• *No counterforce brace*
Medial epicondylitis	Pronator teres, FCR, PL	• Palpation of medial epicondyle • Resisted elbow extension with supination and wrist extension • Repetitive or forceful pronation • Resisted wrist flexion • Passive composite extension (elbow, wrist, digits)	• Cervical radiculopathy • Proximal neurovascular entrapment • Ulnar neuropathy • Elbow ulnar collateral ligament problem	• Volar wrist cock-up splint with wrist in neutral • Counterforce brace on flexor wad • Soft four-finger buddy strap
de Quervain's tenosynovitis	APL and EPB at first dorsal compartment	• Finkelstein's test • Resisted thumb extension or abduction • Pain/thickening at first dorsal compartment	• Osteoarthritis of thumb CMC joint or wrist • Scaphoid fracture • Intersection syndrome • Radial nerve neuritis	• Forearm-based thumb spica cast with IP joint free
Digital stenosing tenosynovitis	Digital flexor tendon at the A1 pulley	• Tenderness at A1 pulley • Possible palpable nodule • Crepitus with active digital flexion • Snapping or locking with active composite digital flexion	• Flexor tendon tumors, ganglia, lipoma	• Hand-based splint with MCP joint in neutral • Digital volar gutter splint with PIP joint in neutral, MCP and DIP joints free

TABLE 14-1

Overview of Tendinitis/Tendinosis of the Upper Extremity—cont'd

DIAGNOSIS	STRUCTURES MOST INVOLVED	PROVOCATIVE TESTS	DIFFERENTIAL DIAGNOSES	SPLINTING CONSIDERATIONS
Intersection syndrome	APL and EPB muscle bellies, approximately 4 cm proximal to wrist where they intersect with ECRB and ECRL	• Swelling locally at muscle bellies • Pain with resisted wrist extension • Similar provocative tests as for de Quervain's tenosynovitis	• de Quervain's tenosynovitis	• Same as for de Quervain's tenosynovitis
EPL tendinitis	EPL at Lister's tubercle	• Pain at Lister's tubercle • Resisted composite thumb extension • Passive composite thumb flexion	• De Quervain's tenosynovitis • Intersection syndrome	• Forearm-based thumb spica cast with composite thumb extension, IP joint included
ECU tendinitis	ECU	• Forearm supination with wrist ulnar deviation • Pain at ulnar wrist	• DRUJ instability • TFCC tear • Ulnocarpal abutment	• Forearm-based ulnar gutter splint • *Ulnar head padded as needed for comfort*
FCR tendinitis	FCR	• Resisted wrist flexion and radial deviation • Pain with passive wrist extension • Pain over proximal wrist crease and at scaphoid tubercle	• Ganglion cysts • Thumb CMC osteoarthritis • Scaphoid fracture • de Quervain's tenosynovitis	• Volar wrist cock-up splint with wrist in neutral or position of comfort
FCU tendinitis	FCU	• Pain with palpation over pisiform • Resisted wrist flexion and ulnar deviation • Passive wrist extension and radial deviation	• Pisiform fracture • Pisotriquetral arthritis	• Forearm-based ulnar gutter splint

APL, Abductor pollicis longus; *CMC,* carpometacarpal; *DIP,* distal interphalangeal; *DRUJ,* distal radioulnar joint; *ECRB,* extensor carpi radialis brevis; *ECRL,* extensor carpi radialis longus; *ECU,* extensor carpi ulnaris; *EDC,* extensor digitorum communis; *EPB,* extensor pollicis brevis; *EPL,* extensor pollicis longus; *FCR,* flexor carpi radialis; *FCU,* flexor carpi ulnaris; *IP,* interphalangeal; *MCP,* metacarpophalangeal; *PIP,* proximal interphalangeal; *PL,* palmaris longus; *TFCC,* triangulofibrocartilage complex.

Modified from Lee MP, Nasser-Sharif S, Zelouf DS: Surgeon's and therapist's management of tendonopathies in the hand and wrist. In Mackin EJ, Callahan AD, Skirven TM et al, editors: *Rehabilitation of the hand and upper extremity,* ed 5, St Louis, 2002, Mosby; Evans RB, Hunter JM, Burkhalter WE: Conservative management of the trigger finger: a new approach, *J Hand Ther* 1:59-68, 1988; Trumble TE: Tendinitis and epicondylitis. In Trumble TE, editor: *Principles of hand surgery,* Philadelphia, 2000, WB Saunders; Lindner-Tons S, Ingell K: An alternative splint design for trigger finger, *J Hand Ther* 11:206-208, 1998; and Verdon ME: Overuse syndromes of the hand and wrist, *Prim Care* 23:305-319, 1996.

AI pulley area. She was seen only once, but she reported 1 week later by phone that she was doing very well clinically.

CASE 14-3

A 38-year-old teacher was referred to hand therapy for lateral epicondylitis of her right-dominant UE. She had considerable point tenderness over the lateral epicondyle (pain rating of 8/10), a positive Cozen's test result, and tenderness of the ECRB muscle belly. The middle finger test result was negative. The client reported that she remembered injuring her arm 3 weeks earlier when lifting boxes right before school started. Her right elbow was particularly sore when she wrote on the overhead projector overlay. She was seen for fabrication of a volar wrist splint with 35 degrees of wrist extension, which she wore for all aggravating activity. She was seen twice a week for 3 weeks for ultrasound therapy to the lateral epicondyle, instruction in biomechanical and positioning guidelines for symptom management, gentle isometrics and isolated short arc AROM for the ECRB, proximal ROM, and conditioning. She used ice as needed. Built-up pens were provided to reduce the force of grip needed to write. When she became pain free, she was given an upgraded home exercise program to strengthen the wrist extensors progressively, followed by icing as needed. ADL were explored to maximize function and prevent pain. After 3 months she came in for a follow-up visit. She was pain free and had regained normal strength in her right forearm. She stated that she had a good understanding of strategies for avoiding a recurrence of the problem and that she had successfully resumed all her activities.

References

1. Carlstedt CA, Nordin M: Biomechanics of tendons and ligaments. In Nordin M, Frankel VH, editors: *Basic biomechanics of the musculoskeletal system*, ed 2, Media, Pa. 1989, Williams & Wilkins.

2. Ashe MC, McCauley T, Khan KM: Tendinopathies in the upper extremity: a paradigm shift, *J Hand Ther* 17:329-334, 2004.

3. Nirschl RP: Elbow tendinosis/tennis elbow, *Clin Sports Med* 11:851-870, 1992.

4. Fedorczyk JM: Therapist's management of elbow tendinitis. In Mackin EJ, Callinan N, Skirven TM, editors: *Rehabilitation of the hand and upper extremity*, ed 5, St Louis, 2002, Mosby.

5. Skirven T, Trope J: Complications of immobilization, *Hand Clin* 10:53-61, 1994.

6. Terrono AL, Millender LH: Management of work-related upper extremity nerve entrapments, *Orthop Clin North Am* 27:783-793, 1996.

7. Khan KM, Cook JL, Taunton JE et al: Overuse tendinosis, not tendinitis. Part 1. A new paradigm for a difficult clinical problem, *Phys Sportsmed* 28:38-48, 2000.

8. Wadsworth TG: Elbow tendinitis. In Mackin EJ, Callinan N, Skirven TM, editors: *Rehabilitation of the hand and upper extremity*, ed 5, St Louis, 2002, Mosby.

9. Lee MP, Nasser-Sharif S, Zelouf DS: Surgeon's and therapist's management of tendinopathies in the hand and wrist. In Mackin EJ, Callinan N, Skirven TM, editors: *Rehabilitation of the hand and upper extremity*, ed 5, St Louis, 2002, Mosby.

10. Evans RB, Hunter JM, Burkhalter WE: Conservative management of the trigger finger: a new approach, *J Hand Ther* 1:59-68, 1988.

11. Saldana MJ: Trigger digits: diagnosis and treatment, *J Am Acad Orthop Surg* 9:246-252, 2001.

15

Common Finger Sprains and Deformities

CYNTHIA COOPER

*Only with the invisible knowledge of the fingers will one ever
be able to paint the infinite fabric of dreams.*

From *The Cave* by Jose Saramago, Harcourt Books, 2002

KEY TERMS

Accessory collateral ligament (ACL)

Bicondylar

Boutonniere deformity

Central extensor tendon (CET)

Collateral ligaments

DIP extensor lag

DIP flexion contracture

Functional stability

Fusiform swelling

Gamekeeper's thumb

Ginglymus joint

Lateral bands (LB)

Mallet finger

Oblique retinacular ligament (ORL)

ORL tightness

Proper collateral ligament (PCL)

Pseudoboutonniere deformity

Skier's thumb

Stener's lesion

Swan neck deformity

Transverse retinacular ligament (TRL)

Volar plate (VP)

Mallet fingers, boutonniere deformities, and swan neck deformities are common finger injuries that can be recognized by a hand therapist with a keen eye. They also can be treated successfully by precise management. The trauma and disease processes that cause these deformities vary, but regardless of the cause, the therapist's detailed knowledge of pathomechanics and therapy guidelines helps to manage and direct the course of treatment.

Some clients may be referred by primary care physicians, who may not have identified serious injuries such as gamekeeper's thumb or a **volar plate (VP)** injury. This may be especially likely in the setting of an occupational medicine clinic. In this situation, the therapist has an opportunity to identify the clinical findings and help arrange for the client to see a physician who specializes in hand problems.

Jamming injuries to the digits occur often in sports. Football players have a high incidence of proximal interphalangeal (PIP) joint injuries. In these sports-related injuries, dorsal dislocations are more common than volar dislocations. Boutonniere deformities frequently occur in basketball players. Mallet injuries occur when the player's fingertip strikes a helmet or ball.[1] Therapists whose clients participate in sports can expect to see these common sprains and finger injuries as part of their caseload.

Many nonathletes enjoy sports activities after work, and these "weekend warriors" often sustain finger injuries that initially go untreated. Clients who later seek medical attention may have chronic pain, edema, and stiffness. More long-term problems, such as persistent residual pain and swelling, can be very challenging to treat.

MALLET FINGER

A finger with drooping of the distal interphalangeal (DIP) joint is called a **mallet finger** (Fig. 15-1).[2] Typically the DIP can be passively corrected to neutral, but the client is unable to actively extend it; this condition is called a **DIP extensor lag.** If the DIP joint cannot be passively extended to neutral, the condition is called a **DIP flexion contracture.** A DIP flexion contracture seldom is present early after injury; however, if the injury goes untreated, this problem may develop.

ANATOMY

The DIP joint of the finger is a **ginglymus joint,** or hinge joint. It is **bicondylar** (it has two condyles) and is similar to the PIP joint in its capsular ligaments. The terminal extensor tendon and terminal flexor tendon attach to the most proximal edge of the distal phalanx. This insertion contributes to the joint's dynamic stability.[3]

DIAGNOSIS AND PATHOLOGY

A mallet injury frequently is caused by a blow to the fingertip with flexion force or by axial loading while the DIP is extended.[4] The terminal tendon is avulsed. An avulsion fracture also may occur and should be ruled out. Laceration injuries are another cause of this deformity. Anteroposterior (AP) and true lateral x-rays typically are obtained. In addition, the PIP joint should be examined for possible injury.[5]

TIMELINES AND HEALING

The DIP joint is splinted in full extension for approximately 6 weeks to allow the delicate terminal tendon to

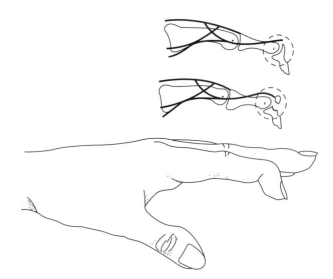

FIGURE 15-1   Mallet finger deformity. A fracture may also occur with this injury. (From *The hand: examination and diagnosis,* ed 2, Edinburgh, 1983, Churchill Livingstone.)

heal. The joint should not be allowed to flex even briefly during this period of immobilization. After 6 weeks, the client is weaned off the splint while the therapist observes for DIP extensor lag.

NONOPERATIVE TREATMENT

The DIP joint is splinted in extension or hyperextension, depending on the physician's preference. If hyperextension is recommended, the therapist should make sure the position of hyperextension is less than that which causes skin blanching. Exceeding tissue tolerance in DIP hyperextension can compromise circulation and nutrition to the healing tissues.[6]

Many types of DIP splints are available, and clients sometimes need more than one type (Fig. 15-2). They may also need a splint designated for showering; the client can carefully remove this type of splint after showering, according to the therapist's instructions, and replace it with a dry splint. In this way, the skin is protected against maceration, which occurs if a wet splint is left on a digit. Casting also can be used when client compliance is a concern. Quick Cast, a waterproof casting material, can be applied and changed weekly.

If the DIP joint cannot be passively extended to neutral, serial adjustments of splinting may be done. If necessary, a small static progressive DIP extension splint can be used.[7] In addition to splinting of the DIP, edema is treated as appropriate, and normal PIP active range of motion (AROM) with the DIP splinted is promoted. Dorsal edema and tenderness over the DIP are common and can interfere with full DIP extension.

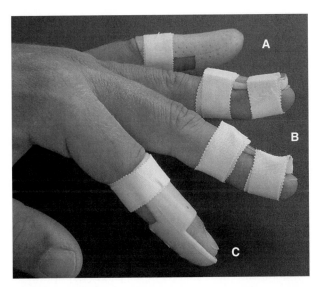

FIGURE 15-2 Mallet splints. **A,** Custom thermoplastic. **B,** Alumafoam. **C,** Stack. (From Burke SL: *Hand and upper extremity rehabilitation: a practical guide,* ed 3, St Louis, 2005, Churchill Livingstone.)

After 6 weeks of continuous splinting, if no DIP extensor lag is present and the physician approves, gentle composite AROM can be started. The therapist should instruct the client to avoid forceful or quick grasping or forceful DIP flexion in the early phase of AROM therapy. At this point, it is very important to watch for DIP extensor lag. If DIP extensor lag occurs, the splinting regimen is adjusted to promote recovery of DIP active flexion while maintaining active DIP extension. Some prefer to splint between gentle AROM sessions initially. Night splinting typically continues for another 2 to 3 weeks. If DIP extensor lag recurs, daytime splinting should be reinstituted. If splinting does not correct the DIP extensor lag, the client is referred to a hand surgeon, because surgery may be needed to correct the problem.

Although splinting is best initiated as soon as possible after injury, even a delayed splinting regimen can be effective.[8] Operative intervention can produce complications; therefore, nonoperative solutions often are well worth the effort.

OPERATIVE TREATMENT

Surgical complications include the possibility of infection and nail deformities. Nonetheless, if the mallet injury has associated large fracture fragments (greater than 30% of the joint surface), surgery may be necessary. A variety of procedures can be performed to treat this injury.[4,9,10]

The client may be sent to therapy with the DIP pinned for instruction in pin site care, edema control as needed, and protective splinting. Protective splinting may also help the client avoid bumping the pins. When

the pins are removed, AROM guidelines, as provided by the physician, are followed. Some physicians may order a DIP extension splint when the pins are removed to assist with the gradual weaning program. As with nonoperative treatment, the therapist should observe for DIP extensor lag.

Questions to Ask the Physician

- *Is a bony injury present?*
- *How long will the DIP need continuous extension support?*
- *Does the physician prefer the DIP in neutral position or in hyperextension?*
- *If a wound is present, what are the dressing guidelines?*
- *If the DIP is pinned, how long will the pin remain in place?*
- *Will a splint be needed after pin removal?*

What to Say to Clients

About the Injury

Information about the injury might be provided as follows:

"Here is a diagram of the anatomy of the distal digit and the terminal tendon. The terminal tendon is very delicate, and in order to heal, it needs continuous, uninterrupted DIP support for about 6 weeks." Reiterate this concept as necessary until the client appears to understand the importance of continuous DIP extension.

About Splinting

Information about splinting might be provided as follows:

"It is important for us to practice techniques for putting the splint on and taking it off while maintaining DIP extension. One technique is to keep the hand palm down on the table and carefully slide the splint forward. A second technique is to use your thumb to provide support under the fingertip while using your other hand to remove the splint, sliding it forward. To reapply the splint, maintain DIP extension with your other hand as you put the splint back on."

Work with the client to devise a schedule for removing the splint four to six times daily to provide airflow. Make sure the client knows the proper techniques for keeping the DIP always supported in extension.

Emphasize the importance of skin care: "Moisture that is trapped inside the splint may lead to skin problems such as maceration, which must be avoided." Teach the client what skin maceration looks like.

About Exercises

Information about exercise might be provided as follows:

"It is important to avoid resistive or powerful gripping or forceful bending or flexion of the injured fingers and of the entire hand, if need be, to prevent any strain on the healing terminal tendon."

Instruct the client in AROM for the unsplinted digits and especially PIP flexion of the injured digit: "It is very important to achieve full PIP active flexion. The injured finger could stiffen at the PIP if it is not exercised gently. It is very important to prevent the uninjured digits from stiffening." Demonstrate and practice gentle PIP blocking exercises and flexor digitorum superficialis (FDS) fisting motions with the DIP splint in place.

EVALUATION TIPS

- The client's finger is likely to be tender and swollen over the dorsal DIP area. Use a gentle touch around this area.
- Circumferential measurements may best be deferred to avoid causing pain by applying or cinching a tape measure or similar measurement device. Also, measuring the DIP joint is difficult while maintaining and supporting the digit in full DIP extension.

Precaution. Avoid volumetric measurement, because this would leave the DIP unsupported, which is contraindicated.

- Assess the client for digital hypermobility. Observe for DIP extensor lag or PIP hyperextension of other digits and treat accordingly (see description of swan neck deformity).
- Check isolated DIP flexion of other digits gently while the injured DIP is splinted, if the client can isolate this without stressing the terminal tendon of the injured digit. This helps prevent the development of a quadriga effect.

DIAGNOSIS-SPECIFIC INFORMATION THAT AFFECTS CLINICAL REASONING

- Individualize the treatment based on your observation and evaluation. If DIP hyperextension has been ordered but the client cannot tolerate it, support the DIP in a tolerable position and see the client every few days for splint modification until the desired position is achieved. Notify the physician if full DIP extension or hyperextension cannot be achieved in the splint.
- If edema is significant, assume that you will need to readjust the splint as this resolves and schedule recheck visits accordingly. Upgrade the interventions as appropriate for edema management.
- A client who is hypermobile and has laxity of the uninjured digits is at greater risk of developing a secondary swan neck deformity. This client needs a splint that prevents PIP hyperextension and supports the DIP in extension. Teach clients the FDS fist exer-

cise with the DIP splint in place. The FDS fist technique is a compatible exercise because it does not stress the mallet injury and it promotes metacarpophalangeal (MP) and PIP flexion AROM.

- Make sure your client is well trained in monitoring skin tolerances to the splint. Consider giving clients a color picture showing maceration. Using more than one style of splint can help prevent skin problems.

Precaution. Clients should call for a recheck if any skin problems occur.

TIPS FROM THE FIELD

Splinting

- Show the client pictures or samples of DIP splints or casts. Explain your recommendation in terms of comfort, effectiveness, and adjustability. Ask clients about their preferences. Advise the client to tape the splint in place at night, because it may slide off during sleep.
- Small splints are not always the quickest to make. Allow time to fine-tune the splint and readjust it as needed.
- Clients often appreciate having a separate splint to use in the shower. Also, they can change into the dry splint after the shower, which helps prevent maceration.

Client Compliance

- In the clinic, does the client demonstrate proper technique for maintaining DIP extension at all times? Is the splint clean? Does it look unused? Are the straps showing wear? Do you see lack of improvement in gaining DIP extension?
- Some clients need more supervision and follow-up than others. Reasons to recheck the client more often include (1) resolving or fluctuating edema, (2) wound care, (3) PIP stiffness, (4) risk of swan neck deformity developing, and (5) questionable technique for putting on and taking off the splint. The therapy note should document whether the client demonstrates good technique in therapy and at follow-up.

Precautions and Concerns

- *Check for skin maceration.*
- *Emphasize the importance of avoiding forceful or resistive gripping or quick flexion motions.*
- *Monitor for the development of PIP hyperextension, especially if the client demonstrates laxity of the digits.*

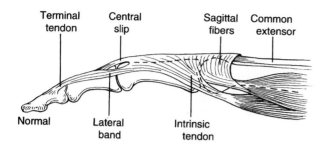

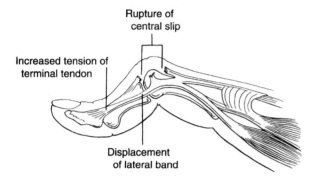

FIGURE 15-3 Boutonniere deformity. (From Burke SL: *Hand and upper extremity rehabilitation: a practical guide*, ed 3, St Louis, 2005, Churchill Livingstone.)

- *If the splint is taped on at night, caution the client to avoid circumferential taping, because this could produce a tourniquet effect.*

BOUTONNIERE DEFORMITY

ANATOMY

With a **boutonniere deformity,** the finger postures in PIP flexion and DIP hyperextension (Fig. 15-3). The injury may be open or closed. With a closed injury, the boutonniere deformity may not develop immediately but may become noticeable within 2 or 3 weeks after the injury.[8] The client may have a PIP extensor lag or, with an older injury, a PIP flexion contracture. This distinction affects the therapy choices.

DIAGNOSIS AND PATHOLOGY

A boutonniere deformity involves disruption of the central slip of the extensor tendon, which normally inserts into the dorsal base of the middle phalanx. The disruption of the central slip causes the **lateral bands (LB)** to slip volar to the PIP joint axis of motion, creating flexor forces on the PIP joint.[11] The imbalance results in hyperextension of the DIP joint.[12] With this DIP posture, the **oblique retinacular ligament (ORL)** of Landsmeer, which is located at the dorsal DIP joint, is at risk of

becoming tight. A **pseudoboutonniere deformity** is actually an injury to the PIP volar plate and is usually the result of a PIP hyperextension injury.

CLINICAL *Pearl*

With a pseudoboutonniere deformity, the damage occurs at the volar surface. With a boutonniere deformity, the damage occurs at the dorsal surface.[1]

TIMELINES AND HEALING

PIP extension splinting or casting may be used day and night for up to 6 weeks. This is followed by 3 weeks of night splinting. Splinting is used during the time needed for the central slip to re-establish tissue continuity and for correction of the deformity.[8]

NONOPERATIVE TREATMENT

The ability to passively extend the PIP may be a good indicator for nonoperative treatment with PIP splinting in extension. The MP and DIP are not splinted. Serial splinting adjustments may have to be made to achieve full passive PIP extension. Different types of splints can be used for this purpose (Fig. 15-4).

While the PIP is being splinted, it is very important that the therapist instruct the client in isolated DIP flexion exercises to recover normal length of the ORL. These exercises are done actively and passively in a gentle fashion (Fig. 15-5). The therapist should watch for normal MP AROM and should exercise this as needed.

Precaution. *After the client has been medically cleared to begin PIP active flexion, initiate restricted amounts of flexion at first and watch for PIP extensor lag.*

It also is important to exercise PIP active extension, which is facilitated by positioning the digit in MP flexion. Splinting is reinstituted as needed if a PIP extensor lag develops.

If exercise fails to recover DIP flexion with the PIP extended, **ORL tightness** (limited passive DIP flexion with the PIP extended) may need to be addressed with splinting. Various small, custom-made splints can be used for dynamic or static progressive DIP flexion with the PIP in full extension.[13]

OPERATIVE TREATMENT

Boutonniere deformity is caused by injury to zone III of the extensor tendons. Various surgical techniques are used to treat these injuries.[8] The therapy protocol is determined by the hand surgeon. The short arc of motion

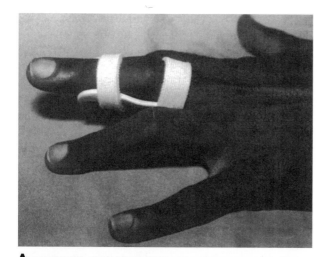

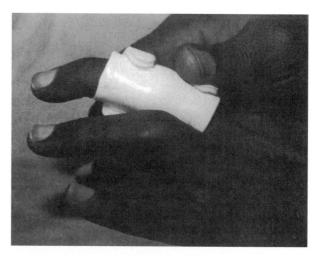

FIGURE 15-5 Oblique retinacular ligament stretch entails isolated DIP flexion with PIP supported in extension. This is done actively and passively. (From Clark GL: *Hand rehabilitation: a practical guide*, ed 2, New York, 1998, Churchill Livingstone.)

- *When can active PIP extension be started?*
- *What are the precautions?*

What to Say to Clients

About the Injury

Information about the injury might be provided as follows:

"Here is a diagram of the area of your finger that is injured. Notice how, as a result of injury to the central slip, the lateral bands have slipped forward (volar) and how they now contribute to the bent posture of the PIP joint. The PIP joint needs to be supported in extension for the injured tendon to heal in proper alignment. Also note how the end of the finger is tipped upward (hyperextended). As the injury at the PIP is corrected, the position at tip of the finger will also improve. In addition, specific exercises can help correct this."

About Exercises

Information about exercise might be provided as follows:

"With this diagnosis, improving DIP flexion while the PIP is extended actually helps improve PIP extension. Therefore, flexing just the DIP helps correct the lack of extension at the PIP. It is very important to exercise by bending the tip gently while the PIP is splinted, because this is corrective for your injury."

EVALUATION TIPS

- Check for hypermobility of the other digits. Do the uninjured digits have a boutonniere-like posture? If so, document this condition.
- Determine whether the PIP joint can be passively corrected to neutral and whether the DIP joint can

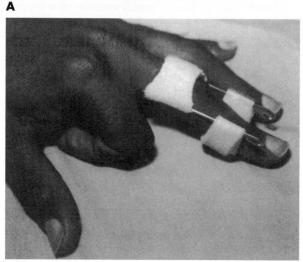

FIGURE 15-4 A, Volar splint for boutonniere deformity. **B,** Wire-foam splint for boutonniere deformity. (From Clark GL: *Hand rehabilitation: a practical guide*, ed 2, New York, 1998, Churchill Livingstone.)

protocol for zone III extensor tendon repairs is appropriate if the client is considered a good candidate for this treatment (see Chapter 16).

Questions to Ask the Physician

- *Nonoperative clients*
  - *How long should the PIP be splinted in extension?*
  - *When can active PIP flexion be started?*
- *Operative clients*
  - *What structures were repaired? (Ask to see the operative report.)*
  - *Does the surgeon prefer an early active motion protocol or more conservative therapy, such as immobilization?*

be passively corrected to normal flexion with the PIP in extension (i.e., check for ORL tightness).

- Check and practice isolated DIP flexion of the other digits. Think ahead about preventing a quadriga effect.
- Check composite flexion of the other digits as you are able.

DIAGNOSIS-SPECIFIC INFORMATION THAT AFFECTS CLINICAL REASONING

- In nonoperative clients, determine whether the injury involves a PIP extensor lag (the PIP can be passively extended to neutral position, but the client cannot actively extend it) or a PIP flexion contracture (the PIP cannot be passively extended to neutral position). This distinction affects splint decisions (see below).
- Determine whether the client has ORL tightness. With this condition, both active and passive DIP flexion with PIP extension are limited.

TIPS FROM THE FIELD
Clinical Picture

- Edema over the area of injury (dorsal PIP) worsens the deforming forces of a boutonniere position. Treat the edema as a high priority, because this helps recover PIP joint passive extension and promotes normalization throughout. Light compression wrapping can help reduce the edema.

Precaution. *If ORL tightness is present, the client may be at risk of losing flexor digitorum profundus (FDP) excursion, and a quadriga effect could develop.*

- Isolating and exercising DIP active flexion of the uninjured digits while protecting the injured finger is a good measure for preventing a quadriga effect. PIP cylindric splints may be helpful for performing isolated blocking exercises for DIP flexion. These splints can be used on all digits to isolate DIP active flexion with varying MP positions.

CLINICAL *Pearl*

- After the client has been medically cleared for active PIP extension exercises, use positioning of the MP in flexion for the exercises. This can help isolate and achieve active PIP extension.
- Check for intrinsic versus extrinsic tightness if composite flexion is limited and prioritize the MP position accordingly for PIP exercise.

Precaution. *As PIP flexion improves, watch closely for PIP extensor lag.*

Splinting

- If the client has a PIP flexion contracture, corrective splinting or casting is needed. Splint and casting choices for recovering PIP extension include serial static splints, serial casts, static progressive splints, and dynamic splints. These may be prefabricated or custom-made and digit based or hand based. Therapists have different preferences, and the client should participate in the selection process. Comfort, fit, and skin tolerance all influence these choices.
- If full passive PIP extension is possible, a small PIP extension gutter splint or cast may be used. Adjust it as needed to accommodate resolution of edema and the client's comfort. The splint may need to be taped in place at night. It is very important to keep the DIP free and to perform frequent exercises for DIP active and passive flexion while the PIP is splinted in extension.
- If ORL tightness is present, a dorsal dropout splint for DIP flexion may be helpful, or a gentle DIP flexion static progressive or dynamic splint may be appropriate. Ease of application and adjustability are criteria that help determine which type should be used.
- If the client has been cleared for active PIP extension and flexion exercises and if ORL tightness is present, try using a dorsal distal splint that maintains DIP flexion while actively exercising PIP extension.

Precautions and Concerns

- *Avoid PIP flexion during the protective splinting phase.*
- *If the client has had surgery, follow the guidelines presented in Chapter 16. Instruct the client in techniques for supporting the digit while putting on and taking off the splint for skin care needs. If surgery was not required, instruct the client in ways to manage splint and skin care while avoiding PIP flexion. If a cast has been applied, change it at least weekly.*
- *ORL tightness contributes to the boutonniere deforming forces. Monitor this condition throughout the program and continue exercising active and passive DIP flexion with the PIP extended.*
- *Monitor for loss of FDP excursion and difficulty isolating the FDS, particularly in the involved digit.*
- *If the client has had surgery, adhesions may occur at the incision sites.*

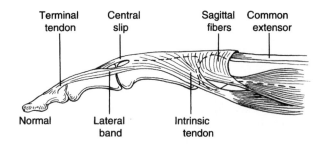

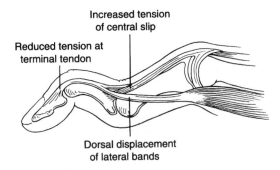

FIGURE 15-6 Swan neck deformity. (From Burke SL: *Hand and upper extremity rehabilitation: a practical guide,* ed 3, St Louis, 2005, Churchill Livingstone.)

SWAN NECK DEFORMITY

ANATOMY

In a **swan neck deformity,** the finger postures with PIP hyperextension and DIP flexion (Fig. 15-6).[5] The MP tends to be flexed, and the finger appears to zigzag when observed from the side. The IP joints may be passively correctable, or they may be fixed in their deformity positions. The IP positions in the swan neck deformity are the opposite of their positions in the boutonniere deformity.

DIAGNOSIS AND PATHOLOGY

The swan neck deformity can be caused by injuries at the level of the DIP, the PIP, or the MP joint. At the DIP level, a mallet injury can lead to swan neck deformity. In this case, the terminal extensor tendon is disrupted (i.e., stretched or ruptured). This allows the extensor force to be more powerful proximally at the PIP joint, leading to PIP hyperextension.[12]

If the cause is primarily at the PIP level, the volar capsule is involved, with hyperextension at the PIP joint. The LB are dorsally displaced, contributing to PIP hyperextension; this minimizes the pull on the terminal extensor tendon; therefore, the DIP joint assumes a flexed position. Normally the FDS helps deter PIP hyperextension. However, if the FDS has been ruptured or lengthened, PIP hyperextension forces are less restricted or controlled. Intrinsic muscle tightness compounds the problem.[12] Painful snapping may be noticed with active flexion. This snapping is caused by the LB at the proximal phalanx condyles.[14]

If the cause of the swan neck deformity is primarily at the MP level, MP volar subluxation and ulnar drift may be the initiating factors, as is seen in rheumatoid arthritis. The MP joint disturbance leads to intrinsic muscle imbalance and tightness, with resulting PIP hyperextension forces.[12]

TIMELINES AND HEALING

Swan neck deformity is a challenging diagnosis. In conservative management of this condition, splinting may be used indefinitely if it promotes improved function and eliminates painful snapping with active flexion.

NONOPERATIVE TREATMENT

Splinting of the PIP in slight flexion may be very helpful functionally. Many different kinds of splints can be used for this type of deformity, including dorsal blocking splints, figure **8** splints, and commercially available splints, such as the SIRIS (i.e., silver ring) splint (Fig. 15-7). The purpose of the splint is to prevent hyperextension at the PIP joint and to promote active PIP flexion.

OPERATIVE TREATMENT

Surgery to correct swan neck deformity may be done in conjunction with other reconstructive procedures for clients with rheumatoid arthritis. Surgical techniques include flexor FDS tenodesis or VP advancement procedures.[14] Some researchers have found that capsulodesis and tenodesis techniques for restoring balance lose effectiveness as a result of attenuation if these issues are stressed over time.[15]

After the surgery, clients may be referred to therapy for protective dorsal PIP splinting in flexion or for pin site care, wound care, or edema control. After they have been medically cleared for them, active DIP extension exercises may be advised. Positioning the digit in PIP flexion helps promote DIP active extension excursion.

Pins often are used postoperatively to maintain PIP flexion. When the pins are removed, digit-based, dorsal PIP splints are used, typically fabricated in approximately 20 to 30 degrees of flexion. This is done to prevent recurrence of PIP hyperextension and imbalance. Active PIP

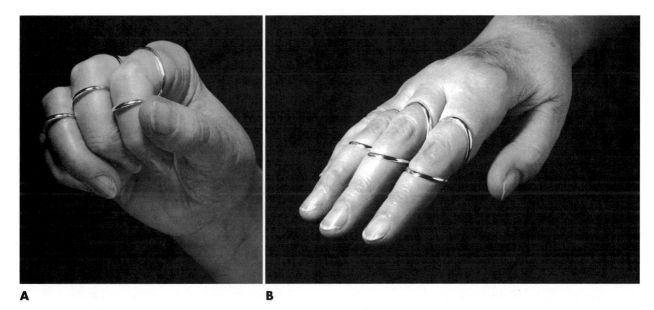

FIGURE 15-7 A SIRIS (silver ring) splint prevents PIP hyperextension and allows PIP flexion. (Courtesy Silver Ring Splint Co., Charlottesville, VA.)

flexion exercises are started when ordered by the surgeon. The PIP dorsal splint can remain in place during PIP AROM. The Velcro strap is removed distally to allow PIP flexion while full extension is blocked.

The therapist should focus on balancing digit and hand function while avoiding stress or PIP hyperextension. DIP caps may be helpful exercise tools to promote ease of flexion at the PIP. As a result of the imbalance associated with swan neck deformities, these clients habitually have made fisting motions with the PIP in hyperextension, visibly initiating motion with DIP flexion while the PIP is hyperextended. Their fisting motions look awkward and difficult to achieve. The therapist should try practicing gentle fisting arcs of motion, with PIP flexion preceding DIP flexion if possible. Gently holding the MPs in flexion may help restore a more natural and balanced fisting motion. Practicing on the contralateral side may also be helpful.

Questions to Ask the Physician

- *Nonoperative clients*
  - *Are particular precautions required?*
  - *Is surgery a possibility?*
- *Operative clients*
  - *What structures were repaired? (Ask to see the operative report.)*
  - *When will the pins be removed?*
  - *When can active PIP flexion be started?*
  - *What specific precautions are in order?*

What to Say to Clients

About the Injury

Information about the injury might be provided as follows:

"Here is a diagram of the deforming forces associated with swan neck deformity. Notice how the lateral bands have slipped upward (dorsally) and how they now contribute to the overextended posture of the PIP joint. The PIP joint needs to be supported in flexion for balance and proper alignment to be restored."

About Exercises

Information about exercise might be provided as follows:

"With this diagnosis, it is most important to avoid extending the PIP joint beyond its newly pinned or corrected position until the doctor upgrades the program. For this reason, we will use protective dorsal splints. When the doctor gives the okay for exercise, it is important to practice gentle bending movements at the PIP joint in a comfortable range."

EVALUATION TIPS

- Check for hypermobility or swan neck posture of uninjured digits. Document this condition if present.
- Determine whether PIP hyperextension is passively correctable or fixed. Does it affect function?
- In a nonoperative client, distinguish between primary injury to the DIP or the PIP:

- Stabilize the PIP in neutral position. If the client cannot actively extend the DIP, the injury is primarily a DIP extensor injury. If the client can actively extend the DIP, the injury is primarily a volar PIP injury.
- When exercise therapy has been medically cleared, observe the quality of active flexion and promote practice of motions that do not elicit snapping.

DIAGNOSIS-SPECIFIC INFORMATION THAT AFFECTS CLINICAL REASONING

- Focus treatment on the primary cause of the deformity. If the client has rheumatoid arthritis (RA), are other digits involved or at risk? Have any tendons ruptured? Is the client receiving medical care for the RA? Consider antideformity splinting for other digits as appropriate. Is MP involvement present? Is intrinsic tightness of other digits a factor? Night splinting or intrinsic stretching (or both) to counteract deforming forces may be valuable. Even if this option was not ordered originally, discuss it with the client and the physician.
- Is PIP flexion splinting likely to be long term? If so, consider a low-profile, long-lasting style of splint, such as a silver ring splint.

TIPS FROM THE FIELD

- Observe the balance of the digit and the hand, and address uninvolved digits unless this is contraindicated. Promote normal range of motion (ROM) throughout the extremity as appropriate.
- If postoperative wound healing is a factor, try to see the client often for splint modifications to accommodate dressing changes and edema reduction.
- If the client's joints are hypermobile, instruct the person in hand use patterns for activities of daily living (ADL) that do not encourage PIP hyperextension. For example, teach the client not to put stress on the digits in PIP hyperextension.

Precautions and Concerns

- *If you are treating a mallet injury, watch closely for signs of PIP hyperextension that occur secondary to DIP splinting (see the section on mallet finger).*
- *Clients do not need to be hypermobile to develop a swan neck deformity after distal digital injury.*
- *Mallet injury is not the only diagnosis that can lead to PIP hyperextension. A distal crush or fracture requiring DIP splinting may also result in PIP hyperextension. Be alert for this and treat it accordingly with PIP splinting in slight flexion to normalize the balance of the digit.*

PIP JOINT INJURIES

Digital PIP injuries occur frequently, yet they can be extremely challenging to treat. Proper management of therapy helps prevent the situation from becoming frustrating.

PIP joint dislocation is a common injury.[15] A client initially may ignore a sprain of the small joints of the hand, not realizing the significance of the injury, and may not seek medical attention for days or weeks after the injury. *By this time, significant edema, fibrosis, and stiffness may be established.* Joint enlargement and flexion contractures are common residual problems.[3,16]

CLINICAL *Pearl*

Therapists are likely to see clients with digital sprains or dislocations quite often. Because clients may not understand the serious clinical implications of this seemingly simple diagnosis, they can become frustrated with the progression of treatment. Early communication with the client about the nature of the PIP joint injury and the likelihood of a prolonged recovery are important.

ANATOMY

PIP Joint Architecture

The PIP joint is a hinge joint with 100 to 110 degrees of motion. At the proximal phalanx are two condyles, and between the condyles is the intercondylar notch. Because of the slight asymmetry of the condyles, about 9 degrees of supination occurs with PIP flexion.[3] At the base of the middle phalanx are two concave fossae and a ridge that separates the phalanx's flat, broad base. Stability is enhanced by the amount of congruence of this joint and by its tongue-and-groove contour. The IP joint of the thumb is architecturally similar to the PIP joint of the other digits.[15]

PIP Joint Stability

The architecture of the PIP joint, along with its ligamentous support, provides joint stability. The **collateral ligaments** are the main restraints on deviation forces at the PIP joint. These ligaments are 2 to 3 mm thick and are extremely important to the joint's stability. The collateral ligaments have two components: the **proper collateral ligament (PCL),** and the **accessory collateral ligament (ACL),** which are differentiated by their areas of insertion.

The PCL originates on the lateral aspect of the proximal phalanx. The fibers of this ligament insert volarly

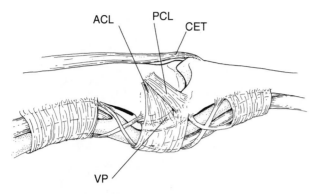

FIGURE 15-8 Structures that provide PIP joint stability include the accessory collateral ligament (ACL), the proper collateral ligament (PCL), the dorsal capsule with the central extensor tendon (CET), and the volar plate (VP). (From Mackin EJ: *Hunter, Mackin & Callahan's rehabilitation of the hand and upper extremity,* ed 5, St Louis, 2002, Mosby.)

and distally, on the lateral tubercles of the middle phalanx. The fibers of the ACL insert in a more volar direction on the VP. The VP is fibrocartilaginous and is situated between the collateral ligaments on the volar aspect of the PIP joint. The convergence of the PCL, ACL, and VP at the middle phalanx is known as the *critical corner,* a term that reflects its importance to PIP joint stability.[3]

The anatomic arrangement of the VP functions to prevent PIP hyperextension. The VP also acts as a secondary PIP joint stabilizer laterally when the collateral ligaments have been injured.[3,15]

The dynamic stability of the PIP joint is enhanced by the tendons that cross the joint. These are the **central extensor tendon (CET),** the LB, the **transverse retinacular ligament (TRL),** and the ORL. The CET is part of the dorsal capsule of the PIP joint and attaches to the middle phalanx at the dorsal tubercle. The LB have intrinsic muscle contributions and lie volar to the MP joint axis; they join dorsal to the PIP joint axis to form the terminal extensor tendon. The TRL originates from the volar surface of the LB and envelops the collateral ligaments and PIP joint, thereby preventing dorsal displacement of the LB. The ORL originates from the flexor sheath, progresses volar to the PIP joint axis, and inserts at the terminal extensor tendon dorsally. The ORL tightens when the PIP joint extends. It provides concomitant PIP and DIP extension and helps prevent hyperextension of the PIP joint (Fig. 15-8).[3]

DIAGNOSIS AND PATHOLOGY

Physical examination of ligament injuries at the PIP joint requires assessment of joint stability. Posteroanterior

BOX 15-1

Grades of Ligament Sprain Injuries

MILD GRADE I SPRAIN
- *Definition:* No instability with active or passive ROM; macroscopic continuity with microscopic tears. The ligament is intact, but individual fibers are damaged.
- *Treatment:* Immobilize the joint in full extension if comfortable and available; otherwise, immobilize in a small amount of flexion. When pain has subsided, begin AROM and protect with buddy taping.

GRADE II SPRAIN
- *Definition:* Abnormal laxity with stress; the collateral ligament is disrupted. AROM is stable, but passive testing reveals instability.
- *Treatment:* Splint for 2 to 4 weeks. The physician may recommend early ROM, but avoid any lateral stress.

GRADE III SPRAIN
- *Definition:* Complete tearing of the collateral ligament, along with injury to the dorsal capsule or volar plate. The finger usually is dislocated by the injury.
- *Treatment:* Early surgical intervention often is recommended.

Modified from Campbell PJ, Wilson RL: Management of joint injuries and intraarticular fractures. In Mackin EJ, Callahan AD, Skirven TM et al, editors: *Rehabilitation of the hand and upper extremity,* ed 5, St Louis, 2002, Mosby; and Glickel SZ, Barron A, Eaton RG: Dislocations and ligament injuries in the digits. In Green DP, Hotchkiss RN, Pederson WC, editors: *Green's operative hand surgery,* ed 4, Philadelphia, 1999, Churchill Livingstone.

(PA) and true lateral x-rays can identify articular involvement, but x-rays alone may not reveal subtle injuries. The critical issue is whether joint stability exists with active motion.[15]

The **functional stability** of the PIP joint is tested actively and passively. If the client demonstrates normal active ROM with no PIP joint displacement, joint stability is adequate despite the injury. A brief period of immobilization can be followed by protected ROM exercises. If the joint is displaced with active ROM, major disruption of the ligaments probably has occurred. In these cases the position of immobilization is determined by the physician, partly by identifying the range at which the displacement occurs (Box 15-1). In grade I and mild grade II injuries, the joints are swollen; they also are painful on palpation and with lateral stress.

BOX 15-2

Directional Types of PIP Joint Dislocation

DORSAL PIP DISLOCATIONS

Dorsal PIP dislocations are classified according to three subcategories:

- *Type I (hyperextension):* Volar plate avulsion and minor split in collateral ligaments longitudinally; if left untreated, this type of dislocation can lead to a swan neck deformity.
- *Type II (dorsal dislocation):* Dorsal dislocation of PIP joint and volar plate avulsion with major split in collateral ligaments bilaterally.
- *Type III (fracture-dislocation):* This type of dislocation may be stable or unstable.

LATERAL PIP DISLOCATIONS

Lateral stability is tested with the PIP joint in extension so that the collateral ligaments and secondary stabilizers, including the volar plate, can be assessed. Complete collateral ligament disruption is suggested by deformity that exceeds 20 degrees of deformity with gentle stress.

VOLAR PIP DISLOCATIONS

Volar PIP dislocations are rare. The injury may have a rotational component, and the central slip may be ruptured.

Modified from Glickel SZ, Barron A, Eaton RG: Dislocations and ligament injuries in the digits. In Green DP, Hotchkiss RN, Pederson WC, editors: *Green's operative hand surgery,* ed 4, Philadelphia, 1999, Churchill Livingstone.

Direction of PIP Joint Dislocation

The direction of dislocation is determined by the position of the middle phalanx at the time of joint injury (Box 15-2).

TIMELINES AND HEALING

CLINICAL *Pearl*

PIP joint sprains usually require a prolonged recovery period, and clients are at risk for long-standing edema. Permanent limitations in ROM and function are not uncommon.

PIP joint sprains initially have **fusiform swelling** (swelling that is fuller at the PIP joint and tapers at both ends), and ligament fibrosis can progress for over a year after injury, resulting in limitations in ROM and function. *Uninjured digits may become stiff, and a quadriga effect can occur.*

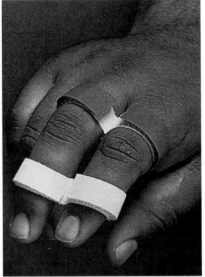
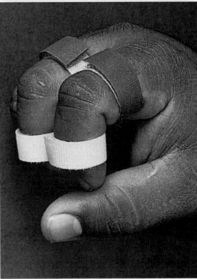

FIGURE 15-9 Buddy straps support the injured digit and facilitate motion. (From Mackin EJ: *Hunter, Mackin & Callahan's rehabilitation of the hand and upper extremity,* ed 5, St Louis, 2002, Mosby.)

NONOPERATIVE TREATMENT

Grade I injuries are treated with edema control and PIP immobilization in extension or possibly slight flexion while acute pain is present, which may be for a week or so. Buddy taping (Fig. 15-9) is very important, because it protects the injured digit by enhancing support from the adjacent digit and allows initiation of early AROM in pain-free ranges. Many different styles of buddy taping can be used.[3]

Grade II injuries are treated with splinting for up to 4 weeks. If early AROM is prescribed, the therapist should take care not to put stress on the joint (i.e., the joint should not be pushed laterally, and loading the tip should be avoided). The client also should be taught to avoid stressing the joint. Edema is treated as possible. Compressive sleeves or wraps may not be tolerated early on, but an attempt can be made to try to use them with light pressure.

Grade III injuries frequently require surgical correction. If joint congruence is present with AROM, conservative treatment may be tried. If the VP has been injured (as in a hyperextension injury), a dorsal blocking splint can be provided to prevent full PIP extension in the first few weeks. The amount of PIP flexion in this splint usually is 20 to 30 degrees, and the physician may specify the degree of flexion.

OPERATIVE TREATMENT

Surgical techniques vary, depending on the injury. VP arthroplasty may be performed on dorsal dislocations. Complications of this procedure can include angulation deformity of the middle phalanx, recurrence of subluxation, or IP joint stiffness. FDS tenodesis techniques may be performed for chronic PIP hyperextension (swan neck) deformities. Complications with the tension of the tenodesis may affect the PIP position after surgery. Collateral ligament repair may be performed for lateral PIP dislocation injuries. Stiffness can be an undesirable sequela of this surgery.[15]

Questions to Ask the Physician

- *Nonoperative clients*
  - *Is surgery a possibility?*
  - *Are precautions required regarding AROM and stability (i.e., a safe range for AROM exercises or VP implications)?*
- *Operative clients*
  - *What structures were repaired? (Ask to see operative report.)*
  - *Is PIP extension to be restricted? If so, to what degree (i.e., is VP involvement a factor)?*
  - *What ROM does the physician expect the client ultimately to achieve?*

What to Say to Clients

About the Injury

Information about the injury might be provided as follows:

"This diagnosis is associated with a long timeline for slow healing, and swelling typically persists for a much longer time than you might expect. It helps to be aware of this so that you won't be discouraged by the persistent swelling or stiffness. Sometimes clients have had to have their rings resized, but time will tell whether this will be necessary. It may be helpful to use sleeves or wraps for the swelling for a considerable time."

"While the tissue is healing over weeks and months, it is very important not to stress the finger with force or high-demand gripping activity. If you do something with your hand and the finger swells or becomes painful, this is a sign that your tissues are not tolerating that much stress. It is best to avoid this response so that the swelling and flexibility can continue to improve."

About Splinting

Information about splinting might be provided as follows:

"Buddy straps are very helpful in providing support to the injured finger. You may find they also help promote more flexibility of the finger. Various splinting options can help with recovering motion, and different types may be tried over time."

Instruct the client in a schedule for wearing the buddy straps and splints between exercises and at night as appropriate.

About Exercise

Information about exercise might be provided as follows:

"Each time your tissue is stimulated by pain-free movement, favorable clinical responses occur, including lubrication and circulation to promote healing. The more this happens, the better the finger will be. However, exercises that result in swelling or pain are not helpful and are actually detrimental."

EVALUATION TIPS

- Ask about previous injuries to this or other digits, because pre-existing stiffness may affect the client's prognosis.
- Be very gentle when evaluating the digit; the client's finger may be quite sore.
- Distinguish between fusiform swelling (swelling localized around the PIP joint) and edema throughout the digit.
- When the client is cleared for AROM exercises, check isolated FDS and FDP function. Also check for ORL tightness (i.e., check for DIP flexion with PIP extension).
- Distinguish between intrinsic, extrinsic, and joint tightness.
- Inquire about daily activities to determine whether some of them may be detrimental to the healing process.

DIAGNOSIS-SPECIFIC INFORMATION THAT AFFECTS CLINICAL REASONING

- The mechanics of the injury and whether the VP was involved are important pieces of information. If the VP was involved, the PIP should be protected in 20 to 30 degrees of flexion to promote VP healing. Also, keep in mind that collateral ligaments are at risk of tightening if full extension is not achieved in a timely fashion.

- Edema management is paramount with PIP joint injuries, which are notorious for persistent swelling. Swelling contributes to pain, shortening or tightening of the collateral ligaments, and loss of joint motion and tendon excursion. Therefore the treatment of swelling should be a clinical priority. Compounding the problem, AROM and all exercises should be limited to the amount of stimulation that does not cause increased swelling.

CLINICAL *Pearl*

- It does no good to gain 10 degrees of motion with exercises if swelling and stiffness also occur in response to those exercises.

- Devise exercises that are tissue specific. Distinguish between intrinsic and extrinsic tightness and position the finger for exercises accordingly. Check FDS and FDP excursion in the uninjured digits and perform isolated FDS exercises, because these promote PIP flexion and prevent the insidious development of limitations.

TIPS FROM THE FIELD

Tissue Tolerances and Client Education

- Monitor tissue tolerances, which dictate the hand therapy intervention. This can be frustrating to clients and therapists. Explain to clients that with this type of injury, they cannot force motion to improve, and strenuous hand movements will only worsen the clinical condition. Despite this instruction, clients may be inclined to perform forceful place and hold exercises to recover flexion, and this may actually be injurious to the tissues. Keep discussing tissue tolerances with clients and teach them how to perform pain-free exercises. Friends may have recommended forceful gripping exercises, such as squeezing a tennis ball or a resistive gripper; explain that the tissues need to be ready for this much stimulation, that negative tissue responses are manifested by swelling and pain after exercise, and that these responses can set back the progression toward recovery.

Buddy Taping

- Include clients in the decision on which adjacent finger to buddy tape to the injured finger. Normally, the finger that supports the injured side is selected. If the right long finger sustained an injury to the PIP radial collateral ligament, it needs protection to avoid ulnar stress. In this instance, buddy tape the long finger to the index finger to promote neutral alignment.

- Buddy tapes may be most helpful when used at two levels (e.g., proximal phalanx and middle phalanx). The important features are support, comfort, and ease of use. Monitor the tightness of the buddy tapes, because tapes that are too tight can worsen the edema by creating a tourniquet effect.

Exercise Guidelines

- Brief, frequent, pain-free exercises are more effective than infrequent sessions. Explain to the client that tissue tolerance dictates the exercise regimen.

- Gentle upward petting or stroking of the skin on the sides of the PIP joint, along with gentle circular motions over the dorsal PIP joint, may promote comfort with exercises. The pressure should be just enough to move the skin (this technique should not be used if tenderness is present).

Precautions and Concerns

- *Avoid exercises that cause increased pain or stiffness.*
- *With PIP joint injuries, the importance of tissue tolerance cannot be overstated.*
- *Persistent edema that is avoidable can lead to serious clinical and functional consequences.*
- *The long healing timeline for this type of injury makes therapy a challenge. Therapists must be very creative in providing factual information about steady progress while preventing the client from becoming disappointed or discouraged.*

THUMB MP JOINT INJURY

Clients with injuries of the thumb MP joint, particularly ulnar collateral ligament (UCL) injuries, frequently are referred for hand therapy. Proper hand therapy can favorably affect the recovery of stable, pain-free function in such cases.

Injury to the thumb MP joint may involve either the ulnar collateral ligament (UCL) or the radial collateral ligament (RCL). The UCL is injured 10 times as often as the RCL. The treatment guidelines described for UCL injury also apply to the RCL.

ANATOMY

The MP joint of the thumb is primarily a hinge joint. Flexion and extension comprise the primary arc of motion. Pronation-supination and abduction-adduction are considered secondary arcs of motion at this joint. Pronation occurs as the thumb MP joint flexes because the radial condyle of the metacarpal head is wider than the ulnar condyle.[3,15]

The thumb MP joint's ROM is unique; it has the most variation in the amount of movement of all the body's joints. ROM at the thumb MP joint ranges from 6 to 86 degrees of flexion. People with flatter metacarpal heads tend to have less motion, and individuals with more spherical metacarpal heads have more motion. Lateral motion at the thumb MP joint ranges from 0 to 20 degrees when the MP is in extension. The stability of this joint comes primarily from ligamentous, capsular, and musculotendinous support.[15]

Laterally, the thumb MP joint displays strong proper collateral ligaments that arise from the metacarpal lateral condyles and progress volarly and obliquely to their insertion on the proximal phalanx. The ACL originates volar to the PCL and inserts on the VP and the sesamoid bones.[17] The sesamoid bones have been described as the convergence point of the thumb MP joint's periarticular structures.[18] The proper collateral ligaments are tightest with MP flexion.

The thumb MP joint receives stability from thenar intrinsic muscles, specifically the adductor pollicis (AP), the flexor pollicis brevis (FPB), and the abductor pollicis brevis (APB). The FPB and the APB insert on the radial sesamoid, and the AP inserts on the ulnar sesamoid.[15]

DIAGNOSIS AND PATHOLOGY

A UCL injury is called **skier's thumb,** because a fall on an outstretched hand with the thumb in abduction is a common skiing injury. The ski pole handle may cause the thumb to abduct. Historically, this injury has also been called **gamekeeper's thumb,** because the term describes an injury that occurred as a result of killing rabbits with a technique that stressed the thumb MP joint radially. Nowadays the term *gamekeeper's thumb* refers to chronic UCL instability at the thumb MP joint.[3]

Acute UCL injuries of the thumb MP joint usually involve detachment of the ligament from its proximal phalanx insertion. Concomitant injury of the ACL, the VP, or the dorsal capsule also may occur. If complete disruption occurs along with forceful radial deviation at the thumb MP joint, displacement of the ligament superficially with interposition of the adductor aponeurosis may result; this condition is called **Stener's lesion** (Fig. 15-10).

Precaution. *Stener's lesion requires surgical correction because the interposition prevents healing of the ligament.[3]*

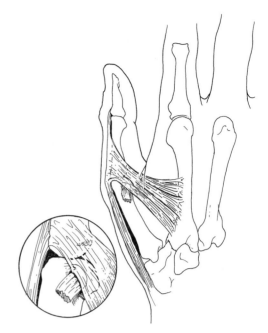

FIGURE 15-10 Stener's lesion. The ulnar collateral ligament is displaced with interposition of the adductor aponeurosis. Surgery is required for this type of injury, because interposition of the adductor aponeurosis prevents healing. (From Mackin EJ: *Hunter, Mackin & Callahan's rehabilitation of the hand and upper extremity,* ed 5, St Louis, 2002, Mosby.)

The thumb MP joint is clinically assessed for UCL injury by providing gentle stress in radial deviation to the thumb with the MP joint in both extension and flexion at 30 degrees. This result is compared with that on the contralateral side. Physicians may use an injection of anesthetic if pain prohibits testing. Varying criteria are used to describe a complete ligament tear: (1) instability greater than 35 degrees or (2) instability 15 degrees greater than on the uninjured side.

CLINICAL *Pearl*

Stress testing may be more painful on a partial tear than on a complete tear.

X-rays in the PA, lateral, and oblique views are taken to rule out the possibility of an avulsion fracture. Stress x-rays may also be helpful. Additional imaging techniques, such as ultrasound studies, magnetic resonance imaging (MRI), and arthrograms, may be ordered as necessary. An overlooked and untreated injury can lead to pain and instability.

TIMELINES AND HEALING

The thumb is immobilized for approximately 4 to 6 weeks to allow healing. Thumb IP joint ROM should be encouraged throughout the immobilization stage. It can take a few months after injury for resistive pinch or axial loading of the thumb to be comfortable and safe to perform.

NONOPERATIVE TREATMENT

If the ligament injury is a partial tear, the thumb is immobilized in a hand-based thumb spica cast (with the IP joint left free) for 2 to 4 weeks. After this, treatment is upgraded to a splint, and AROM exercises are begun with medical clearance. A variety of splints may be used.[19,20] Progression to active assistive range of motion (AAROM) occurs gradually over a few weeks. Light key pinch exercises are started early, but tip pinch and thumb tip loading exercises are not performed until medically approved, which may be 8 weeks or longer after injury. This restriction is necessary in preventing stress on the ligament.[3]

OPERATIVE TREATMENT

Surgical procedures may include open reduction with internal fixation (ORIF) to reduce fracture fragments. The UCL may be reattached to its insertion. The MP joint may be pinned, and this often may be done with a slight overcorrection ulnarly to prevent stress on the repaired ligament. A thumb spica cast is used for 4 weeks, at which time the pin usually is removed.[3]

After the cast is removed, AROM of the thumb carpometacarpal (CMC) and MP joints is started. Scar management and edema control are helpful for minimizing the possibility of adherence of the extensor pollicis longus (EPL) at the incision scar. As in the nonoperative program, lateral pinch may be initiated sooner than tip pinch, which should be avoided for about 8 weeks after surgery to prevent stress on the repair. Protective splinting with a hand-based thumb spica splint may be used for up to 6 to 8 weeks after the repair. The therapist should inform the client that some tenderness at the ulnar MP joint is normal for a few months after this surgery.[3]

Questions to Ask the Physician

- *Nonoperative clients*
  - *Are any precautions indicated for AROM?*
  - *How long should axial loading or resistive tip pinch be avoided?*
- *Operative clients*
  - *What structures were repaired? (Ask to see the operative report.)*
  - *How much ROM does the physician expect the client to achieve at the MP joint?*

- *How long should axial loading or resistive tip pinch be avoided?*
- *Should any other precautions be taken?*
- *How long should protective splinting be used?*

What to Say to Clients

About the Injury

Information about the injury might be provided as follows:

"With this diagnosis, it is more important to achieve a pain-free, stable thumb MP joint than it is to achieve full MP motion. You may not recover full MP motion, but achieving functional, pain-free motion for pinching and resistive hand use usually is considered a successful result."

About Splinting

Information about splinting might be provided as follows:

"You may need to wear your protective splint to prevent forceful use of or stress on the injured thumb. It may also help signal others to be careful when shaking your hand or interacting with you in public."

About Exercises

Information about exercise might be provided as follows:

"It is important to focus on the motion at the last joint [the IP joint] and to prevent stiffness at this site. However, be careful not to put pressure on the end of the thumb tip or to use a powerful pinching motion against the tip of the thumb until the doctor permits this."

EVALUATION TIPS

- Observe the client's contralateral thumb for laxity (including laterally).
- Assess the contralateral thumb for MP and IP AROM.
- Is tightness of the injured thumb's web space present?
- In clients who have had surgery, observe for scar adherence and test for full excursion of the EPL, which also may be adherent.
  - Is full IP active extension present with MP extension? If not, is IP active extension present with the MP in some flexion?
  - Is IP extensor lag present?
- Explore the client's ADL needs and discuss any adaptations needed to protect the injured tissue.

DIAGNOSIS-SPECIFIC INFORMATION THAT AFFECTS CLINICAL REASONING

- Be careful to avoid radial stress on the thumb when splinting and exercising. Some therapists overcorrect the splint position with slight thumb MP ulnar deviation for this reason.

- Fabricate the splint with a good web space opening and with the thumb positioned to prevent loading of the tip. Placing the thumb CMC in abduction/extension may be more protective for preventing loading than placing it in opposition.

TIPS FROM THE FIELD

- The location of the incision scar can put the EPL at risk for developing adherence at that point. If EPL adherence is present, splinting the IP joint in extension at night or when not exercising may help. Work on scar management and, at that site, position the MP or other proximal joints in some flexion to promote active IP extension.
- The flexor pollicis longus (FPL) is easier to isolate than the FPB. Because of this, and because immobilization contributes to MP stiffness, clients often have difficulty isolating active flexion at the thumb MP. If they override with IP flexion, try using a volar IP extension gutter splint to isolate for MP flexion active exercises. Simultaneous proximal support of the metacarpal also may help.

Precautions and Concerns

- *Be alert for and take steps to prevent the development of a thumb web space contracture. Although a typical approach is to splint in overcorrection (slight ulnar deviation), don't allow thumb abduction or tightness of the thumb web space to occur.*
- *Avoid tip loading and resistive pinching.*
- *Assess and problem-solve ADL to protect injured structures. Try building up the girth of implements (e.g., construct padded pens) to reduce the load on the thumb MP joint.*
- *Instruct clients to avoid painful use of the thumb.*

Roles of Therapy Assistants

Therapy assistants may be assigned the following tasks:

- Managing edema
- Modifying and refurbishing splints
- Instructing clients in a home program, splint application, and splint and skin care
- Assisting in skin inspection and wound care
- Supervising clients' home exercise program as identified by the therapist
- Providing modifications and adaptations that assist the client in activities of daily living (ADL)
- Reinforcing precautions as identified by therapists

CASE *Studies*

CASE STUDY 15-1

RP, a 48-year-old, left-dominant warehouse worker, had a work-related accident that resulted in a soft tissue mallet injury (i.e., no bony involvement). He was seen for medical care 2 weeks after injury. He had not been splinted after the injury.

Treatment

RP was referred to hand therapy for DIP splinting in neutral position. He had moderate localized edema and tenderness over the dorsal DIP. He had a 30-degree DIP extensor lag but could be passively positioned to neutral. He did not demonstrate signs of hypermobility of the other digits.

RP was shown the typical splint options. He also was taught the importance of maintaining PIP flexion while avoiding any DIP flexion for approximately 6 weeks. He stated that he preferred a splint that supported both the PIP and the DIP for use at work. He said he would not be well enough protected in just a DIP splint. He agreed to use a DIP splint with the PIP free when not at work. He stated that he understood the importance of PIP flexion AROM and that he understood the blocking exercises he had been shown. All this information was documented.

RP was seen again 7 days later. His long splint was dirty, indicating good use of it, but his shorter DIP splint was not dirty. He had limited PIP flexion AROM. He was adamant about continuing to use the full digit-based splint for protection at work. He agreed to exercise more to recover PIP flexion. The physician was consulted and agreed to this plan only if RP demonstrated normal PIP flexion at the next therapy visit in 7 days. All this information was documented.

Result

When seen at the third therapy appointment 7 days later, RP had achieved full PIP flexion. He demonstrated a good understanding of his home splint regimen. The rest of his therapy program was uneventful. He made a good recovery, with full AROM at the DIP in flexion and extension over time.

CASE STUDY 15-2

AR, a 73-year-old, retired, right-dominant man was a winter visitor to the southwest. He attended therapy with his wife and his daughter, who was a physician. AR fell while playing tennis and sustained an ulnar dislocation of the right small finger PIP joint. He initially was seen in the emergency department (ED) of a local hospital. He reported no medical problems that would affect his recovery.

The ED physician splinted the finger in a full-digit alumifoam splint, but the client removed it immediately because it was uncomfortable and he did not want to be restricted in function. He was referred to hand therapy 10 days later with significant edema of the involved digit. Circumferential measurements were deferred because of tenderness. He reported his pain to be localized to the radial PIP joint area; he rated the pain as 4/10 with motion (i.e., 4 on a scale of 1 to 10, 10 being the worst pain) and 1/10 at rest. No sensory problems were reported. AROM of the digit was MP 0/90, PIP 0/45, and DIP 0/17. No dislocation was noted with AROM.

Treatment

AR and his family were instructed in the concepts of tissue tolerance and in balancing rest and gentle stimulation with AROM. AR initially was seen for edema control and fabrication of a hand-based protective splint with the right ring and small fingers in intrinsic-plus position with slight PIP flexion of the small finger. The splint was hand based to provide radial support to the small finger with the ring finger. AR and his family were instructed in splint and skin care. He was instructed to wear the splint when not exercising and at night. He was also instructed in pain-free AROM with gentle blocking for IP flexion. Offset buddy straps were provided for the ring to small finger.

AR was highly motivated and tended to perform strenuous exercises. Further discussion revealed that he was eager to return to playing tennis, and he believed that more aggressive exercising would be helpful. The hand therapist emphasized the importance of tissue tolerances and the significance of edema control in his functional recovery. Manual edema mobilization pump points, digital compressive sleeves, gentle frequent PIP blocking exercises, and FDS and FDP fists were very helpful. After five visits over 3 weeks, AR's pain was 0/10, edema at the PIP had been reduced from 6.7 to 5.9 cm (the uninvolved digit measured 5.4 cm), and he demonstrated good PIP alignment with AROM at MP 0/88, PIP 0/76, and DIP 0/48. He had begun to hold a tennis racquet without pain, and doing this had been his favorite exercise. He used buddy straps occasionally for support. A small, soft, ring-style Velcro strap was fabricated for use around the proximal phalanx of the small finger, and this facilitated active IP flexion without pain. AR also liked using a very small volar PIP gutter in flexion as an exercise tool with composite flexion AROM to promote supported DIP flexion with composite fisting.

Result

AR was a highly motivated client. He did not "comply" with the initial splinting provided by the ED, although he may not have understood the medical rationale for resting

the injured digit, or he might have tolerated a better-fitting or more comfortable splint. This client was determined to return to playing tennis quickly, and he did, despite having sustained a complicated injury.

CASE STUDY 15-3

RG was a 20-year-old, right-dominant female who worked as a nanny. She enjoyed playing softball and exercising. She fell and sustained an injury to the UCL of the left thumb MP joint; the injury was surgically repaired. RG was referred to hand therapy when the pin was removed 4 weeks later. She had been taking pain medications that day and had difficulty staying awake during the therapy session for splint fabrication.

Treatment

A protective forearm-based thumb spica splint was fabricated with the IP free. All instructions were provided in writing and reviewed with the client. She was instructed to wear the splint at all times except for skin care and for gentle AROM to the wrist and thumb CMC and IP. She had not been medically cleared to begin thumb MP AROM at that time.

RG did not attend her next three therapy appointments. Attempts were made to call her, messages were left, and the physician was notified. When seen 2 months later, she reported that she had stopped wearing her splint after about a week. Her incision scar had healed, but she demonstrated EPL adherence at the incision site.

AROM was thumb MP 0/14 and IP 11/35. Passive IP extension was full. Passive MP flexion was 0/14 and was equal to active MP flexion. RG had thumb IP extensor lag and also MP joint tightness. She was not tender over the ulnar MP joint area, nor was she tender with radial stress. CMC motion was normal. Wrist AROM and index through small finger AROM were normal. RG expressed concern primarily about the droop of her thumb at the IP and secondarily about MP joint stiffness.

Therapy focused on scar softening with silicone gel, gentle scar mobilization, and AROM. The client was instructed in thumb IP extension AROM with available (limited) MP flexion to promote EPL function. Place and hold exercises also were performed. For MP flexion, she was fitted with a removable volar gutter in IP extension, and this was used for MP flexion AROM with self-stabilization at the metacarpal joint. Medical clearance was provided to begin gentle passive MP flexion, and she was instructed in this. Use of a dynamic thumb MP flexion splint was planned if passive MP flexion did not improve quickly.

Active flexion exercises progressed from isolated MP to composite motions. Active IP extension exercises were upgraded with the wrist and thumb MP in varying positions of flexion and in extension. Emphasis was placed on promoting flexibility of the EPL and on gaining thumb MP flexion if able. The client was reminded that the goals of surgery were to have a pain-free, stable MP joint and that some stiffness might linger.

Result

RG did not attend any therapy or medical appointments thereafter. The EPL adherence probably could have been prevented completely if timely therapy visits had been made earlier on.

References

1. Wright HH, Rettig AC: Management of common sports injuries. In Mackin EJ, Callahan AD, Skirven TM et al, editors: *Rehabilitation of the hand and upper extremity*, ed 5, St Louis, 2002, Mosby.

2. Brzezienski MA, Schneider LH: Extensor tendon injuries at the distal interphalangeal joint, *Hand Clin* 11:373-386, 1995.

3. Campbell PJ, Wilson RL: Management of joint injuries and intraarticular fractures. In Mackin EJ, Callahan AD, Skirven TM et al, editors: *Rehabilitation of the hand and upper extremity*, ed 5, St Louis, 2002, Mosby.

4. Hofmeister EP, Mazurek MT, Shin AY et al: Extension block pinning for large mallet fractures, *J Hand Surg* 28A:453-459, 2003.

5. *The hand: examination and diagnosis*, ed 2, Edinburgh, 1983, Churchill Livingstone.

6. Evans RB: Clinical management of extensor tendon injuries. In Mackin EJ, Callahan AD, Skirven TM et al, editors: *Rehabilitation of the hand and upper extremity*, ed 5, St Louis, 2002, Mosby.

7. Biernacki SD: A flexion contracture splint for the distal interphalangeal joint, *J Hand Ther* 14:302-303, 2001.

8. Doyle JR: Extensor tendons: acute injuries. In Green DP, Hotchkiss RN, Pederson WC, editors: *Green's operative hand surgery*, ed 4, Philadelphia, 1999, Churchill Livingstone.

9. Tetik C, Gudemez E: Modification of the extension block Kirschner wire technique for mallet fractures, *Clin Orthop Relat Res* 404:284-290, 2002.

10. Takami H, Takahashi S, Ando M: Operative treatment of mallet finger due to intraarticular fracture of the distal phalanx, *Arch Orthop Trauma Surg* 20:9-13, 2000.

11. Coons MS, Green SM: Boutonniere deformity, *Hand Clin* 11:387-402, 1995.

12. Alter S, Feldon P, Terrono AL: Pathomechanics of deformities in the arthritic hand and wrist. In Mackin EJ, Callahan AD, Skirven TM et al, editors: *Rehabilitation of the hand and upper extremity*, ed 5, St Louis, 2002, Mosby.

13. Saleeba EC: Dynamic flexion splint for the distal interphalangeal joint, *J Hand Ther* 16:249-250, 2003.

14. Catalano LW, Skarparis AC, Glickel SZ et al: Treatment of chronic, traumatic hyperextension deformities of the proximal interphalangeal joint with flexor digitorum superficialis tenodesis, *J Hand Surg* 28A:448-452, 2003.

15. Glickel SZ, Barron A, Eaton RG: Dislocations and ligament injuries in the digits. In Green DP, Hotchkiss RN, Pederson WC, editors: *Green's operative hand surgery*, ed 4, Philadelphia, 1999, Churchill Livingstone.

16. Chinchalkar SJ, Gan BS: Management of proximal interphalangeal joint fractures and dislocations, *J Hand Ther* 16:117-128, 2003.

17. Mohler LR, Trumble TE: Disorders of the thumb sesamoids, *Hand Clin* 17:291-301, 2001.

18. Rotella JM, Urpi J: A new method of diagnosing metacarpophalangeal instabilities of the thumb, *Hand Clin* 17:45-60, 2001.

19. Galindo A, Suet L: A metacarpophalangeal joint stabilization splint, *J Hand Ther* 15:83-84, 2002.

20. Ford M, McKee P, Szilagyi M: Protecting the ulnar collateral ligament and metacarpophalangeal joint of the thumb, *J Hand Ther* 17:64-68, 2004.

Tendon Injury

LINDA J. KLEIN

Bowstringing

Extension outrigger splint

Extensor tendon adhesion

Fibroplasia phase

Flexor tendon adhesions

Immediate active motion

Immediate passive motion

Inflammatory phase

Juncturae tendinum

Place and active hold

Proximal interphalangeal flexion contracture

Quadriga effect

Reverse blocking exercises

SAM protocol

Synovial bursa

Tensile strength

Work of flexion

Tendon repair and rehabilitation have posed challenges to surgeons and therapists for decades. Tendons in the hand are long and thin compared with tendons elsewhere in the body. They glide large distances to allow the digits full composite flexion and extension, running under tight pulley systems to maximize their efficiency (Fig. 16-1). Following repair, the tendon quickly becomes adherent to surrounding tissue because of scar formation, especially when repaired within the pulley systems. Once adherent, the tendons do not glide as needed to perform active motion, resulting in functionally limiting deficits in range of motion. Prevention of adhesions to the repaired tendon would be possible if the tendon were allowed to glide immediately after surgery, but this approach historically resulted in rupture of the tendon repair. For this reason, a large number of solutions have been attempted over the past 50 years, resulting in numerous approaches to repair and rehabilitation. The goal of the evolving approaches has been to improve tendon gliding by minimizing adhesion formation to the tendon while avoiding rupture of the repaired tendon.

This chapter helps the therapist gain an understanding of the rationale behind the various approaches to tendon management and when each may be appropriate to apply to the individual client. Generally, the physician determines the approach to be used.

DIAGNOSIS AND PATHOLOGY

Traumatic injury to the tendons may be by open or closed means. Open lacerations most often occur from a sharp object cutting externally, deep enough to include the tendons, and occasionally from an injury that causes a bone to be forced through the tendon and skin as it fractures. Open tendon injuries are diagnosed at the time of injury as the wound is explored for tendon, nerve, and ligament damage. Injury to the tendon may be a partial

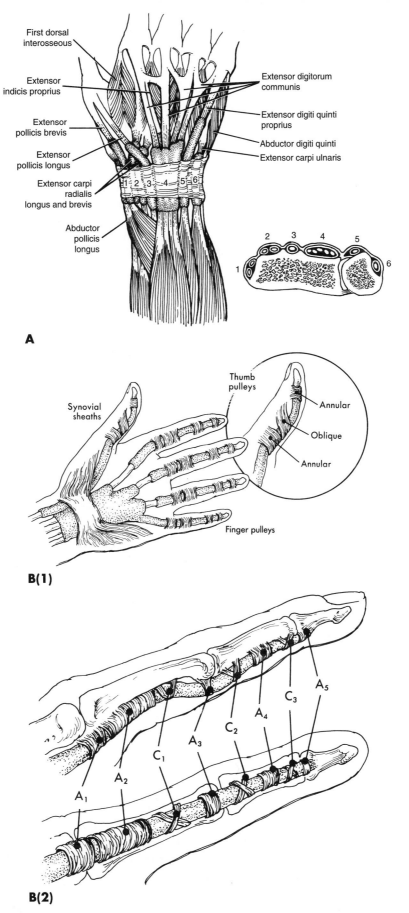

FIGURE 16-1 Pulley systems of the tendons. **A,** Arrangement of the extensor tendons in the compartment of the wrist. **B,** Flexor tendon anatomy illustrating the synovial lining around the tendons within the pulley systems at the wrist and within the digits. (**A** from Fess EE: *Hand and upper extremity splinting: principles and methods,* ed 3, St Louis, 2005, Mosby; **B** from Chase RA: *Atlas of hand surgery,* vol 2, Philadelphia, 1984, WB Saunders.)

laceration, may include loss of length of the tendon, or may be a clean laceration or a jagged tear or cut with frayed ends. The wound may be clean or dirty. Associated pulley injuries and ligament, nerve, or vessel injuries may have occurred, increasing the complexity of repair. Repair of the tendon and associated structures is performed as soon after the injury as possible, often in the emergency room.

Closed traumatic injuries of a tendon occur as a rupture of the tendon from its attachment, from friction of the tendon across a rough bony prominence, or from disease that weakens the tendon, such as rheumatoid arthritis. Closed injuries occur most often in the digit. Extensor tendon closed injuries include mallet and boutonniere injuries, and closed injury to the flexor tendon occurs most often to the flexor digitorum profundus (FDP) tendon and is referred to as jersey finger. This injury occurs as the flexed fingertip is extended forcefully, causing rupture of the FDP from the bone or an avulsion fracture.

This chapter focuses on surgical repair, postoperative healing, and rehabilitation approaches following tendon repair. Closed injuries to the tendon that do not require surgical repair, such as mallet and boutonniere injuries, are discussed in the chapter on common sprains and finger deformities.

SURGICAL REPAIR OF TENDONS

Surgical repair of the extensor tendon is considered to be simpler than flexor tendon repair. Extensor tendons in the hand are flat and thin, and in the digit they do not run under the same type of tight pulley system as do the flexor tendons. A variety of suture techniques for extensor tendons are available.[1] The therapy protocols discussed in this chapter have been applied to a variety of suture techniques, thus they do not depend on the type of surgical technique used.

Precaution. *The therapist must know, however, whether the surgeon considers the repair to be sufficiently strong to tolerate immediate motion protocols before considering their use.*

Flexor tendon repair techniques have been changing for the past decade. Historically, outcomes of flexor tendon repairs in the digit have been plagued by poor results because of adhesions or, if early active motion were attempted, rupture. Research and clinical studies have investigated suture materials and techniques to determine the best way to create a repair strong enough to tolerate immediate stress on the flexor tendon and obtain gliding while minimizing adhesions, without rupture. A large number of suture techniques are available for flexor tendon repair. Research has shown that in

general, the more strands of suture material that cross the tendon repair, the stronger the repair.[2,3] The traditional suture repair technique consists of a two-strand repair. This type of repair has been shown to tolerate application of an immobilization protocol or **immediate passive motion** protocol in the early phase of tendon healing but is not shown to be sufficiently strong to tolerate **immediate active motion** protocols following a flexor tendon repair. A four-strand repair has been shown to tolerate gentle active motion. A repair of six or more strands certainly will tolerate gentle active motion; however, this repair is technically demanding and may become so bulky as to not glide under the pulleys, creating friction, possible wearing, and eventual rupture. Thus a four-strand suture technique is seen most commonly in the literature. This procedure allows an immediate active motion protocol to be applied following flexor tendon repair, although some surgeons are electing to perform repairs with six or more strands.

Precaution. *The therapist must know the number of strands used in the repair of a flexor tendon before determining what type of motion protocol may be appropriate.*

TIMELINES AND HEALING

We now know that repaired tendons have the ability to heal by nutrition from direct blood supply and from diffusion of nutrients in the synovial fluid that surrounds the tendons as they run under the pulley systems.[4] This information, combined with new surgical techniques and materials, has led to a renewed attempt to move the repaired tendon earlier to avoid adhesions that limit tendon gliding and resulting motion.

Three basic approaches to rehabilitation of the repaired tendon in the hand are (1) immobilization, (2) immediate passive motion in the direction of the repaired tendon, and (3) immediate active motion in the direction of the repaired tendon. The main difference in these approaches is within the early phase, or first month, of tendon healing.

The early phase of tendon healing consists of the **inflammatory phase** and early **fibroplasia phase** of tendon healing, when the tendon is at its weakest and collagen is just beginning to be laid down at the repair site. This phase is also the time when adhesions begin to occur. The intermediate phase of tendon healing includes the period from 4 weeks to approximately 7 or 8 weeks after repair, during which time the tendon repair gains **tensile strength.** The late phase of tendon healing includes the period from 7 or 8 weeks to 12 weeks after repair. During this period, the tendon repair continues to gain tensile strength and begins to remodel in alignment with the tension placed on it. The repaired tendon is considered to have nearly full tensile strength at 12 weeks after the repair.

Individuals with a repaired flexor tendon are allowed normal use of the hand at 12 to 14 weeks after repair. Those with extensor tendon repairs usually are allowed normal use of the hand earlier, at approximately 6 to 8 weeks after repair because the normal use of the hands consistently offers resistance to the flexor tendons while rarely offering resistance to the extensor tendons. Grasp or pinch of objects greatly increases tension within the flexor tendons and therefore is to be avoided in the early phase of flexor tendon rehabilitation and in the intermediate phase unless adhesions limit gliding. However, the function of the extensor tendon is for release of objects. Thus the client with an extensor tendon repair is allowed to grasp or pinch objects much earlier, beginning at 6 weeks after repair.

Knowledge of tendon healing is the basis for determining safe advancement to resistive exercises of the repaired tendon.

CLINICAL *Pearl*

The better the active motion that is present early in the rehabilitation process, the longer resistance to the tendon is deferred.

This is an important concept to understand. This guideline affects clinical decisions about strengthening of grip or pinch following a flexor tendon repair or applying resistance to digital extension following an extensor tendon repair. Resistance is introduced appropriately to motion of a tendon when adhesions limit active motion more than passive motion, in an effort to place tension on the scar to improve proximal gliding of the tendon. *This same resistance, however, may overcome the tensile strength of the repair and result in a rupture.* When there is good active motion of the repaired tendon, it indicates lack of adhesions that would prevent proximal gliding of the repaired tendon. Tension develops in the tendon when the muscle pulls against added resistance. Without the support and restriction of surrounding adhesions, all this tension is transferred directly through the tendon, and the risk of tendon rupture greatly increases when resistance is introduced. Thus all timelines in this chapter must be individualized, and advancement to resistance of the repaired tendon that is showing good to excellent gliding is done at the later of the timelines discussed or is deferred until the referring surgeon determines the tendon is near or at full tensile strength.

PRECAUTIONS FOR MINIMIZING TENSION ON A REPAIRED TENDON

Tendon repairs are never at their full strength when motion is initiated. The precaution always exists regarding gapping or potential rupture of a tendon until 12 weeks after repair. Two things cause gapping or rupture of a repaired tendon. The first of these is overstretch of the repair by moving too far into extension following a flexor tendon repair or too far into flexion following an extensor tendon repair. The second is an excessive internal pull on the tendon by the muscle during active or resisted motion in the same direction as the repaired tendon. This would include active or resisted flexion following a flexor tendon repair or active or resisted extension following an extensor tendon repair before the tendon is strong enough to tolerate the amount of internal tension on the tendon.

Precaution. *When initiating active motion, do it gently, with a gradual increase in tension applied to the tendon as healing advances.*

As we encourage tendon gliding for active motion, we must consider the amount of tension the muscle is placing on the repaired tendon to achieve the active motion. Our goal in tendon rehabilitation is to achieve tendon gliding while minimizing tension on the repair during the healing process. We can minimize resistance or tension on the tendon when mobilizing the tendon by decreasing edema and joint stiffness, performing motion slowly and gently, and using optimal positions of proximal joints during active motion. When we mobilize stiff joints associated with the tendon repair in the first 6 weeks after repair, we must do it with the tendon in a protected position.

CLINICAL *Pearl*

The protected position of a tendon is with all proximal joints held to provide slack to the tendon.

For instance, following a flexor tendon repair, when a **proximal interphalangeal flexion contracture** (proximal interphalangeal joint is passively limited into extension) exists at 4 weeks after repair, support the wrist and metacarpophalangeal joint in flexion while applying gentle joint mobilization or passive proximal interphalangeal (PIP) extension. This will prevent overstretch of the repaired flexor tendon while providing assistance to improve extension of the joints.

Questions to Ask the Doctor

Because of the large number of variables that exist in the type and complexity of injuries to tendons, it is important for us to have a good understanding of the injury and surgery before beginning treatment. Questions to ask the doctor may include the following:

- *Which tendons were lacerated? (This is not always obvious from the laceration).*
- *What other structures were included in the injury (nerve, ligament, vessel, bone)?*
- *Were all structures able to be repaired strongly, or are there concerns with strength or healing of certain structures?*
- *If referred immediately after repair, is the client being placed into an immobilization protocol or immediate passive or immediate active motion protocol? Clarify the approach you are planning to use for this client.*
- *For an extensor tendon repair, if not immediately apparent, in which zone is the injury?*
- *Which joints should be included in the splint?*
- *If the injury was to a flexor tendon, what type of suture repair (how many strands) was used?*

What to Say to Clients

"A tendon connects the muscle to the bone and is what makes your [finger/thumb] move in this direction" (illustrate with your hand). Use a picture or diagram to show the client how the muscle becomes tendon, and how the tendon must be pulled or glide proximally to result in active motion.

"When your tendon was injured, it could no longer do this motion. Now that the surgeon has repaired it, it needs time to heal. A flexor tendon takes twelve weeks to heal, and an extensor tendon takes six to eight weeks to heal. We will increase what you do with your repaired tendon gradually, but if you do too much too soon, it will tear apart. The two things that will cause your tendon to tear apart, or rupture, are a stretch on the tendon in this direction [illustrate on your hand how a stretch into extension would place excessive stretch on a repaired flexor tendon, or how a stretch into flexion would place excessive stretch on a repaired extensor tendon] or a pull from the muscle on the inside that is too strong for the tendon repair to tolerate. For this reason, you must keep your splint on at all times for the first month. It will prevent the tendon from over-stretch. We will take the splint off in therapy only, to clean your hand and the splint, and to do some additional exercises. If you follow the directions carefully, you also will avoid having the muscle pull too hard on the tendon."

"Under no circumstances should you do more than we instruct you to do with your hand through this healing process, or the tendon may rupture. If it ruptures, it may not be able to be repaired again, or if further surgery is done, the results are not likely to be as good."

EXTENSOR TENDON INJURIES

Anatomy

Extrinsic extensor tendons to the digits include the extensor digitorum communis (EDC), extensor indicis proprius, extensor digiti minimi, extensor pollicis longus, extensor pollicis brevis, and abductor pollicis longus. Each of these tendons crosses the wrist dorsally, passing under the extensor retinaculum, which is separated into various compartments to maximize mechanical efficiency of the extensor tendons as they cross the wrist, preventing **bowstringing** (Fig. 16-1, *A*).

Proximal to the metacarpophalangeal joints, the **juncturae tendinum** fibers separate from the EDC tendon, providing a cross-connection to the adjacent EDC tendon. This cross-connection of fibers exists to a variable extent in each individual but most consistently occurs between the EDC to the ring finger and the EDC tendons to the small and middle fingers. The juncturae tendinum fibers assist in extension of the neighboring finger and help maintain the EDC in midline over the metacarpal head during finger flexion.

The extrinsic extensor tendons serve the primary purpose of extending the metacarpophalangeal joints of the fingers and the thumb metacarpophalangeal and interphalangeal joints. The extrinsic extensor tendons also assist in extension of the finger interphalangeal joints by their anatomic contribution to the lateral bands and by assisting PIP extension through the EDC attachment just distal to the PIP joint.

Extension of the finger PIP and distal interphalangeal (DIP) joints is performed primarily by the lateral bands, which consist of a merging of fibers from the EDC with fibers from the lumbrical and interossei tendons (Fig. 16-2). The lateral bands on both sides of the fingers pass dorsal to the axis of motion at the PIP and DIP joints and merge over the DIP joint to form the terminal extensor tendon. Extension at the PIP and DIP joints is delicately balanced by this combination of tendon fibers and ligamentous support in an uninjured finger to prevent excessive dorsal or volar migration (subluxation) of the lateral bands. The transverse retinacular ligament supports the lateral bands volarly, and the triangular ligament supports the lateral bands dorsally. The oblique retinacular ligaments run along the sides of the finger and cross the PIP and DIP joints volar to the PIP axis of motion and dorsal to the DIP axis of motion. Thus when the PIP joint extends, it places tension on, or stretches,

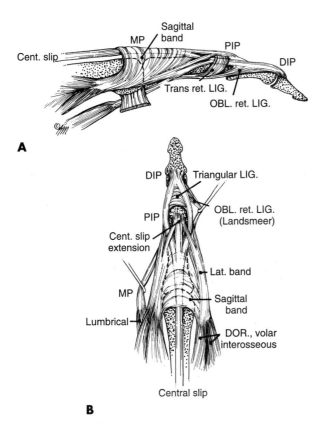

A

B

FIGURE 16-2 A, The extensor tendon at the metacarpophalangeal *(MP)* joint level is held in place by the transverse lamina or sagittal band, which tethers and centers the extensor tendons over the joint. This sagittal band arises from the volar plate and the intermetacarpal ligaments at the neck of the metacarpals. Any injury to this extensor hood or expansion may result in subluxation or dislocation of the extensor tendon. **B,** The intrinsic tendons from the lumbrical and interosseous muscles join the extensor mechanism at about the level of the proximal and midportion of the proximal phalanx and continue distally to the distal interphalangeal *(DIP)* joint of the finger. The extensor mechanism at the proximal interphalageal *(PIP)* joint is best described as a trifurcation of the extensor tendon into the central slip, which attaches to the dorsal base of the middle phalanx, and two lateral bands. The lateral bands continue distally to insert at the dorsal base of the distal phalanx. The extensor mechanism is maintained in place over the proximal interphalangeal joint by the transverse retinacular ligaments. (From Doyle JR: Extensor tendons: acute injuries. In Green DP, Hotchkiss RN, Pederson WC, editors: *Green's operative hand surgery,* ed 4, New York, 1999, Churchill Livingstone.)

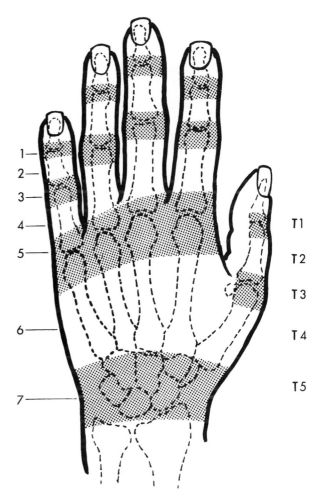

FIGURE 16-3 Extensor tendon zones as defined by the Committee on Tendon Injuries for the International Federation of the Society for Surgery of the Hand. (From Kleinert HE, Schepel S, Gill T: *Surg Clin North Am* 61:267, 1981.)

the oblique retinacular ligament. This causes the ligament to tighten across the DIP joint, placing a passive extension assist on the DIP joint by this tenodesis effect.

The interphalangeal joint of the thumb is extended primarily by the extensor pollicis longus tendon, and the metacarpophalangeal joint is extended by a combination of the extensor pollicis longus and the extensor pollicis brevis. The abductor pollicis longus, extensor pollicis brevis, and extensor pollicis longus tendons extend the carpometacarpal joint.

Injuries to the extensor tendon are discussed in relation to the zone of injury, for there are different protocols for the extensor tendon in each set of zones. Extensor tendon zones are reviewed in Fig. 16-3. Splints used for extensor tendon repairs in the early phase of tendon healing are reviewed in Table 16-1.

Zones I and II Extensor Tendon Injuries

Injuries to the extensor tendon in zones I and II result in a mallet finger. Closed injuries may be caused by a tendon rupture or avulsion, resulting in a drooped distal phalanx of the digit. Treatment of the closed mallet finger is covered in the chapter on common finger sprains and

TABLE 16-1

Overview of Splints Used for Extensor Tendon Repairs in the Early Phase of Tendon Healing

ZONE OF INJURY	IMMOBILIZATION	IMMEDIATE PASSIVE EXTENSION	IMMEDIATE ACTIVE EXTENSION
I and II	DIP extension splint (Fig. 16-4)	None available	None available
III and IV	Finger gutter, taped in place (Fig. 16-5)	Hand-based outrigger allowing 30 degrees of PIP flexion (Fig. 16-6)	Finger gutter, taped in place between exercises (Fig. 16-5) Exercise template with 30 degrees of PIP flexion, 20 degrees of DIP flexion (Fig. 16-7)
V, VI, and VII	Full-length resting pan (Fig. 16-8)	Dynamic metacarpophalangeal extension outrigger allowing 30 degrees of metacarpophalangeal flexion (Fig. 16-9, A, B)	Immediate active extension splint using wrist support and yoke (Fig. 16-10)

DIP, Distal interphalangeal; *PIP*, proximal interphalangeal.

deformities. Management of an open laceration of an extensor tendon in zones I and II is managed by surgical repair, often with additional support of a pin to hold the DIP joint in extension. Therapy following surgical repair of an extensor tendon in zones I and II is similar to that for closed treatment, which includes immobilization for 6 to 8 weeks (Fig. 16-4) followed by a gradual increase in flexion of the DIP joint. Details regarding treatment of the mallet finger are covered in the chapter on common finger sprains and deformities.

Zones III and IV Extensor Tendon Injuries

Diagnosis and Pathology
Injuries in this region may result from closed ruptures or open lacerations. Closed ruptures are often caused by a direct blunt force to the dorsal PIP joint, resulting in rupture of the EDC tendon from its attachment on the middle phalanx. Closed ruptures result in weakened active PIP extension, with a limited amount of active PIP extension still present because of the intact lateral bands. Over time, development of a larger PIP extension lag results in a boutonniere deformity. Treatment of this injury is covered in detail in the chapter on common finger sprains and deformities.

Open lacerations of the extensor tendon in zones III and IV are common from sharp objects of any kind at the level of the PIP joint and proximal phalanx. Following primary repair of the extensor tendon in this zone, three types of protocols are available from which to choose to apply in the early phase of tendon healing:

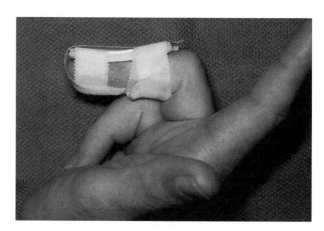

FIGURE 16-4 Distal interphalangeal extension splint.

immobilization, immediate passive extension, and immediate active extension. Immobilization commonly is applied, but in the presence of a complex injury such as a deep laceration that includes a partial bony injury, the physician may prescribe an immediate motion protocol to prevent dense adhesions. The three types of protocols vary in application of splinting and exercises in the early phase of tendon healing for the first 4 weeks following repair. After that time the client is advanced according to the amount of limitation present. Usually, the physician determines the protocol.

Rehabilitation: Early Phase
The early phase of tendon healing occurs in the first 3 to 4 weeks following repair.

Immobilization Protocol

SPLINTING. When the repaired extensor tendon is treated with immobilization in the initial phase of tendon healing, a postoperative splint, a finger length cast, or a thermoplastic splint made in therapy is applied to hold the PIP joint in full extension. If the lateral bands were injured in addition to the EDC tendon, the DIP is held in full extension as well. The splint is worn full time until 3 to 4 weeks postoperatively (Fig. 16-5).

EXERCISES. In an immobilization protocol in the early phase of tendon healing, the client moves only the joints that are not splinted. The repaired tendon is protected in extension at all times during the first 3 to 4 weeks.

Immediate Passive Extension Protocol

INDICATIONS. When dense adhesions are expected to limit gliding of the tendon, the referring surgeon may prefer an immediate passive extension approach to rehabilitation to achieve 3 to 5 mm of extensor tendon glide distally.

SPLINTING. Within the first 3 days following repair, fabricate a hand-based **extension outrigger splint** that supports the metacarpophalangeal joint and provides passive extension of the PIP joint (Fig. 16-6). The PIP joint is allowed to flex 30 degrees, with an elastic extension sling bringing the PIP joint back to 0 degrees following the limited amount of flexion.[5] The outrigger holds the finger in full PIP extension at rest, between exercises. The wrist is not included in this splint.

EXERCISES. Instruct the client to exercise hourly with the splint on at all times with 10 repetitions of 30 degrees of PIP flexion followed by passive extension provided by the sling attachment. Flexion is limited at 30 degrees by an attachment on the outrigger line that blocks further distal migration of the outrigger line at that point. The outrigger splint is left in place for the first 3 to 4 weeks. Some protocols allow a gradual increase in the number of degrees that the PIP is flexed during the 3 to 4 week period.[6] At that time, the splint is removed and the client is allowed to flex to tolerance as discussed in the intermediate phase exercises below.

Precaution. *It is important to educate the client not to flex further than instructed to avoid rupture of the repair.*

Immediate Active Extension Protocol

INDICATIONS. An immediate active extension protocol is appropriate for the same situations as an immediate passive extension protocol and has the added benefit of more definitive proximal tendon gliding and the distal tendon gliding that the passive extension protocol exercises provide. Apply the protocol within the first 3 days after repair. An immediate controlled active extension approach titled the short arc motion protocol or **SAM protocol**, as described by Evans,[7] follows.

SPLINTING. The SAM protocol splints the finger in full interphalangeal extension at all times except exercise. Fabricate a second splint with 30 degrees of PIP and 20 degrees of DIP flexion that is used as an exercise template (Fig. 16-7). Fabricate a third, shorter finger gutter splint that holds the PIP joint in full extension and allows the DIP to flex to tolerance. If the lateral bands also were injured and repaired, the DIP joint is limited to 30 degrees of flexion during this exercise, which the client visually monitors.

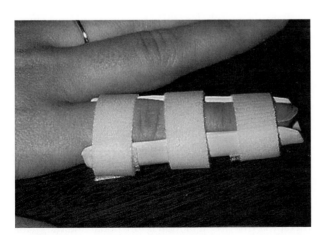

FIGURE 16-5 Finger gutter, taped in place.

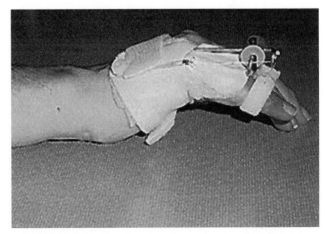

FIGURE 16-6 Hand-based outrigger allowing 30 degrees of proximal interphalangeal flexion.

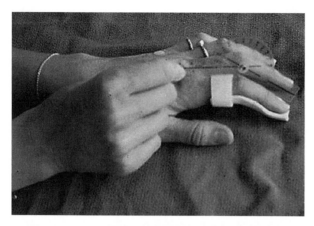

FIGURE 16-7 Exercise template with 30 degrees of proximal interphalangeal flexion and 20 degrees of distal interphalangeal flexion.

EXERCISES. Hourly, the exercise template is placed on the finger that allows 30 degrees PIP and 20 degrees DIP flexion. The wrist is placed in 30 degrees of flexion to give slack to the flexor tendons, resulting in less resistance to active extension of the interphalangeal joints. With the finger gutter exercise template in place, the finger is allowed to flex to the exercise template splint and then perform active extension of the interphalangeal joints. If the lateral bands are uninjured, the third exercise splint is applied, and while holding the PIP joint in full extension, the DIP is flexed to tolerance. Brief but frequent exercises (10 to 20 repetitions hourly) are performed. At 2 weeks after repair, the exercise template is increased to 40 degrees of PIP flexion. At 3 weeks after repair, the exercise template is increased to allow 50 degrees of PIP flexion, and at 4 weeks, 70 degrees of PIP flexion. The exercises then progress into the intermediate phase of exercises.

Rehabilitation: Intermediate Phase

At 4 weeks, discontinue splinting and begin active flexion with individual joint flexion. Active flexion is likely to be most limited in the client who has been immobilized in the early phase of tendon healing, as described before. At 5 weeks, advance to gentle composite flexion. Heat may be used to warm the tissues before active exercises.

Precaution. *Client education is important, for early overaggressive flexion of the PIP joint may result in reinjury of the extensor tendon.*

The tendon that has not been moved in the early phase of tendon healing often is limited by adhesions, and the temptation is immediately to apply force to help it move. The immobilized tendon, however, is not stronger than the mobilized tendon, and motion must be initiated gradually.

What to Say to Clients

"We are now going to be moving the finger in a way that places a limited amount of stress on the repaired tendon. Because the tendon is not at full strength yet, it is important to do the motions slowly and to aim for a gradual increase in ability to bend the middle and tip joints. You don't want to force the finger down using an outside force such as your other hand, or you may reinjure your tendon. We hope to see about thirty degrees of improvement each week, and make sure that you can keep straightening your finger. It is easier to get better at bending the finger, but harder to regain the ability to straighten the finger once it is lost."

At 6 weeks, if active flexion is not showing steady, gradual progress, therapy may advance to use of passive flexion. Heat with support in flexion may assist in regaining composite flexion. Initiate grip strengthening at this time. A gentle dynamic or static progressive flexion splint may be used after 6 weeks after repair if flexion remains significantly limited.

Diagnosis-Specific Information That Affects Clinical Reasoning

When an immediate passive or active extension protocol is used in the initial phase of healing, less limitation in flexion is expected in the intermediate phase of tendon healing.

Precaution. *If steady, gradual progress is being made into flexion, passive flexion or dynamic splinting to increase flexion is deferred until a plateau occurs.*

Limited extension of the interphalangeal joints caused by **extensor tendon adhesion** (passive extension is better than active extension) is treated with night extension splinting, an emphasis on active extension exercises during the day, and less emphasis on strong flexion.

Because interphalangeal extension is performed most strongly by the lateral bands, it increases efficiency of the extensors to hold the metacarpophalangeal joint in flexion while performing active interphalangeal extension. This is called reverse blocking. Metacarpophalangeal hyperextension is to be avoided when performing interphalangeal extension because metacarpophalangeal hyperextension limits the ability of the EDC to assist in interphalangeal extension and decreases efficiency of the lateral bands.

The individual with an extensor tendon repair often is allowed to return to full use of the hand without restriction after 6 weeks and may be discharged from therapy at this time if motion is functional and the client is advancing with a home exercise program. However, the finger may not achieve a functional level of motion within the intermediate phase of healing when strong adhesions are present, requiring further therapy.

Rehabilitation: Late Phase

From 8 to 12 weeks following extensor tendon repair, the client is allowed full normal use of the injured hand. In therapy, limited flexion continues to be treated with heat that may be combined with stretch, passive and active flexion, blocking exercises, and composite flexion exercises and grip strengthening. Static progressive or dynamic flexion splints can be used to supplement the home exercise program to increase flexion. Limited active interphalangeal extension continues to be treated with **reverse blocking exercises,** night interphalangeal extension splinting, and the addition of resistance to the repaired tendon. Resistance to extension facilitates a stronger proximal pull on the adherent extensor tendon to improve active extension. This is performed by applying reverse blocking with manual resistance, or the client may extend the fingers against a loop of putty, resistive band strip, or rubber band. However, these exercises are only effective in improving gliding of the extensor tendon in zones III and IV if metacarpophalangeal hyperextension is blocked during the exercise. If passive interphalangeal extension is limited, dynamic interphalangeal extension splinting intermittently during the day and night static extension splinting are indicated.

Zones V, VI, and VII Extensor Tendon Injuries

Diagnosis and Pathology

Injuries in zones V, VI, and VII are most often due to lacerations. Another cause of injury to the extensor tendons in zone VII is rupture from disease such as rheumatoid arthritis or bony abnormality resulting in fraying and rupture. Tendon injuries in these zones require surgical repair for healing. Following surgical repair in these extensor tendon zones, there are protocols for all three approaches of immobilization, immediate passive extension, and immediate active extension from which to choose in the early phase of tendon healing.

Rehabilitation: Early Phase
Immobilization Protocol

Immobilization of extensor tendon repairs at the metacarpophalangeal joints and proximally is in the form of a full-length resting cast or splint (Fig. 16-8). Some surgeons keep the client in a postoperative slab for the full 4 weeks; others have a thermoplastic splint fabricated. The position of the splint is in partial wrist extension and full digit extension. Some surgeons prefer slight metacarpophalangeal flexion (20 degrees) in the splint;

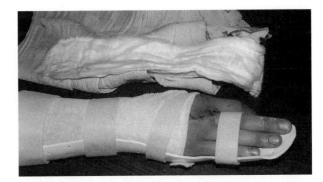

FIGURE 16-8 Full-length resting pan splint.

however, this may result in an metacarpophalangeal extension lag.[7] If the repair is proximal to the juncturae tendinum in the dorsum of the hand, the tendons on either side of the injured tendons must be supported in extension along with the injured tendon. If the repair is over the metacarpophalangeal joint, distal to the juncturae tendinum, the injured finger with the repaired tendon may be held in full extension, with the adjacent fingers placed in 30 degrees of metacarpophalangeal flexion or allowed to flex to tolerance. Flexion of the adjacent fingers, when the repair is distal to the juncturae tendinum, pulls the proximal portion of the repaired tendon distally, relieving tension from the repair. Exercises begin in the intermediate phase of tendon healing in the immobilization protocol, at approximately 4 weeks after repair.

Immediate Passive Extension Protocol

INDICATIONS. Immediate passive extension may be used for complex injuries, multiple tendon injuries, injuries under the extensor retinaculum at the wrist, or by surgeon preference. In her most recent publication, Evans[7] recommends immediate motion for all extensor tendon repairs proximal to zones I and II. Injuries in zone VII of the finger extensor tendons or zone TV of the thumb are in the area of the extensor retinaculum. Repairs in this area are considered complex, for dense adhesions to the tendon occur that are difficult to overcome following immobilization. Initiation of this protocol is within the first 3 days following repair.

SPLINTING. The splint for immediate passive extension consists of an extension outrigger that supports the wrist in extension and the injured fingers in full extension at rest, allowing 30 degrees of metacarpophalangeal flexion during exercise (Fig. 16-9). The metacarpophalangeal flexion may be blocked at 30 degrees by a volar splint or by a stop bead placed on the outrigger line that stops the flexion at 30 degrees. The splint is worn full time for the

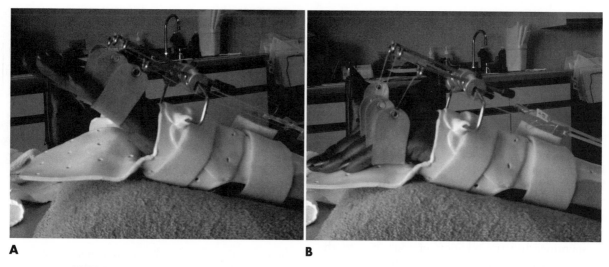

A   **B**

FIGURE 16-9 A, Dynamic metacarpophalangeal extension outrigger allowing 30 degrees of metacarpophalangeal flexion. **B,** Active flexion within the immediate passive extension splint is blocked at 30 degrees by a volar portion of the splint base.

first 3 weeks after repair and is removed in therapy only for exercises and cleansing of splint and skin.[7]

EXERCISES. Instruct the client to flex the fingers using only metacarpophalangeal flexion, to 30 degrees, and then to relax the fingers. When the fingers are relaxed, the outrigger and sling attachments move the fingers passively back to 0 degrees of extension. Flexing to 30 degrees at the metacarpophalangeal joint results in 3 to 5 mm of distal glide of the extensor tendon, which decreases the dense adhesions that occur with immobilization. The interphalangeal joints of the fingers can be flexed gently with the metacarpophalangeal joints supported in full extension. The exercises are performed for 10 to 20 repetitions hourly. At 3 weeks after repair, remove the flexion block from the splint, and allow the client to flex the fingers to tolerance, with extension continuing to be assisted by the dynamic slings for another 2 to 3 weeks.

This protocol can be applied to the repaired extensor pollicis longus tendon of the thumb following repair in zone TV.[7] The splint holds the wrist and the thumb metacarpophalangeal and carpometacarpal joints in extension and applies an outrigger support to the interphalangeal joint. The interphalangeal joint is allowed to flex 60 degrees to attain 3 to 5 mm of tendon gliding in zone TV (under the retinaculum). The exercises progress along the same timelines as the extensor repair of the finger.

Immediate Active Extension Protocol

INDICATIONS. Evans[7] has described a program that is performed in therapy only that includes an active com-

ponent for repairs in zones V to VII in the early phase of tendon healing. She suggests its use for any extensor tendon repair, especially repairs that are considered complex, such as those under the extensor retinaculum at the wrist. Howell, Merritt, and Robinson[8] describe another immediate controlled active extension protocol that is applied for zones IV to VII extensor tendon repairs.

SPLINTING AND EXERCISE. The following describes two methods of splinting and exercise for the injured tendon:

1. *Evans' program.* The immediate active rehabilitation approach described by Evans and Thompson[9] uses an outrigger splint as described in the immediate passive extension program for the client to wear at all times except therapy. In therapy only, the splint is removed for the active motion portion of the exercises. Results described by Evans that compare immobilization to the immediate passive and active extension approaches show a significant improvement in tendon gliding using the immediate motion programs.
2. *Howell, Merritt, and Robinson's program.* Within the first 10 days, preferably within the first 3 days after repair, a two-piece splint is fabricated. One component of the splint is a volar wrist support that holds the wrist in 20 to 25 degrees of extension. The second component of the splint is a yoke that is made from a long, thin piece of thermoplastic material that is the width of the proximal phalanx and 1.5 times the length of the dorsum of the hand across the metacarpals. This yoke is wrapped under the

injured fingers and over the uninjured fingers to support the injured fingers in slight metacarpophalangeal hyperextension compared with the adjacent fingers (Fig. 16-10).

Full active composite flexion and extension are performed as soon as possible with the splint in place on an ongoing basis. The client wears the splint full time for 3 weeks. At 3 weeks, the therapist removes the wrist splint to allow wrist range of motion (ROM) with the yoke splint in place. The client continues to wear the wrist and yoke splint combination for moderate to heavy activities until 5 weeks after repair. Between 5 and 7 weeks, the client wears only the yoke portion of the splint. Most clients were discharged from therapy at 7 weeks postoperatively with better than 90% excellent and good results.[8]

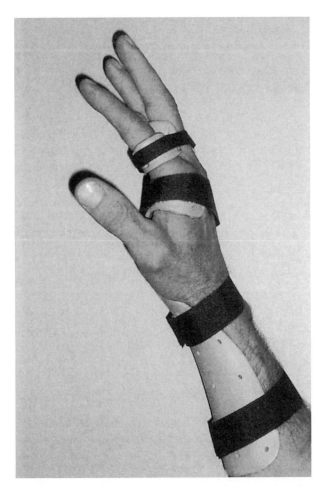

FIGURE 16-10 Immediate active extension splint using wrist support and yoke. (From Howell JW, Merritt WH, Robinson SJ: *J Hand Ther* 18[2]:182, 2005.)

Rehabilitation: Intermediate Phase
Splinting
At 4 weeks after repair, protective splinting is decreased to intermittent use during work and heavy or risky activities and gradually is discontinued. If extension is limited, a night resting pan splint in full extension is indicated. With use of an immediate active or passive extension protocol, the dynamic extension splint described under those protocols may be continued until 6 weeks after repair, allowing flexion of the metacarpophalangeal joints to tolerance with assistance of the slings into extension from 3 to 6 weeks after repair.

Exercises
At 4 weeks after repair of extensor tendons in zones V, VI, VII, a gradual increase in active flexion for individual joints is allowed as follows:

- Metacarpophalangeal flexion with interphalangeal joints extended
- Interphalangeal flexion with metacarpophalangeal joints extended
- Wrist flexion with fingers extended

Modalities may include heat of choice to decrease stiffness if not otherwise contraindicated.

At week 5 or 6, begin composite flexion of fingers. Gentle passive flexion may be added if flexor is limited significantly. Support the fingers in a flexion wrap to tolerance, and apply heat as appropriate. At week 7, composite flexion of wrist/fingers may be added.

Diagnosis-Specific Information That Affects Clinical Reasoning
When active metacarpophalangeal extension is limited because of adhesions in zone V, VI, or VII, an extensor lag results in which passive extension is better than active extension. In addition to an extension splint at night, active extension exercises are important to place proximal tension on the adhesion to improve proximal gliding of the adherent tendon.

Regaining full composite extension, which is a balance of EDC and intrinsic muscle function, may be even more challenging. Supporting the finger in full passive extension such as on a table, and attempting to lift the limited finger up from the table can facilitate this motion. When the repaired EDC is adherent, although clients are unsuccessful in lifting the finger up from the table, clients often can feel the proximal tugging of the extensor tendon on the dorsal hand. This is necessary to facilitate proximal gliding of the tendon and provides feedback to clients that they are using the correct muscle/tendon. If clients flex the metacarpophalangeal joints

CLINICAL *Pearl*

The most effective way to improve active metacarpophalangeal extension is with the interphalangeal joints flexed or relaxed. When the metacarpophalangeal joint is limited in active extension and the client attempts to lift the unsupported finger actively, the intrinsic muscles often work first, for they are not limited by adhesions. Because the intrinsic muscles perform interphalangeal extension with metacarpophalangeal flexion, when they work to extend the finger without effective EDC gliding, strong interphalangeal extension and metacarpophalangeal flexion result, defeating the purpose of the exercise. Isolated metacarpophalangeal extension is achieved with the interphalangeal joints relaxed in flexion and is the most successful way to begin to attain proximal gliding of the adherent EDC proximal to the metacarpophalangeal joint.

during this exercise, rather than using the EDC to attempt to lift the metacarpophalangeal joint, they will feel increased pressure on the table from the fingertip, providing feedback that they are using the wrong muscles. It may be helpful to perform the composite extension lift bilaterally. To do this, have clients use the uninjured hand to hold the injured hand gently flat on the table while performing the composite extension lift with the injured hand. This allows them to feel and possibly see the tug on the adherent extensor tendon.

Precaution. *This exercise should be done only 6 weeks or more after repair because the uninjured hand may be offering resistance to the repaired extensor tendon while supporting the hand downward on the table.*

Rehabilitation: Late Phase

Continue with exercises to maximize proximal and distal gliding of the extensor tendon as described for the intermediate phase exercises. Add grip strengthening and gradual increase in functional upper extremity exercise beginning at 6 weeks after repair. For deficits in flexion, add dynamic or static progressive flexion splinting intermittently during the day beginning at 6 to 8 weeks after repair, as approved by the referring surgeon.

FLEXOR TENDON INURIES

Anatomy

The flexor tendons to the digits enter the hand through the carpal tunnel. They are comprised of the flexor digitorum superficialis (FDS) for each finger, FDP for each finger, and flexor pollicis longus to the thumb. The FDP

tendons are deep to the FDS tendons in the forearm, wrist, and hand. At the level of the proximal phalanx, the FDS tendon separates, becoming two separate slips, which then reconverge just before attachment on the middle phalanx (Fig. 16-11). The FDS flexes the metacarpophalangeal and PIP joints. The FDP tendon emerges through the separation of the FDS tendon at the level of the proximal phalanx and continues distally to insert on the distal phalanx. The FDP tendon is the sole tendon responsible for DIP flexion of the finger. In the thumb, the flexor pollicis longus tendon inserts on the distal phalanx and is the sole flexor of the thumb interphalangeal joint.

As the flexor tendons run under the retinaculum and transverse carpal ligament at the wrist and palm, they are surrounded by a **synovial bursa,** which is a sheath filled with synovial fluid that allows tendon gliding without excess friction. A synovial sheath also surrounds the flexor tendons in the digit, where they run under a series of pulleys that prevent the flexors from bowstringing as active flexion occurs (Fig. 16-1, *B*). Under the pulleys, dense adhesions occur following repair of the flexor tendons.

Precaution. *In addition to lacerations of the flexor tendons in the digit, it is common to see digital nerve lacerations because of their proximity to the flexor tendons.*

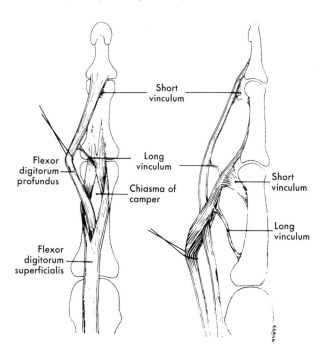

FIGURE 16-11   Flexor digitorum profundus and flexor digitorum superficialis anatomy in the digit illustrating the split in the superficialis tendon that allows the profundus tendon to continue distally to its insertion on the distal phalanx. (From Schneider LH: *Flexor tendon injuries,* Boston, 1985, Little, Brown.)

Flexor Tendon Rehabilitation

Flexor tendon rehabilitation following repair poses more of a challenge than extensor tendon rehabilitation because of dense adhesions that occur within the flexor pulley system of the digit of zones I and II. Flexor tendon zones are reviewed in Fig. 16-12. An immobilization approach rarely is applied following repair of the flexor tendon in the digit, but there are certain situations for which it is appropriate. Immediate passive flexion protocols were developed in the 1960s and were the treatment of choice for decades in an attempt to minimize dense adhesions that resulted under the pulley system in the digit. Results were inconsistent in regaining active flexion using immediate passive flexion, and controlled active flexion approaches were developed using stronger surgical repair techniques, beginning in the 1990s. Numerous researchers have found significantly improved outcomes with better flexor tendon gliding with use of immediate active flexion rehabilitation approaches in the early phase of flexor tendon healing.[9-12]

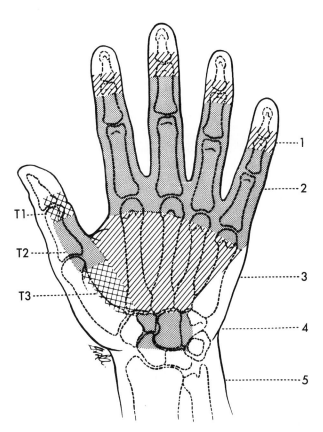

FIGURE 16-12 Flexor tendon zones in the hand. (From Kleinert HE, Schepel S, Gill T: *Surg Clin North Am* 61:267, 1981.)

Early Phase of Tendon Healing
Immobilization Protocol

Immobilization following repair of a flexor tendon in the digit has been reserved for those individuals unable to participate in an immediate passive or immediate active flexion rehabilitation program. Immobilization is used for young children, who are unable to adhere to a motion protocol with its specific precautions. Children younger than age 12 most often are placed in immobilization for the first 3 to 4 weeks, but each child should be evaluated related to their maturity level. Other individuals who may be placed in immobilization after a flexor tendon repair are those who have cognitive limitations such as Alzheimer's and noncompliant clients. Sometimes, it is difficult to know the client's compliance abilities at the first therapy session. When a client demonstrates inability to comply appropriately with the precautions and exercises within a certain approach, it may become necessary to change the rehabilitation approach to one allowing less motion, or a cast may be needed instead of a removable splint in the first 4 to 5 weeks postoperatively. When there is a concomitant fracture or significant loss of skin requiring a skin graft, a period of immobilization may be necessary to allow the bone or skin to heal adequately before beginning motion. Not all fractures require immobilization. Stable fractures or those that have had open reduction and internal fixation may tolerate immediate controlled motion, as determined by the surgeon.

Table 16-2 summarizes general guidelines for splinting and exercises within an immobilization protocol. Box 16-1 gives an overview of splints used for flexor tendon repairs in the early phase of flexor tendon healing.

SPLINTING. When splinting is used, the immobilization approach places the client's hand in a dorsal blocking cast or a dorsal blocking splint wrapped securely in place, with instructions not to remove the splint at home (Fig. 16-13). The position of the cast or splint in the early phase of immobilization is 20 to 30 degrees of wrist flexion and 40 to 50 degrees of metacarpophalangeal flexion, with interphalangeal extension. This position keeps the flexor tendons on slack yet prevents the most difficult joint problems (i.e., PIP flexion contractures). The cast or splint stays in place for 3 to 4 weeks.

EXERCISES. The client generally remains immobilized in the dorsal blocking splint or cast during the early phase of the immobilization approach. When the client is referred to therapy during the early phase, the therapist may perform passive flexion to prevent joint stiffness. The therapist may teach a significant other, such as a parent, to perform passive flexion at home if that person is reliable.

TABLE 16-2

Immobilization Protocol Following Flexor Tendon Repair

	EARLY PHASE	INTERMEDIATE PHASE	LATE PHASE
Splint	Dorsal blocking cast or splint • Wrist 20–30 degrees of flexion • Metacarpophalangeal joints 50–60 degrees of flexion	• Adjust dorsal blocking splint for wrist neutral • Remove for exercises	• No protective splint • Splint for extension at night, if needed
Exercises	• Immobilized • Passive flexion by therapist if referred early	• Passive flexion • Active extension with wrist flexed • Wrist tenodesis • Gentle active tendon gliding Assess tendon gliding at 3 weeks • If adherent, begin blocking	Add the following: • Full active flexion and extension • Blocking • Light resistance

BOX 16-1

Overview of Splints Used for Flexor Tendon Repairs in the Early Phase of Tendon Healing

IMMOBILIZATION
Dorsal blocking splint or cast (Fig. 16-13)

IMMEDIATE PASSIVE FLEXION
Dorsal blocking splint with static interphalangeal positioning (Fig. 16-14)
Dorsal blocking splint with elastic traction (Fig. 16-15)

IMMEDIATE ACTIVE FLEXION
Indiana protocol
    Dorsal blocking splint with static positioning for protection (Fig. 16-17, A)
      Wrist hinge splint for exercise (Fig. 16-17, B)
      Dorsal blocking splint with elastic traction, wrist neutral for protection and exercise (Fig. 16-18)

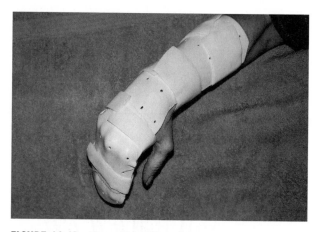

FIGURE 16-13 Dorsal blocking splint or cast.

Goals in the early phase of the immobilization approach include protecting the repaired flexor tendons from rupture with full-time splinting and client education, obtaining passive flexion when allowed, edema control, and obtaining full active motion of the upper extremity proximal to the wrist.

Immediate Passive Flexion Protocols

INDICATIONS. Until recently, immediate passive flexion has been the most commonly used type of protocol for the past 4 decades. Immediate passive flexion approaches apply passive flexion and active interphalangeal extension to the fingers within 3 or 4 days after surgery. The wrist and metacarpophalangeal joints are splinted in partial flexion to prevent stretch and potential rupture. These guidelines were developed to decrease the dense adhesions that followed immobilization in the early phase of flexor tendon healing. Immediate passive flexion protocols have been applied to the traditional two-strand flexor tendon repair.

The benefits of an immediate passive flexion approach over immobilization are improved circulation to the digit and tendon for healing, prevention of extreme stiffness, partial distal gliding of the flexor tendon, and in some cases, a limited amount of proximal gliding of the repaired tendon. Reports indicate a wide variety of results with use of the immediate passive flexion approach, and there are frequent problems with tendinous adhesions.[13,14] Table 16-3 summarizes the general splinting and exercise guidelines of immediate passive flexion protocols.

Many variations of immediate passive flexion protocols exist that are separated into two main categories. These two categories include approaches that use a splint that holds the interphalangeal joints statically between exercises during the early phase of tendon healing or a splint with elastic traction to flex the interphalangeal joints dynamically between exercises.[15] The rationale for holding the interphalangeal joints in flexion between exercises in the early phase of tendon healing is potentially to increase proximal tendon gliding, in part by allowing more time for the tendon to be resting proximally in relation to the repair site and to the pulley system. Holding the digits in flexion also decreases stiffness of the digits by applying passive flexion for a greater portion of time. Placement in passive flexion with elastic traction to the fingers between exercises also decreases the potential for even inadvertent active flexion of the fingers in the early phase of flexor tendon healing, protecting the tendon from rupture. The negative effect of elastic traction is the increased potential to develop interphalangeal flexion contractures and the increase in complexity perceived by the client in having a dynamic splint on the hand as opposed to a less complicated static splint. Clients are placed into the approach preferred by the surgeon/therapist team. Immediate passive flexion protocols with elastic traction are an option for those clients who are not showing signs of interphalangeal flexion contracture, who can be compliant with the rehabilitation program, and who have no soft tissue healing complications.

SPLINTING. Both aforementioned approaches use a dorsal blocking splint with the wrist at 20 to 30 degrees of flexion and the metacarpophalangeal joints at 50 to 60 degrees of flexion, with the interphalangeal joints allowed full extension within the splint unless a digital nerve is repaired.

TABLE 16-3

Immediate Passive Flexion Protocols Following Flexor Tendon Repair

	EARLY PHASE	INTERMEDIATE PHASE	LATE PHASE
Static positioning splint	Dorsal blocking splint: • Wrist 20–30 degrees of flexion • Metacarpophalangeal joints 50–60 degrees of flexion • Interphalangeal joints straight	• Remove splint for bathing and exercises	• No protective splint • Add night extension splint if loss of extension
Elastic traction splint	Same as static positioning splint, but add the following: • Elastic traction to fingertips during day	• Remove elastic traction from fingertips • Remove splint for bathing and exercises	• No protective splint • Add night extension splint if loss of extension
Exercises	• Passive flexion • Active interphalangeal extension	Remove splint, but add the following: • Wrist tenodesis • Place/active hold flexion • Gentle active flexion • Finger extension with wrist flexed, gradual wrist to neutral Assess tendon gliding • If adherent, add gentle blocking and tendon gliding	Add the following: • Finger extension with wrist neutral • Light resistance if adherent; if minimal adhesions, delay resistance until 8 to 10 weeks • Passive interphalangeal extension if needed

Precaution. *If a digital nerve is repaired, the PIP joint is limited to 15 degrees less than full extension or as specified by the surgeon for the first 2 to 3 weeks after repair.*

The difference between the two approaches is the positioning of the fingers in dynamic flexion or static interphalangeal extension in the splint in the early phase of healing. The dorsal blocking splint is fabricated and applied within the first 3 days after surgery.

Prepare the splint for either approach as follows:

Static positioning approach: The static splint base is fabricated with positions as described previously. Passive digit flexion is performed manually and is described in the following section on exercises. Between exercises, the fingers remain strapped to the dorsal hood of the splint (Fig. 16-14).

Dynamic positioning approach: When a dynamic traction approach is preferred, the same splint base is fabricated, with the addition of elastic traction applied from the fingertip of the injured fingers, passing under a distal palmar pulley and connected at the mid-forearm level to the proximal splint strap on the volar forearm (Fig. 16-15). The splint base is the same as that for the static finger positioning approach, with the wrist in 20 to 30 degrees of flexion, the metacarpophalangeal joints in 50 to 60 degrees of flexion, and the interphalangeal joints straight. The elastic traction may consist of rubber bands, rubber band and monofilament line combination, or other elastic thread. Traction can be attached to the tip of the finger by a suture placed by the surgeon through the fingernail, a dress hook glued to the fingernail, or other attachment. The line is threaded through a

pulley at the level of the distal palmar crease and is attached at the level of the forearm, generally to the proximal splint strap, around a safety pin.

CLINICAL *Pearl*

The distal palmar pulley concept is important, for it achieves passive DIP flexion in an attempt to create a better proximal glide of the flexor tendon.

A safety pin in the strap across the palm is a simple method to obtain the distal palmar pulley.

EXERCISES. Perform exercises for either approach as follows:

Static positioning approach: Exercises should be performed in therapy and at home, 10 repetitions every hour. Within the splint, the client may perform passive PIP flexion to tolerance, passive DIP flexion to tolerance, and then composite passive flexion of metacarpophalangeal, PIP, and DIP joints to tolerance. Use specific passive exercises as described by Duran and Houser (Fig. 16-16).[16] Active interphalangeal extension exercises to the hood of the dorsal blocking splint also are performed.

Dynamic positioning approach: Exercises should be performed in therapy and at home, 10 repetitions every hour. Passive flexion of the fingers is performed within the splint. Full passive PIP flexion, DIP flexion, and composite finger flexion are performed passively to the palm. Full active PIP and DIP extension are performed within the splint to the dorsal hood of the splint. Maintenance of full interphalangeal extension is important, especially within this protocol, unless there is a digital nerve repair.

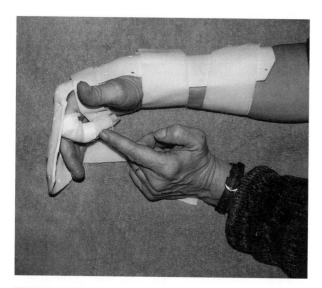

FIGURE 16-14 Dorsal blocking splint with static interphalangeal positioning.

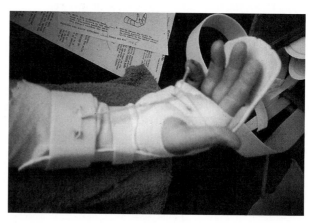

FIGURE 16-15 Dorsal blocking splint with elastic traction.

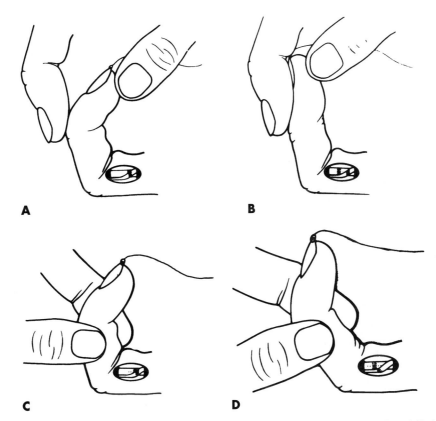

FIGURE 16-16   Duran and Houser's exercises for passive flexor tendon gliding. **A** and **B,** With the metacarpophalangeal and proximal interphalangeal joints flexed, the distal interphalangeal joint is passively extended. This moves the flexor digitorum profundus repair distally, away from the flexor digitorum superficialis repair. **C** and **D,** Then, with the distal interphalangeal and metacarpophalangeal flexed, the proximal interphalangeal joint is extended passively. This moves both repairs distally away from the site of repair and any surrounding tissues to which they might otherwise form adhesions. (From Duran RJ, Coleman CR, Nappi JF et al: Management of flexor tendon lacerations in zone 2 using controlled passive motion postoperatively. In Hunter JM, Schneider LH, Mackin EJ et al, editors: *Rehabilitation of the hand,* ed 3, St Louis, 1990, Mosby.)

Goals in the early phase of the immediate passive flexion approaches include attaining full passive flexion and active interphalangeal extension, tendon gliding as may occur within the limits of the exercises as described, edema control, protecting the repaired flexor tendon from rupture with appropriate splinting and client education, and attaining full upper extremity motion proximal to the wrist.

Immediate Controlled Active Flexion Protocols

Immediate active flexion protocols are the most recent advancement in rehabilitation following flexor tendon repairs. These protocols have been developed following the onset of surgical advancements with stronger repair techniques described earlier in this chapter. Active flexion approaches have been developed to minimize **flexor tendon adhesions** (limited active flexion caused by scar tissue) in the early phase of tendon healing and have

been successful in improving outcomes of flexor tendon repairs.[9-12]

Precaution. *Immediate active flexion approaches are reserved for clients who have had a strong enough surgical repair to tolerate the additional stress placed on the tendon by active flexion and for those who can be compliant to the splinting and exercise program. The presence of severe edema or joint stiffness or health factors that would slow tendon healing may prohibit placement of a client in an active flexion approach.*

DIAGNOSIS-SPECIFIC INFORMATION THAT AFFECTS CLINICAL REASONING. Minimization of the stress on the tendon during active flexion is important, especially in the early phase of tendon healing, to prevent rupture. Edema and stiffness present increased resistance to active flexion, thereby requiring the flexor muscles to pull harder on the tendon, increasing the **work of flexion** within an immediate flexion protocol. *Work of flexion* is a term that describes the amount of tension created within the tendon during active flexion.[17] Work of flexion increases with swelling, stiffness, or any internal friction encountered by the tendon because of bulk of repair, tight pulleys, or swelling of the tendons, in addition to the tension normally developed during active flexion. Our goal as therapists is to minimize the work of flexion, thereby minimizing stress on the repaired tendon, when active motion is initiated immediately following repair. This is achieved by minimizing edema and joint stiffness and by using optimal joint positions that minimize the amount of tension developed within the tendon during active flexion.

Studies have shown that the wrist position that results in the least tension within the flexor tendon during active flexion is that of partial wrist extension and metacarpophalangeal flexion.[18] When the wrist is flexed, a significantly increased amount of work is required by the flexor muscles to flex the fingers compared with when the wrist is slightly extended. By placing the wrist in slight extension, the extensor tendons are given slack at the wrist, allowing the fingers to relax into partial flexion. It requires only a slight pull by the muscle to flex the digits further and actively into a light fist. Thus, most immediate active flexion protocols use a position of wrist neutral to slightly extended during the active flexion exercises and avoid active digit flexion with the wrist flexed. Attaining tight end-ranges of flexion also significantly increases tension within the flexor tendon and is avoided in the early phase of tendon healing.

Precaution. *Our goal in the early phase of flexor tendon healing in an active flexion protocol is to attain a light fist that includes DIP flexion, not a tight fist that is made with force. Education of the client placed in this protocol is important, for those clients who attempt to do more than allowed are much more likely to have tendon ruptures.*

INDICATIONS. Indications for placing a client into an immediate active flexion protocol are essential to understand. The first consideration is the type of suture repair that has been performed. When a four or more strand flexor tendon repair has been performed, it is appropriate to consider use of an immediate controlled active flexion protocol with surgeon approval. Once the surgeon and therapist are convinced that the repair is adequately strong to tolerate active flexion, one must take into account the level of swelling and joint stiffness, for these factors increase resistance to flexor tendon gliding. Another strong consideration is the client's compliance level, because doing any more than is allowed within the protocol has a strong chance of causing a rupture. The

therapist's level of experience is important to consider as well. It is recommended that the therapist have a good understanding of flexor tendon healing, suture technique strengths, risks, and precautions before placing a client into an immediate active flexion protocol. Although an active flexion protocol exists for clients with a two-strand repair, the active flexion portions of the exercises are performed in therapy only and have been designed by an experienced therapist.[9]

Precaution. *An immediate active flexion protocol generally is not recommended in the following situations: a client with a traditional flexor tendon repair of less than four strands, excessive swelling or joint stiffness, a noncompliant client, or an inexperienced therapist in the area of flexor tendon management without appropriate supervision.*

Table 16-4 summarizes guidelines for some immediate active flexion protocols described in this chapter.

SPLINTING. A variety of splints have been designed for use when placing a client into an immediate active flexion protocol following flexor tendon repair. The Indiana protocol places the client in a protective static dorsal blocking splint with the wrist and metacarpophalangeal joints flexed (Fig. 16-17, A) and has them remove that splint to apply a wrist hinge splint for exercises.[10] The wrist hinge splint moves at the wrist from flexion to 30 degrees of extension (Fig. 16-17, B). This splint is applied for exercises only on an hourly basis. The partial wrist extension position is desirable during active flexion of the fingers to reduce tension on the flexor tendons.

Silfverskiold and May[11] casted their clients following repair, with the wrist in neutral, and applied elastic traction to all fingers. The wrist neutral position decreases tension on the flexor tendons during active motion compared with wrist flexion, but not as well as the slightly extended wrist position. Silfverskiold and May did not experience an increase in ruptures when applying active flexion with the wrist neutral, and using this position did not require changing a splint for hourly exercises.

I have modified this approach and applied a thermoplastic splint with the wrist neutral, metacarpophalangeal joints flexed 50 to 70 degrees, with elastic traction to all fingers, used for protection and exercises (Fig. 16-18).[12] Evans and Thompson[9] applied an immediate active flexion protocol to their clients in therapy only, removing the traditional dorsal blocking splint to allow slight wrist extension during the active portion of exercises. At home the clients did not perform the active portion of the exercises and remained in a dorsal blocking splint with the wrist flexed.

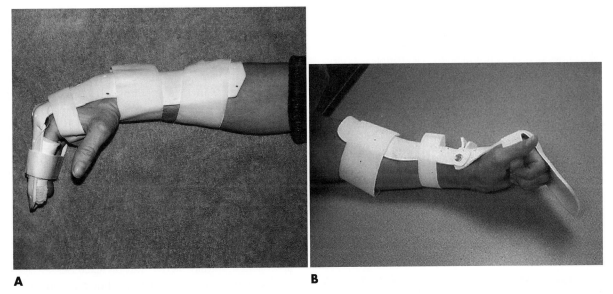

FIGURE 16-17   A, Dorsal blocking splint with static positioning for protection. **B,** Wrist hinge splint for exercise.

TABLE 16-4

Immediate Active Flexion Protocols Following Flexor Tendon Repair

	EARLY PHASE	INTERMEDIATE PHASE	LATE PHASE
Splint options	• Wrist tenodesis splint and static dorsal blocking splint • Dorsal blocking splint wrist neutral, with or without elastic traction	• Continue splint wear to 6 weeks; discontinue elastic traction if used	• No splint, or hand-based dorsal blocking splint during heavy activities, work • Dynamic interphalangeal extension splinting after 10 weeks if interphalangeal flexion contracture is present
Exercises	• Wrist tenodesis • Passive flexion • Active interphalangeal extension with metacarpophalangeal joints flexed • Place and active hold in flexion	Continue with early phase exercises, add the following: • Gentle active flexion • Straight fist • Composite fist • Blocking if adhesions present • Passive interphalangeal extension if needed	Continue with intermediate phase exercises, and add the following: • Hook fist • Light gripping at 8 weeks if adhesions present, at 10–12 weeks if good to excellent tendon gliding

EXERCISES. All of the foregoing protocols use similar exercises in the initial phase of tendon healing for the first 4 weeks. Passive flexion is performed fully. Active extension of the interphalangeal joints is performed fully within the splint unless a digital nerve has been repaired. The additional exercise that is present within this pro-tocol and is not present in any others is an active flexion component, which is performed as a **place and active hold** in flexion. Gentle passive flexion is done using the client's other hand gently to flex the fingers, followed by an active hold of the fingers in the flexed position (Fig. 16-19). This results in a proximal glide of the flexor tendon, which prevents formation of dense adhesions to the flexor tendon from surrounding tissue in the early phase of tendon healing. In therapy, the splint is removed for skin checks and skin and splint cleansing. Exercises in therapy include wrist tenodesis exercises in addition to the passive flexion, active interphalangeal extension, and place/hold flexion exercises. Wrist tenodesis exercises are modified for flexor tendon repair as follows:

- Passive finger flexion to tolerance is followed by wrist extension to 30 degrees.
- Return the wrist to neutral, release the fingers.
- Flex the wrist to tolerance, allowing the fingers to remain relaxed. The relaxed fingers, when the wrist is flexed, extend partially.

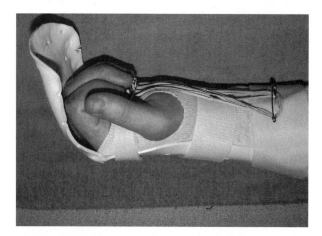

FIGURE 16-18 Dorsal blocking splint with elastic traction, wrist neutral for protection and exercise.

These exercises are performed for approximately the first 4 weeks following repair. Each protocol varies slightly as to when the client is advanced to the intermediate phase of exercises.

Goals in the early phase of an immediate active flexion protocol include attaining full passive flexion, the ability actively to hold in a light fist including at least 75 degrees of PIP flexion and 45 degrees of DIP flexion, full PIP and DIP extension, edema control, protecting the flexor tendon from rupture with appropriate splinting and client education, and obtaining full upper extremity motion proximal to the wrist.

Intermediate Phase of Tendon Healing (3 to 7 Weeks after Surgery): Exercises

Within the immobilization and immediate passive flexion approaches, initiate active flexion exercises at 3 to 4 weeks after surgery. Adjust the splint position to bring the wrist to neutral, and remove the splint for exercises hourly. Initiate passive flexion first to loosen stiff joints created by immobilization, swelling, and scar. For all protocols, when beginning active finger flexion outside of a protective splint, it is appropriate to begin with a wrist tenodesis exercise, performed passively, then actively, as follows:

- Wrist extension to 30 degrees with finger flexion
- Wrist flexion to tolerance with finger extension

Initiate tendon gliding exercises by having the client perform a straight fist, hook fist, and composite fist (Fig. 16-20).[15] Assess flexor tendon adhesions after 3 to 4 days of these exercises by comparing passive flexion to

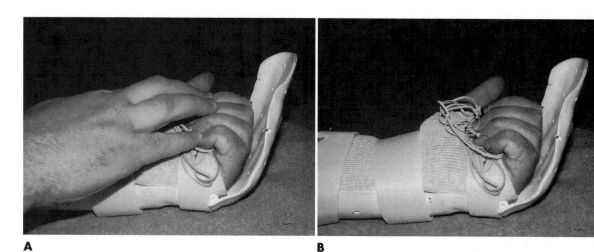

A   **B**

FIGURE 16-19 Place and active hold in flexion following a four-strand flexor tendon repair begins with gentle passive placement of the fingers in flexion using the client's other hand (**A**), followed by release of the fingers while they are held in place actively (**B**).

There are three ways of making a fist:

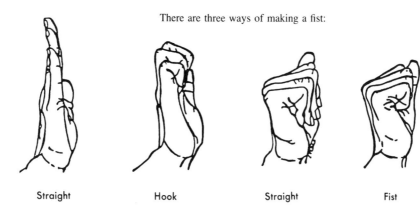

Straight   Hook   Straight   Fist

FIGURE 16-20   The three different positions of tendon gliding exercises: hook fist, straight fist, and full fist. (From Stewart Pettengill K, van Strien G: Postoperative management of flexor tendon injuries. In Mackin EJ, Callahan AD, Skirven TM et al, editors: *Rehabilitation of the hand and upper extremity,* ed 5, St Louis, 2002, Mosby.)

active flexion of the digits. When active flexion is significantly more limited than passive flexion (50 degrees or more total difference between passive and active flexion of the finger joints), add blocking exercises of the PIP and DIP joints. Additional flexor tendon gliding can be obtained with isolated tendon gliding exercises. Isolation of the FDP tendon is achieved by blocking the metacarpophalangeal and PIP joints in extension while performing active DIP joint flexion. Isolate the FDS tendon with blocking of the FDP tendon by holding all other fingers in complete extension and allowing the injured finger to flex at the PIP joint. *These exercises must be done with caution, for the blocking of motion inadvertently may provide resistance to the repaired tendon and thus could result in rupture. These exercises are reserved for the significantly adherent tendon.* If improvement is noted in tendon gliding 1 week later, continue these exercises until 6 weeks postoperatively. If there is no improvement in active flexion with blocking and tendon gliding exercises, initiate light resistance of gripping with very soft putty at 5 or 6 weeks after surgery.

Precaution. *Resistance is initiated in the intermediate phase of healing only in the presence of significant flexor tendon adhesions that prevent active flexion more than passive flexion. If active flexion is not limited significantly, resistance is deferred until the late phase of tendon healing or until the surgeon has determined the tendon is near or at full tensile strength. Resistance has resulted in rupture of the repaired flexor tendon, even in the late phase of tendon healing, when there are minimal to no adhesions.*

Extension of the fingers in this phase initially is performed with the wrist flexed. When PIP joint flexion contractures are present, limiting the PIP and/or DIP

joints from full extension, splint the joints in a volar extension splint at night beginning at approximately 5 to 6 weeks postoperatively or as approved by the surgeon. Passive extension with the flexor tendon in a protected position (with proximal joints in flexion) may be performed cautiously.

Goals in the intermediate phase of tendon healing include obtaining full passive flexion and partial to full active flexion, full interphalangeal extension, and protecting the repaired tendon from rupture with appropriate splinting between exercises and client education, and scar management.

Late Phase of Tendon Healing: Exercises

Discontinue protective splinting unless there is good to excellent tendon gliding. In this case, a small dorsal blocking splint may help remind the client to avoid activities that result in strong use or resistance to the repaired tendon. When passive flexion continues to be limited by joint stiffness and swelling, continue therapeutic techniques such as heat and passive ROM. Active flexion, joint blocking, and tendon gliding exercises continue in an attempt to bring active flexion to match the level of passive flexion. Resistance can be introduced or advanced during this phase when adhesions that limit active flexion are present. Light resistance can be provided with putty or light manual resistance from the therapist. If flexor tendon adhesions are minimal, initiate gentle resistance only after 8 weeks after surgery, with strong resistance restricted until after 12 weeks after surgery.

Goals in the late phase of tendon healing include obtaining full passive and active flexion and extension of the injured fingers, increasing strength to obtain a light fist, and protecting the repaired tendon from rupture with client education.

Regardless of the goals, especially following use of an immobilization or an immediate passive flexion protocol, active flexion of a repaired flexor tendon may be limited because of adhesion formation. Limited active flexion of the repaired digit, especially the DIP joint, frequently occurs, and there may be difficulty actively flexing the adjacent digits because of the common muscle belly of the FDP to the last three digits **(quadriga effect)**. Grip strength is diminished because of loss of active flexion. Flexor tendons with adhesions commonly require a more prolonged time of therapy, with a strong emphasis on a home program of blocking exercises and resistance even longer than the 12-week healing period to continue to facilitate tendon gliding during the long remodeling process. Further surgical procedures are available for the repaired flexor tendon with significant adhesions that limit functional use of the hand. If needed, these procedures most often are performed between 3 and 6 months after repair. Outcomes for the flexor tendon that is allowed immediate passive flexion are improved over those that have been immobilized. Outcomes for the flexor tendon following immediate active flexion protocols are even better, but application of this type of protocol is limited to the strong repair, preferably an experienced therapist, and a compliant and responsible client.

Protocols are numerous in literature for flexor tendon repairs in zone II. Repairs in other areas of the hand receive less attention. Evans[19] has designed a specific protocol for flexor tendon repairs in zone I. Flexor tendon repairs proximal to zone II result in less limiting adhesions and respond better to exercises. I use the same splints and general time guidelines and exercises for repairs in all zones of the repaired flexor tendon unless the surgeon decides to advance the therapy sooner for a client with a strong repair proximal to zone II.

TIPS FROM THE FIELD

Splinting Tips

When applying a splint within a few days following a tendon repair, therapists often need to remove postsurgical dressings and to apply a light dressing to the surgical incision.

Precaution. *The client may want to stretch or move the hand when the postoperative dressings and splint are removed, and it is essential to instruct the client to stay in the position in which he or she is placed during splint fabrication.*

During splint fabrication, place the hand in the tendon-protected position. For an extensor tendon, this is one of passive extension. This can be attained using folded or rolled towels to support the wrist and fingers in extension. For a flexor tendon repair, this is one of being relaxed in flexion, which is attained easily by relaxing the wrist and fingers over the edge of a bolster.

Precaution. *As therapists fabricate the splint, it is essential that they avoid placing a stretch on the repaired tendon because this could cause tendon rupture.*

Evaluation Tips

The first therapy session for a client with a repaired tendon includes removal of dressings and postoperative splint, fabrication of the splint described within the protocol chosen, instruction in a home exercise program, and an abbreviated evaluation. The evaluation portion of the session consists of observation of the wound or surgical incision for drainage, bleeding, or signs of infection, and observation of the amount of swelling in the digits and upper extremity. A verbal description of pain is obtained. Sensation is discussed, and because of the need to fabricate a splint at the first appointment, specific sensory testing may be deferred to a later session.

Precaution. *When sensory testing is done, it is important that the hand and digits be maintained in a tendon-protected position.*

Range of motion is not assessed in the usual manner immediately following a tendon repair. The healing tendon cannot safely be moved through its full excursion in the early phase without rupture. See Box 16-2 for methods to assess motion following tendon repair. Box 16-3 describes the method of final assessment of motion following a flexor tendon repair.

No strength assessment is appropriate during an evaluation immediately following a tendon repair. Limited evaluation of ROM is appropriate as indicated in Box 16-2.

Treatment of tendon repairs in the hand is challenging, requiring us to stay abreast of current changes and gain the experience necessary to understand the process of tendon healing. Box 16-4 summarizes the important concepts of which we must be aware when treating a client with a repaired tendon.

Precaution. *It is strongly recommended that you have supervision when beginning to treat tendon repairs to ensure proper hands-on management and an understanding of these important concepts related to the treatment of an individual with a tendon repair in the hand.*

BOX 16-2

Evaluation of Range of Motion Following Tendon Repair

EXTENSOR TENDON REPAIR

1. When initiating therapy in the early phase of healing after an extensor tendon repair, assess passive extension to 0 degrees at all finger joints and wrist extension passively as tolerated.
2. Do not assess active extension immediately following an extensor tendon repair unless an immediate active extension protocol is being used.
3. Do not assess finger flexion in the early phase of tendon healing, with the exception of 30 degrees of flexion when an immediate passive or active extension protocol is used. Awareness of the position that protects the tendon is essential when allowing controlled motion in the direction that will place tension on the repair.
4. In the intermediate phase of tendon healing, first evaluate the extensor tendon for flexion at each individual finger joint while supporting the other joints in extension. One to 2 weeks later, evaluate composite flexion of the fingers with the wrist in extension, and evaluate the wrist for flexion with the fingers relaxed.
5. At the completion of treatment, composite flexion of the fingers, subtracting any loss of active extension, gives the total active motion results for the injured digits.

FLEXOR TENDON REPAIR

1. In the early phase following a flexor tendon repair, immediately assess passive flexion of all finger joints.
2. When using an immediate active flexion protocol, assess the amount of composite flexion attained in a place and hold in flexion position. With the wrist and metacarpophalangeal joints flexed, assess active interphalangeal extension to 0 degrees if no digital nerve injuries are present. *Do not assess composite extension until the intermediate phase of flexor tendon healing because this could cause tendon rupture.*
3. In the intermediate phase following a flexor tendon repair, evaluate active flexion within all types of protocols. Assess composite finger extension with the wrist flexed and, 1 to 2 weeks later, with the wrist in neutral. *Do not assess grip and pinch strength until after the full 12 week tendon healing process because this requires maximal tension on the repaired tendon.*
4. When healing of the flexor tendon and rehabilitation is complete, calculate the end result of the motion of the injured finger(s) by adding active flexion of the interphalangeal joints and subtracting any loss of extension. Metacarpophalangeal joint motion is not used in this calculation. The formula designed by Strickland and Glogovac[20] commonly is used and can be found in Box 16-3.

BOX 16-3

Classification of Motion Results Following Flexor Tendon Repair[20]

FORMULA

[(PIP + DIP flexion) - (loss of PIP extension + loss of DIP extension)] × 100 = % of normal
175

CLASSIFICATION

Excellent: 85-100%
Good: 70-84%
Fair: 50-69%
Poor: Less than 50%

The Role of the Therapy Assistant

Because of the complex nature of the acute tendon injury, the role of the therapy assistant is limited in the early and intermediate phases of tendon healing unless additional educational opportunities have been provided to the assistant. When a client with a tendon repair is in the late phase of tendon healing or beyond the weeks of tendon healing described in this chapter, the client may be determined by the referring surgeon to have no restrictions on activity of the hand. At this point, strengthening, tendon gliding, blocking exercises, and retraining in functional use of the injured digits and hand may be done by the assistant to overcome residual deficits. In a specialty setting that deals primarily with hand injuries, a therapy assistant may have additional training, and the determination of their intervention is best done within the individual setting.

BOX 16-4

Concepts to Remember When Treating the Repaired Tendon in the Hand

- Initial splints are designed to protect the repaired tendon by preventing tension of the tendon.
- Repaired tendons rupture from stretch or from active motion by the muscle of the repaired tendon that is too strong for the repair to withstand.
- Three types of protocols are designed for all tendon repairs with the exception of extensor tendon zones I and II. These are, from the most conservative to least conservative, immobilization, immediate passive motion, and immediate active motion protocols.
- Motion, when initiated, is done gently. Motion is begun when the surgeon determines the repair and tensile strength of the tendon can withstand gentle motion.

- The better the active motion in the early to intermediate phase of tendon healing, the fewer adhesions are present. The fewer adhesions present, the longer resistance to the repaired tendon is delayed.
- Passive motion in the direction that would stretch the tendon repair is done for joint stiffness only with the tendon supported on slack, in a protected position.
- Advancement from one phase of exercises to the next is done with the awareness of the referring surgeon.
- Resistance to the repaired tendon is deferred unless active motion is limited by adhesions in the intermediate phase of tendon healing.

CASE *Studies*

CASE 16-1

E.E. is a 53-year-old meat cutter who sustained a work-related saw injury of the dorsal right small finger while cutting meat. He was seen at an emergency room at a workmen's compensation clinic associated with the workplace. He developed an infection, was treated with intravenously administered antibiotics, and was referred to the hand surgeon 8 days after injury. Surgery was performed 9 days after injury, and exploration showed a ragged laceration extending into the extensor mechanism, including the central slip. The saw also had removed part of the dorsal condyle and articular surface of the proximal interphalangeal (PIP) joint. The central slip was repaired, and the PIP joint was pinned in almost full extension (see Fig. 16-21 on the CD).

E.E. was referred to therapy 10 days after repair for fabrication of a thermoplastic splint to support the wrist in neutral and the ring and small fingers in extension and to protect the pin (see Fig. 16-22 on the CD). The surgeon chose full support and immobilization because of the combination of bone and tendon injury, history of infection, and questionable level of understanding and compliance by the client.

The pin was removed 4 weeks after surgery, and active therapy was initiated 3 times per week. For the first week, splint use was continued between bathing and exercises, and then the splint was used only when E.E. was out of the house until 6 weeks after surgery. Initial range of motion (ROM) of individual joints was 0 to 50

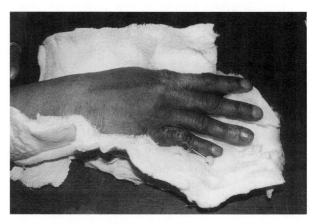

FIGURE 16-21 Complex extensor tendon injury in zones III and IV requiring repair and pin support.

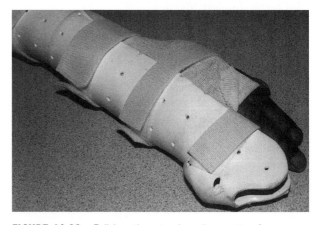

FIGURE 16-22 Full-length extension ulnar gutter for protection of pin and tendon repair.

degrees for metacarpophalangeal joints, −15 to 20 degrees for PIP joints, and 0 to 5 degrees for distal interphalangeal (DIP) joints. Wrist motion was present through 75% of normal range. E.E. was instructed in home exercises for active individual joint flexion, reverse blocking extension exercises, and passive extension. Because of extreme limitations in motion, exercises were advanced to include active composite flexion and gentle passive flexion of individual joints within a week of starting therapy. After 1 week, active ROM was 0 to 60 degrees for metacarpophalangeal joints, −25 to 40 degrees for PIP joints, and 0 to 10 degrees for DIP joints. Passive extension was to −5 degrees at the PIP joint.

The client returned to light duty wrapping meat at 5 weeks after surgery while wearing the protective splint. Therapy consisted of wrapping the fingers in flexion to tolerance with a heat application, followed by active and passive flexion and extension exercises, and functional grasp and release activities. Buddy straps from small to ring finger were provided in an attempt to improve motion of the small finger. ROM at 6 weeks after repair was 0 to 75 degrees for metacarpophalangeal joints, −30 to 55 degrees for PIP joints, and 0 to 10 degrees for DIP joints. Passive extension was available to −5 degrees at the PIP joint, indicating extensor tendon adhesions. Active motion improvements stalled at this time. Improvements of 10 degrees of flexion at each joint would be made in therapy; however, the client would arrive in therapy with the same limitations in motion as the previous session. At 8 weeks after injury, functional strengthening was initiated, and putty was provided for resistance exercises at home in addition to active and passive home exercises.

The diagnosis of posttraumatic arthritis of the PIP joint was made by radiographic evaluation 11 weeks after surgery. Therapy was discontinued at this time with ROM of 0 to 90 degrees for metacarpophalangeal joints, −25 to 60 degrees for PIP joints, and 0 to 25 degrees for DIP joints at the end of a session. The surgeon will continue to follow the client for motion and function of the small finger and hand and will make a determination in the future regarding potential benefit of further surgery, including extensor tenolysis to remove tendinous adhesions.

This case demonstrates the difficulty of regaining flexion and extension of the interphalangeal joints with a complex injury when dense adhesions form between the extensor tendon, surrounding tissue, and bone in zones III and IV. An immediate motion protocol, which may have prevented the limiting adhesions, was not considered because of the involvement of injury to the bone at the articular surface and because of client understanding and compliance issues. This case shows that when this combination of factors exists, it may be necessary to immobilize the digit and accept an intact tendon with adhesions, recognizing the potential need for further surgery to improve motion and function.

CASE 16-2

J.P. is a 23-year-old man employed as a bartender. He suffered an injury to the volar surface of the small finger, lacerating the flexor digitorum profundus and flexor digitorum superficialis tendons in zone II when a glass that he was washing broke in his hand. The surgeon performed a four-strand repair to the tendons and requested an immediate active flexion protocol.

Three days after repair a dorsal blocking splint with the wrist in neutral, metacarpophalangeal joints flexed, and interphalangeal joints allowed full extension was fabricated, with elastic traction to all four fingers (Fig. 16-13). J.P. was instructed in a home exercise program of passive flexion, place and active hold in flexion, and interphalangeal extension within the splint (Fig. 16-19). He was instructed to keep the splint on at all times at home. The splint was removed in therapy for cleansing of skin and the splint, dressing changes, wrist tenodesis exercises of 30 degrees of wrist extension with gentle passive flexion and wrist flexion as tolerated with fingers relaxed. Passive flexion and place and hold flexion with the wrist in 20 to 30 degrees of extension were performed in therapy, and the client did the same at home within the splint, keeping the wrist in neutral. Interphalangeal extension was performed to 0 degrees with the metacarpophalangeal joints supported in flexion.

Initial evaluation revealed moderate swelling in the small finger, mild swelling in the hand, no drainage from the incisional line. Pain was moderate with range of motion on the date the splint was fabricated. Range of motion was evaluated for passive finger flexion and interphalangeal extension within the splint and place and active hold in flexion gently. Passive finger flexion was 70 degrees for metacarpophalangeal joints, 70 degrees for proximal interphalangeal (PIP) joints, and 50 degrees for distal interphalangeal (DIP) joints. Place and active hold in flexion was evaluated at 70 degrees for metacarpophalangeal joints, 65 degrees for PIP joints, and 45 degrees for DIP joints. Interphalangeal extension was evaluated as −10 degrees for PIP joints and −5 degrees for DIP joints with the metacarpophalangeal joints supported in flexion. The client attended therapy 2 times per week. Gradual gains were made in passive and place and active hold flexion.

At 4 weeks after surgery, the client was able to attain equal passive and place and hold flexion of 75 degrees for metacarpophalangeal joints, 85 degrees for PIP joints, 55 degrees for DIP joints with interphalangeal extension

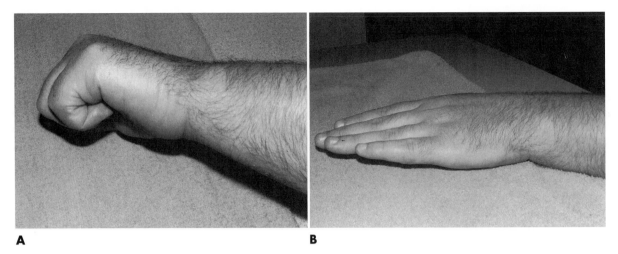

A   **B**

FIGURE 16-23   Case study results at 8 weeks after flexor tendon repair for (**A**) flexion and (**B**) extension.

to −5 degrees for PIP joints and −5 degrees for DIP joints. At 5 weeks postoperative, the elastic traction was removed from the splint. J.P. was allowed to remove the splint for active flexion and extension of the fingers with wrist tenodesis and for bathing. At 8 weeks the splint was cut at the wrist to allow wrist motion, and J.P. was instructed to use the splint at work or during heavy activities to prevent resistance to DIP flexion. Range of motion at 12 weeks after surgery was 0 to 90 degrees for metacarpophalangeal joints, 0 to 90 degrees for PIP joints, and 0 to 70 degrees for DIP joints (Fig. 16-23).

J.P. returned to regular duty and unrestricted use of the hand at 12 weeks after repair, with instructions to avoid resisted fingertip resistance, such as a hook grasp with weight, for another 1 to 2 weeks. The motion results were calculated as $[(90 + 70) - 0] \div 175 = 92\%$, which falls into the excellent result category.

References

1. Newport ML, Williams CD: Biomechanical characteristics of extensor tendon suture techniques, *J Hand Surg* 17A:1117, 1992.
2. Shaeib MD, Singer DI: Tensile strengths of various suture techniques, *J Hand Surg* 22B(6):764, 1997.
3. Strickland JW: The scientific basis for advances in flexor tendon surgery, *J Hand Ther* 18(2):94, 2005.
4. Lundborg G, Rank F: Experimental intrinsic healing of flexor tendons based upon synovial fluid nutrition, *J Hand Surg* 3(1):21, 1978.
5. Walsh MT et al: Early controlled motion with dynamic splinting versus static splinting for zones III and IV extensor tendon lacerations: a preliminary report, *J Hand Ther* 7:232, 1994.
6. Thomes LJ: Early mobilization method for surgically repaired zone III extensor tendons, *J Hand Ther* 8:195, 1995.
7. Evans RB: Clinical management of extensor tendon injuries. In Mackin EJ, Callahan AD, Skirven TM et al, editors: *Rehabilitation of the hand and upper extremity*, ed 5, St Louis, 2002, Mosby.
8. Howell JW, Merritt WH, Robinson SJ: Immediate controlled active motion following zone 4-7 extensor tendon repair, *J Hand Ther* 18(2):182, 2005.
9. Evans RE, Thompson DE: The application of force to the healing tendon, *J Hand Ther* 6:262, 1993.
10. Strickland JW, Cannon NM: Flexor tendon repair: Indiana method, *Indiana Newsletter* 1:1-12, 1993.
11. Silfverskiold KL, May EJ: Flexor tendon repair in zone II with a new suture technique and an early mobilization program combining passive and active flexion, *J Hand Surg* 19A:53, 1994.
12. Klein L: Early active motion flexor tendon protocol using one splint, *J Hand Ther* 16(3):199, 2003.
13. Silfverskiold KL, May EJ, Tornvall AH: Flexor digitorum profundus tendon excursions during controlled motion after flexor tendon repair in zone II: a prospective clinical study, *J Hand Surg* 17A:122-133, 1992.
14. Manske PR: Flexor tendon healing, *J Hand Surg* 13B:237-245, 1989.
15. Stewart Pettengill K, van Strien G: Postoperative management of flexor tendon injuries. In Mackin EJ, Callahan AD, Skirven TM et al, editors: *Rehabilitation of the hand and upper extremity*, ed 5, St Louis, 2002, Mosby.

16. Duran RJ, Coleman CR, Nappi JF et al: Management of flexor tendon lacerations in zone 2 using controlled passive motion postoperatively. In Hunter JM, Schneider LH, Mackin EJ et al, editors: *Rehabilitation of the hand,* ed 3, St Louis, 1990, Mosby.

17. Halikis MN, Manske PR, Kubota H et al: Effect of immobilization, immediate mobilization, and delayed mobilization on the resistance to digital flexion using a tendon injury model, *J Hand Surg* 22A:464, 1997.

18. Savage R: The influence of wrist position on the minimum force required for active movement of the interphalangeal joints, *J Hand Surg* 13B:262, 1988.

19. Evans RB: Zone I flexor tendon rehabilitation with limited extension and active flexion, *J Hand Ther* 18(2):128, 2005.

20. Strickland JW, Glogovac SV: Digital function following flexor tendon repair in zone II: a comparison of immobilization and controlled passive motion techniques, *J Hand Surg* 5:537, 1980.

17

Arthritis

JEANINE BIESE

More than 100 diseases and conditions fall into the category of rheumatic diseases.[1] **Osteoarthritis,** one of these conditions, affects more than 20 million Americans, most of whom are over the age of 45. Osteoarthritis is the most common joint disorder throughout the world.[2] Osteoarthritis is defined as a gradual loss of articular cartilage caused by degenerative joint disease and chemical factors. Clients from all corners of the world report similar patterns of joint involvement.[3] **Rheumatoid arthritis** affects more than 2 million Americans.[4] Rheumatoid arthritis is defined as a systemic disease characterized by **synovial** inflammation. The therapist also may treat other rheumatic diseases such as **systemic lupus erythematosus** (a systemic autoimmune disease characterized by inflammation and blood vessel abnormalities), **gout** (a disorder caused by uric acid or urate crystal deposition), **bursitis** (inflammation of the **bursa**), and **fibromyalgia** (diffuse widespread pain often with specific tender points). In the late 1990s, nearly 43 million Americans were affected with rheumatic diseases.[5,6] Clearly, with this level of prevalence, many therapists at some time will find these clients on their caseload. The therapist must have an understanding of the disease process and how it can affect the clients' activities of daily living. Client education about the disease and awareness of treatment options are also critical aspects of the treatment process.

OSTEOARTHRITIS

Osteoarthritis often is called the wear-and-tear disease, but research demonstrates that the breakdown in the articular cartilage is due to mechanical and chemical factors.[7] Affected persons have a genetic susceptibility, and osteoarthritis occurs more frequently in women over age 50 than in men of the same age. In addition to the breakdown in the cartilage, new bone formation (or **osteophytosis**) can occur, resulting in pain and limitations of joint movement.

CLINICAL *Pearl*

In the upper extremity the joints that are most symptomatic are the distal interphalangeal (DIP) joints and the first carpometacarpal joints.[8]

Additional involvement can occur at the proximal interphalangeal (PIP) joints, the metacarpophalangeal joints, and at the wrist. **Osteophytes,** or bone spurs, occurring at the metacarpophalangeal joints can contribute to **triggering** (limited digital range of motion caused by dragging of the tendon as it passes through a pulley) of the flexor tendons.[4] The client also may demonstrate reduced range of motion, pain, **crepitus** (**grating** or popping as the digit flexes and extends), **locking** (the digit locks into flexion as the tendon fails to pass through a pulley), and signs of inflammation.[9] In the lower extremity the knees and hips commonly are affected.

Precaution. *If the client needs to use a walker or crutches because of lower extremity pain, this can put additional stress on the joints of the hands.*

Pathology

The pathogenesis of osteoarthritis involves an alteration of the normal wearing down and repair of the articular cartilage. The deterioration of the joint cartilage in osteoarthritis begins at the superficial layer and gradually progresses to the point that fissures and lesions develop. The cartilage eventually tears, releasing fragments into the joint space. Enzymatic wearing down of the cartilage also occurs. The cartilage gradually becomes thinner and over time may wear away completely. Osteophytes (bony outgrowths) and synovial (tissue that lines the joints, tendons, and bursa) inflammation also may occur.[3,10] This synovial tissue is what produces lubrication and lines the joints and tendon sheaths. Synovial inflammation is called **synovitis**. Synovial inflammation is discussed further in the section on rheumatoid arthritis.

Timelines and Healing

Currently, no cure is available for osteoarthritis. The therapist can help manage the symptoms as the disease progresses with client education, modalities, splinting, joint protection, and adaptive equipment. Some activities can increase pain. Most commonly, clients report that heavy pinch activities can increase pain at the thumb carpometacarpal joint. Regarding postoperative care, the following timelines are for some specific surgeries.

Nonoperative Treatment

Nonoperative treatment includes a complete evaluation to determine the client's specific needs. Treatment can include joint protection principles, modalities, exercise, splinting, and adaptive equipment as outlined subsequently.

Evaluation

The evaluation should include an assessment of pain, active range of motion, joint stability, joint inflammation, palpation, and ability to do activities of daily living. Pain is measured best with a 10 cm visual analog scale with 0 being no pain and 10 being severe pain. This scale can be used to determine pain at rest and with activities. Document areas of inflammation by specifying which joints are involved. If the joint is warm and red, it may be in an acute inflammatory stage, and this should be noted. Take active range of motion measurements of the upper extremity.

Precaution. *Passive range of motion measurements usually are not recommended, especially if there is a lack of joint stability. Not applying passive stretch to a joint that lacks stability is important because of the osteoarthritis disease process, for passive stretch can be injurious.*

The evaluation of activities of daily living should include home, work, and avocational activities. Difficulties with work and avocational activities are what most commonly bring the client to the clinic. We, as a society, often seek help when the activities that are most meaningful to us are threatened.

Evaluate thumb joint stability by having the client attempt a tip pinch. If the thumb metacarpophalangeal and interphalangeal joints are unable to maintain a near-neutral position during pinch, ligament stability is questionable. Assessing lateral joint stability is important at the PIP and DIP joints. Test the involved joint by stabilizing the proximal phalanx and gently moving the distal phalanx laterally in each direction. A greater degree of joint play is evident when joint stability is decreased. Lateral deviation of the interphalangeal joints at rest also is noted if evident. Also advisable is to document fixed deformities such as deformities that cannot be corrected passively when the joint is positioned by the therapist. Fixed joint deformities in osteoarthritis can include DIP flexion or angulation, carpometacarpal adduction, and thumb metacarpophalangeal joint extension or flexion.

Grating or crepitus evident at a joint can indicate damaged cartilage. The **grind test** for degenerative joint disease at the carpometacarpal joint involves compressing the joint while gently rotating the head of the metacarpal on the trapezium[11] (Fig. 17-1). Pain and crepitus at the carpometacarpal joint generally are considered positive findings.

General Joint Protection Principles

Joint protection principles ideally are initiated early in the disease process in hope of decreasing stress to the involved joints.[12] Box 17-1 provides a simple overview.

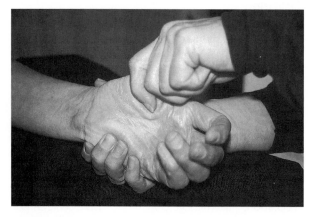

FIGURE 17-1 The grind test as described by Swanson[11] for crepitus at the carpometacarpal joint involves compressing the joint while gently rotating the metacarpal at the carpometacarpal joint. (From Biese J: Therapist's evaluation and conservative management of rheumatoid arthritis in the hand and wrist. In Mackin EJ, Callahan AD, Skirven TM et al, editors: *Rehabilitation of the hand and upper extremity,* ed 5, St Louis, 2002, Mosby.)

With the thumb, joint protection focuses on decreasing the amount of force used for pinching activities. Adaptive equipment that can help to increase leverage and also distribute pressure in the hand includes larger-diameter pens, broad key holders, large plastic tabs on medicine bottles, and car door openers. In clients who demonstrate involvement of the PIP and DIP joints, joint protection is accomplished by avoiding activities that have prolonged and forceful PIP and DIP flexion. This can include avoiding a tight three-jaw chuck pinch when writing and using larger handles to reduce and relax the client's grip. Moving objects out of the hand (e.g., using a shoulder strap tote bag instead of a brief case with a handle) can be helpful in avoiding prolonged interphalangeal joint flexion. Plastic grocery bags held by the handle also should be replaced with bags that can be carried closer to the body.

The therapist must look at all aspects of the client when treating the osteoarthritic hand. Clients often place strong forces on the hands when lifting themselves from one position to another. In some cases, adaptive equipment also can reduce the effort on the lower extremities (such as a lift chair, a shower chair, or elevated toilet seat) and may help to reduce the stress placed on the hands.

In addition, the therapist should take into consideration the individual needs of each client, including the client's sociocultural context. The client may or may not have insurance coverage or finances for adaptive equipment or splints. Carefully discuss options with the client and weigh them in terms of cost versus value in meeting the client's specific needs. The therapist should be aware of resources in the community that may assist clients in obtaining specific adaptive equipment (e.g., grab bars and elevated toilet seats) if they exceed the client's ability to purchase them. Civic, community, or religious organizations also may offer resources. For further information on joint protection, the reader is encouraged to review the work *Rheumatic Disease in the Adult and Child: Occupational Therapy and Rehabilitation* by Jeanne L. Melvin.[4]

Modalities
Thermal Agents

Superficial thermal agents such as heat and cold commonly are used in the treatment of osteoarthritis to decrease pain, but further research is needed to determine their effectiveness.[16] Decreasing pain and maintaining or improving joint range of motion is a primary goal in the application of these agents. Types of superficial heating agents include paraffin, fluidotherapy, hot packs, microwave packs, hydrotherapy, and electric mitts. Clinically, clients report decreased pain and less muscle guarding following superficial heat application.[17]

BOX 17-1

Overview of Joint Protection Principles[4,12-15]

RESPECT PAIN
- Stop activities before the point of discomfort.
- Decrease activities that cause pain that lasts more than 2 hours.
- Avoid activities that put strain on painful or stiff joints.

BALANCE REST AND ACTIVITY
- Rest before exhaustion.
- Take frequent, short breaks.
- Avoid activities that cannot be stopped.
- Avoid staying in one position for a long time.
- Alternate heavy and light activities.
- Take more breaks when inflammation is active.
- Allow extra time for activities—avoid rushing.
- Plan your day ahead of time.
- Eliminate unnecessary activities.

EXERCISE IN A PAIN-FREE RANGE
- Consider warm-water pool exercise programs.
- Use exercises specific to each deformity.

REDUCE THE EFFORT
- Avoid excessive loads with carts, getting help, and appliances.
- Keep items near where they are used.
- Use prepared foods.
- Avoid low chairs.

- Maintain proper body weight.
- Freeze leftovers for an easy meal later.
- Try to eliminate trips up and down the stairs by completing work on each floor.
- Sit to work when possible.

AVOID POSITIONS OF DEFORMITY
- Avoid bent elbows, knees, hips, and back while sleeping.
- Have good posture during the day.
- Obtain a workstation evaluation for proper posture.
- See text for specific hand deformities.

USE THE LARGER JOINTS
- Slide heavy objects on kitchen counters.
- Use palms, rather than fingers, to lift or push.
- Use a backpack instead of handheld purse.
- Keep packages close to the body—use two hands.
- Push swinging doors open with side of body instead of the hands.

USE ADAPTIVE EQUIPMENT
- Use items such as jar openers and button hooks that are specific to each patient's needs.

DISTRIBUTE PRESSURE
- Use both hands for leverage and carts.

Precaution. *When clients benefit from superficial heat and cold modalities and use them in their home program, the therapist must instruct them carefully to avoid the possibility of burns.*

Ultrasound is a deep heat modality that often is used in the clinic to treat osteoarthritis, and use of this modality also requires additional research.

Exercise

General principles of exercise include avoiding painful active range of motion (AROM) and passive range of motion (PROM) and working within the client's comfort level. General AROM exercises for the hand include wrist flexion and extension, gentle digit flexion and extension, and thumb opposition.

Precaution. *Keep range of motion exercises pain free to prevent stretching of joint structures. Use strengthening programs for the osteoarthritic hand with caution to avoid aggravation of deformities.*

For example, even light putty-pinching exercises impart large forces[18] to an unstable carpometacarpal joint

and might aggravate a potential deformity. Stability must not be sacrificed for a possible increase in strength. A stable pain-free thumb provides a post against which the digits can grip and pinch effectively. Grip strengthening is a common example of an exercise that can aggravate inflamed flexor tendons. A digit that is triggering or locking will not be improved with grip strengthening exercises, and strengthening usually increases these symptoms.

Precaution. *Therapy exercises should never create deforming forces or cause pain in the osteoarthritic client.*

The Thumb

Osteoarthritis can affect all of the joints of the thumb but most commonly is seen at the carpometacarpal joint. As the disease progresses, sometimes the carpometacarpal joint partially dislocates off the trapezium, and the first metacarpal can progress into an adduction deformity. The client then develops a metacarpophalangeal hyperextension position while trying to open the hand around an object (Fig. 17-2). Pinch is often painful because

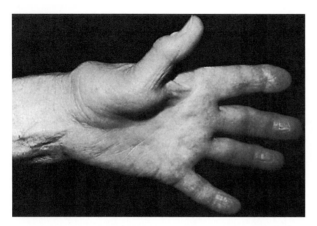

FIGURE 17-2 The type III thumb deformity involves subluxation of the carpometacarpal joint, metacarpophalangeal joint hyperextension, and distal joint flexion. (From Terrono AL, Nalebuff EA, Phillips CA: The rheumatoid thumb. In Mackin EJ, Callahan AD, Skirven TM et al, editors: *Rehabilitation of the hand and upper extremity,* ed 5, St Louis, 2002, Mosby.)

the carpometacarpal subluxation becomes more pronounced during heavy pinch activities. The thumb interphalangeal joint sometimes assumes a flexed position. This has been categorized as a **type III deformity.**[19] Box 17-2 gives a complete description of these deformities. The reader is encouraged to see *Rehabilitation of the Hand and Upper Extremity*[19] for more information. When evaluating the thumb, determine the specific pattern of deformity so that treatment can be more exacting in terms of splint support and prevention.

Questions to Ask the Doctor

- *What joints of the thumb are involved (as seen on the x-ray film)?*
- *Is there also joint involvement of the wrist?*
- *Is the client using any medications for this condition?*

What to Say to Clients

About the Condition

"Here is a picture (x-ray film) of a thumb with osteoarthritis. The problem often starts at this joint (the carpometacarpal joint). With wearing down of the cartilage and weakening of the joint ligaments and capsule, this joint has a tendency to dislocate partially or slide out of place. Over time, this results in a thumb that has difficulty abducting or moving away from the palm of the hand (at the carpometacarpal joint). The next joint of the thumb (metacarpophalangeal joint) then has to do extra work, and it often stretches out and hyperextends."

BOX 17-2

Deformities of the Rheumatoid Thumb

The original categorization by Dr. Edward Nalebuff in 1968 gives six types of deformities[19]:

Type I: This sometimes is referred as to the boutonniere deformity and includes metacarpophalangeal flexion and interphalangeal joint hyperextension. The carpometacarpal joint is not involved. This type is one of the most common deformities.

Type II: This uncommon deformity includes carpometacarpal flexion and adduction, metacarpophalangeal flexion, and interphalangeal joint hyperextension.

Type III: This sometimes is referred to as the swan neck deformity and includes metacarpophalangeal joint hyperextension, interphalangeal flexion, and carpometacarpal joint subluxation with adduction and flexion. This deformity also commonly is seen in osteoarthritis.

Type IV: This deformity is similar to a gamekeeper's thumb in that the metacarpophalangeal joint is hyperextended and the metacarpophalangeal ulnar collateral ligament is unstable. Metacarpal adduction also develops as the deformity progresses.

Type V: The metacarpophalangeal joint is hyperextended because of a lax volar plate.

Type VI: This deformity is seen in arthritis mutilans and involves collapse resulting from bone loss.

About Splinting

"We are going to try a couple of splints that may help to give the thumb some stability. We have several options, but we need to see what works best for you and your daily activities. Some people like one type of splint for night wear, and some like a less restrictive splint for day wear. We are going to see what gives you the type of support you need without getting in the way of your daily activities."

About Exercise

"Heavy pinch activities and exercises really put a lot of stress on this (the carpometacarpal) joint and can decrease joint stability. The splint will help give your thumb more stability, and you may feel like you have more strength with less pain. For your general conditioning, warm-water pool exercises may be helpful in managing your osteoarthritis."

Evaluation Tips

- Determine whether the thumb deformity is passively correctable. This involves gentle pressure with your thumb to support the carpometacarpal joint while gently placing the first metacarpal in palmer abduction (Fig. 17-3). Place the thumb metacarpophalangeal joint in slight flexion. This is the proper position for your splint for a type III deformity.

- Determine how the disease process is affecting the client's activities of daily living and what the client is seeking regarding therapy. This allows you to determine whether the client will be compliant with the splinting program and will help to determine the adaptive equipment needs.

Diagnosis-Specific Information That Affects Clinical Reasoning

If the splint is fabricated and fits well, the client will report decreased pain with pinch activities with the splint in place because the splint is helping to hold the carpometacarpal joint in position and is helping to distribute the forces. It may be helpful, if available, to have an x-ray film taken with the splint in place and the client pinching.[20] This allows you to see whether the splint is holding the joints in proper alignment.

CLINICAL *Pearl*

If the thumb deformity is not passively correctable, the splint can help provide support but cannot change the deformity.

Tips from the Field

The goal of the splint is gently to position the thumb opposite to the developing deformity. For example, a type III deformity is splinted with the carpometacarpal joint stabilized, the metacarpal in gentle palmer abduction, and the metacarpophalangeal joint in slight flexion. The DIP joint usually is left free to allow for activities in the splint. This splint can be made of lightweight thermoplastics, or in some cases a soft material (e.g., Neoprene) can be used if the strapping is applied properly, to counteract the deforming forces (Figs. 17-4 and 17-5). Clients often report decreased pain and increased joint stability when using their splints during pinching activities. This stability often is misinterpreted by the client as an

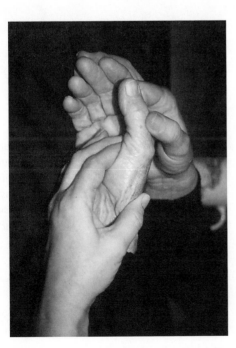

FIGURE 17-3 When the thumb deformity is passively correctable, the placement of the therapist's hands often determines the forces that are needed to apply the splint correctly. Concept courtesy Judy Leonard, OTR, CHT. (From Biese J: Therapist's evaluation and conservative management of rheumatoid arthritis in the hand and wrist. In Mackin EJ, Callahan AD, Skirven TM et al, editors: *Rehabilitation of the hand and upper extremity*, ed 5, St Louis, 2002, Mosby.)

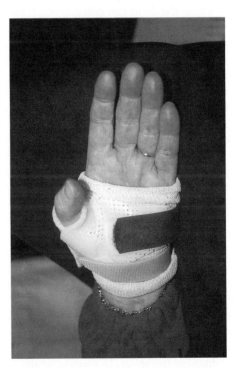

FIGURE 17-4 The hand-based thumb spica splint for deformities that are passively correctable can help decrease pain. The splint places the metacarpal in gentle palmar abduction and the metacarpophalangeal joint in slight flexion. The wrist strap gives the splint additional stability to stabilize the joint. (From Biese J: Therapist's evaluation and conservative management of rheumatoid arthritis in the hand and wrist. In Mackin EJ, Callahan AD, Skirven TM et al, editors: *Rehabilitation of the hand and upper extremity*, ed 5, St Louis, 2002, Mosby.)

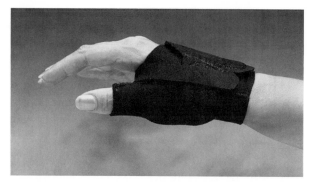

FIGURE 17-5 Comfort Cool Thumb carpometacarpal restriction splint has an additional strap to support and gently compress the carpometacarpal joint. The splint also gently positions the metacarpal in abduction. (Photo and splint courtesy of North Coast Medical, Inc, Morgan Hill, Calif. In Biese J: Therapist's evaluation and conservative management of rheumatoid arthritis in the hand and wrist. In Mackin EJ, Callahan AD, Skirven TM et al, editors: *Rehabilitation of the hand and upper extremity,* ed 5, St Louis, 2002, Mosby.)

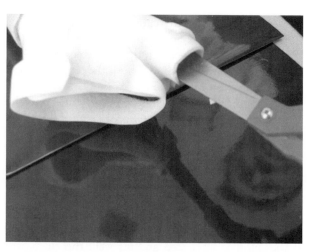

FIGURE 17-6 One easy way to enlarge the splint thumbhole, when it is nearly cool, is to insert a closed scissors into the thumb portion of the splint and gently open the scissors.

increase in strength. A stable, pain-free thumb provides a post to which the digits can grip and pinch effectively. This thumb stability is important to hand function.

In some cases, the client has a large thumb interphalangeal joint that makes donning and removing the splint difficult. The splint must be large enough to fit over this joint while still supporting the proximal phalanx. One easy way to enlarge the splint thumbhole when it is nearly cool is to remove the splint from the client and then insert a closed scissors into the thumb portion of the splint and gently open the scissors (Fig. 17-6). Another technique is to pry open the splint seam that would be supporting proximal phalanx, after the splint has cooled (and the splint has been removed from the client). The unsecured seam then can be expanded partially open when the splint is applied. Then secure this seam with a Velcro strap to cinch the splint comfortably and support around the proximal phalanx. Another solution is a splint that has been cut down but incorporates a dorsal proximal phalanx flap (Fig. 17-7), as described by Colditz.[21] This splint may be recommended to help position the metacarpophalangeal joint in flexion in clients demonstrating metacarpophalangeal hyperextension and also helps in donning the splint. In cases in which the joint of other bones of the wrist are involved, the splint needs to incorporate the wrist.[4] This then requires a forearm-based thumb spica splint (Fig. 17-8).

The client usually responds favorably to wearing the splint if it is comfortable and fits correctly. Many clients wear the soft splint during the day and the more rigid splint at night.[20] Other clients feel that the rigid splint supports the thumb more completely, and they often

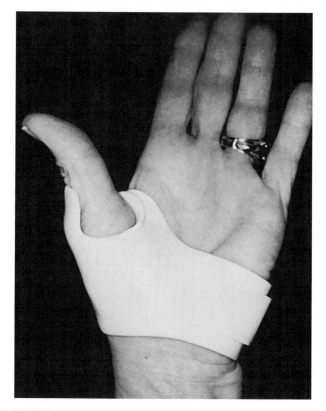

FIGURE 17-7 This splint designed by Judy Colditz for carpometacarpal joint subluxation has a metacarpophalangeal block to prevent metacarpophalangeal hyperextension. This splint makes donning and doffing easier when there is a large thumb interphalangeal joint. (From Colditz J: Anatomic considerations for splinting the thumb. In Mackin EJ, Callahan AD, Skirven TM et al, editors: *Rehabilitation of the hand and upper extremity,* ed 5, St Louis, 2002, Mosby.)

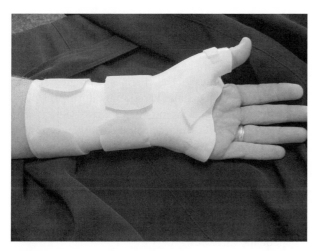

FIGURE 17-8 A thumb spica splint for use when the arthritic process also involves the wrist.

report decreased pain with its use. These clients often reject the soft splints.

In clients with bilateral involvement, only one rigid splint should be fabricated at the first visit to determine how the client responds. This helps one to make the proper decisions about the contralateral extremity. Once the client has decided on a soft splint or rigid splint for one hand, the client will have a preference for the other hand. In many cases the client will want both. The client may have one splint for part time during the day and another for night wear.

Precautions and Concerns

- *The most troubling problem with any splint is the development of pressure areas. The client should return for at least one follow-up visit to make any necessary splint adjustments.*
- *Remember, a splint that is clean is not being worn. Usually, a clean splint is one that is uncomfortable to wear and needs adjustment. Some clients hesitate to ask for splint adjustments for fear of offending their therapist.*

Operative Treatment
Therapy after Carpometacarpal Interposition Arthroplasty

Carpometacarpal interposition arthroplasty involves resection of carpometacarpal joint that allows the metacarpal to assume an abducted position.[19] A donor tendon is rolled up and interpositioned in the joint space. The ligaments usually are reconstructed and help to give the carpometacarpal joint stability. In some cases the hyperextension of the metacarpophalangeal joint may be cor-

rected as well. In most cases the client is in a cast for 4 to 5 weeks and then is referred for a splint. The postoperative course varies from surgeon to surgeon. When the surgeon allows carpometacarpal AROM, it is important to help the client learn how to move the carpometacarpal joint again. These clients have been compensating before surgery by only moving their thumb interphalangeal and metacarpophalangeal joints. One technique for this is having the client flex the thumb interphalangeal and metacarpophalangeal joints and try to keep them flexed while moving the carpometacarpal joint in gentle flexion and extension. The splint may be worn anywhere from 6 to 12 weeks from the date of surgery.

Precaution. *Many surgeons recommend waiting at least 3 months before any heavy pinching activities are allowed.*

Questions to Ask the Doctor

- *May we see the client while the client is still in the cast for thumb interphalangeal, digit, elbow, and shoulder active range of motion, as well as edema management?*
- *When will the cast be removed?*
- *At the time of cast removal, should we apply a hand-based or forearm-based splint?*
- *At what point may we begin gentle active range of motion of the carpometacarpal joint?*
- *At what point may we discontinue the splint?*
- *How long would you prefer that we have the client wait before doing heavy pinch activities of daily living?*

What to Say to Clients

About the Condition

"The surgery helped to correct the joint deformities you were having as a result of your osteoarthritis. The two little scars on your arm (or leg) are where they got your tendon graft. The tendon was rolled up and placed in the joint between the trimmed bones."

About Splinting

"Now that your cast has been removed, we need to make you a splint to maintain the proper position and stability of the joint that has been reconstructed. To get the best result, we need to maintain a good balance between mobility and stability. You will need to wear your new splint between exercise sessions and at night until it is okay with your surgeon to discontinue it. It is important that your splint be comfortable and not cause any pressure areas."

About Exercise

"When it is approved by your surgeon, we will start gentle exercises of your new carpometacarpal joint. It is a joint that you have not moved in a long time. Before the surgery, you mainly moved the end and middle joints of your thumb. We will begin by gently trying to touch the tip of each finger and move your thumb in a small circle. I will show you an exercise where you try to keep your thumb end and middle joint (the metacarpal) bent while you try to move the base of your thumb in and then away from your hand (carpometacarpal flexion and extension). We may have you doing grip-strengthening exercises that do not involve the thumb. The thumb is a stable post for the digits. We usually do not do pinch-strengthening exercises because they put too much stress on a repair that we want to be stable. Doing pinch activities too soon will compromise the surgical repair."

EVALUATION TIPS

- Many clients who arrive for therapy are surprised at how long the recovery is for this surgical procedure.
- Most clients are usually not in much pain. Those that have pain may have had a tight cast or pressure on the superficial branch of the radial nerve. These clients complain of burning pain.

Precaution. *When making the splint, take care to avoid any pressure to the base of the thumb where the superficial branch of the radial nerve is very sensitive.*

- After being in a cast for several weeks, the skin will be very dry and the scars very sensitive. The client will appreciate a gentle cleaning of the skin and an application of lotion. If the scars can tolerate it, initiate gentle scar massage. Show the client how to do scar massage a couple of times each day.
- Be aware and look for signs of complex regional pain syndrome with this population (see chapter on pain syndromes).

DIAGNOSIS-SPECIFIC INFORMATION THAT AFFECTS CLINICAL REASONING. Most clients gain AROM quickly and want to resume activities as soon as possible. Many activities of daily living require a strong pinch and must be delayed until approved by the physician. Decisions to return to work depend on the type of activities that are done at work. Some clients, after being cleared to return to work, wear a soft neoprene splint (see Fig. 17-4) to help make the transition. This splint supplies gentle support while allowing range of motion.

TIPS FROM THE FIELD

- *Splinting.* The splinting tips previously outlined for the thumb spica splint apply after surgery for carpometacarpal interposition arthroplasty as well. An additional area of concern following this surgery is that special attention should be paid to splinting near

the incision site at the base of the thumb near the superficial branch of the radial nerve. This area can be very sensitive in some clients. The surgeon should specify a forearm-based or hand-based thumb spica splint. In some cases the client may progress from a forearm-based to a hand-based splint during the postoperative program. Some clients prefer a soft neoprene splint after the rigid splint is discontinued for gentle support as they return to their activities of daily living. In clients with persistent pain from the superficial branch of the radial nerve, the neoprene splints (see Fig. 17-5) can provide gentle padding to the hand.[22] This padding helps to prevent accidental bumping or irritation as the client's activity level gradually increases.

- *Client compliance.* Client compliance is usually not an issue because this is an elective surgery. A more common problem is that clients may do too much too soon after surgery. The therapist must stress the need for joint stability to maximize the postoperative outcome for these clients.

Precautions and Concerns

- *Avoid heavy pinch activities for up to 3 months after this surgery.*
- *Avoid splint pressure areas especially over the base of the thumb and incision sites.*
- *The splint should position the thumb opposite of the preoperative deformity but should not force the thumb into position.*
- *Be alert for signs of complex regional pain syndrome, including persistent pain and sympathetic nervous system responses.*
- *If the superficial branch of the radial nerve is irritated, some clients report relief with a transcutaneous electrical nerve stimulation unit. A silicone gel pad also may be helpful.*

Therapy after Carpometacarpal Fusion

In the past the carpometacarpal fusion or arthrodesis had been reserved for the treatment of traumatic arthritis in younger clients with high-demand occupations. The carpometacarpal arthroplasty with ligament reconstruction and tendon interposition was used more often on clients with less demanding activities of daily living.[23] A comparative study done by Hartigan et al.[24] found that the two procedures had similar results regarding pain, function, and client satisfaction. The group receiving arthrodesis had a significantly stronger lateral pinch, but the thumb opposition range of motion was better in the group receiving ligament reconstruction and tendon interposition. The postoperative course for the carpometacarpal fusion usually consists of a thumb spica

splinting for at least 6 weeks after surgery or until radiographic fusion is evident.

Questions to Ask the Doctor

- *May we see the client while still in the cast for thumb interphalangeal, digit, elbow, and shoulder active range of motion, as well as edema management?*
- *When will the cast be removed?*
- *At the time of cast removal, should we apply a hand-based or forearm-based splint?*
- *At what point may we discontinue the splint?*
- *How long would you prefer that we have the client wait before doing pinch activities of daily living?*

What to Say to Clients

About the Condition

"The joint at the base of your thumb is called the carpometacarpal joint. It is made up of the metacarpal and the trapezium. Your surgeon removed the bone surfaces and trimmed them so they would fit together. A pin was placed to hold the bones snug until the joint is stable."

About Splinting

"After your cast is removed, you will be put in a thumb spica splint. This is usually a forearm-based splint. Your surgeon will determine how long you need to wear your splint, but it is usually in place for at least six to eight weeks after surgery. You should remove the splint only for cleaning the hand and changing the stockinet liner."

About Exercise

"While in your cast and also in your splint, you will be shown exercises for the very end joint of your thumb, fingers, elbow, and shoulder. We will wait to start gentle movement of the middle joint of your thumb until it is okay with your surgeon."

EVALUATION TIPS. Evaluation tips are the same as for thumb carpometacarpal interposition arthroplasty.

DIAGNOSIS-SPECIFIC INFORMATION THAT AFFECTS CLINICAL REASONING. Most clients want to resume activities as soon as possible. Many activities of daily living require a strong pinch and must be delayed until the fusion is complete. Decisions to return to work depend on the type of activities that are done at work. Avoiding a **nonunion** (failure of a bone to heal or fuse) and obtaining good movement of the thumb metacarpophalangeal and interphalangeal joints are the initial goals of this postoperative course. Some clients in more

demanding jobs may wear a hand-based thumb spica splint for additional protection even after there is radiographic evidence of fusion.

Clients who are progressing slowly may be experiencing complications. These can include complex regional pain syndrome (previously called reflex sympathetic dystrophy) or a troublesome irritation of the superficial branch of the radial nerve. (See the chapter on complex regional pain syndrome.)

TIPS FROM THE FIELD.

- *Splinting.* The splinting tips previously outlined for the thumb spica splint also apply to the client who has had a carpometacarpal fusion. The carpometacarpal joint is fused, but most clients need to be placed in a slight degree of metacarpophalangeal joint flexion because the metacarpophalangeal joint has a tendency to hyperextend in the preoperative deformity. The surgeon should specify a forearm-based (Fig. 17-8) or hand-based thumb spica splint (see Fig. 17-4). In some cases, the client may progress from a forearm-based to a hand-based splint during the postoperative course.
- *Client compliance.* Client compliance is usually not an issue because this is an elective surgery. The more common problem is that clients may do too much too soon after surgery. It is important to stress to the client that the fusion needs to heal for maximum joint stability and the best postoperative outcome.

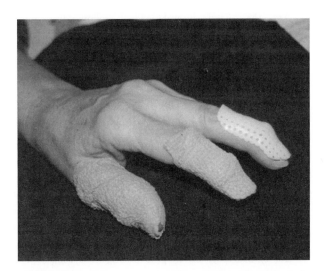

FIGURE 17-9 Splints to the distal interphalangeal joints usually only are used with patients who are demonstrating a painful flare-up, those patients who are considering a surgical fusion, or following surgical fusion.

Precautions and Concerns

See precautions and concerns under the section on thumb carpometacarpal interposition arthroplasty.

Distal Interphalangeal Joint

Anatomy and Pathology

Clients with osteoarthritis at the DIP joints often have enlargements called **Heberden's nodes.** These nodes appear because of osteophytes or bony outgrowths near where the extensor tendon inserts on to the distal phalanx. When these nodes are present at the PIP joints, they are called **Bouchard's nodes.**[8]

Timelines and Healing

Osteoarthritis at the DIP joints can be painful initially, but pain usually decreases over time.

Nonoperative Treatment

Some clients are referred for splinting of the DIP joints during this painful time. The splints can help support the joints and are helpful in decreasing pain. The client also may be referred for joint protection and modalities (see the previous discussion). Some clients are referred to therapy for splints that may help mimic a DIP fusion before a possible surgery. These splints help the client determine whether to accept a surgical fusion of the DIP joint.

Questions to Ask the Doctor

- *Is the client a candidate for a distal interphalangeal fusion?*
- *Are the distal interphalangeal splints for pain management?*

What to Say to Clients

About the Condition

- "The end joints of the fingers are one of the most common sites of osteoarthritis."
- "These joints can be painful for a time, but usually the pain gradually goes away."

About Splinting

- "If you are having pain, splints on the end joints of the fingers can give some relief (see Fig. 17-9). Most clients do not have pain for an extended period, but the splints can be helpful during this temporary painful time."
- "If you are considering a surgery to fuse your distal interphalangeal joints, the splints may help you decide on this elective surgery."

About Exercise

- "Many clients with morning stiffness use heat to increase mobility. They usually apply it about twenty minutes a day when stiffness is a problem."
- "It is helpful to avoid holding objects tightly for a long time. This position keeps the joint bent and under stress and can increase pain."

Evaluation Tips

Determination of the client's specific needs before providing treatment is important. Some clients are not responsive to splinting, whereas others are at the clinic only for the splints. Be aware of the client's activities of daily living and adaptations that may need to be recommended (see the section on joint protection).

Diagnosis-Specific Information That Affects Clinical Reasoning

Splints usually are used only with clients who are in a painful acute inflammatory stage or those who are considering surgical fusion.

Tips from the Field

SPLINTING. Because of the presence of Heberden's nodes and joint inflammation, splints to the DIP joints need to conform well and provide even pressure distribution. Thin or "light" splinting material is recommended, and the material should have excellent drape characteristics, such as polyform light. These splints usually are made on the dorsal surface to allow for tactile input of the volar surface. To hold these splints in place, a nonadhesive wrap such as Coban or Co-Wrap is recommended.

CLIENT COMPLIANCE. Client compliance is good if the splint fits well and decreases pain during the acute inflammatory flare-up. Many clients report that pain is not an issue after the flare-up and reject the splints. Other clients report they have no pain at the DIP joints, but joint inflammation is observed during the evaluation.

Precautions and Concerns

- *During an acute flare-up, the skin is very sensitive at the dorsal DIP level. Splints should conform well to prevent any pressure areas or should be lightly padded to prevent any pressure. Comfort is the key to splinting the DIP joints.*
- *The splints should fit snugly so that they do not slide on the digit but should not be so snug as to feel constricting. The dorsal design allows the client to feel objects more easily on the volar surface.*

- *Edema changes may necessitate splint modifications as the swelling decreases.*

Operative Treatment: Therapy after Distal Interphalangeal Joint Fusion

Fusion of the DIP joints is a procedure that is reserved for cases of severe pain, instability, and deformity. The type of fixation varies in the literature, but the joint usually is fused in neutral to slight (5 degrees) of flexion. Splints are used to protect the arthrodesis until radiographic evidence of fusion occurs.

Questions to Ask the Doctor

- *What type of fixation was used?*
- *Does the client need to wear the splint(s) for protection in the shower?*
- *At what point may we discontinue the splint?*
- *When can the client begin to use the digits for daily living activities?*

What to Say to Clients

"The pain and joint involvement you are having at the ends of your fingers will be reduced with the distal interphalangeal joint fusion. The joints will be placed in a neutral or slightly bent position to help you use your fingers without pain and with greater stability."

About Splinting

"After surgery, you will be in a bulky surgical dressing. When that is removed in the doctor's office, you will be sent to therapy and will be fitted with splints that immobilize only the end joints of your fingers. You will be shown how to remove and reapply the splints to clean your skin and your surgical scar. You must wear the splints to help the fusions heal. Your surgeon will tell you if you need to wear your splints while showering. You should be aware of any red areas and report them to the therapist."

About Exercise

"You will be shown how to exercise the joints in your hand that were not part of the fusion. This will keep these joints from getting stiff. You should wear your splints on the end joints of your fingers during the exercises."

Evaluation Tips

- Tenderness over the dorsal incision site is common and should be monitored to avoid any possible skin breakdown.

- The splints should be well conformed over a light stockinet dressing to avoid pressure areas.
- If the dressing is too thick, the splints will slide around as the edema changes.
- If redness or irritation occurs, the dorsal splint should be changed to a volar splint.

Diagnosis-Specific Information That Affects Clinical Reasoning

Postoperative edema changes affect the splint fit and should be monitored at every visit. Skin breakdown is a complication that needs to be avoided by frequent inspections by the clinician and the well-trained client. PIP joint stiffness also can be a complication in clients who hesitate to move their proximal joints after surgery.

Tips from the Field

SPLINTING. Dorsal-based splints should extend from the joint axis of the PIP joint to the very distal end of the digit. This allows the splint to have a long lever arm and helps to distribute the forces along the digit. The splint will not interfere with PIP joint motion when placed on the dorsal surface. It also allows the client greater volar digit sensation than some of the other designs. If there is a dressing still in place, it should be a light dressing to prevent slipping of the splint. In most cases, light stockinet on the finger after the physician has removed the stitches is an adequate liner under the splint. Secure the splint with tape, Coban, or Co-Wrap. Velcro tends to slide with these small splints. Some therapists make a splint with a dorsal/volar design. Take care to account for edema changes with this splint, for it is less forgiving to edema than the dorsal design. In clients who are demonstrating dorsal skin tenderness, fabricate a volar splint, but this splint has a tendency to slide as the client flexes the PIP joint because of volar proximal phalanx skin contact.

CLIENT COMPLIANCE. Clients who are not compliant with the PIP joint exercise program may develop stiffness. If the client does not wear the splints and is overly aggressive too early, the risk of nonunion is a concern. In the clinic the client should demonstrate the ability to don and doff the splints independently or with the help of a caregiver. Some clients have difficulty learning how to wrap on the splints with the tape, Coban, or Co-Wrap. Tape is the most difficult choice for a self-splinting application because once it is removed, it leaves the splint tacky, and it can be difficult to reapply.

Precautions and Concerns

Possible complications include nonunion, dorsal skin irritation, dorsal skin necrosis, cold intolerance, pain, infec-

tion, numbness, and hardware that occasionally may work its way out to the surface of the skin.[25]

RHEUMATOID ARTHRITIS

Rheumatoid arthritis is a chronic systemic disease characterized by synovial inflammation (synovitis). It affects all racial and ethnic groups and is evident worldwide. Incidence estimates in North America vary in the literature[26] from 0.3% to 1.5%. Women are affected more frequently than men with the peak onset of adult rheumatoid arthritis usually occurring between the ages of 40 and 60. Evaluation and treatment of the hand of the client with rheumatoid arthritis can be challenging for even the most experienced therapist. The disease can affect the intricate balance of the hand when joints and soft tissue structures become compromised.

Therapeutic treatment is individualized and specific to the client's deformity or potential deformity, stage of the disease (Table 17-1), and daily living needs. Only after a complete evaluation are goals and treatment methods selected to meet the needs and expectations of these clients. Client education about the disease and treatment options is critical in the treatment process.

Diagnosis and Pathology

Early clinical signs of rheumatoid arthritis are joint swelling and inflammation of the PIP and metacarpophalangeal joints and of the wrists.[27]

CLINICAL *Pearl*

With RA, the joint involvement is often symmetric and bilateral.

Onset of symptoms can be abrupt, but more commonly a slower progression occurs over several weeks. The synovial lining increases, forming granulation tissue that is called **pannus.**[26] This pannus destroys joint tissue, weakens the joint capsule, and causes adhesions, resulting in joint deformities.

The therapist must have an understanding of the stages of the disease process, as well as potential deformities. This knowledge will assist in determining the appropriate treatment options (Table 17-1). The therapist also must note that the client may return to earlier stages during the clinical course and will have remissions and exacerbations as the disease progresses.

During the acute phase, or stage I as classified by Steinbrocker et al.,[28] the client demonstrates joint swelling and inflammation that is warm when palpated. This is the most painful phase, and it is also when most clients seek medical care.

The subacute, or stage II phase, often is marked by a decrease in symptoms.[13,14] The inflammatory synovium forms a pannus that extends beyond the cartilage and invades ligament attachments and tendons.[29] **Nodules** (small rounded lumps) may be evident at the joint bursa

TABLE 17-1

Stages of Rheumatoid Arthritis[13,14,26-29]

STAGE	SYMPTOMS	RADIOGRAPHIC CHANGES	SPLINTING
Stage I: • Early • Acute • Inflammatory	Joint swelling, heat, redness, and pain are most severe	No destructive changes, but osteoporosis may be present	Resting splits as needed for pain
Stage II: • Moderate • Subacute • Proliferation	Synovium begins to invade the soft tissues, causing decreased mobility Tenosynovitis Less pain Decreased mobility	May have slight bone and cartilage destruction No obvious deformity	Night splints in an attempt to prevent potential deformity and to decrease pain
Stage III: • Severe • Destructive • Chronic active	Joint deformity and soft tissue involvement	Bone, joint, and cartilage destruction, with osteoporosis	Night splints and functional day splints
Stage IV: • Skeletal collapse and deformity • Chronic	Joint disorganization and severe deformities	Severe bone, joint, and cartilage destruction with joint instability, dislocation, and/or fusion	Splinting at this stage cannot reverse deformities but may provide joint stability during activities and comfort at night

(a fluid-filled sac that decreases friction) or along the tendons. Joint range of motion is usually less painful, and there are no obvious deformities.

In the destructive, chronic active stage III, the client often reports less pain, but irreversible joint deformities have progressed.

Stage IV has been referred to as chronic inactive or skeletal collapse and deformity. The joint deformities are considerable and may include instability, dislocation, spontaneous fusion, and bony or fibrous **ankylosis** (stiffening of a joint).

Timelines and Healing

Unfortunately, there is no cure for rheumatoid arthritis at this time. The therapist can help manage the symptoms as the disease progresses, with client education, modalities, splinting, joint protection, and adaptive equipment. The postoperative timelines for specific surgeries follow.

Nonoperative Treatment

Evaluation
A complete evaluation of the client is necessary and includes range of motion, activities of daily living, joint deformities, stage of the disease process, previous surgeries, expectations of therapy, and pain.

Range of Motion
Measurements of AROM of the rheumatic hand varies daily, with increased stiffness often noted in the morning.[30] Goniometric measurement should be done when possible, but deformities make this difficult in the later stages. Measurement of composite digit flexion, active digit extension, and thumb opposition often gives more functional information. Some clients are able to complete only a lateral pinch and are unable to perform palmar pinch because of a pronation deformity of the index digit,[31] and this should be noted. The degree of ulnar deviation at the metacarpophalangeal joints can provide helpful information for measuring progression of joint deformity but should be done with the digits extended and not supported by a table. Friction from the table changes the degree of ulnar deviation when measured.

CLINICAL *Pearl*

Ulnar deviation often varies in metacarpophalangeal flexion and available extension because of ligament laxity, and therefore the position of the metacarpophalangeal joint should be reported in combination with the ulnar drift measurement.

Loss of AROM can be caused by tendon rupture. Rupture occurs as the tendon glides over roughened and irregular bone areas.

Precaution. *The extensor pollicis longus and the extensor digitorum communis tendons of the third, fourth, and fifth digits are particularly vulnerable to rupture.*

The tendon, which may be weakened by the inflammatory synovium, can fray and eventually rupture, resulting in loss of motion.[13] The extensor tendons are more vulnerable to rupture than the flexor tendons because of their proximity to the distal radius, ulna, and carpal bones. Extensor tendon rupture at the wrist level most often is seen with extensor pollicis longus at **Lister's tubercle** (a boney prominence) and with extensor digitorum communis at the distal end of the ulna. The extensor digiti quinti is often the first extensor to rupture and may signal the possible rupture of the other extensor tendons.[15]

Strength
Phillips[14] reports that a grip of 20 psi is necessary for most daily activities. The standard Jamar dynamometer has good reliability[32] but is often painful to use in a rheumatic client. The **sphygmometer** (which measures grip strength with a soft pressure gauge bulb) is more comfortable for these clients, but further study is needed to determine reliability of this instrument. Pinch strength can be obtained with the pinch meter, but some clients will be unable to complete tip or three-jaw chuck pinch, and therefore they perform many daily tasks with a key or lateral pinch. Joint instability, rather than weakness, is usually more problematic during activities of daily living. Even with good muscle strength, clients will be unable to maintain a grip on an object if their joints collapse into deformities.

Activities of Daily Living
Evaluation of the client's functional level begins as the client enters the clinic. Observation as the client removes a coat and sits at a table can be invaluable in understanding the client's ability to pinch and grasp, complete simple functional activities, and even use the hand for mobility (such as using crutches). Joint deformities can be observed and may be accentuated with simple activities. The speed of the client entering the clinic often reveals the level of pain that the client is having and the involvement of the lower extremities. The therapist must gain an understanding of the client's home situation and support system when planning the home program and potential splint designs. For example, if the client is unable to don a splint independently, a caregiver will be needed. The therapist needs to evaluate the client's goals for therapy carefully to make sure that they are realistic. A client diary, as described by Devore,[15] can give insight

into the needs of the client and make the client an active participant in the treatment process. The diary helps the client to determine problem areas with activities of daily living, including which joints are involved and also whether the joint difficulties are because of pain, power, or position.

Pain

Pain caused by acute inflammation is usually greater in the early stages of the disease than in the end stages, when severe deformities are evident. Pain analog scales can be used to determine the effectiveness of treatment, but clinical observation suggests that these clients, in the later stages, rate their pain much lower than anticipated by the therapist. Splinting may be helpful in decreasing pain but should be balanced with the daily living requirements of each client. **Rheumatoid nodules** can be painful when palpated, and should be noted in the evaluation because they may affect splint design or strap placement (Fig. 17-10). Pain from nerve compression caused by synovitis also may be evident. Compression of the median nerve, or carpal tunnel syndrome, is one of the most commonly seen conditions at the wrist. Also, the ulnar nerve can be compressed at Guyon's canal (a canal adjacent to the hook of the hamate) at the wrist and at the **cubital tunnel** (the groove between the medial epicondyle and the olecranon of the ulna) at the elbow.

Diagnosis-Specific Information That Affects Clinical Reasoning
Joint Deformities

Palpate joint deformities to help determine whether they are fixed or passively correctable, dislocated, or partially dislocated. Note this information in your evaluation. Common wrist and hand deformities are listed next.

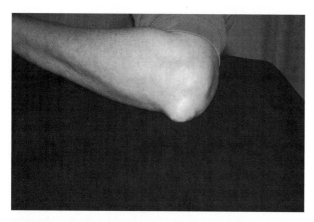

FIGURE 17-10 Rheumatoid nodules near the elbow joint. (From Biese J: Therapist's evaluation and conservative management of rheumatoid arthritis in the hand and wrist. In Mackin EJ, Callahan AD, Skirven TM et al, editors: *Rehabilitation of the hand and upper extremity,* ed 5, St Louis, 2002, Mosby.)

SWAN NECK DEFORMITY. The **swan neck deformity** is characterized by flexion of the DIP joint and hyperextension of the PIP joint (see Fig. 15-6). Synovitis of the flexor tendons can erode the PIP joint **volar plate,** which normally helps prevent PIP joint hyperextension. The flexor tendon synovitis also limits PIP joint flexion and causes the client primarily to use the metacarpophalangeal joints for digit flexion.[29] This results in an **intrinsic plus position** (metacarpophalangeal flexion with interphalangeal joints extended) during grasping activities, causing an altered pull of the intrinsic muscles. This altered pull tends to facilitate dorsal subluxation of the lateral extensor tendons and PIP joint hyperextension. The DIP joint then flexes reciprocally by action of the flexor digitorum profundus tendon. The action of the extensor mechanism thus is concentrated at the PIP joint, resulting in PIP hyperextension, if the PIP volar plate (a thick fibrocartilaginous structure on the volar aspect of the PIP joint) is lax or disrupted. Splinting techniques for the swan neck deformity are outlined under nonoperative treatment.

BOUTONNIERE DEFORMITY. The **boutonniere deformity** is characterized by PIP joint flexion and DIP joint hyperextension. Synovitis causes the central tendon to become weakened, lengthened, or disrupted from the bony and capsular attachments allowing the PIP joint to rest in flexion. The lateral bands then rest volar to the axis of the PIP joint, resulting in PIP joint flexion and DIP joint hyperextension (see Fig. 15-3). Splinting techniques for the boutonniere deformity are outlined in the chapter on sprains.

METACARPOPHALANGEAL JOINT ULNAR DEVIATION AND PALMAR SUBLUXATION.

CLINICAL *Pearl*

Ulnar deviation of the metacarpophalangeal joints is the most common deformity seen in rheumatoid arthritis.

The metacarpophalangeal joints, unlike the PIP hinge joints, have more planes of movement in that they also can abduct, adduct, pronate, and supinate. With this degree of mobility, the hand collapses into deformity if the restraining system of tendons, ligaments, or bony structures is disrupted by synovitis. Factors that can contribute to the development of the ulnar deviation deformity include an anatomic susceptibility and ulnar and volar forces applied during daily activities.[29] The flexor tendons, during functional activities, exert strong ulnar and volar forces at the metacarpophalangeal joint. These forces, in the presence of weakened and diseased joint ligaments and capsules, contribute to the development of the deformity of metacarpophalangeal volar subluxation and ulnar drift. Lateral pinch activities, gripping an object, writing, and even gravity, tend to place ulnarly and volarly deviating forces to the metacarpophalangeal joints (Table 17-2). The deformity also may include radial deviation of the wrist[33] (Fig. 17-11). Splinting techniques for this deformity are outlined in the nonoperative treatment section.

VOLAR SUBLUXATION OF THE CARPUS ON THE RADIUS. Ligament laxity caused by chronic synovitis at the wrist and the natural volar tilt of the distal articular surface of the radius can result in volar subluxation of the carpus on the radius (Fig. 17-12). Splinting of this condition usually includes a volar component to support the wrist.[34]

DISTAL ULNA DORSAL SUBLUXATION. The arthritic client commonly demonstrates instability of the distal ulna. The distal ulna is normally less prominent in supination and more prominent in pronation. The rheumatoid arthritic disease process often weakens the ligamentous structures causing dorsal prominence of the distal ulna, pain, and crepitation with pronation and supination.[29] This instability and dorsal prominence of the ulna also may lead to extensor tendon disruption at the wrist level.

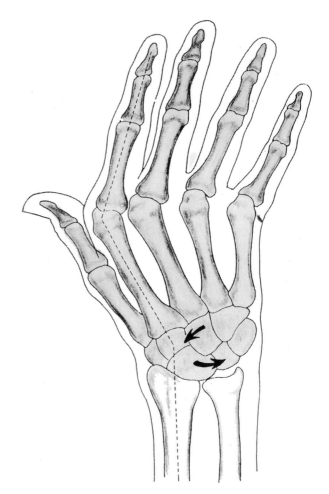

FIGURE 17-11   The zigzag deformity with wrist radial deviation and metacarpophalangeal joint ulnar deviation. (Redrawn with permission from Melvin JL: *Rheumatoid disease: occupational therapy and rehabilitation,* ed 3, Philadelphia, 1989, FA Davis.)

TABLE 17-2

Joint Protection Principles for the Metacarpophalangeal Joints with Rheumatoid Arthritis[4,12,14,15]

ACTIVITIES THAT AGGRAVATE METACARPOPHALANGEAL ULNAR DEVIATION	JOINT PROTECTION TECHNIQUE
Closing a jar with the right hand	Use the heel of the hand to close the jar or use a jar opener with two hands.
Smoothing a sheet with shoulder adduction	Use shoulder abduction to smooth the sheet.
Stirring with a spoon using forearm pronation and lateral pinch on spoon	Stir with the forearm in neutral and without thumb pinching.
Resting the hand on the chin, with ulnar forces to the digits	Avoid resting the hand on the chin or place the chin in the palm.
Lifting a cup of coffee	Use two hands and a lightweight cup.
Cutting foods	Hold the knife like a dagger or use a pizza cutter or electric knife.
Lateral pinch to turn the key in the car door or ignition	Use a built-up key turner.
Carrying a purse strap with a lateral pinch	Use a fanny pack, back pack, or shoulder bag.

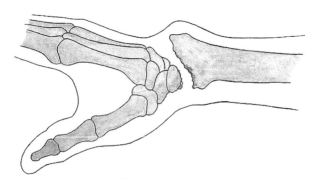

FIGURE 17-12 The natural volar tilt for chronic synovitis can result in volar subluxation of the carpus on the radius. (Redrawn with permission from Melvin JL: *Rheumatoid disease: occupational therapy and rehabilitation*, ed 3, Philadelphia, 1989, FA Davis.)

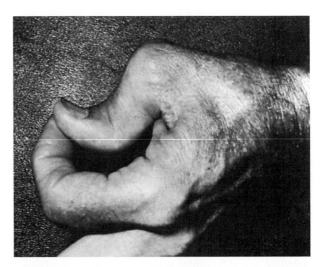

FIGURE 17-13 The type I deformity with metacarpophalangeal joint flexion and distal joint hyperextension. (From Terrono AL, Nalebuff EA, Phillips CA: The rheumatoid thumb. In Mackin EJ, Callahan AD, Skirven TM et al, editors: *Rehabilitation of the hand and upper extremity*, ed 5, St Louis, 2002, Mosby.)

CARPAL TRANSLOCATION AND WRIST RADIAL DEVIATION. With ligament instability, the carpal bones can shift into a variety of deformities. Ulnar displacement of the proximal carpal row results in radial deviation of the hand.[4,35] The metacarpophalangeal joints may be affected secondarily and demonstrate ulnar deviation (see Fig. 17-11). Techniques for splinting this condition are outlined in the section on nonoperative treatment.

THUMB DEFORMITIES. Terrono et al.[19] have identified common patterns of thumb deformity in the rheumatoid thumb. Type I is common with metacarpophalangeal joint flexion and distal joint hyperextension (Fig. 17-13). Type III is also common with carpometacarpal subluxation, metacarpal adduction, metacarpophalangeal joint hyperextension, and distal joint flexion (see Fig. 17-2). The deformity is comparable to the osteoarthritic thumb deformity described previously. The reader is referred to Terrone et al. for further information on rheumatoid thumb deformities.

Crepitus
Grating or crepitation during AROM may be palpated or heard. It will sound like a crunching or popping sound. Volar inspection of the hand should include palpation of the **A-1 pulley** (at the volar aspect of the metacarpophalangeal joints) as the client flexes and extends the digits. A thickening of the flexor tendons, triggering, or periodic locking of the digit in flexion indicates flexor **tenosynovitis** (inflammation of the synovial lining of the tendon sheaths).

Skin Condition
Evaluation of the skin condition should include color, temperature, and areas of swelling. In the initial stage, the skin often is red and warm. In the later stages the

skin may be very thin and bruise easily, which may be due to the long-term use of steroids and/or antiinflammatory medications. Fragile skin characteristics can affect postoperative healing and tolerance to splints.

Precaution. *Skin tears may occur with only minimal shearing, such as rubbing from dressings or from the edge of a table.*

Symptom Management and Joint Protection
Joint protection principles ideally are initiated early in the disease process in hope of decreasing stress to the involved joints.[4,12,14,15] Box 17-1 includes a simple overview. Specific joint protection principles for metacarpophalangeal ulnar deviation (see Table 17-2) include avoiding activities that aggravate the deformity, such as activities that place or push the digits into metacarpophalangeal joint ulnar deviation. With the thumb, joint protection principles focus on decreasing the amount of force used for pinching activities. The joint protection principles outlined previously for the osteoarthritic client also apply in this case. In clients demonstrating a swan neck deformity, emphasize joint protection principles that avoid the intrinsic plus position (metacarpophalangeal flexion and interphalangeal extension) during activities of daily living.

Modalities
Thermal Agents
Superficial thermal agents, such as heat and cold, commonly are used in the treatment of the rheumatoid arthritic hand and were described in the section on

osteoarthritis. Decreasing pain and maintaining or improving range of motion are primary goals in the application of these agents. The stage of the arthritic process is also a determining factor.

Precaution. *During the acute inflammatory phase when joint temperatures are elevated, heat is contraindicated.*

Cryotherapy—which lowers joint temperatures, reduces pain, and decreases inflammation—is more appropriate during the acute phase. Many clients cannot tolerate cooling treatments. During the subacute and chronic phases, heat may be more applicable to decrease pain, encourage relaxation, improve range of motion, and increase functional use of the hand.

Exercise

General principles of exercise include avoiding painful AROM and PROM and working within the client's comfortable range of motion. General exercises for the hand include AROM of the wrist, gentle digit flexion and extension, and thumb opposition. Keep range of motion exercises pain free to prevent overstretching of joint structures that may be vulnerable or distended by the inflammatory process. Shoulder and elbow AROM in the supine position is also beneficial for preventing stiffness. Clients often obtain increased shoulder motion in the supine position because this position lessens the effects of gravity during the exercise. Many clients report benefits from pool exercise programs for general conditioning while reducing strain on the weight-bearing joints. The temperature of the pool should be comfortably warm to avoid muscle guarding, joint stiffness, and increasing pain. The psychological benefits of this social interaction and the informal support group that this type of exercise provides should not be underestimated.

Strengthening

Precaution. *Strengthening programs for the rheumatic hand should be used with caution to avoid aggravation of deformities.*

Stability must not be sacrificed for a possible increase in strength. Grip strengthening is a common example of an exercise that can place the digits in increased ulnar deviation during flexion if the position of the digits is left unchecked.

Precaution. *Therapy exercises should never create deforming forces or cause pain.*

Remedies

Most therapists treating the client with rheumatoid arthritis are approached for advice on a variety of home remedies. These can include copper bracelets, magnets, nutritional supplements, diets, homeopathy, topical preparations, and many others. Although the medical community often has disregarded the claims for these remedies, it is important that the therapist use care in addressing these questions. The therapist should scrutinize research on nontraditional treatments carefully. As therapists, we cannot act as advocates working outside our scope of practice, nor can we refuse to review nontraditional methods of treatment. When evaluating the effectiveness of any treatment, we should remember that rheumatoid arthritis is a disease of remissions and exacerbations. Many clients report improvement with a variety of home treatments. Asking oneself whether the client might have improved even without the treatment is always reasonable. Of course, the therapist should advise the client against any nontraditional therapy that has the potential for harm.

Wrist and Metacarpophalangeal Joint Deformities

With ligament instability, the carpal bones can shift into a variety of deformities. Ulnar displacement of the proximal carpal row results in radial deviation of the hand.[35,36] The metacarpophalangeal joints may be affected secondarily and demonstrate ulnar deviation (see Fig. 17-11).

Questions to Ask the Doctor

- *Is the splint primarily for night wear?*
- *Are there any tendon ruptures?*
- *Is surgery an option for this client in the future?*

What to Say to Clients

About the Condition

- "Your hand is demonstrating a deformity in which the fingers go in one direction and the wrist goes in another. This can look like a zigzag deformity."
- "When you have rheumatoid arthritis, the lining of the joint becomes active and moves outside of the joints. This stretches out the area around the joint and also can affect the tendons."

About Splinting

- "The splint is designed to be worn at night to keep your fingers and wrist in good alignment. It should be comfortable and can help decrease your pain."
- "Some clients like to wear soft splints during the day for heavier activities. This keeps your fingers in position but lets you do some activities."

About Exercise and Joint Protection

- "It can be helpful to learn some ways that you can protect your joints and avoid positions of deformity."

- "Sometimes adaptive equipment can be helpful to decrease the stress on the joints as you do some activities. I can help you determine the best options for you."
- "Any exercise that you do should be pain free and should avoid positions of deformity."
- "It is important to be gentle with the exercises and not force the hand into uncomfortable positions."

Evaluation Tips

Even with severe deformities, clients are able somehow to do a great deal with their hands during their daily activities. Be sure to find out whether the client really wants, and will wear, a splint before fabrication. Adaptive equipment also should be used with the client's individual needs and desires in mind.

Tips from the Field

SPLINTING. If the digits alone are aligned radially in the splint without correction for the wrist position, the wrist can be pulled into further radial deviation in the resting pan splint. This is undesirable because the goal of splinting this deformity is gently to position all involved joints. In the splint a metacarpophalangeal strap provides a necessary stop to counterbalance the long lever arm alignment pull of the digital straps or spacers (Fig. 17-14). The resting pan splint also places the metacarpophalangeal joints in gentle extension. The hand should never be forced into a position, for you cannot correct a severe deformity. Small foam spacers provide a soft but forgiving alignment to the metacarpophalangeal joint and yield to changes in digit size caused by edema or inflammation. The spacers are cut from a sheet of self-adhesive contour foam. A second method for applying ulnar pull to the wrist is to secure a beta pile strap to the inside of the splint at the index metacarpal joint. The gentle pull of this strap helps keep the wrist from its tendency to follow the digits into radial positioning when aligned in the splint.

Some clients also wear soft neoprene digit alignment splints[22] during the day to protect their hands during more active activities of daily living. The gentle pull of

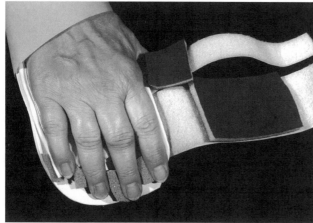
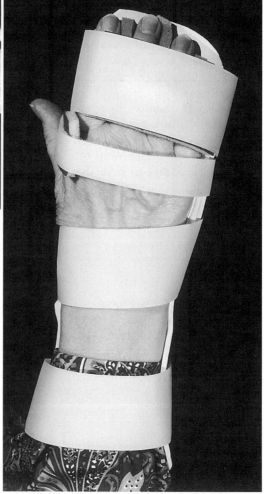

FIGURE 17-14 When splinting the zigzag deformity, the therapist needs to avoid forcing digits into alignment with a splint that leaves the wrist positions unchecked. The long lever arm involved in placing the digits into alignment can cause the wrist to go into additional radial deviation. This night splint helps to guide the wrist into gentle ulnar alignment and the metacarpophalangeal joints into radial alignment. This splint also is used for night splinting following metacarpophalangeal implant resection arthroplasty. (From Boozer JA: *J Hand Ther* 6:46, 1993.)

the radial alignment straps helps to keep the digits in proper position, counteracting the ulnar deviation forces.

CLIENT COMPLIANCE. A client will wear a splint that fits well and is comfortable for an extended time. Some clients return for new splints every year because of wear and tear. If the client returns with a clean splint, it is most likely not being worn. Most clients need splints for both hands, which can make nighttime trips to the bathroom difficult. Alternating a splint on the right hand and the left hand every other night can be helpful in managing this situation.

Precautions and Concerns

- *The digits and wrist should never be forced into an aligned position.*
- *According to Brand et al.,[18] it is important to avoid the use of the long lever arm of the digit to extend the metacarpophalangeal joint. If the proximal phalanx tilts rather than glides into position, it can wear away at the dorsal lip of the phalanx. This results in a splint that actually increases pain and in absorption of the joint surface.*
- *Clients who are fitted with night splints should be made aware of proper application techniques to avoid this joint tilting, and the splint should be formed properly, allowing the joint to glide into position.*

Swan Neck Deformity
Swan neck deformity is characterized by flexion of the distal DIP joint and hyperextension of the PIP joint.

Questions to Ask the Doctor

- *"Is surgery an option for this client in the future?"*
- *"What is the condition of the joints as observed on the x-ray film?"*

What to Say to Clients

About the Condition
- "Rheumatoid arthritis can loosen the stability of your joints and ligaments. Sometimes as the joints lose their stability, the fingers go into a swan neck deformity."
- "As you use your hand, the middle (proximal interphalangeal) joints of your fingers tend to buckle backward and your end joints (distal interphalangeal joints) bend. This makes it difficult to grasp objects."

About Splinting
- "Splints can help keep the middle joints (proximal interphalangeal) flexed. This has a secondary effect on the end joints (distal interphalangeal joints), helping them to straighten. This is the position opposite your deformity."
- "There are several styles of splints that can work for you. These splints allow your fingers to bend but prevent your middle joints (proximal interphalangeal) from buckling backward."
- "Some of the splints are made out of plastic, and some are made out of metal to look like special rings on your fingers."

About Exercise
- "It is important that you maintain the bending ability (flexion) of the middle joints. This is done by taking your other hand and gently bending it toward the palm."
- "Activities like holding a book can keep your middle joints straight while bending your knuckles (metacarpophalangeal joints). This can aggravate this deformity. You should avoid activities that keep your middle joints straight for a long time."

Evaluation Tips
Take care to measure the active and PROM of the PIP joints and DIP joints. If the joints are passively correctable, the client is usually a good candidate for the swan neck splints.

Tips from the Field
SPLINTING. In clients demonstrating a swan neck deformity, splinting techniques that prevent PIP joint hyperextension, yet allow flexion, are often effective. These splints are needed long term and therefore should be durable. Many of the low-temperature plastic splints can wear out and need to be replaced frequently. A high-temperature plastic option, the Oval-8 splint, is available in a variety of sizes and can be obtained from 3-Point Products, Inc. (Stevensville, Maryland). This is a prefabricated splint available in many sizes. The client is fitted in the clinic by trying on the different sizes. Minor one-time changes can be made to this high-temperature plastic using a heat gun. For clients who are between sizes, the rings can be worn with the smaller ring proximal to make the fit more snug. Clients may enjoy using this fit option because their fingers naturally change in size from day to day because of edema. A metal custom-sized splint, the SIRIS splint, is available from the Silver Ring Splint Co. (Charlottesville, Virginia). The therapist measures these splints with ring sizers. Measure the middle phalanx and proximal phalanx to determine the proper size. When measuring for the Silver Ring splints,

it is important that the sizers be placed on the finger at the angle that the actual splint will have. This helps to ensure accuracy in measuring. These splints are well tolerated by clients because they allow most daily living activities and do not need to be removed for hand washing. The Silver Ring splints are adjustable at the solder. They are designed to tolerate multiple (even daily) adjustments to account for differences in finger size caused by edema. If the ring is opened, it is tighter on the finger. Conversely, if the two rings are brought closer together, the splint is looser on the finger.

CLIENT COMPLIANCE. Client compliance with both of the aforementioned swan neck splints is excellent if the splints fit well. With the splint in place, the client is able to do most activities of daily living, which helps facilitate the full-time wearing schedule.

Precautions and Concerns

- *Take care to ensure that the splints are not too tight or too loose. If they are too loose, the client often loses them; if they are too tight, they can cause pressure areas.*
- *In the case of the Silver Ring splints, the client should have a good understanding of how to adjust them to make the splints tighter and looser to account for changes in finger size from day to day.*
- *Some clients with sensitive skin may react to the metal or plastic. For this reason, with the metal splints, a coating is available from the manufacturer.*

Operative Treatment

Metacarpal Phalangeal Implant Resection Arthroplasty

Implant resection arthroplasty for the metacarpophalangeal joint is performed in cases of rheumatoid arthritis to eliminate pain, restore motion, provide joint alignment, and improve functional use. Postoperative management requires an organized program of dynamic splinting and range of motion to remodel the capsular structures properly. This allows good joint alignment and an adequate arc of motion. Many types of implants are available for treatment of this condition. Materials include silicone, pyrocarbon, cobalt chrome, and polyurethane implants. Some implants come equipped with their own postoperative programs from the manufacturer. Discuss these programs and protocols with the surgeon. The new metacarpophalangeal joint implant acts as a spacer, and the joint encapsulation process begins to form in the first 3 to 5 days after surgery. A careful postoperative program of early motion and splinting is important to remodel the capsular structures properly.[37-40] The joint still may need

to be protected with night splinting for 3 to 12 months and beyond while the tissues continue to remodel.[41] Postoperative protocols vary from hand center to hand center according to the preferences of physicians and therapists. Good communication with the surgeon is important to help determine the postoperative course and the specific protocol, as well as to evaluate the individual needs of each client.

Timelines and Healing

IMMEDIATELY FOLLOWING SURGERY (0 TO 3 DAYS): INFLAMMATORY STAGE. The client leaves surgery in a bulky conforming hand dressing. Edema is treated with elevation. The client is instructed in AROM exercises of the elbow and shoulder.

FIRST POSTOPERATIVE WEEK (1 TO 5 DAYS). The therapist's presence with the surgeon at the initial dressing change to discuss the specifics of the surgical procedures is optimal. Some protocols for pyrocarbon implants delay application of the dynamic splint for 3 to 4 weeks. In most protocols for silicone implants, the bulky dressing is removed and a dynamic metacarpophalangeal joint extension splint is fabricated over a light dressing at this time.

Precaution. *Clients who are taking steroids or immunosuppressant medication may have sensitive skin that heals slowly, and the splint application may be delayed until wound healing has progressed.*

In these cases, apply a bulky dressing and re-evaluate the wound in 5 to 7 days for application of the dynamic splint. The dynamic splint usually is worn full time for the first 6 weeks postoperatively (Fig. 17-15). A static splint is worn at night.

SECOND TO THIRD POSTOPERATIVE WEEKS. The client's sutures usually are removed, and scar massage is initiated if the tissues are well healed. If the client has good extension but is not achieving the goals of flexion, use dynamic flexion techniques with physician approval. Secure flexion slings to a volar outrigger so that a 90-degree line of pull is achieved in the direction of the scaphoid bone.[37,40] Dynamic flexion generally is applied for 20 to 30 minutes, 2 to 3 times a day. In the case of a client with rheumatoid arthritis who has received pyrocarbon implants, the dynamic extension splint usually is delayed until this time.[41]

SIXTH POSTOPERATIVE WEEK. If the client is demonstrating good extension and digit alignment, discontinue the dynamic metacarpophalangeal extension splint.[37,40] If extension or alignment problems persist, continued day

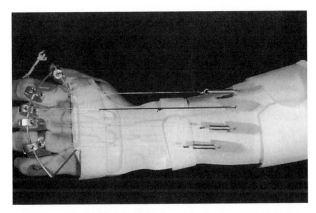

FIGURE 17-15 The low profile dynamic metacarpophalangeal splint fabricated with a Phoenix outrigger. The outrigger is curved to account for the differing lengths of the proximal phalanges. (From Biese J, Goudzwaard P: Postoperative management of metacarpophalangeal implant resection arthroplasty, *Orthop Phys Ther Clin North Am* 10(4):595-616, 2001.)

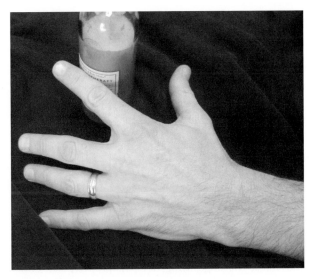

FIGURE 17-16 Strengthening of the first dorsal interosseous muscle can be done by having the patient push a glass with the index digit while the rest of the hand is stabilized.

splinting is needed. Static night splinting (see Fig. 17-14) continues for at least 3 months to 1 year and beyond. The client is allowed to use the extremity for light activities. Reinforce instruction in joint protection principles to help the client avoid positions that aggravate ulnar deviation. A good pad-to-pad pinch (avoiding lateral or key pinch) with the thumb is important in preventing pressure that can aggravate ulnar deviation of the digits. Initiate strengthening exercises, paying careful attention to maintain good joint position. Resistive exercises also should include strengthening of the first dorsal interosseous muscle. One activity that strengthens this muscle is to push a glass (Fig. 17-16) by abducting the index finger while the rest of the hand is stabilized.

THREE MONTHS AFTER SURGERY. Night splinting usually continues. If the client is employed, an evaluation for return to work may be necessary. The client should follow joint protection principles for all activities. Some clients use hand-based digit alignment splints[22] for joint protection during heavier activities.

Questions to Ask the Doctor

- *"At what point would you like to have the dynamic splint applied?"*
- *"At what point would you like the dynamic splint discontinued?"*
- *"How severe was the preoperative deformity?"*
- *"Can you send me an operative report so that I have a better understanding of what other structures may have been involved?"*

- *"Does the client have a long history of steroid or immunosuppressant use that might affect the skin integrity after surgery?"*

What to Say to Clients

About the Condition

"Before your surgery, your fingers were going over to the side. This is called ulnar deviation. Your surgery put the fingers back into proper alignment. Here is a picture of the implant that is in your joint. The surgeon trimmed the bone ends and put the implant in place. Some of the soft tissues around the joint were rebalanced to place the finger in proper alignment and position. We need to keep this balance yet allow protected motion of the finger during your postoperative healing."

About Splinting

"You need to wear a splint during the day for at least 6 weeks. This allows your fingers to move gently in a way that allows for proper alignment. You need to learn to put your splint on and take it off and to take care of your skin. You may need help to do this. You will have a different splint for night wear that holds your fingers in proper position. This night splint will be worn for several months after the surgery. You should not have much pain. If you do, tell us where it is, so we can adjust your splint. We will change your dressing every time you come in for therapy."

About Exercise

"You will have exercises to do every hour while you are awake. This includes bending and straightening your fingers in your splint as a group and individually. At six to eight weeks after surgery, you will be shown some grip-strengthening exercises and exercises that strengthen the small muscles between your fingers."

Evaluation Tips

The proper position of the digits in the dynamic splint includes full metacarpophalangeal extension and neutral digit alignment avoiding ulnar deviation.[37] The splint should allow adequate active metacarpophalangeal flexion during AROM. The splint may need to be adjusted frequently during the postoperative course to evaluate and adjust the finger slings for this proper positioning. Inspect the incision at every visit, which will require dressing changes. Avoid skin breakdown and irritation by using appropriate padding over the sensitive incision area. Evaluate to determine whether the client or the client's family member is applying the splint correctly.

Diagnosis-Specific Information That Affects Clinical Reasoning

At each therapy visit, inspect the skin for wound healing, edema, and possible pressure points. Sometimes it is necessary to see the client frequently because repositioning of the digits may be necessary. Check rubber bands for wear. Active and PROM measurements are recommended to be taken during each visit to identify any flexion or extension lags. If the client is not obtaining good metacarpophalangeal flexion (usually 70 degrees), increase the frequency of PROM.

Tips from the Field

SPLINTING. The base of the dynamic splint extends from the metacarpal heads to two thirds of the forearm for adequate support of the outrigger. The base should conform well and be free of pressure points. The base will need to be adjusted for dressing and edema changes as the client progresses throughout the postoperative course. In many cases the wrist has a tendency for radial deviation; this often is seen preoperatively as the zigzag deformity (see Fig. 17-11). Strap the wrist in a neutral position to avoid radial deviation. Take special care to apply appropriate padding at the incision site to prevent pressure areas.

The palmar arch should be well supported with a volar hand component to prevent flattening of the transverse arch, which ultimately would limit flexion of the ring and small digits. Phillips[14] prefers to use a separate piece of splinting material formed to the palmar arch. Having this piece detach prevents pressure at the first

web space and makes the splint more adjustable for changes in edema.

Apply the outrigger to achieve a 90-degree line of pull[18,37,40,42] when the finger slings are placed on the proximal phalanges (see Fig. 17-15). Also, angle the outrigger to account for the differing lengths of the proximal phalanges. High-profile (Fig. 17-17) and low-profile splints may be used, but Boozer et al.[43] reported that the low-profile splint required more force to initiate and flex the metacarpophalangeal joints during AROM exercises than the high-profile splint. Therefore in cases in which the client is demonstrating weak flexors, a high-profile splint may be preferred to facilitate ease of range of motion.

In most cases, apply a lateral outrigger radially to the index finger for the supination force couple described subsequently. Position this outrigger to provide a 90-degree line of pull to the middle phalanx.[12,40] In general, the sling application should align the digits in a slight radial direction to achieve metacarpophalangeal extension and to avoid metacarpophalangeal ulnar deviation, but each digit will have individual rotational, alignment, and tension needs (see Fig. 17-17).

The tension of the rubber bands should be tight enough to support the digits in 0 degrees of extension yet allow 70 degrees of active flexion.[44] The digits respond

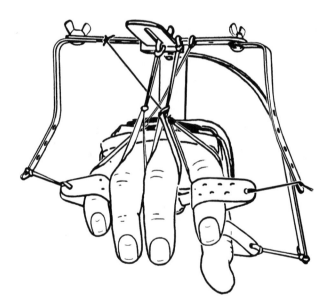

FIGURE 17-17 The high-profile Swanson hand splint with outriggers in place to supinate the index digit with a force couple and to pronate the small finger to avoid having it tuck under the ring finger. The thumb outrigger may be needed with some patients to abduct the thumb and avoid lateral thumb pressure to the index digit during active flexion. (From Boozer J, Leonard J, Swanson AB et al: *Postoperative care for patients with Silastic finger joint implants (Swanson's design)*, Arlington, Tenn, 1988, Wright Medical Technology. Used with permission.)

quickly to the dynamic forces applied during the first few days following dynamic splint application, so it is important to use only gentle tension.

The index digit has a tendency for a pronation deformity,[31] which makes it difficult for the thumb to perform a pad-to-pad pinch. Swanson et al.[44] recommends correcting this deformity in surgery with a capsule and radial collateral ligament reconstruction and by positioning the implant to place the digit in supination. This position is maintained in the dynamic splint by the application of the proximal sling rotating the digit into supination, while the distal sling guides the digit into radial alignment. The combined pull of these slings completes the force couple (see Fig. 17-17). Boozer et al.[43] describe the increased effectiveness of the force couple in high-profile splinting compared with low-profile splinting. Devore et al.[31] described additional splinting techniques that can be effective in positioning the digit in supination. These include various adhesive materials that are applied directly to the digit, rotating it into gentle supination and terminating at the radial outrigger.

In addition to the dynamic splint, most clients are fit with a static night splint[37,40] (see Fig. 17-14). Receiving the static night splint during the first postoperative visit just as the client usually is getting adjusted to the dynamic splint is often overwhelming to the client. Fabrication of the static splint is best done at a subsequent therapy visit. The night splint places the digits in 0 degrees of metacarpophalangeal extension and proper alignment. If the PIP joints have a tendency toward a swan neck deformity, place them in slight flexion. Place the wrist in neutral alignment or slight ulnar deviation when possible, with a strap or pad[45] to prevent aggravation of wrist radial deviation.

Precaution. *When one is switching from one splint to the next, the metacarpophalangeal joints must be supported in extension.*

For more information on fabricating this night splint, see the section on splinting the wrist and metacarpal joints.

EXERCISES. The goals as outlined by Swanson et al.[44] for AROM at the metacarpophalangeal joints are full extension with flexion as follows:

Index: 45 to 60 degrees
Middle: 60 degrees
Ring: 70 degrees
Small: 70 degrees

Exercises usually are performed with 10 repetitions every waking hour in the dynamic splint and include flexion of the digits as a group and individually. If the goals are not being achieved, initiate PROM with medical clearance.[37,42,44] The client applies gentle pressure to the proximal phalanx to flex the metacarpophalangeal joints. Family members also can be instructed in PROM. In some cases, the client has a tendency to flex the PIP joints during AROM instead of the metacarpophalangeal joints. Small PIP extension splints may be applied to limit the movement of the PIP joints and allow all of the flexion force during exercise to be directed to the metacarpophalangeal joints. When swan neck deformities are present, the splints should place the PIP joints in slight flexion.

CLIENT COMPLIANCE. The client must be prepared for the postoperative course with a good preoperative education program. The client needs to understand his or her responsibility as an active participant; surgery is only the beginning of the process.[31] Stress the importance of wearing the dynamic splint after surgery, completing the exercise program, and the needed commitment to attending hand therapy.

CLINICAL *Pearl*

Assistance at home and with driving during the postoperative course is extremely helpful to the client.

Precaution. *The involved extremity should not be used for function during the first 6 weeks after surgery.*

The client can complete many activities using one-handed techniques, provided the client maintains elevation of the operated extremity. Adaptive equipment can be used in some cases, but assess this temporary expense for true need, for function will improve as the postoperative program progresses. Instruct the client in joint protection principles for the nonoperative extremity as the workload increases during one-handed activities.

This elective surgery and postoperative course require a significant commitment from the client. To develop good rapport with the client is important to provide the support and encouragement necessary for the postoperative course. Good communication between the client, therapist, and the surgeon facilitates the best possible outcome. The program and protocols presented in this chapter are to be used only as a guideline. The therapist should constantly re-evaluate the client to determine when modifications are necessary in order to meet individual needs and desired goals.

Precautions and Concerns

- *Monitor pressure areas from the splint, wound breakdown, and delayed wound healing.*
- *Clients who are taking steroids or immunosuppressant medication may have sensitive skin that heals slowly, and the splint application may be delayed until wound healing has progressed. In these cases, apply a bulky dressing and re-evaluate the wound in 5 to 7 days for application of the dynamic splint.*

The Role of the Therapy Assistant

The therapy assistant (occupational therapy assistant or physical therapy assistant) can assist the hand therapist (occupational therapist or physical therapist) in obtaining information during the evaluation such as discussing daily living activities, measuring joint range of motion, obtaining information about pain, making observations about deformities, and learning the client's expectations from therapy. The hand therapist determines goals for the client based on the evaluation. Regarding treatment, the hand therapist can have the therapy assistant implement the treatment program based on the goals established by the therapist. This can include instruction in joint protection, specific adaptive equipment, application of specific modalities, home programs, and gentle active range of motion. Based on their level of splinting skills, assistants can fabricate or fit splints as determined by the hand therapist. The treatment roles of the hand therapist and the assistant are based on the experience level of each, as well as their experience with the specific diagnosis.

CASE *Studies*

CASE 17-1: NONOPERATIVE TREATMENT OF RHEUMATOID ARTHRITIS

B.L. is a 53-year-old nurse with rheumatoid arthritis. She works 40 hours a week on the cardiac care unit of a local hospital and reports that her pain is largely under control with medication. She has two children in college and likes to play the organ at church. She reports that with some activities such as playing the organ, her right hand proximal interphalangeal (PIP) joints buckle backward at her right index and ring digits. This requires her to push even harder on the organ keys and is sometimes painful. She

would like some support that would give her index and ring finger (PIP) joints stability yet allow her to do her activities.

B.L. was fit with size 5 and 6 Oval 8 splints (from 3-Point Products, Inc.). She was shown the proper way to apply the splints to prevent PIP joint hyperextension yet to allow full PIP joint flexion. She was instructed that the splints would be tighter when applied in the opposite direction and that this might be useful if her swelling were to decrease. She was instructed in joint protection principles including avoiding the intrinsic plus position as she held a book or played cards. She was shown passive range of motion to the PIP joints to help maintain PIP flexion.

B.L. returned to the clinic 1 week later with her husband. She reported increased stability as she played the organ, and she even felt the splints increased the stability of her PIP joints at work and during various other activities. Her husband wanted to purchase a Silver Ring splint for her ring finger with a blue stone for their anniversary. She was measured for the Silver Ring splint using the ring sizers. Care was taken when measuring to be sure that the two ring sizers could be applied and removed when held together at the volar aspect by the therapist. This would be how the new splint would fit, with the two rings soldered together at an angle. The correct size was determined and the form was completed. Her husband had a blue stone that was given to him by his mother, and this was included for placement on the ring with the order. The couple mailed in the form and the stone. The form stated the ring was to be delivered to the hand clinic for fitting by the therapist.

The Silver Ring splint arrived 8 days later and was fit to the client. She was instructed in how to make adjustments to the splint fit by bending the rings together (for a looser fit) or apart (for a tighter fit). This would help with fit despite daily edema fluctuations. B.L. continued to wear her Oval 8 splint on her index finger.

B.L. stopped by the clinic 2 weeks later. She had lost her Oval 8 splint and needed a replacement. She reported decreased pain and increased stability with her splints and was wearing the splints day and night. They allowed full PIP joint flexion but prevented PIP hyperextension. She also felt she needed less pain medicine with the splints in place during activities. Her lost Oval 8 splint was replaced, and she was encouraged to contact the therapist if further assistance was needed.

CASE 17-2: OPERATIVE TREATMENT OF RHEUMATOID ARTHRITIS

J.B. is a 64-year-old retired school teacher who has had rheumatoid arthritis for the past 10 years. She has reported a gradual loss of range of motion and strength in her hands during activities of daily living. She has metacarpophalangeal joint ulnar deviation bilaterally combined with palmar subluxation of joints 2 to 5. Her right thumb metacarpophalangeal joint had been fused by the surgeon 2 years ago. She also has proximal interphalangeal joint swan neck deformities at digits 2 to 5.

She arrives at the hand clinic today in a bulky dressing. Three days ago she underwent surgery on her right (dominant) hand for metacarpophalangeal joint implant resection arthroplasty on digits 2 to 5. The order from the physician indicates that Swanson silicone implants were used and that a dynamic metacarpophalangeal extension splint was to be applied. The order also indicated that the therapist was to contact the physician when the client arrived so he could see how she is progressing. This physician visit will take place in the hand therapy clinic (the physician's office conveniently is located next door to the therapy office).

The physician was contacted, and the bulky dressing was removed. The wound had only minimal swelling, and the incision sight was clean and dry. The skin was cleaned with sterile water per physician orders. The physician arrived and evaluated the wound and digit position. The decision was made to proceed with the standard protocol.

The wound was dressed with sterile gauze, and the dynamic splint was fabricated. The pull of the slings was slightly radial at digits 3 to 5 because of slight postoperative metacarpophalangeal ulnar deviation. The index digit was placed in slight supination with a force couple (see Fig. 17-17) because of the tendency for index digit pronation. The client was instructed to do gentle metacarpophalangeal active range of motion every waking hour, to elevate the hand, and was instructed (with the help of her husband) to don and remove the splint for clothing changes.

J.B. returned to the clinic 3 days later. She had 50 degrees of metacarpophalangeal active range of motion at digits 2 to 5. The alignment of her digit slings was adjusted to maintain the slight radial pull on digits 3 to 5 and apply slightly more supination with the force couple to the index digit. The wound was cleaned, and the dressing was reapplied. A night splint was fabricated (see Fig. 17-14) to place the metacarpophalangeal joints in neutral alignment, the wrist in slight ulnar deviation, and her proximal interphalangeal joints in slight flexion because of the swan neck deformities. The client continued with this program and attended therapy 2 to 3 times a week until she reached the sixth postoperative week. She followed up with the physician at the 2 week point and had her stitches removed.

At 6 weeks after surgery, she was demonstrating full (0 degrees) metacarpophalangeal extension and 60 to 70 degrees of metacarpophalangeal active range of motion in flexion at digits 2 to 5. The day splint was discontinued,

but the night splint was continued. She was instructed in scar massage to the incision site, strengthening exercises for the first dorsal interosseous (see Fig. 17-16), gentle grip-strengthening exercises, and joint protection principles (see Table 17-2).

At 7 weeks after surgery, the therapist asked J.B. whether she was using her hand for activities of daily living. She said she missed playing the piano. J.B. was instructed in a finger-walking exercise. The hand was placed flat on the table, and she was instructed to have her digits "walk" (one at a time) into radial deviation in the direction of the thumb. This helped J.B. to increase control of her intrinsic muscles. She also was encouraged to begin to use her right hand for simple tunes on the piano for a short duration. She was encouraged gradually to increase her time on the piano, as she felt she could tolerate, avoiding fatigue.

At 12 weeks after surgery, J.B. had returned to doing all of her activities of daily living. She was cooking, doing laundry, and playing the piano. She had a good understanding of the joint protection principles and felt the surgery was a success. She is considering having the other hand done next year.

References

1. Callahan LF, Yelin EH: The social and economic consequences of rheumatic disease. In Kippel JH, Crofford LJ, Stone JH et al, editors: *Primer on the rheumatic diseases*, ed 12, Atlanta, 2001, Arthritis Foundation.
2. Brandt KD, Doherty M, Lohmander S, editors: *Osteoarthritis*, New York, 1998, Oxford University Press.
3. Berenbaum F: Osteoarthritis A: epidemiology, pathology, and pathogenesis. In Kippel JH, Crofford LJ, Stone JH et al, editors: *Primer on the rheumatic diseases*, ed 12, Atlanta, 2001, Arthritis Foundation.
4. Melvin JL: *Rheumatic disease in the adult and child: occupational therapy and rehabilitation*, ed 3, Philadelphia, 1989, FA Davis.
5. Lawrence RC, Helmick CG, Arnett FC et al: Estimates of the prevalence of arthritis and selected musculoskeletal disorders in the United States, *Arthritis Rheum* 41:778-799, 1998.
6. Centers for Disease Control and Prevention: Prevalence and impact of chronic joint symptoms: seven states, *MMWR Morb Mortal Wkly Rep* 47:345-351, 1998.
7. Kuttner KE, Goldberg V, editors: *Osteoarthritic disorders*, Rosemont, Ill, 1995, American Academy of Orthopedic Surgeons.
8. Hochberg MC: Osteoarthritis B: clinical features. In Kippel JH, Crofford LJ, Stone JH et al, editors: *Primer on the rheumatic diseases*, ed 12, Atlanta, 2001, Arthritis Foundation.
9. Moratz V, Muncie HL Jr, Miranda-Walsh H: Occupational management in the multidisciplinary assessment and management of osteoarthritis, *Clin Ther* 9:24, 1986.

10. Bozenthka DJ: Pathogenesis of osteoarthritis. In Mackin EJ, Callahan AD, Skirven TM et al, editors: *Rehabilitation of the hand and upper extremity*, ed 5, St Louis, 2002, Mosby.

11. Swanson A: Disabling arthritis at the base of the thumb: treatment by resection of the trapezium and flexible (silicon) implant arthroplasty, *J Bone Joint Surg* 54A:456, 1972.

12. Haviland N, Kamil-Miller L, Sliwa J: *A workbook for consumers with rheumatoid arthritis*, Rockville, Md, 1978, American Occupational Therapy Association.

13. Melvin JL: Therapist's management of osteoarthritis in the hand. In Mackin EJ, Callahan AD, Skirven TM et al, editors: *Rehabilitation of the hand and upper extremity*, ed 5, St Louis, 2002, Mosby.

14. Phillips CA: The management of patients with rheumatoid arthritis. In Hunter JM, Schneider LH, Mackin EJ et al, editors: *Rehabilitation of the hand: surgery and therapy*, ed 3, Philadelphia, 1990, Mosby.

15. Devore GL: Preoperative assessment and postoperative therapy and splinting in rheumatoid arthritis. In Hunter JM, Schneider LH, Mackin EJ et al, editors: *Rehabilitation of the hand: surgery and therapy*, ed 3, Philadelphia, 1990, Mosby.

16. Biundo JJ, Rush PJ: Rehabilitation of patients with rheumatic diseases. In Kelley WN, Harris ED, Ruddy S, et al, editors: *Textbook of rheumatology*, ed 5, Philadelphia, 1997, WB Saunders.

17. Michlovitz S: *Thermal agents in rehabilitation*, Philadelphia, 1986, FA Davis.

18. Brand P, Hollister AM, Agee JM: Transmission. In Brand PW, Hollister AM, editors: *Clinical mechanics of the hand*, St Louis, 1985, Mosby.

19. Terrono AL, Nalebuff EA, Phillips CA: The rheumatoid thumb. In Mackin EJ, Callahan AD, Skirven TM et al, editors: *Rehabilitation of the hand and upper extremity*, ed 5, St Louis, 2002, Mosby.

20. Biese J: Therapist's evaluation and conservative management of rheumatoid arthritis in the hand and wrist. In Mackin EJ, Callahan AD, Skirven TM et al, editors: *Rehabilitation of the hand and upper extremity*, ed 5, St Louis, 2002, Mosby.

21. Colditz J: Anatomic considerations for splinting the thumb. In Mackin EJ, Callahan AD, Skirven TM et al, editors: *Rehabilitation of the hand and upper extremity*, ed 5, St Louis, 2002, Mosby.

22. Biese J: Soft splints: indications and techniques. In Mackin EJ, Callahan AD, Skirven TM et al, editors: *Rehabilitation of the hand and upper extremity*, ed 5, St Louis, 2002, Mosby.

23. Ryan GM, Young BT: Ligament reconstruction arthroplasty for trapeziometacarpal arthrosis, *J Hand Surg* 22:1067-1076, 1997.

24. Hartigan BJ, Stern PJ, Kiefhaber TR: Thumb carpometacarpal osteoarthritis: arthrodesis compared with ligament reconstruction and tendon interposition, *J Bone Joint Surg* 83A(10):1470-1478, 2001.

25. Stern PJ, Fulton DB: Distal interphalangeal joint arthrodesis: an analysis of complications, *J Hand Surg* 17(6):1139-1145, 1992.

26. Goronzy JJ, Weyand CM: Rheumatoid arthritis: A. epidemiology, pathology, and pathogenesis. In Kippel JH, Crofford LJ, Stone JH et al, editors: *Primer on the rheumatic diseases*, ed 12, Atlanta, 2001, Arthritis Foundation.

27. Calabro JJ: Rheumatoid arthritis: diagnosis and management, *Clin Symp* 38(2):1-32, 1986.

28. Steinbrocker O, Traeger CH, Batterman RC: Therapeutic criteria in rheumatoid arthritis, *JAMA* 140(8):659-662, 1949.

29. Swanson AB: Pathomechanics of deformities in hand and wrist. In Hunter JM, Schneider LH, Mackin EJ et al, editors: *Rehabilitation of the hand: surgery and therapy*, ed 3, Philadelphia, 1990, Mosby.

30. Anderson RJ: Rheumatoid arthritis: B. Clinical and laboratory features. In Kippel JH, Crofford LJ, Stone JH et al, editors: *Primer on the rheumatic diseases*, ed 12, Atlanta, 2001, Arthritis Foundation.

31. Devore GL, Muhleman CA, Sasarita SG: Management of pronation deformity in metacarpophalangeal implant arthroplasty, *J Hand Surg* 11A(6)859-861, 1986.

32. Fess EE: A method for testing Jamar dynamometer calibration, *J Hand Ther* 1(1):28-32, 1987.

33. Flatt A: *Care of the arthritic hand*, ed 4, St Louis, 1983, Mosby.

34. Colditz JC: Arthritis. In Malick MH, Kasch MC, editors: *Manual on management of specific hand problems*, Pittsburgh, 1984, AREN Publications.

35. Shapiro JS, Heijna W, Nasatir S, et al: The relationship of wrist motion to ulnar phalangeal drift in the rheumatoid patient, *Hand* 3:68-75, 1971.

36. Shapiro JS: The wrist in rheumatoid arthritis, *Hand Clin* 12(3):477-498, 1996.

37. Biese J, Goudzwaard P: Postoperative management of metacarpophalangeal implant resection arthroplasty, *Orthopedic Physical Therapy Clinics of North America* 10(4):595-616, 2001.

38. Madden MD, Devore G, Arem MD: A rational postoperative management program for metacarpophalangeal joint implant arthroplasty, *J Hand Surg* 2(5):385-366, 1977.

39. Kirkpatrick WH, Kozin SH, Uhl RL: Early motion after arthroplasty, *Hand Clin* 12(1):73-86, 1996.

40. Swanson AB, deGroot Swanson G, Leonard J et al: Postoperative rehabilitation programs in flexible implant arthroplasty of the digits. In Hunter J, Schneider LH, Mackin EJ, et al, editors: *Rehabilitation of the hand*, ed 3, St Louis, 1990, Mosby.

41. Beckenbaugh RD: The development of an implant for the metacarpophalangeal joint of the fingers, *Acta Orthop Scand* 70(2):107-108, 1999.

42. Cannon N et al: MP implant arthroplasties: postoperative management (for rheumatoid arthritis). In Cannon N et al, editors: *Diagnosis and treatment manual for physicians and therapists*, ed 3, Indianapolis, 1991, Hand Rehabilitation Center of Indiana.

43. Boozer JA, Sanson MS, Soutas-Little RW et al: Comparison of the biomechanical motions and forces involved in high-profile versus low profile dynamic splinting, *J Hand Ther* 7(3):171-182, 1994.

44. Swanson AB, deGroot Swanson G, Leonard J: Postoperative rehabilitation programs in flexible implant arthroplasty of the digits. In Hunter JM, Schneider LH, Mackin EJ et al, editors: *Rehabilitation of the hand,* ed 4, St Louis, 1995, Mosby.

45. Boozer JA: Splinting the arthritic hand, *J Hand Ther* 6:46-48, 1993.

18

Pain-Related Syndromes: Complex Regional Pain Syndrome and Fibromyalgia

ROMINA P. ASTIFIDIS

Pain-related syndromes can be among the most difficult to treat, causing fear and apprehension in therapists and clients. The clinical and psychosocial presentation may vary from client to client, and often you, as the therapist, are the first person to realize that healing is not progressing as expected. If you suspect that symptoms are atypical, with abnormal persistent pain and/or any uncharacteristic response of the sympathetic nervous system, it is critical that you contact your physician, monitor symptoms closely, and modify your treatment plan. The most successful treatment of pain syndromes involves a team approach with the physician providing medical intervention as appropriate, the therapist managing clinical symptoms, and possibly other team members (anesthesiologist, social worker/psychologist, psychiatrist, nurse manager) providing their services as needed.

Complex regional pain syndrome (CRPS), previously described as reflex sympathetic dystrophy, is a disorder that can affect all the extremities, but when it affects the arm and hand, it can lead to incredible loss of function. The causes of CRPS are not clearly understood, although most theories assume that there is some abnormality in the processing of pain by the neurologic system and/or an exaggerated sympathetic nervous system response to the posttraumatic inflammatory stage.[1] Although CRPS can be provoked by inappropriate or aggressive medical or therapeutic treatment, it often has no apparent cause. For this reason, it is important that the team and the clients realize that often no one is at fault or responsible for the disorder. Therapists frequently see CRPS diagnosis associated with mild or severe injuries and/or surgeries of the upper extremity. CRPS is most often seen after carpal tunnel release, Dupuytren's release, and distal radius fracture.[1,2] The clients may be referred for therapy for the associated diagnoses and may develop CRPS during the course of treatment, or they may be referred by the physician because a diagnosis of CRPS is suspected. In either case, appropriate and timely treatment is critical.

COMPLEX REGIONAL PAIN SYNDROME

Definition and Anatomy

The two types of CRPS[3] are type I, which develops after an initiating noxious event, and type II, which develops after a nerve injury. Both types must have spontaneous pain that is disproportionate to the initial event, evidence of edema, skin blood flow abnormality, or abnormal **sudomotor** (sweating) activity. The symptoms must be exclusive of an alternative diagnosis. Also, the pain can be described as sympathetically maintained or sympathetically independent based on the response to treatment to the sympathetic system. Often the hand is involved, although many clients describe involvement of specific digits, specific nerve distribution (ulnar nerve, median nerve), or of entire upper extremity and shoulder referring into the cervical area (**shoulder-hand syndrome**).

Diagnosis and Pathology

Diagnosis of CRPS often is based on clinical symptoms and may include diagnostic testing such as vascular studies, electrodiagnostic studies, radiographic studies, bone scans, and blood tests. These tests are done initially to rule out other conditions. Other tests such as **thermography** (heat mapping test), **sweat testing** (test to show sweating response), and **sympathetic blocks** (procedure in which sympathetic system is numbed temporarily) can be used to aid in the diagnosis of CRPS, although they may have false positives or false negatives. Most often, diagnosis is based purely on clinical findings. Box 18-1 lists the most common symptoms you may note or the client may describe.[4]

BOX 18-1

Common Symptoms of Complex Regional Pain Syndrome

Pain that spreads beyond the area of original injury and most commonly is described as burning, searing, or stabbing and may include the following:

Allodynia: pain from sources that do not typically cause pain
Hyperalgia: increased response to a painful stimulus
Hyperpathia: pain that continues after painful stimulus is removed
Swelling that can become permanent and thick and can lead to joint stiffness
Stiffness of joints, contractures, palmar nodules, and thickening; usually facilitated by pain with motion and edema limiting motion
Discoloration often described by clients or noted in clinic; usually bluish coloring, mottling, and redness; and often associated with abnormal temperature of extremity and caused by specific activities
Abnormal hair growth and texture and abnormal nail growth
Abnormal sweating (also called *hyperhidrosis*), which can be seen along nerve distribution or in an atypical place
Motor dysfunction, which includes tremor, dystonia, increased muscle tone, muscle spasms, and loss of strength and endurance

Timelines and Healing

Onset of CRPS can be immediately after injury/surgery or weeks after.

Precaution. *It is critical that treatment for CRPS begin immediately, even if the diagnosis is only suspected and is not yet confirmed. Delay in treatment, medically and therapeutically, ultimately can lead to a less functional outcome.[5]*

Timelines for improvement are individualized to the clients. In most cases, the sooner appropriate treatment begins, the quicker the improvement occurs. If the symptoms have progressed and significant soft tissue contracture is visible, the prognosis is not as good.[5] Some clients have chronic pain symptoms that persist and require long-term treatment.[4]

Nonoperative Treatment

The goal of therapy is to manage pain and other symptoms, maximize motion, and restore function with activities of daily living and job duties. Therapy often requires a combination of various techniques based on clinical reasoning with modifications as needed if symptoms worsen (Fig. 18-1).

Precaution. *It is imperative to note that aggressive treatment without consideration of worsening symptoms may lead to exacerbation of CRPS, poor client compliance, and poor outcome.*

Pain

The first symptom to treat is pain. Pain is managed most easily through superficial heating modalities, especially moist heat. Most clients, especially those with **sympathetically maintained pain,** prefer elevated moist heat because their limb is more often in a cold, cyanotic state.[6] A trial of **fluidotherapy** (a heating device that provides a dry whirlpool using sandlike material) is an option, but be sure to ask the clients to perform active range of motion (AROM) in the unit, for the limb is in a dependent position. Lower the fluidotherapy temperature to 98 degrees if possible.[7] *Also with fluidotherapy, be cautious not to overstimulate hypersensitive areas.[6]* If the clients have a warm, reddened limb, use ice packs and monitor them closely; however, *few clients with CRPS tolerate ice well.* Some therapists prefer to use contrast baths combined with AROM or squeezing a sponge.

Precaution. *Contrast baths may increase the instability of an already unstable vasomotor state and therefore should be monitored closely.[6,7]*

Ultrasound as a thermal modality also can be used because it is effective in heating soft tissues that contrib-ute to contracture. Pain also can be treated using transcutaneous electrical nerve stimulation (TENS), which can be applied at the site of pain or along the peripheral nerve or dermatome. Some clients tolerate TENS better on the contralateral limb if they are too hypersensitive on the involved limb. If TENS is effective, arrange to send a unit home with the client if possible for self-management of pain.[6,8,9]

Edema

Precaution. *Immediately start treatment of swelling in the limb because prolonged swelling can increase pain, decrease movement, and lead to permanent joint stiffness.*

Edema management should include simple elevation with or without gentle pain-free AROM.[6] Be cautious when clients position their limb in constant protected elevation or when they use a sling. This position limits active motion of the hand, stiffens the shoulder and neck, and prohibits use of the arm—all of which are necessary for good functional outcome. Other edema management techniques include sensory level high-voltage pulsed current,[10] intermittent pneumatic compression,[7] **manual edema mobilization** (a massage technique developed by Sandra Artzberger to reduce swelling in clients with intact lymphatic systems), compression gloves/stockings, and massage.

CLINICAL *Pearl*

Monitor massage because the cyclic stimulation provided in retrograde massage may increase **allodynia.** Also, be aware that if the massage pressure is too heavy, it can collapse rather than stimulate the lymphatic system and lead to worsening of edema.[6]

Sensation

Treatment of sensory issues is also important, for a hypersensitive hand is not be able to function with activities of daily living. Initiate a frequent **desensitization** (decreasing sensitivity using frequent, mildly irritating stimulus) program at least 5 to 6 times a day. This can include textures, tapping, pressure, and vibration as tolerated.[6,8] Always start the desensitization outside the sensitive area and work slowly toward the sensitivity. However, if desensitization is poorly tolerated, use a TENS unit concurrently to help with pain management.[11]

Precaution. *Sometimes intermittent tactile touch increases allodynia, so make an effort to maintain contact with the skin during desensitization, especially with massage.[6]*

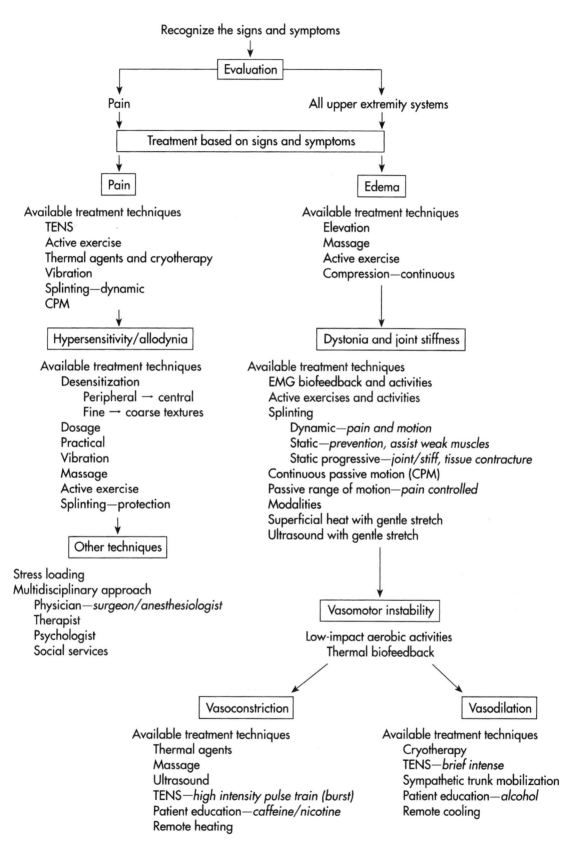

FIGURE 18-1   Algorithm for evaluation and treatment. *EMG,* Electromyograph; *TENS,* transcutaneous electrical nerve stimulation. (From Walsh MT, Muntzer E: Therapist's management of complex regional pain syndrome [reflex sympathetic dystrophy]. In Mackin EJ et al, editors: *Rehabilitation of the hand and upper extremity,* ed 5, St Louis, 2002, Mosby.)

Attempt vibration at 100 Hz for 45 minutes at modest pressure using a 2 inch diameter probe for added desensitization and pain management.[6] Also important is to protect sensitive parts between stimulation sessions using appropriate gloves, **gel sheets** (silicone-based pads), or other protective measures.

Vasomotor Changes

Clients often describe abnormal vasomotor changes, although these may not always appear during the course of treatment in the clinic. Encourage the clients to participate in a generalized aerobic exercise routine to increase circulation[6,8,9] and oxygenation to the body and to the affected arm. Dietary changes should include avoidance of caffeine (causes vasoconstriction) and alcohol (causes vasodilation). Instruct clients to self-manage a cold cyanotic limb at home using moist heat and/or paraffin and to be sure to keep the limb warm and covered when exposed to cold external temperatures. Clients can purchase small gel-heating devices from most sporting goods stores that can be activated by squeezing or shaking, and these can be used if needed when not at home. If the area of vasoconstriction is extremely sensitive and does not tolerate direct heat, attempt heating the contralateral limb or the entire body in a bath.[6] TENS also can be used to treat vasodilation and vasoconstriction. In some cases, temperature biofeedback is taught so that the clients can self-regulate vasomotor changes.

Range of Motion

> ## CLINICAL *Pearl*
>
> Educate the clients that frequent gentle AROM of the entire limb without increasing pain helps to decrease swelling, increase motion, and decrease pain.

Passive range of motion (PROM) to include stretching must be used with care and often is contraindicated because it increases pain and swelling, which in turn causes the clients to have less motion. Some clients tolerate **blocked exercises,** in which each joint is isolated individually, and **tendon gliding**[5] exercises that move the tendon through its full range. Others, however, perform better with functional activities including dressing, manipulation, grasping, pushing, and pulling. Include the uninvolved limb in the exercises to encourage bilateral use and provide normal input to the central nervous system. Exercises can include dressing simulation, reach-

ing tasks including ball toss, **proprioceptive neuromuscular facilitation,** a neurologically based exercise routine using diagonal patterns, and weight-bearing activities. Assess posture and movement; direct exercises toward postural normalization and stabilization, and address any myofascial disturbances that change movement patterns.

> ## CLINICAL *Pearl*
>
> Be sure to assess trigger points in the scapular and thoracic region because they can limit normal scapular motion.

Stress Loading

The most recognized therapeutic treatment associated with CRPS is a stress loading program, usually with modifications as needed, based on the type of injury.[12] Instruct the clients in weight bearing in the form of scrubbing a table/floor or rolling a ball starting with 3 to 5 minutes for 3 times a day working up to 10 minutes. Follow each of these upper extremity compression sessions with distraction techniques including carrying weights, water bottles, and bags starting with 1 lb and increasing to 5 lb as tolerated for up to 10 minutes. Sometimes the injury prevents the ability to bear weight. If so, add weight bearing when the client is medically cleared.[8] Although not researched, clinically clients have had success with aquatic therapy; the warmth of the water, weightlessness, and resistance with motion encourages increased use in painful and weak limbs.

Splinting

If the client needs it, a **thermoplastic splint** positioned in resting/safe position at night can help rest the limb and decrease potential contractures.[7,9] The resting position usually incorporates wrist neutral, metacarpal joint flexion, and interphalangeal joint extension. The splint should be used only if it decreases pain, and the hand should be positioned in the splint comfortably. Sometimes a stretching splint (**static progressive or dynamic**) can be fabricated or ordered to increase motion; however, continue to monitor pain and limit time in the splint because AROM is more functional than passive stretching. Add strengthening only if symptoms are minimal and the clients have returned to functional use.

Joint Protection

Always discuss joint protection techniques, including **energy conservation,** with clients. Recommend assistive devices and alternative methods to do activities to encourage clients to use their arms in a purposeful and functional way. Some examples of assistive devices include pen build-ups, enlarged handles for hygiene and kitchen tools, and alternative keyboards or work tools. Support groups can help clients by allowing them to discuss their symptoms and coping techniques with other persons who have similar problems. Not only is this a forum to share information, but also it often helps for clients to know that they are not alone. Often, psychological counseling including relaxation techniques, imagery, hypnosis, and coping skills can be helpful in symptom management and should be encouraged.[5]

Regional Anesthesia

Medically, the clients are treated with pharmacologic agents (Box 18-2) initially or concurrently with regional anesthesia techniques. The most common anesthesia technique is the **stellate block**/sympathetic block, which blocks the sympathetic efferent impulses into the extremity without blocking the somatic nerve.[13,14] The clients do not experience anesthesia or paralysis. The block is performed by injecting an anesthetic into the cervical sympathetic trunk in the anterior neck (Fig. 18-2). If the block is successful, the clients usually experience general warming, drying, and normal color restoration to the affected extremity. Motion may improve and pain usually is lessened. However, the block also may cause **Horner's sign** (drooping eyelid, constriction of the pupil, and redness and warming of the ipsilateral side of the face), and most clients have difficulty swallowing and have a hoarse voice. In most cases, it is critical that therapy is scheduled after the block to take advantage of the decrease in pain and symptoms to perform exercises

better.[6] A successful stellate block sometimes is used as a diagnostic tool; however, CRPS cannot be confirmed or ruled out absolutely based on this procedure, for pain can be **sympathetically independent pain** or the block may not have been done appropriately. Educate clients and families about what to expect during the block and afterward, for many clients are nervous about the procedure.

Other regional anesthesia treatments include **somatic blocks, bier blocks,** and **intrathecal/epidural blocks.**[13] Be cautious of performing aggressive passive manipulation after a block because tissue structures can be damaged without the normal pain feedback loop.[5]

Operative Treatment

Sometimes, surgical treatment is aimed toward management of the mechanical or neurologic causes of the pain, including **neuroma, compression neuropathy,** and removal of hardware (Box 18-3). Surgical treatment also may include **neuromodulation,** which is often beneficial if there is persistent, chronic pain not relieved by conservative measures. With **spinal cord stimulation,**[2] an electric current is introduced through an implanted battery and helps to suppress pain. Usually a testing period occurs before the permanent implant is inserted. **Peripheral nerve stimulation**[1,2] is similar to spinal cord simulation, but the electrode is positioned in the peripheral nerve instead. Finally, intrathecal analgesia[2] decreases painful symptoms, allowing therapy to focus on improvement of motion and function. Therapy after surgical neuromodulation is similar to nonoperative therapy.

BOX 18-2

Pharmacologic Agents Used to Treat Complex Regional Pain Syndrome

Oral steroids: usually used in early cases with signs of inflammation[1,2]
Nonsteroidal antiinflammatory drugs[5,13]: decrease inflammation of joint and tendons
Antidepressant agents (amitriptyline [Elavil], fluoxetine [Prozac], sertraline [Zoloft]): affect neuropathic pain, decrease depressive symptoms, and can improve sleep, mood, and anxiety[1,2,5]
Anticonvulsants (gabapentin [Neurontin], phenytoin [Dilantin])[2]: decrease spontaneous firing of neurons to decrease neuropathic pain
Lidocaine transdermal patches[5]: topical analgesics
Opiates: decrease pain, used with caution[5,13]
Calcium channel blockers: assist with blood profusion[1]

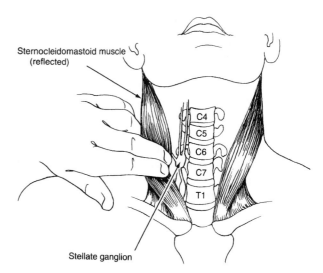

FIGURE 18-2 Location of stellate ganglion block, generally volar to the sixth cervical transverse process. (From Burke et al, editors: *Hand and upper extremity rehabilitation*, ed 3, St Louis, 2006, Churchill Livingstone.)

BOX 18-3

Definitions

> *Neuroma:* spontaneously firing growth buds from damaged peripheral nerves; tapping produces a radiating electric shock sensation in the distribution of the nerve
>
> *Compression neuropathy:* compression of a peripheral nerve in the limb that may cause motor or sensory problems
>
> *Neuromodulation:* altering transmission of nerve impulses
>
> *Spinal cord stimulation:* placement of an electrode in the epidural space on the spinal cord at the level of the nerve innervating the painful area through which electric current is introduced through an implanted battery to help suppress pain
>
> *Intrathecal analgesia:* indwelling or intermittent boluses of local anesthetic and opioid combinations directly into the spine

Questions to Ask the Doctor

Communicate with the physician as soon as you notice abnormal symptoms. Ask the following questions:

- *When do you want to see this client?*
- *How often do you want the client to have therapy?*
- *Do you want me to do any passive range of motion/stretching?*
- *Do you want a resting splint?*
- *Can I add modalities? Isotoner gloves? Home TENS unit?*

What to Say to Clients

About Their Symptoms

"I am concerned that you have swelling, pain, and stiffness that are worse than they should be at this time in your recovery. Pain, swelling, and stiffness are normal after an injury/surgery: that is the natural way your body heals. However, sometimes it goes a little haywire and the symptoms persist. I am recommending that you see your physician as soon as possible to see whether there are any medical treatments he or she would like to add."

About Exercises and Use

"It is important that you continue to exercise and use your [hand/arm], but you should try to stay in a comfortable and pain-free range. If you take it too far, your body will respond by increasing the pain and swelling, causing you not to be able to use your hand at all."

About Pain Management

"Decreasing your pain is important to help improve your symptoms. I will be asking you questions about your pain as you do activities and after you finish therapy to make sure that our treatment does not increase your pain significantly. At home, I will give you some options to help decrease your pain, and you can do whatever combination helps most to decrease your pain."

Evaluation Tips

Determine which areas are hypersensitive by asking the clients before you examine or measure the extremity. Sensory evaluation such as Semmes-Weinstein monofilament test and Two-Point Discrimination Test may point to a specific nerve involvement that could be diagnostic of symptoms (i.e., neuroma).[10]

Explain all measurements before doing them. Instruct clients to do only as much as is comfortable.

Precaution. *Avoid PROM measurements unless absolutely indicated because they may increase symptoms.*

Only do tests that are absolutely necessary and nonprovocative for the evaluation. Defer tests such as grip and pinch strength to a later date if the client's extremity is stiff, swollen, or painful.

Take a thorough pain assessment and be sure to note the location of pain, type of pain, what worsens and improves the pain, how long pain lasts after a painful activity, and how limiting to function the pain is. Use a variety of scales including body diagram and verbal and visual analog scales. This will help you understand how acute the symptoms are and the clients' level of tolerance.

If taking volumetric measurements, make sure to use warm water and avoid the dependent position for a prolonged time. Monitor circulatory (cold or hot) changes and sympathetic (skin color, hair growth, sweating) changes during evaluation and at each session, for treatment may change based on the clients' current signs and symptoms.

Diagnosis-Specific Information That Affects Clinical Reasoning

No typical treatment protocol works for all clients with CRPS. *Individualize* the treatment based on the clients' level of pain, current symptoms, response to treatment, and tissue tolerance. Fig. 18-1 is an algorithm for evaluation and treatment based on clinical reasoning.

Precaution. *Avoid aggressively manipulating a hand that is treated medically with anesthesia techniques because clients have altered pain perceptions and there may be a rebound pain with worsening afterward.*

Tips from the Field

Diagnosis and Treatment

You are the client's advocate. If the symptoms appear atypical and there is not good communication with the physician, it may be necessary to discuss alternative medical intervention with clients.

CLINICAL *Pearl*

Remember that immediate treatment is critical to improving outcome.

Education

Educate your clients about CRPS and symptom management because this will increase compliance. Be empathetic regarding symptoms and their effects on the clients' home and work activities; sometimes you are the only person willing to listen. Encourage the clients to use the limb as much as possible if tolerated. Help clients find a support group or counseling if needed, but caution them about Internet searches because some of the information is inaccurate or conveys dramatic worst-case scenarios that can increase fear in clients. Clients with long-standing pain and dysfunction may begin to feel hopeless and discouraged with their persistent symptoms. Often clients can dwell on their limitations and how their life is restricted. Be sure to encourage the clients with examples of their progress in motion or function and rejoice in each small improvement.

Precautions and Concerns

- *Communicate worsening symptoms with physician immediately.*
- *Avoid activities that increase pain and swelling.*

The Role of the Therapy Assistant

- *Communicate with therapist and physician if treatment is not progressing as expected and if complex regional pain syndrome symptoms are noted.*
- *Monitor symptoms during treatment and adjust accordingly.*
- *Communicate with the therapist on the goals of therapy and expectations related to treatment.*
- *Discuss maximal pain limits and which pain reduction techniques are most effective with clients.*
- *Supervise and adjust home exercise program as appropriate.*
- *Provide activities of daily living and work-related assistive devices and adaptations.*
- *Modify and adjust splints.*

FIBROMYALGIA

Fibromyalgia is a pain syndrome that affects the entire musculoskeletal system. Symptoms include chronic widespread musculoskeletal pain, sleep disturbances, morning stiffness, fatigue, anxiety, and depression.[15] This syndrome is more common in women than men. The causes of fibromyalgia are not clear, but theories include that clients have a lowered mechanical and thermal pain threshold, high pain ratings for noxious stimuli, and altered temporal summation of pain stimuli.[16]

Treatment, which should be team-based, often includes education, medication, and therapies to include cognitive/behavioral therapy, exercise, and alternative therapies. Often the primary focus should be educating the clients to promote self-management and, in the case of a concurrent upper extremity injury, making progress in treatment without worsening existing pain symptoms. This section is devoted to treatment of fibromyalgia in the context of an existing upper extremity injury or surgery.

Diagnosis

The diagnosis of fibromyalgia is based on the criteria established by the American College of Rheumatology in 1990, which includes a history of widespread (entire body) pain and excessive tenderness to at least 11 out of 18 specific muscle-tendon sites.

Precaution. *Clients who complain of generalized chronic pain and stiffness and appear to have multiple abnormally tender points in the cervical and upper back area should be referred to a rheumatologist or physiatrist familiar with fibromyalgia for further assessment and management.*

Timelines and Healing

Fibromyalgia is a chronic pain condition, and the symptoms can wax and wane. Although the symptoms are not progressive and usually can be managed with a combination of education, medication, and therapy, the condition generally persists throughout the client's lifetime.

Nonoperative Treatment

Fibromyalgia is difficult to treat, and symptoms can flare up with an injury to the upper extremity. More than likely, healing may take more time than normal, with abnormal pain responses to exercise and activities and a rapid fatigue response.[15]

One of the most effective treatment techniques for fibromyalgia is regular gentle exercise, especially aerobic exercise. Aerobic exercise can be in the form of walking, exercise bike, or pool therapy. Regular exercise provides improvement in pain and fitness and minimizes tender points.

Teaching clients about the condition, the importance of exercise, ways to improve sleep patterns, and energy conservation is important, especially if clients have had no formal education. Client-centered informational handouts can be obtained from several sources on the Internet and books on the topic. Cognitive behavioral therapy is also effective to improve pain, fatigue, mood, and function.[16]

Consider some alternative therapies if fibromyalgia symptoms interfere with appropriate healing of an upper extremity injury. Trigger point treatments, massage, relaxation techniques, biofeedback, acupuncture, and hypnoses have been shown to improve symptoms temporarily.[16]

No specific medications are approved to treat fibromyalgia; however, physicians often prescribe the following medications: (1) tricyclic antidepressants especially amitriptyline (Elavil) and cyclobenzaprine (Flexeril, cycloflex) for sleep, fatigue, and pain management; and (2) analgesic medications including tramadol (Ultram) with or without acetaminophen to decrease pain. Nonsteroidal antiinflammatory drugs are often not effective for treatment of fibromyalgia; however, they may be used if the upper extremity symptoms include inflammation.[16]

Questions to Ask the Doctor

- *Can I add massage and/or other modalities to help with muscular pain as needed?*
- *Discuss with physician that progress may be slower than normal and that flare-ups may be more frequent.*

What to Say to Clients

About Exercise Management

"It is very important that you continue to exercise the rest of your body because that helps you minimize your fibromyalgia symptoms. Frequent exercises with low repetitions are more beneficial than only exercising infrequently. You may have to keep up an exercise program indefinitely."

About Getting Enough Sleep

"It is very important to get enough sleep to allow your body time to heal. If you are having trouble sleeping, you may need to see your doctor or change your sleep habits."

About Activities of Daily Living and Work Activities

"If you are having a hard time doing your home and work activities, we can discuss some alternatives, including

changing your home and work habits, using different tools, or finding other ways to get everything done."

Evaluation Tips

- Avoid evaluation techniques initially that exacerbate the pain, such as strength testing, stretching of musculotendinous units, or other painful positioning.
- Take a thorough pain assessment, being sure to note location of pain, type of pain, what worsens and improves the pain, how long it lasts after a painful activity, and how limiting to function the pain is. Note at every session the amount of activity tolerated before symptoms worsen to help you determine an effective home program.

Diagnosis-Specific Information That Affects Clinical Reasoning

Fibromyalgia is a pain syndrome that affects the musculoskeletal system.

Precaution. *Be aware of increasing activities or treatment techniques quickly or aggressively because this may increase overall pain and further limit activity.*

Use the client's report of symptoms to modify your treatment with the understanding that treatment also may need to include therapy techniques to other parts of the body if they are currently painful. Be respectful of the clients' symptoms and pain during and after the treatment.

Tips from the Field

Pain Management

It may be helpful to instruct clients to keep a pain diary. This helps them remember how they responded to therapy and to their home exercise program so that the program can be adjusted as needed.

Exercise

Start off a new exercise program with very low repetitions.

Precaution. *Too little exercise is better than too much because a flare-up in symptoms can take a long time to calm down.*

An example would be to start an aerobic exercise routine at 3 minutes or a range of motion routine at 5 repetitions.

Avoid increasing the exercise routine if the clients report they are "feeling good." Clients may have days with minimal symptoms, and increasing exercises optimistically can lead to a flare-up and an increase in pain.

Expected Progress

Often, progress in symptoms may be slower than expected, and the clients may have frequent regressions or increases in pain. Expectations may need to be lowered, and progress in exercises and activities may need to be slower.

Splints

Clients may need to wear a resting splint for longer periods during the day or for a longer period because symptoms may flare up more frequently.

Precautions and Concerns

- *Avoid or modify activities that increase pain in the musculature.*
- *Lower the number of repetitions and slow down the pace of exercise upgrades.*

The Role of the Therapy Assistant

- *Communicate with therapist and physician if treatment is not progressing as expected or is slower than expected.*
- *Monitor symptoms during treatment and adjust accordingly.*
- *Communicate with the therapist on the goals of therapy and expectations related to treatment.*
- *Supervise and adjust home exercise program as appropriate.*
- *Provide activities of daily living and work-related assistive devices and adaptations.*
- *Modify and adjust splints.*
- *Listen attentively and offer empathy to clients as appropriate.*

CASE *Studies*

CASE 18-1: COMPLEX REGIONAL PAIN SYNDROME

L.H. is a 54-year-old right-handed man who tripped and fell and sustained a distal radius fracture. He underwent placement of external fixator and Kirschner wire pinning 3 days later. He was referred to therapy 2 weeks after surgery for range of motion, edema, and pain management. L.H. had swollen fingers, inability to extend or flex fingers, pain levels of 3/10 to 4/10, and inability to use right hand for any functional activity including writing or driving (Fig. 18-3, *A*). Therapy included elevated heat, compressive garments for swelling, and active and passive

range of motion including blocked exercises and tendon gliding. He was encouraged to position fingers in extension while at rest to decrease flexion positioning and to use hand for light activities. L.H. frequently admitted to not doing exercises at home, so his wife was instructed on the home program, which led to improvement in motion and swelling. The external fixator was removed, and the client presented 1 week later with severe swelling, shiny skin, worsened contractures, and pain levels of 8/10 (Fig. 18-3, *B*). The physician recommended stellate blocks, and L.H. was seen for a series of three blocks (in 10-day intervals) with therapy at least 3 times a week and after blocks. He used a transcutaneous electrical nerve stimulation unit at home and was given a light rubber-band hand gripper, which he gripped in elevation throughout the day. He also started a program of flattening putty (for weight bearing) and carried his water bottle (for distraction) throughout the day. Using his arm as much as possible for functional activities was a priority: a built-up pen was given for writing, driving was simulated in the clinic, and dressing and hygiene activities were simulated. L.H.'s family was encouraged to remind him to use his upper extremity and to exercise frequently in minimal pain range. After 5 months of therapy, L.H. had full use with his daily activities, he returned to work as an insurance salesman, and his range of motion and strength were functionally restored except for a 15-degree flexion contracture in the little finger proximal interphalangeal joint (Fig. 18-3, *C*).

CASE 18-2: COMPLEX REGIONAL PAIN SYNDROME

C.O. is a 47-year-old woman who had a motor vehicle accident while employed as a school bus driver. She had persistent pain for 2 to 3 years and had no success with conservative management. Three years after the original injury, with a history of thumb pain, numbness in median nerve distribution, and wrist pain, C.O. underwent a thumb carpometacarpal joint arthroplasty with tendon interposition, an endoscopic carpal tunnel release, and a wrist arthroscopy to determine whether there was any ligamentous injury (there was none). C.O. presented for therapy 5 weeks after surgery with limited wrist and thumb motion, swelling in the wrist and hand, and intermittent pain at 5/10 to 6/10. C.O. did some cooking and cleaning at home and reported severe pain and increased swelling that continued to worsen without relief. C.O. was referred back to the physician, and she began a series of three stellate blocks and began taking an antidepressant and oral steroids. The first stellate block was effective, with excellent decrease in pain although C.O. continued to report tingling along the distribution of the radial sensory nerve. The next two blocks were not as effective, although the client reported continued improve-

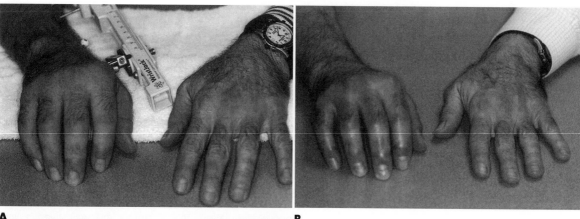

A

B

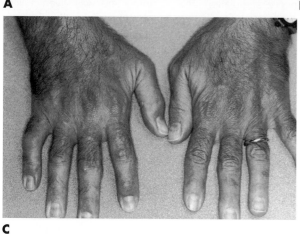

C

FIGURE 18-3 **A,** Hand has swollen fingers and inability to close or open fingers fully. **B,** External fixator removed and hand swelling increased with redness, shiny skin, and limited motion. **C,** At discharge, client had full range of motion and strength except for a persistent proximal interphalangeal joint contracture in the little finger.

ment in swelling, stiffness, and pain. In the clinic the client was seen for active range of motion, scar, and edema massage, Kinesio taping, a trial of transcutaneous electrical nerve stimulation (with mild improvement), and functional manipulation. She also did weight bearing on putty, which allowed her to bear weight without full wrist extension, which she avoided because it was painful (Fig. 18-4). At home, the client performed pain-free active range of motion 6 to 8 times a day, performed weight-bearing exercises 3 times a day, and carried around a purse with weights in it for distraction. She was encouraged to do any activity that caused minimal or no pain. Three months after starting therapy, C.O. was able to do all activities of daily living except some heavy housework, and she tolerated simulated bus driving. She still had difficulty cutting with scissors, knives, and turning doorknobs. At last visit, she had 50% of grip strength and 25% of pinch strength compared with the opposite side, and functional range of motion. She was discharged at the physician's request and was scheduled for a functional capacity evaluation to determine whether she could return to work. At a follow-up phone call, she stated that she was not going to be driving the bus any longer but would return to work in a clerical position.

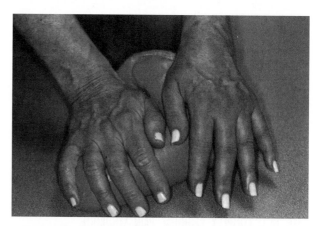

FIGURE 18-4 Simulated weight bearing initiated on putty to allow weight bearing without full wrist extension. Note swelling in fingers and wrist as evidenced by decreased wrinkles in skin of involved joint.

CASE 18-3: FIBROMYALGIA

R.M. is a 57-year-old woman with a 12-year diagnosed history of fibromyalgia and osteoarthritis of both knees and the right carpometacarpal joint worsened by using her cane on the right. She underwent a carpometacarpal joint soft tissue arthroplasty with tendon interposition, was casted for 2 weeks, and then was put into a thermoplastic thumb spica splint to immobilize her wrist and thumb. Four weeks after surgery she was referred to therapy to initiate wrist motion. R.M. presented to therapy with pain in the entire right upper extremity at a 6/10 pain rating with stiffness and soreness in her neck. She reported that she was using her cane in her left hand, which made it hurt more. Range of motion in the wrist was limited and increased pain to 8/10; although shoulder and elbow range of motion was full, the client described pain and stiffness with all motions. R.M. was encouraged to soak her hand and have a family member or herself perform a very gentle massage over the scar and wrist area. Home exercise program included removal of the splint for 3 to 4 times a day with gentle massage or range of motion exercises. R.M. called the day after therapy to report increased overall pain and more stiffness. It was recommended that she decrease the number of exercise sessions out of the splint and rest her upper extremity more to decrease inflammatory pain. At 6 weeks after surgery, attempts to discontinue the use of the splint (per protocol) were unsuccessful because pain increased without support of the splint. To encourage more motion, the client was given a neoprene splint to alternate with her thermoplastic splint for support. Her therapy program was upgraded to include short sessions of manipulation exercises followed by rest. Some days she only tolerated two sessions, and some days she was able to do more. She also was encouraged to perform these manipulation exercises at home. At 8 weeks, R.M. called and cancelled 10 days worth of sessions because of a flare-up of her knee arthritis. Upon her return, aquatic therapy was discussed as a way to increase her aerobic exercise without the weight on her knees. She agreed to try but wanted to wait until her hand was stronger. Gentle strengthening exercises were added to her home program, and she was able to wean to the neoprene splint only. Goals were to obtain 50% to 75% of her left hand grip and pinch strength, but R.M. reported being functional at approximately 30% to 40% strength; therefore she was discharged to a home program and to aquatics. Six weeks later at a follow-up visit with her physician, her strength had increased to 50% to 60% of her left hand, and she stated that her neck, shoulder, and knee pain were significantly better with the aquatic program. She was planning to switch to independent exercises in the pool at least 2 to 3 times a week.

References

1. Turner-Stokes L: Reflex sympathetic dystrophy: a complex regional pain syndrome, *Disabil Rehabil* 24(18):939-947, 2002.
2. Koman LA et al: Reflex sympathetic dystrophy (complex regional pain syndromes: types 1 and 2). In Mackin EJ et al, editors: *Rehabilitation of the hand and upper extremity*, ed 5, St Louis, 2002, Mosby.
3. Stanton-Hicks M et al: Reflex sympathetic dystrophy: changing concepts and taxonomy, *Pain* 63:127-133, 1995.
4. Rho RH et al: Complex regional pain syndrome, *Mayo Clin Proc* 77:174-180, 2002.
5. Stanton-Hicks et al: Consensus report—complex regional pain syndromes: guidelines for therapy, *Clin J Pain* 14:155-166, 1998.
6. Walsh MT, Muntzer E: Therapist's management of complex regional pain syndrome (reflex sympathetic dystrophy). In Mackin EJ et al, editors: *Rehabilitation of the hand and upper extremity*, ed 5, St Louis, 2002, Mosby.
7. Bengston K: Physical modalities for complex regional pain syndrome, *Hand Clin* 13(3):443-454, 1997.
8. Hardy M, Hardy S: Reflex sympathetic dystrophy: the clinician's perspective, *J Hand Ther* 10:137-150, 1997.
9. Hareau J: What makes treatment for reflex sympathetic dystrophy successful, *J Hand Ther* 9:367-370, 1996.
10. Fedorczyk J: The role of physical agents in modulating pain, *J Hand Ther* 10:110-121, 1997.
11. Lankford LL: Reflex sympathetic dystrophy. In Hunter JM, Mackin EJ, Callahan AD, editors: *Rehabilitation of the hand: surgery and therapy*, St Louis, 1995, Mosby.
12. Watson HK, Carlson L: Treatment of reflex sympathetic dystrophy of the hand with an active "stress loading" program, *J Hand Surg* 12A(5):779-785, 1987.
13. Curran MJ, Astifidis R: Complex regional pain syndrome type 1 (formerly reflex sympathetic dystrophy), *Orthopedic Physical Therapy Clinics of North America* 10(4):649-665, 2001.
14. Manning DC: Reflex sympathetic dystrophy, sympathetically maintained pain, and complex regional pain syndrome: diagnoses of inclusion, exclusion, or confusion? *J Hand Ther* 13:260-268, 2000.
15. Redondo JR et al: Long-term efficacy of therapy in clients with fibromyalgia: a physical exercise-based program and a cognitive-behavioral approach, *Arthritis Rheum* 51(2):184-192, 2004.
16. Goldenberg DL et al: Management of fibromyalgia syndrome, *JAMA* 292(19):2388-2395, 2004.

19

Burns

LISA DESHAIES

KEY TERMS

Autograft

Deep partial thickness burn

Dermis

Donor site

Epidermis

Flap

Full thickness burn

Full thickness burn with subdermal injury

Full thickness skin graft (FTSG)

Heterograft (xenograft)

Homograft (allograft)

Hypertrophic scars

Scar contraction

Scar contracture

Split thickness skin graft (STSG)

Superficial partial thickness burn

Total body surface area (TBSA)

Wound contraction

According to the American Burn Association, a burn of any depth to the hand is classified as a major injury that requires treatment at a specialized burn center.[1] However, therapists may see clients with burns in a variety of clinical settings after acute management of the injuries. Burn injuries are caused by thermal, chemical, or electrical action. The causes are numerous and include house fires, motor vehicle accidents, and contact with an electrical current or hot objects or liquids at home or at work.[2]

CLINICAL *Pearl*

Thermal injuries are the most common type of burn injuries, and dorsal hand burns occur more often than palmar burns.[3]

Along with their effect on hand function, burns can have a significant impact on a person's social and psychologic functioning. Scarring, perceived disfigurement, and loss of control over the body and the environment may lead to significant body image changes, social avoidance, anxiety about the future, and hopelessness.[4] Other psychologic symptoms that commonly develop after a burn injury are sleep disturbances, depression, anxiety disorders, and posttraumatic stress.[5] Related cognitive, emotional, and physiologic problems, such as lack of concentration, apathy, pain, and low energy, can influence the client's recovery, making it difficult for the client to comply fully with treatment.[6]

To plan the appropriate intervention, therapists who treat burn injuries must thoroughly understand the related anatomy and the wound healing and scar maturation processes. Emotional support for the client and family is crucial to a positive outcome.

ANATOMY

The skin is the largest organ of the human body. Its essential functions include providing protection against bacterial invasion, preventing excessive loss of body fluids, regulating body temperature through perspiration, shielding deep structures from injury, absorbing certain substances (e.g., vitamin D), and receiving sensory feedback from the environment.[7,8] Without the protection skin affords, exposed underlying tissues (e.g., muscle and tendon) become desiccated and nerve endings are exposed. An important nonphysiologic function of the skin is to provide a cosmetic covering of the body that is unique to each individual.

Normal skin is composed of two basic layers, the epidermis and the dermis. The **epidermis** is the thin, avascular, outermost layer, which accounts for only about 5% of the skin's thickness. The **dermis,** which is much thicker, contains blood vessels, nerves, hair follicles, sweat and sebaceous glands, and the epithelial bed from which the skin regenerates. The thickness of the skin varies according to its location.

CLINICAL *Pearl*

On the hand, the dorsal skin is much thinner than the palmar skin.

The structure and function of the skin also vary. Dorsal hand skin contains hair follicles and sebaceous glands, whereas palmar skin does not. Palmar skin contains a greater number of sensory end organs.

CLINICAL *Pearl*

For the hand to function fully, the dorsal skin must be nonadherent and elastic, allowing hand closure, and the palmar skin must be thick enough to withstand forces arising from daily use.[8,9]

The delicate balance of the intrinsic and extrinsic musculotendinous systems also can be affected by a burn injury.[8]

DIAGNOSIS AND PATHOLOGY

The temperature and duration of exposure to heat and the characteristics of the skin burned determine the amount of tissue destruction. Burn injuries are classified by both depth and extent. The larger and deeper the burn, the worse the prognosis.[10] Burn depth is assessed by visual examination to determine the extent of damage to or the destruction of anatomic structures. Depth can be described by degree (i.e., first, second, third, or fourth)

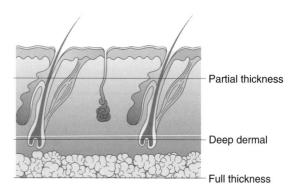

FIGURE 19-1 Classification of burns by thickness. (From Leveridge JE: Burns. In Prosser R, Conolly WB, editors: *Rehabilitation of the hand and upper limb,* Edinburgh, 2003, Butterworth Heinemann.)

or by thickness (superficial partial thickness, deep partial thickness, full thickness, and full thickness burn with subdermal injury); thickness is the more descriptive and contemporary method (Fig. 19-1). Because skin thickness varies, a burn to the hand may involve tissues at different depths.

A **superficial partial thickness burn** (which corresponds to first and second degree burns) involves the epidermis and possibly portions of the upper dermis. This type of burn is red or bright pink, blistered, soft, and wet. Sensation is intact, and the exposure of nerve endings results in pain and sensitivity to temperature, air, and light touch. Because the epithelial bed is intact, this type of burn can re-epithelialize spontaneously in 2 weeks or earlier, therefore skin grafting is not necessary.

A **deep partial thickness burn** (which corresponds to a deep second-degree burn) involves the epidermis and a deeper portion of the dermis. Hair follicles, sebaceous glands, and epithelial elements remain intact. This type of burn is mottled red or waxy white, soft, wet, and elastic. Sensation may or may not be present, depending on the extent to which nerve endings have been exposed or damaged. Re-epithelialization can occur in approximately 3 to 6 weeks, but skin grafting may be done to expedite wound closure.

Precaution. *A deep partial thickness burn may convert to a full thickness burn.*

A **full thickness burn** (which corresponds to a third-degree burn) involves the epidermis and the entire dermis, including hair follicles, nerve endings, and the epithelial bed. Sebaceous glands may be involved if the burn extends to the subcutaneous fat layer. Sensation is absent because nerve endings have been destroyed. This type of burn is white or tan, waxy, dry or leathery, and rigid. Spontaneous re-epithelialization is impossible, and skin grafting is required.

A **full thickness burn with subdermal injury** (which corresponds to a fourth-degree burn) involves deep tissue damage to fat, muscle, or possibly bone. Electrical burns often cause this type of injury. These burns require extensive debridement of necrotic tissue, followed by skin grafting. Amputation may be necessary if the damage is too extensive and severe.[7,11]

The extent of a burn is determined by estimating the percentage of the body surface burned. The two methods used for this are the rule of nines and the Lund-Browder chart. The extent of injury is described as the percentage of the **total body surface area (TBSA)** burned. A rough estimation is that the palm of the client's hand represents approximately 1% of the client's body surface. Each side of the hand is considered 1.5% of the body surface, therefore a person with circumferential burns to both hands would have a 6% TBSA burn.[1,12]

TIMELINES AND HEALING

The objective with any wound, including a burn, is to obtain quick healing to minimize scar formation and associated sequelae. The length of time required for wound closure is the most important determinant of scar development. Age, race, and burn depth are other variables.[13]

Wound healing is a dynamic cellular process that consists of three overlapping phases. Phase 1, the inflammatory (or exudative) phase, is characterized by inflammation and the presence of neutrophils and macrophages, which are responsible for clearing debris and preparing the wound for repair. This phase begins when the wound occurs and lasts 3 to 5 days. Phase 2, the fibroblastic (or proliferative or reparative) phase, lasts 2 to 6 weeks. It is characterized by the presence of fibroblasts, which lay down collagen and myofibroblasts, which cause **wound contraction.** The newly formed epithelium is very thin and fragile, and the tensile strength of the wound increases with collagen proliferation. Collagen is deposited in a random, disorganized fashion. Wound contraction continues even after epithelialization but to a lesser degree. Phase 3, the maturation (or remodeling) phase, may last for years. Collagen continues to cross-link, and tensile strength increases progressively. Typically, 50% of normal tensile strength has been regained by 6 weeks, and the ultimate tensile strength is only about 80% of that of normal skin.[13-15] As scars mature, collagen deposition slows, and the breakdown of excessive collagen proceeds until scar maturity is reached.

Hypertrophic scars may develop in wounds that take longer than 3 weeks to close. These scars are raised, thick, red, tight, and itchy. They also contract, often with deforming force. Scars that cross joints are the most problematic, because **scar contraction** can lead to loss of functional joint mobility. Scar hypertrophy and contraction are most active for the first 4 to 6 months.[11] Clients with full range of motion (ROM) early on may lose motion in the ensuing months, therefore long-term follow-up therapy is needed. As long as scars are active, they may be responsive to intervention with conservative therapy. Once scars have matured, surgical intervention is required to improve ROM or cosmetic appearance.

PHASES OF BURN RECOVERY

Four overlapping phases of recovery have been described for burn injuries: (1) emergent, (2) acute, (3) skin grafting, and (4) rehabilitation.[11] The emergent phase comprises the first 2 to 3 days after injury. The acute phase is considered to be the interval from day 2 or 3 to wound closure, which can occur by spontaneous healing or surgical intervention. The skin grafting phase is the period during which grafting is performed to cover wounds in the acute phase or as a component of reconstructive surgery in the rehabilitation phase. The rehabilitation phase lasts from wound closure to scar maturity.

CLINICAL *Pearl*

Edema is the primary deforming force in the emergent and acute phases. After the wound has been closed in the skin grafting and rehabilitation phases, scar contraction becomes the major deforming force.

NONOPERATIVE TREATMENT

The course of treatment is influenced by the depth and extent of the burn injury, the client's medical status, the stage of wound healing, and the physician's plan of care. Nonsurgical management is an option for partial thickness burns, because they are able to regenerate epithelium.[7,11] Treatment is aimed at preventing infection, promoting healing, and minimizing complications.

Dressings

Dressings are used to protect the wound and provide an optimum environment for healing. Dressings may be the adherent or nonadherent type, and they can serve a number of purposes, including infection control, comfort, wound immobilization, fluid absorption, debridement, and early pressure.[15] Numerous dressing products and wound care/dressing change schedules are available. The selection of dressings and topical agents depends on the type and status of the wound; it also is often influenced by the physician's preference. Therapists must work closely with the physician so that they fully understand the dressing program and the reasons for it.

Positioning

Positioning is important in the early phases of burn recovery to minimize edema, because edema can cause ischemia, intrinsic muscle tightness, deforming positions, loss of motion, adhesions, and fibrosis. Edema is a natural component of the wound healing process. Postburn edema peaks up to 6 hours after injury and usually resolves within 7 to 10 days.[16] Edema still present in later stages is a matter of great concern.

Precaution. *To prevent a decrease in arterial flow to the hand, elevate the hand to heart level only in the emergent phase.*[11]

In addition to elevation, use pressure techniques (e.g., compression wraps, sleeves, or gloves) as needed, taking care to monitor circulation and skin integrity, because fragile wounds and scars break down easily.

Positioning is also used to prevent loss of motion from soft tissue shortening. The position of comfort typically is that of shoulder adduction and internal rotation, elbow flexion, and wrist flexion. Loss of motion can occur in joints not even involved in the burn injury. Facilitate proper positioning out of the expected pattern using pillows, bulky dressings, or splints.

CLINICAL *Pearl*

Remember a burn treatment adage: the position of comfort is the position of deformity.

Splints

Splints can be used to facilitate wound healing by immobilizing the wound and protecting key structures in the hand. It is important to note that not all hand burns need to be splinted. The decision to splint or not to splint depends on the depth and extent of the burn and the client's ability to tolerate positioning, exercise, and function. Most superficial partial thickness burns do not require splinting, because healing is completed within 3 weeks. In some cases a splint may be indicated for a client who is unable to actively move the hand or for a client who may move too aggressively.[11] Splints are used more often with deeper burns.

CLINICAL *Pearl*

In the emergent and early acute phases, edema can lead to poor positioning and the classic burn deformity of wrist flexion, MCP hyperextension, IP flexion, thumb adduction, and a flattened palmar arch.

Unless otherwise indicated, immobilize the hand with the wrist in extension, the metacarpophalangeal joints (MCPs) in flexion, the interphalangeal joints (IPs) in extension, and the thumb in abduction.[11,17] Slight wrist extension encourages MCP flexion by means of a tenodesic effect, and MCP flexion in turn puts tension on the collateral ligaments to prevent shortening. Proximal interphalangeal (PIP) joint extension protects the vulnerable extensor mechanism, and thumb abduction maintains the first web space. Considerable variation in ideal joint angles can be found in the literature.[17] A consensus calls for wrist extension of 20 to 30 degrees, MCP flexion of 50 to 70 degrees, full IP extension, thumb abduction midway between radial and palmar abduction, MCP flexion of 10 degrees, and full thumb IP extension (Fig. 19-2).[7,11,18] *Never force joints into the ideal position.* Although prefabricated splints are available, custom splints made from perforated material are preferable because they allow a more precise fit and can be adjusted to accommodate changes in edema and joint mobility.

Precaution. *Apply the splint with gauze wraps for the first 3 to 5 days after injury to prevent vascular compromise.*[11]

For clients with significant involvement of the IP joints, the surgeon may opt to place Kirschner wires across the joints to obtain complete immobilization and protection of the extensor mechanism.[3]

Splints may also be used in the later phases of recovery to prevent or correct **scar contracture**. To prevent contracture, use static splinting, placing joints in positions opposite the direction the scar will pull. Common burn scar contractures in the hand are wrist flexion from volar burns, wrist extension or flexion from dorsal burns, thumb adduction from a burn to the first web space, MCP and IP extension from dorsal hand burns, and MCP and IP flexion from volar hand burns. Have the client wear the static splint at night only, if possible, to avoid compromising functional hand use during the day. Use serial static dynamic splinting (also known as *elastic mobilization*) or static progressive splinting (also known as *inelastic mobilization*) to regain ROM with joint and/or scar contracture. Place scars under tension in an elongated position to promote new cell growth, collagen remodeling, and tissue lengthening.[8,19]

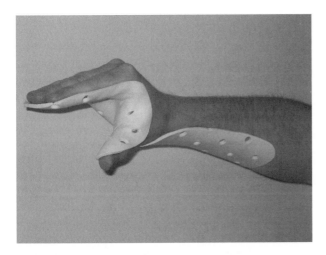

FIGURE 19-2 Positioning a splint for an acute hand burn.

Exercise

Exercise is important in the early phases of burn recovery to control edema, promote tendon gliding, and help maintain ROM and strength. Have the client perform active motion with the dressings removed while you carefully monitor the status of the wound. Muscle pumping exercises with a low number of repetitions can help with edema. Include lumbrical position exercises and adduction/adduction of the fingers to contract intrinsic muscles.[20] If the client is unable to move effectively through full ROM, perform *gentle* active assistive or passive motion. It is important to stay within wound and pain tolerance; take care to put your hands on the most stable and least painful areas of the wound.

Precaution. *Aggressive motion at this stage is harmful to fragile tissue and will result in more scarring.[11] To prevent tendon rupture, do not perform IP motion if extensor tendon involvement is known or suspected.*

In the later phases of recovery, emphasize exercises to achieve full active and passive wrist and hand motion. Include gentle passive exercises for individual joint tightness. Composite wrist and finger flexion or extension exercises may also be needed for scars that cross several joints (commonly seen with dorsal hand burns). Resistive exercises can help with regaining strength and muscle endurance. Stronger muscles are better able to move against tightening scars. Have the client perform resistive exercises in both directions to address scar and tendon adhesions. Use exercises and therapeutic activity to promote strength, dexterity, coordination, and hand function.

Joint mobilization for stiff joints can begin during the scar maturation phase once the scar has adequate tensile strength to tolerate the friction caused by mobilization techniques.[21]

Continuous passive motion (CPM) has been reported to be an effective adjunct to therapy in the treatment of hand burns for clients who show little active motion because of pain, anxiety, or edema.[22]

Precaution. *Be very careful using CPM if extensor tendon injury is involved or suspected, because this technique might be too forceful for the delicate extensor mechanism.*

Functional Hand Use

Functional hand use in daily activities should be encouraged as much as possible throughout all phases of recovery. Assistive devices, such as built-up handles, can facilitate functional use if limitations exist. Using the hand has important physical and psychologic benefits; it facilitates motion, strength, endurance, tendon glide, and edema reduction, and it gives the client a sense of self-control and sufficiency. However, keep in mind that improvement in pain, healing, motion, and strength does not always lead to spontaneous reintegration of the hand into tasks. Clients may be fearful of pain or of injuring fragile tissues. Acknowledge these concerns and provide support to help the client overcome them.

Scar Management

The goal of scar management is to modulate scars as much as possible to achieve a flat, smooth, supple, and cosmetically acceptable scar. Because scar formation is an unavoidable component of wound healing, the best we can hope to accomplish is to minimize scarring by altering its physical and mechanical properties through interventions such as compression, silicone products, massage, and physical agent modalities. The exact mechanisms by which these interventions work are not well understood, and objective support of their efficacy is less than adequate, but they have produced positive clinical effects.

Compression can be provided in a variety of ways, including splinting, compression wraps, and pressure garments. The processes of hypertrophic scarring and scar contraction begin shortly after injury, therefore early application of pressure is advised (i.e., within 2 weeks of wound closure).[11,23] As a rule of thumb, use interim compression bandages and gloves until the hand is ready to be measured for a custom-fitted pressure garment. Pressure from self-adherent elastic wraps is effective in both edema and scar management, and these wraps can be used over light dressings as needed (Fig. 19-3).[23,24] Grade the amount of pressure to make sure it is tolerable. Prefabricated digital sleeves and gloves are an option once the scar is able to tolerate the shear forces created by putting them on, taking them off, and motion while

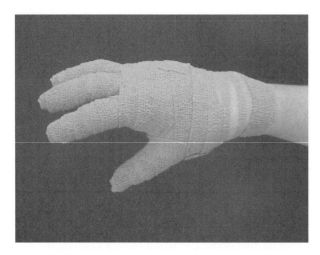

FIGURE 19-3   Self-adherent compression wrap.

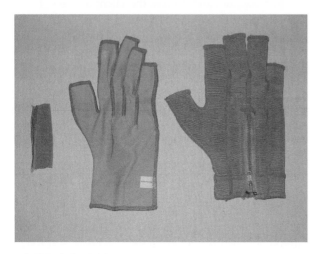

FIGURE 19-4   Prefabricated digital sleeve, prefabricated glove, and custom pressure glove.

wearing them. Measure for a custom glove only after edema has plateaued, wounds are smaller than a quarter, and the scar is ready to tolerate the heavier pressure and friction custom gloves impose (Fig. 19-4).[11] To be most effective, compression devices should be worn continually except during skin hygiene routines and exercise.

Silicone products are available in many forms, including sheets and putty. Some silicone gel sheets are self-adherent, whereas others must be held in place. Silicone can be effective when used alone, but better results usually are obtained when it is used with pressure devices.[11] Some manufacturers make pressure garments with a thin silicone lining, but these may be more difficult for a client to put on and remove because of increased friction from the silicone. The recommended wearing time is a minimum of 12 to 24 hours a day, and increased use enhances the efficacy of these products.[25-27]

Precaution. *Do not apply silicone over open wounds or fragile skin.*

Massage, delivered manually or with a vibrator, may be helpful for freeing restrictive fibers, reducing itching, and relieving pain. Begin with gentle massage of newly healed skin to avoid blister formation and skin breakdown. As tensile strength improves, progress to greater pressure and massage with circular motions to work the scar in all directions. Lubricate the scar before massage to precondition the tissue. Massage should be performed at least twice a day.[11,28]

Physical agent modalities (e.g., paraffin and ultrasound) have been used for burn scars. Paraffin combines the benefits of heat and skin lubrication, both of which are useful before exercise. Dense burn scars are best heated by ultrasound. The use of ultrasound to modulate scar tissue, relieve pain, and increase ROM has been reported,[29,30] but studies to date have been inconclusive or contradictory with regard to the effectiveness of this treatment.[11]

Precaution. *Care must be taken with paraffin and ultrasound treatments, because scars may have diminished sensation and heat tolerance. Never use paraffin or ultrasound on open wounds or broken skin.*

OPERATIVE TREATMENT

Full thickness burns require surgical intervention because re-epithelialization is not possible. Deep partial thickness burns that would require prolonged spontaneous healing (generally longer than 2 to 3 weeks) may be treated surgically to improve functional and cosmetic results.[3,11]

Early excision of nonviable burned skin (known as *escharotomy* or *fasciotomy*) may be needed to establish a healthy wound bed and to maintain blood perfusion.[3,31] The wound then can be covered with tissue transfers, cultured epithelial skin, or skin substitutes. A **heterograft (xenograft)** is skin taken from another species, such as a pig. A **homograft (allograft)** is human skin, most often taken from a cadaver. Heterografts and homografts are used as a temporary wound covering until the client's own skin can be used. An **autograft** is the client's own skin, taken as a graft harvested from a **donor site** and placed on the recipient wound site.[9,12] It may be a **split thickness skin graft (STSG)** or a **full thickness skin graft (FTSG).** The thicker the graft, the more dermal appendages it will contain. Thinner STSGs typically are used to cover the dorsal hand. Thicker STSGs or FTSGs commonly are used for the palmar surface because they provide better sensibility and durability.[9] STSGs may be applied as is (known as a *sheet graft*), perforated to allow drainage of fluid (known as a *meshed graft*), or meshed and expanded to cover more surface area. A **flap** may be needed for deep wounds with exposed tendon or bone.[3,11] Grafts and flaps require time to heal and leave scars at both the recipient and donor sites.

CLINICAL *Pearl*

Scar contraction of grafts occurs; the thinner the graft, the more it will shrink.[32]

Grafts that are meshed and expanded tend to produce more scarring and contraction than sheet or unexpanded mesh grafts.[11] Cultured epithelial grafts are composed of sheets of epidermal cells grown in a laboratory. These very thin, fragile grafts are used for clients who do not have adequate donor sites.[11]

Postoperative therapy for burn wounds treated surgically is crucial for maximizing functional outcomes. Postoperative protocols vary according to the surgical procedure and the surgeon's preference. STSGs and FTSGs typically are immobilized for several days after surgery to allow establishment of vascularity and graft adherence. Cultured skin grafts are progressed more slowly than standard STSGs because of their fragile nature. Flaps usually are immobilized for slightly longer than grafts because they do not take as readily. Grafts and flaps are like any other healing wound in that time is required for collagen deposition and improvement of tensile strength. Initiate and cautiously progress positioning, splinting, exercise, and scar management as soon as graft or flap stability allows.

Precaution. *Healing tissues are very susceptible to injury in the first 3 weeks, especially from shearing forces.[3,9] Monitor carefully for signs of blistering or breakdown. Discuss with the surgeon whether therapy can proceed or should be discontinued temporarily.*

Surgery is an integral part of the rehabilitation phase for contracture release and reconstruction. Surgical intervention also may be used after the scar has reached maturity. In children, surgery may be needed periodically until growth is complete because of a discrepancy between the rapid rate of bony growth relative to the slower rate of scar tissue growth. Scar contracture release involves introducing more skin in areas where tight scarring has caused ROM limitations. Tissue transfers as described above are common, as are local rotational and advancement flaps (e.g., Z-plasties).[3,31,33] Postoperative treatment follows guidelines and timelines similar to those for wound coverage.

Questions to Ask the Physician

Nonoperative Clients

- *What are the wound care and dressing guidelines?*
- *Will a splint be needed?*
- *Are there any known or suspected problems with tendon or joint integrity?*
- *Are any precautions necessary with regard to elevation, motion, or compression?*

Operative Clients

- *What surgery was performed? (Obtain a copy of the operative report if possible.)*
- *What type of graft or flap was used?*
- *What was the intraoperative ROM?*
- *How well had the graft or flap taken when postoperative dressings were removed?*
- *What are the wound care and dressing guidelines?*
- *Are there any problems with tendon or joint integrity?*
- *Will a splint be needed?*
- *Are any precautions required with regard to elevation, motion, or compression?*
- *What postoperative protocol would you like followed?*

What to Say to Clients

About the Injury

"A burn causes serious injury to the skin. Skin is important for preventing infection and for protecting deeper structures in our hands. Here is a diagram showing the layers of the skin and key anatomic features, such as hair follicles, sweat glands, oil glands, and nerve endings. The burn you sustained injured your skin to this depth, and this is how your skin will be affected."

Customize your information according to the client's level of injury and the symptoms related to pain and sensation.

About Wound Care and Healing

"The primary concern is to help you heal as quickly as possible to prevent infection and to minimize scarring. This is the wound care and dressing program that has been designed for you. It is important that you understand it, feel comfortable with it, and follow it closely."

Clients may have less pain and anxiety if they perform or assist with their wound care. Educate and practice with the client and family as often as needed to increase their comfort level. If a tissue transfer will be or was used, explain the purpose of it and what the client can expect at the recipient and donor sites.

About Scar Management

"Wounds heal with a process of scar formation. It may take several months or years for your active scars to complete the process of becoming mature. Active scars are red and may become thick, raised, and firm. Active scars also tend to become tight and may get very itchy, especially in the first 2 or 3 months. As the scars mature, you'll see the redness fade to your more normal skin color and the scars will be flatter, softer, and less itchy. Scars are more sensitive to sunlight, therefore you should use sunscreen or gloves to protect them. You should wash your hands with mild soap; don't use anything with a strong detergent, which can dry your skin. Dry scars crack or injure more easily, and they may itch more. Over time your scars will become more durable, but they will never be quite as resilient as your normal skin. Because the feeling in your scars may not be normal, you'll have to rely more closely on visually inspecting them for signs of injury. Scars also don't have the natural ability to stay moist, therefore you will need to lubricate your skin frequently throughout the day to keep it healthy. Avoid moisturizers with a high perfume or alcohol content, which can cause dryness. Although we can't prevent scarring, we can try to keep your scars as flat, soft, and mobile as possible using interventions such as massage, pressure, and silicone."

Educate the client and family so that they understand the scar management program, how to monitor for skin problems, and how to care for pressure and silicone devices properly.

About Splinting

"Splints are used to help keep your active scars from becoming tight and causing loss of joint motion. They can also be used to regain motion you may have lost since your burn injury. It is important to follow the splinting schedule we set and to watch out for any problems with your skin that the splint may cause."

Make sure that the client and family understand the purpose of the splint, the wearing schedule, and how to care for the splint.

About Exercise

"Exercise is important to keep your joints and scars mobile. The exercises designed for you include some for stretching your scars, some to help your tendons glide, and some to make your hand stronger. Always make sure to moisturize your scars well before you start your exercises so that they don't crack."

Educate the client and family about the purpose of each exercise and when and how each should be performed.

About Function

"One of the best ways to keep your hand moving is to use it as much as possible during all your normal daily activities. Although it may be a little awkward at first,

using your hand will help your scars to stay supple, your joints to remain loose, and your muscles to become strong. You may have to be a little more careful to protect your scars from injury by monitoring for signs of pressure or blistering."

If assistive devices are used, explain, "These devices will help you use your hand better right now until it becomes easier for you to hold things or to do more with your hand."

EVALUATION TIPS

- Be careful and gentle when placing your hands or tools (e.g., a goniometer) over healing wounds, fragile scars, and insensate or hypersensitive areas.
- Contractures may be caused by scar tightness, joint tightness, or both. Differentiate between a scar contracture and a joint contracture by watching for blanching and by palpating the scar.

CLINICAL *Pearl*

If the joint reaches maximum end-range and the scar blanches, scar tightness is contributing to the limitation. If the scar does not blanch at end-range, the limitation is caused by joint or other soft tissue tightness.

- Scars that cross several joints need to be assessed closely. Assess individual joint active range of motion (AROM) and passive range of motion (PROM) with the scar in a relaxed position to measure the true joint motion. Tension on the scar may limit motion and make it appear that joint mobility is affected. For example, in a client with dorsal hand burns, place the wrist and MCP in full extension while measuring PIP flexion. Once you have determined individual joint mobility, assess composite active and passive motion to determine if and how the scar is limiting motion.
- Use photographic images to help track wound healing and scar appearance. Quantify open wounds by measuring their size in centimeters and by describing their features (e.g., color, integrity, drainage, and odor).[34] Quantify scars using scar assessment tools such the Vancouver Burn Scar Scale, which rates pigmentation, vascularity, pliability, and height.[35] Assessing the client's subjective rating of the scars through visual analog scales is also beneficial, because the client's perception may not match yours. Despite the objective improvement you see, the client may not share your opinion that the scars are better.[36] Remember also to evaluate donor sites.

- Use hand tracings to evaluate and track changes in web spaces. You can obtain the most accurate representation by using a thin ballpoint refill without the pen body.
- Do not use volumetric measurement if open wounds are present without first obtaining the physician's permission. *Always disinfect the volumeter after use.*
- Watch for signs and patterns of peripheral nerve involvement. Nerve damage can be caused by direct injury, infection, or neurotoxicities. Localized compression caused by tight scars, poor positioning, or edema is also common.[37]
- Discuss how the burn is affecting the client's overall ability to function. Ascertain which activities are most important for the client to resume, and determine the factors that are most interfering with the client's ability to function.

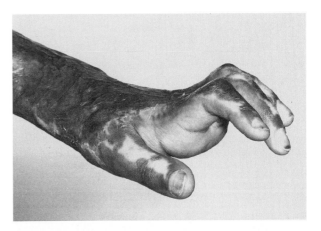

FIGURE 19-5 Dorsal hand burn resulting in the intrinsic minus deformity position. (From Thornes N: Therapy for the burn patient. In Prosser R, Conolly WB, editors: *Rehabilitation of the hand and upper limb,* Edinburgh, 2003, Butterworth Heinemann.)

DIAGNOSIS-SPECIFIC INFORMATION THAT AFFECTS CLINICAL REASONING

Each client has unique clinical, functional, psychologic, social, and cultural needs. Individualize treatment based on your evaluation results and an understanding and appreciation of each person. Empower the client and family to be involved throughout therapy through education and an open approach that fosters active participation. Provide the client with a sense of control by presenting choices whenever possible. Because the scar maturation process may take several years, make sure you give clients all the tools they need to manage their own care. Teach clients how to perform interventions for themselves at every possible opportunity rather than doing the treatment for them; this facilitates better long-term outcomes. Treatment needs also are dictated by the depth and location of the burn, the timing of injury and surgical procedures, the stage of wound healing, and the phase of burn recovery. Anticipate potential scar contractures and direct treatment at preventing or correcting them. The principles of hand burn treatment can be applied to burns on any area of the body.

Precaution. *Work closely with the physician on the plan of care and report any new problems promptly.*

Dorsal burns to the hand commonly result in a thumb web space contracture that limits functional positioning of the thumb and finger web space contractures that limit digital abduction and possibly MCP flexion. Loss of MCP, IP, and composite finger flexion is also typical. In some cases the hand may have assumed an intrinsic minus position from poor early positioning, edema, or scar contraction (Fig. 19-5). A boutonniere deformity also may be present if the extensor mechanism was damaged. Palmar burns often cause limited thumb, finger, and composite extension.

Keep in mind that every scar is unique, and clients will have a variety of clinical problems; therefore perform a thorough evaluation to identify needs. The treatment of burn injuries is a dynamic process. Prioritize treatment based on the scars that are most active and the most functionally limiting. Re-evaluate often and shift treatment in response to changing needs. Circumferential scars are especially challenging, because they involve scars that pull in both directions of flexion and extension.

TIPS FROM THE FIELD

Edema

If open wounds or fresh grafts are present, obtain the physician's permission before taking volumetric measurements. When elevating the hand, keep the elbow as straight as possible to aid flow. To provide more even pressure, use foam inserts placed in the palm, between the fingers, or on the dorsum of the hand under compressive wraps and prefabricated gloves.

Wound Care

When applying a dressing to the hand, make sure to wrap the digits individually and separately from the hand so as not to restrict motion unnecessarily and impede hand function (Fig. 19-6). If the thumb is involved in the dressing, pay attention to thumb positioning and wrap it to facilitate functional palmar abduction. Wrap dressings over gauze pads in finger web spaces to provide early

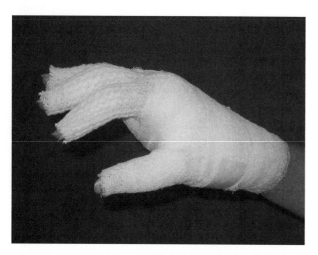

FIGURE 19-6 Hand dressing that allows unimpeded motion.

pressure. Keep the thickness of dressings consistent if a splint or interim garment is to be worn over them.

Scar Management

Scar hypersensitivity is a common problem that often must be addressed before the client is able to tolerate other interventions such as splinting, pressure, or massage. Hypersensitive scars on the palmar surface can also significantly impede hand function. Use graded stimuli to lessen sensitivity, taking care to stay within the scar's pressure and shear force tolerances to avoid injury.

CLINICAL *Pearl*

To be effective, compression must conform to the scar.

Use inserts under compression devices to augment pressure in difficult areas such as the web spaces and the palmar arch. Inserts can be made from products such as silicone or foam (Fig. 19-7).[11,17,23,28] Rubber tubing also has been reported to be an effective insert for finger web spaces.[38]

Grade pressure to the tolerance of the scar. A graded sequence may be compressive wraps using self-adherent elastic materials, progressing to a prefabricated glove made from soft material, progressing to a custom-fitted pressure glove. Order custom garments with the client's specific needs in mind. Zippers or Velcro closures make it easier for the client to put on and remove gloves, with less trauma to fragile skin. Open tips allow for better finger sensation and hand function. Most manufacturers

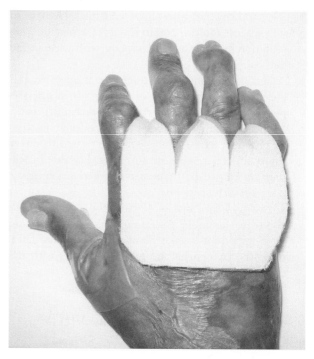

FIGURE 19-7 Silicone gel sheet in the thumb web space and foam inserts in the finger web spaces augment pressure under the glove.

offer different grades of fabric from which the glove can be made. Select the material based on scar tolerance and functional demands. Very fragile scars may need a glove made of soft material; scars with good tolerance in a very active client may require a more durable material. Panels of soft material can be strategically placed in areas prone to discomfort or scar breakdown, such as bony prominences and the thumb web space (Fig. 19-8). Suede patches and strips can be sewn onto the palmar surface to increase the glove's durability and prevent objects from slipping on slick fabric.[39]

Compression materials stretch as the client wears them throughout the day. Laundering the garments helps materials return to their original state. Provide the client with two sets of all garments so that each day a clean one can be put on that provides the appropriate amount of pressure. Custom garments generally last 2 to 4 months under normal wearing conditions. Some clients struggle to keep to the wearing schedule because these garments are tight, they can be uncomfortably hot to wear, and they may limit dexterity and functional sensation. To improve follow-through, provide clients with a choice of design and color and teach them the purpose of the garments.[40]

Precaution. *Watch for allergic reactions, skin maceration or breakdown, and circulation or sensory impairments caused by compression garments, silicone, and inserts.*

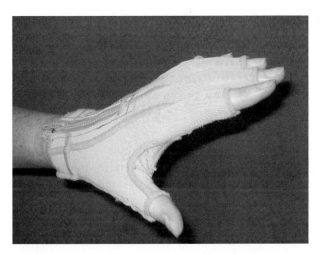

FIGURE 19-8 *Custom pressure glove with dorsal zipper, open tips, and a soft panel in the thumb web space.*

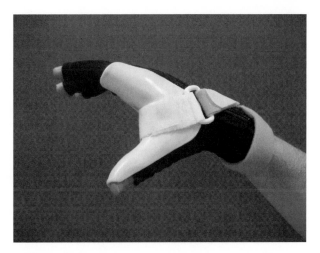

FIGURE 19-9 *Thumb abduction splint for scar contracture of the first web space.*

Splinting

Make sure to fabricate splints over any dressings, inserts, or garments the client will be wearing underneath them to ensure optimal fit. If you are molding a splint directly over scars that may be hypersensitive or heat sensitive, apply a thin cotton sleeve or a light dressing before placing warm material on the client. Relieve pressure over bony prominences or other areas of concern by temporarily placing padding over them before molding the splint; this will "bubble out" the material. Avoid lining or padding the splint itself unless absolutely necessary, because this makes the splint very difficult to keep clean. If lining or padding is used, place it on the splint material before molding.

Because wounds and scars are fragile, it is critical to smooth splint edges completely. Select thermoplastic splinting material based on the type of splint and its intended purpose. A material with full memory is well suited for a serial static splint that will be remolded numerous times. A material with excellent conformability is appropriate for a splint designed to apply pressure to uneven scars. A material with good rigidity is desirable for a splint that must withstand the force of a strongly contracting scar. The choice and placement of strapping also must be carefully considered to prevent the creation of pressure or shear forces.

To prevent unnecessary stiffness or disuse, design splint wearing schedules that leave the hand free for function and motion as much as possible.

Precaution. *With very active scars, just a few hours without a splint may result in significant loss of motion.*

As scars become more mature, splint time can gradually be reduced, especially if the client's activity level or pressure devices are sufficient to control scar shortening.

Serial casts, serial static splints, dynamic splints, and static progressive splints all can be used to treat the wrist and hand. The type of splint used depends on the location of the scar, the direction of scar contraction, and the therapist's preference. Splinting to apply stress to burn scars often involves placing joints in positions not commonly used for other hand conditions, such as the wrist in flexion, the MCPs in extension, the thumb in radial abduction, or all joints in composite extension. Think creatively to design a splint that provides the most benefit. Leave uninvolved joints free whenever possible. Consider using a less restrictive splint during the day and a more restrictive splint at night. Splints may require frequent remolding or modification as edema diminishes, the shape of the scar changes, or scar tightness improves or worsens.

Thumb web space contractures respond well to serial static splinting. A splint that conforms completely to the web space often is most effective. Position the thumb in the plane of abduction where you can achieve maximal stretch (as noted by scar blanching). Strapping can be anchored around the wrist to apply pressure in the desired direction and to keep the splint firmly in place (Fig. 19-9).

Serial casts or gutter splints can be used for IP flexion contractures. Casting may be a better choice for severe contractures, because plaster conforms better than thermoplastics. Gutter splints can be secured with self-adherent compression wrap for a more secure and conforming fit.

MCP extension contractures can be treated with serial static, dynamic, or static progressive MCP flexion splinting. In some cases, use of a simple wrist extension splint or a hand-based lumbrical bar splint during the day

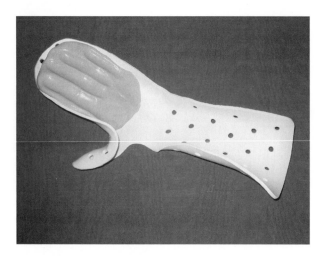

FIGURE 19-10 Full contact splint with silicone elastomer putty insert for palmar scar contracture.

combined with functional use of the hand can encourage MCP flexion. This can be complemented by use at night of a more restrictive splint designed to apply sustained stress to the scar. A full contact palmar splint can be effective for flexion contractures caused by palmar hand burns (Fig. 19-10).

Exercise

Include exercises for scar stretching, ROM, and tendon gliding as appropriate. Strengthening exercises are also useful, because strong muscles are better able to pull against tight scars. Gripping and putty exercises are effective for encouraging composite flexion of the hand. Scars should be well lubricated before exercising. Exercises for nonburned areas may be needed to regain motion or strength lost through immobilization or disuse.

Promoting Function

Use assistive devices to help promote functional use through all phases of burn recovery. Build up handles on utensils or use universal cuffs to assist with grasp. Tight scars can limit dexterity and slow speed of performance. Improvement in skin integrity, pain, motion, and strength does not automatically equate with spontaneous return to functional hand use. Integrate therapeutic activities (e.g., woodworking or leather crafts) and meaningful functional tasks into the therapy program to help clients see their functional potential and gain confidence in their hand use. Discuss self-care, home, community, leisure, or vocational demands with each client and address specific interfering factors. Reintegrating into social activities can be especially difficult for clients with scarring. Work with the client to figure out ways to return to activities as independently, safely, and comfortably as

possible. Keep in mind that the ultimate goal is a return to the client's prior level of function.

Psychosocial Adjustment

Recovery from a burn injury goes beyond the healing of anatomic structures. Be aware of factors that may interfere with treatment and recovery, such as pain, anxiety, and depression. Take time to establish rapport and trust with your client. Provide encouragement, understanding, and emotional support throughout therapy. Facilitate client involvement and a sense of self-control during the therapeutic process to the fullest extent possible. Refer the client to other health care providers as appropriate to help address problems. Educate the client and family about resources for support. Many national and local organizations offer information, peer counseling, support groups, and recreational activities for burn survivors and their families. Find information through the American Burn Association and the Phoenix Society for Burn Survivors.

Reassessment

Reassess scar activity and ROM frequently, because the scar's status can change quickly for the better or worse. Adjust the treatment program, goals, and priorities according to these assessments. Share the results with the client and family, to serve as positive reinforcement if improvements are noted or to motivate them to adhere to therapy recommendations if no gains are seen or the scar's status has deteriorated.

Precautions and Concerns

- *Facilitate wound healing and control edema to reduce the extent of scarring.*
- *Follow appropriate infection control procedures during wound care and dressing changes.*
- *When splinting an edematous hand, never force joints into the ideal position. Instead, position the joints as close to the ideal as possible and modify the splint gradually over time as edema diminishes.*
- *Be especially careful with PIP joints when extensor tendon injury is known or suspected; mobilize these joints only with permission from the physician.*
- *When splints and pressure devices are used, monitor closely for signs of skin breakdown.*
- *Be cautious with the use of thermal treatments over newly healed wounds or scars.*
- *Carefully assess the client's work environment. Clients with a large-percentage body burn have a decreased tolerance for hot temperatures. Chemicals also may pose an increased risk to scars.*

The Role of Therapy Assistants

- Edema management
- Wound care and scar management
- Splint modifications
- Exercises
- Modifications and adaptations for activities of daily living
- Instructing clients in home program designed by therapist
- Reinforcing education and precautions identified by therapist

CASE *Study*

CASE 19-1

D.L. is a 24-year-old, right-hand dominant auto mechanic who sustained 8% TBSA circumferential burns to his right hand in a small explosion at work. The palmar wound was a mix of superficial and deep partial thickness burns that crossed the wrist into the forearm; the dorsal injury involved deep partial thickness burns. The client was admitted to a local burn unit, where he underwent early excision and grafting of the dorsal hand injury with STSGs from his right thigh. The palmar burn was treated with nonsurgical management. D.L. was referred to the outclient hand clinic for therapy 3 weeks after surgery.

Treatment

D.L. arrived at the therapy clinic with his hand wrapped in a bulky dressing, even though he had no open wounds. He stated that it was "too painful" to leave his hand uncovered. He had mild edema, most notably on the dorsum of the hand. The following values were recorded for the right hand:

	AROM (DEGREES)	PROM (DEGREES)
Index finger MCP	30/55	25/60
PIP	35/65	30/85
Distal interphalangeal (DIP)	5/40	0/50
Middle finger MCP	25/40	15/50
PIP	40/70	40/80
DIP	10/50	5/60
Ring finger MCP	25-55	20-65
PIP	40/75	45/80
DIP	15/36	10/35
Small finger MCP	10/30	10/40

	AROM (DEGREES)	PROM (DEGREES)
PIP	55/70	35/75
DIP	20/55	10/60
Thumb MP	20/45	20/55
IP	−30/5	−20/15
Abduction	0-30	0-35

The scars were not hypertrophic but were very red, dry, and tight, as noted by blanching at end-ranges of motion. The hand did not appear to have been recently washed. Grip strength measured 15 lb. All motor function was intact. Touch-pressure sensation was normal with monofilament testing, but hypersensitivity of the palmar surface was noted throughout the evaluation. D.L. lived with his girlfriend, who accompanied him to therapy. He was able to perform his basic activities of daily living using his left hand only.

The immediate treatment priorities were determined to be reducing hypersensitivity, resolving edema, and improving ROM for both hand opening and closing. Hypersensitivity and a fear of pain or damage to his skin were limiting D.L.'s ability to care for his hand and to want to move it or use it. This issue initially was addressed by having him gently wash his hand and apply lotion to scars at the beginning of therapy sessions. D.L. was reluctant to do this for the first few sessions, and he needed a lot of encouragement to do a thorough job. After the third session, his hand consistently appeared clean upon his arrival for therapy. He also was able to tolerate having the therapist massage his scars after he performed massage for the first few minutes.

D.L. felt unable to leave his hand unbandaged, but he did agree to try a self-adherent compressive wrap to help manage edema and provide some light pressure to his scars. Foam inserts were placed in the palm and web spaces and on the dorsum of the hand. The wrap was applied with very light pressure at first, and D.L. was able to tolerate a little more pressure each time as hypersensitivity diminished and his trust of his therapist increased. Two weeks into therapy, the edema had almost resolved and the hypersensitivity had improved enough that D.L. felt he could wear a soft, prefabricated pressure glove. This allowed him to move more freely and to remove the glove often for skin hygiene, massage, and progressive desensitization with textures. When the edema had resolved completely, D.L. began wearing a custom-fitted pressure glove.

Increasing ROM was addressed through a combination of splinting, exercise, and functional use. D.L. lacked motion in both flexion and extension, and the therapist had to prioritize which joints and motions to focus on first. Gaining MCP flexion and PIP extension were selected as priority concerns. Gutter splints were made for each finger and worn over the compression wrap. The aim was to serially gain IP extension ROM and transfer flexor forces to the MCPs to improve active MCP flexion ROM. A volar wrist splint with the wrist in extension was also fabricated for use during the day to encourage MCP flexion and prevent contraction of the volar forearm scar that crossed the wrist. Night splinting was geared toward improving composite extension ROM. A volar wrist-hand splint was fabricated with the wrist and fingers in maximum extension and the thumb in maximum abduction. Because each finger IP needed to be positioned at a different angle, the wrist-hand splint was fabricated over the existing gutter splints for a more precise fit. Once IP extension had improved, lacking only about 15 degrees to neutral, and active MCP flexion also had improved (in about 2 weeks), gutter splints were weaned off during the day to facilitate IP flexion and functional use of the hand. The daytime wrist splint was discontinued shortly thereafter.

Active and gentle passive exercises for all joints were initiated and had to be progressed slowly. As D.L.'s hypersensitivity and edema improved, so did his ability to tolerate more vigorous exercises. Strengthening exercises were graded from squeezing a large, soft foam ball to putty. Later in the program, D.L. was able to perform weight well exercises with progressive resistance.

To help D.L. begin to integrate functional use of his hand at the beginning of therapy, soft, large-diameter tubing was used on his eating utensils and toothbrush. Because he was able to do tasks easily using his left hand, he was reluctant to consider trying with his right hand "until it got better." Once he understood the therapeutic value of active daily use for reducing the edema, hypersensitivity, and scar tightness, he was willing to integrate functional use as part of his home program. When he saw that his hand looked and felt better after he began using it, he became eager to do more at home. D.L. shared with the therapist that he was a drummer who occasionally performed with a band made up of friends. The therapist was able to tap into this interest as a means to motivate D.L. by making drumming a focus of his home program. He was asked to bring in a small drum and his drumsticks, and together D.L. and the therapist were able to devise modifications for his right drumstick. Soft padding was wrapped around the proximal end of the stick to a diameter large enough to allow him to hold it. As composite finger flexion improved, the diameter of the padding was reduced. Therapeutic activities were performed in the therapy clinic to improve fisting and strength. These included leather stamping and a woodworking project in which he fabricated a weight well for himself to use at home. The final activities involved tool use simulating work tasks. D.L. was concerned about being able to wear his pressure glove at work without getting it dirty. He brought in vinyl gloves that he typically wore on his hands at work and found that a larger size fit well over his pressure glove. He began doing some work on his car at home.

Result

Throughout the therapy program, D.L. was educated in all aspects of his injury and care. Building trust, fostering his sense of control over his care, providing him with choices, allowing him to see his progress by continually sharing re-evaluation results, and tapping into motivating interests were keys to his successful rehabilitation. Upon discharge from therapy, D.L. had regained full AROM and hypersensitivity had resolved. Grip strength was 75 lb. He was wearing his pressure glove full time. He returned to using his right hand as dominant for all activities, which was enough to maintain full composite flexion without requiring splinting. He continued to wear a night splint that positioned his wrist and hand in composite extension whenever he felt his scars were tightening. He felt confident about managing his scars long term and knew how to progress his hand strengthening exercises at home. His physician cleared him to return to work shortly after therapy ended.

References

1. Mlcak RP, Buffalo MC: Prehospital management, transportation, and emergency care. In Herndon D, editor: *Total burn care*, ed 2, New York, 2002, WB Saunders.
2. Pruitt BA, Goodwin CW, Mason AD: Epidemiological, demographic, and outcome characteristics of burn injury. In Herndon D, editor: *Total burn care*, ed 2, New York, 2002, WB Saunders.
3. Achauer BM: The burned hand. In Green DP, Hotchkiss RN, Pederson WC, editors: *Green's operative hand surgery*, ed 4, Philadelphia, 1999, Churchill Livingstone.
4. Blakenly PE, Fauerbach JA, Meyer WJ et al: Psychosocial recovery and reintegration of patients with burn injuries. In Herndon D, editor: *Total burn care*, ed 2, New York, 2002, WB Saunders.
5. Thomas CR, Meyer WJ, Blakenly PE: Psychiatric disorders associated with burn injury. In Herndon D, editor: *Total burn care*, ed 2, New York, 2002, WB Saunders.
6. Wiechman SA, Ptacek JT, Patterson DR et al: Rates, trends, and severity of depression after burn injuries, *J Burn Care Rehabil* 22:417-424, 2001.
7. Malick MH, Carr JA: *Manual on management of the burn patient*, Pittsburgh, 1982, Harmarville Rehabilitation Center Educational Resource Division.
8. Richard RL, Staley MJ: Biophysical aspects of normal skin and burn scar. In Richard RL, Staley MJ, editors: *Burn care and rehabilitation: principles and practice*, Philadelphia, 1994, FA Davis.
9. Browne EZ: Skin grafts. In Green DP, Hotchkiss RN, Pederson WC, editors: *Green's operative hand surgery*, ed 4, Philadelphia, 1999, Churchill Livingstone.

10. Hartford CE: Care of outpatient burns. In Herndon D, editor: *Total burn care,* ed 2, New York, 2002, WB Saunders.

11. deLinde LG, Knothe B: Therapist's management of the burned hand. In Mackin EJ et al, editors: *Rehabilitation of the hand and upper extremity,* ed 5, St Louis, 2002, Mosby.

12. Miller SF, Richard RL, Staley MJ: Triage and resuscitation of the burn patient. In Richard RL, Staley MJ, editors: *Burn care and rehabilitation: principles and practice,* Philadelphia, 1994, FA Davis.

13. Greenhalgh DG, Staley MJ: Burn wound healing. In Richard RL, Staley MJ, editors: *Burn care and rehabilitation: principles and practice,* Philadelphia, 1994, FA Davis.

14. Peacock EE: *Wound repair,* ed 3, Philadelphia, 1984, WB Saunders.

15. Smith KL, Price JL: Care of the hand wound. In Mackin EJ et al, editors: *Rehabilitation of the hand and upper extremity,* ed 5, St Louis, 2002, Mosby.

16. Lund T: Edema following thermal injury: an update, *J Burn Care Rehabil* 20:445-452, 1999.

17. Richard R, Staley M, Daugherty MB et al: The wide variety of designs for dorsal hand burn splints, *J Burn Care Rehabil* 15:275-280, 1994.

18. Daugherty MB, Carr-Collins JA: Splinting techniques for the burn patient. In Richard RL, Staley MJ, editors: *Burn care and rehabilitation: principles and practice,* Philadelphia, 1994, FA Davis.

19. Brand PW, Hollister A: *Clinical mechanics of the hand,* ed 2, St Louis, 1993, Mosby.

20. Howell JW: Management of the burned hand. In Richard RL, Staley MJ, editors: *Burn care and rehabilitation: principles and practice,* Philadelphia, 1994, FA Davis.

21. Humphrey CN, Richard RL, Staley MJ: Soft tissue management and exercise. In Richard RL, Staley MJ, editors: *Burn care and rehabilitation: principles and practice,* Philadelphia, 1994, FA Davis.

22. Covey MH, Dutcher K, Marvin JA et al: Efficacy of continuous passive motion devices with hand burns, *J Burn Care Rehabil* 9:397-400, 1988.

23. Staley MJ, Richard RL: Scar management. In Richard RL, Staley MJ, editors: *Burn care and rehabilitation: principles and practice,* Philadelphia, 1994, FA Davis.

24. Lowell M, Pirc P, Ward RS et al: Effect of 3M Coban self-adherent wraps on edema and function of the burned hand: a case study, *J Burn Care Rehabil* 24:253-258, 2003.

25. Ahn ST, Monafo WW, Mustoe TA: Topical silicone gel for the prevention and treatment of hypertrophic scar, *Arch Surg* 126:499-504, 1991.

26. Loeding LA, Guccione JM, Mustoe TA et al: Effects of silicone gel on scar tissue in hand injuries, *J Hand Ther* 6:59, 1993.

27. So K, Umraw N, Scott J et al: Effects of enhanced patient education on compliance with silicone gel sheeting and burn scar outcome: a randomized clinical trial, *J Burn Care Rehabil* 24:411-417, 2003.

28. Serghiou MA, Evans EB, Ott S et al: Comprehensive rehabilitation of the burn patient. In Herndon D, editor: *Total burn care,* ed 2, New York, 2002, WB Saunders.

29. McDiarmid T, Ziskin MC, Michlovitz SL: Therapeutic ultrasound. In Michlovitz SL, editor: *Thermal agents in rehabilitation,* ed 5, Philadelphia, 1996, FA Davis.

30. Ward RS: The use of physical agents in burn care. In Richard RL, Staley MJ, editors: *Burn care and rehabilitation: principles and practice,* Philadelphia, 1994, FA Davis.

31. Simpson RL, Gartner MC: Management of burns of the upper extremity. In Mackin EJ et al, editors: *Rehabilitation of the hand and upper extremity,* ed 5, St Louis, 2002, Mosby.

32. Greenhalgh DG: Wound healing. In Herndon D, editor: *Total burn care,* ed 2, New York, 2002, WB Saunders.

33. Levin LS, Moorman GJ, Heller L: Management of skin grafts and flaps. In Mackin EJ et al, editors: *Rehabilitation of the hand and upper extremity,* ed 5, St Louis, 2002, Mosby.

34. Baldwin JE, Weber LJ, Simon CLS: Wound/scar assessment. In Casanova JS, editor: *Clinical assessment recommendations,* ed 2, Chicago, 1992, American Society of Hand Therapists.

35. Sullivan T, Smith J, Kermode J et al: Rating the burn scar, *J Burn Care Rehabil* 11:256-260, 1990.

36. Martin D, Umraw N, Gomez M et al: Changes in subjective versus objective burn scar assessment over time: does the patient agree with what we think? *J Burn Care Rehabil* 24:239-244, 2003.

37. Dutcher K, Johnson C: Neuromuscular and musculoskeletal complications. In Richard RL, Staley MJ, editors: *Burn care and rehabilitation: principles and practice,* Philadelphia, 1994, FA Davis.

38. Gorham K, Hammond J: An improved web space pressure technique to prevent burn scar syndactyly, *J Burn Care Rehabil* 12:157-159, 1991.

39. Weinstock-Zlotnick G, Torres-Gray D, Segal R: Effect of pressure garment work gloves on hand function in patients with hand burns: a pilot study, *J Hand Ther* 17:368-376, 2004.

40. Stewart R, Bhagwanjee AM, Mbakaza Y et al: Pressure garment adherence in adult patients with burn injuries: an analysis of patient and clinician perceptions, *Am J Occup Ther* 54:598-606, 2000.

Common Infections

CYNTHIA COOPER

Hand therapists are in a front-line position to notice early signs of inflammation or infection, such as redness (**rubor**), swelling (**tumor**), heat (**calor**), and pain (**dolor**). Prompt attention may make the difference between a surgical solution and nonsurgical one. Understandably, clients are grateful when the hand therapist recognizes the signs of infection and facilitates care by alerting the client and the physician.

Several types of infections can develop in the hand. Cellulitis and lymphangitis are superficial infections. Subcutaneous abscesses include paronychias, felons, and subepidermal abscesses. Infection also may occur in the flexor sheaths, joint spaces, and fascial spaces. Hand infections can be caused by human bites, animal bites, intravenous drug use, mycobacteria, and viruses. When the synovial spaces are involved, the infection can be extremely damaging. An infection of the palmar surface may manifest clinically with more edema dorsally than palmarly because of the anatomy and direction of flow of the lymphatic system.[1,2]

Infections start out as **cellulitis,** a superficial infection of the skin and subcutaneous tissue that normally does not produce an **abscess** (a localized collection of pus) (Fig. 20-1). The client usually reports receiving a puncture wound, cut, or scratch before the cellulitis develops. The involved area is tender and warm and marked by **erythema** (redness).[1] Incision and drainage are not routinely performed for cellulitis, but the procedure is done if an abscess develops.[3,4]

A trivial injury left untreated may lead to a very serious hand infection that progresses rapidly, called **lymphangitis.** Although much less common than cellulitis, lymphangitis can lead to a generalized infection within a few hours.

Red streaking up the hand and forearm and along the lymphatic pathways is noted, and an abscess may form at the elbow or axilla if the condition goes untreated. The cause typically is a *Streptococcus* organism. Because this is not a closed-space infection, surgical drainage is not performed unless there is localized pus and abscess formation or necrosis.[1]

ANATOMY AND PATHOLOGY

Perionychium

The **perionychium** is composed of the nail bed and the paronychium (the nail fold) (Fig. 20-2). (Note the

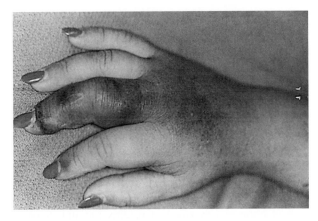

FIGURE 20-1 Cellulitis with redness and edema. (From Mackin EJ, Callahan AD, Skirven TM et al, editors: *Rehabilitation of the hand and upper extremity,* ed 5, St Louis, 2002, Mosby.)

similar spellings of the terms *perionychium, paronychium,* and *paronychia.*) The nail fold is the proximal depression into which the proximal nail fits. The nail fold has a dorsal roof and a volar floor, with the nail in between. Between the nail bed and the distal nail is the hyponychium, which is quite resistant to bacterial contamination.

The nail bed is highly vascularized. If this area is injured but the nail does not break, a **hematoma** (a confined mass of blood) develops. A **subungual hematoma** (i.e., a hematoma beneath the nail) causes throbbing and pain, and associated tuft fractures may be present. Typically, sterile technique is used to evacuate the hematoma to prevent infection.[5]

The fingernails protect the highly sensitive fingertips. They also help regulate temperature and peripheral circulation, facilitate sensory perception in the finger pad, and promote dexterity. An injury in the area of the fingernail may be dismissed as trivial, but it should not be. Deformity or loss of a fingernail has functional and aesthetic implications that may be very important to clients.[6,7]

Paronychia

Paronychia is an infection of the nail fold or nail plate. In acute paronychia the causative organism usually is *Staphylococcus aureus;* in chronic paronychia the organisms involved usually are *Candida albicans* and pyogenic bacteria.[4]

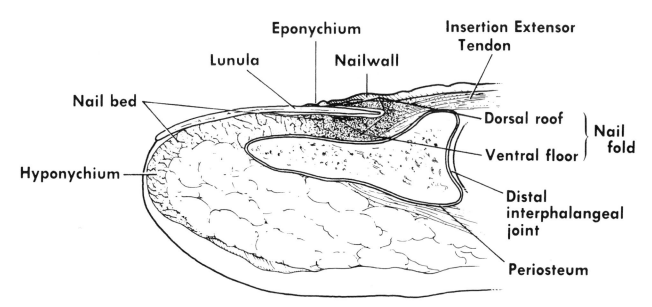

FIGURE 20-2 Anatomy of the nail bed. (From Zook EG, Brown RE: The perionychium. In Green DP, Hotchkiss RN, Pederson WC, editors: *Green's operative hand surgery,* ed 4, Philadelphia, 1999, Churchill Livingstone.)

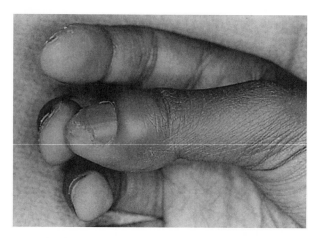

FIGURE 20-3 Acute paronychia with erythema, swelling, and pain at the base of the fingernail. (From Mackin EJ, Callahan AD, Skirven TM et al, editors: *Rehabilitation of the hand and upper extremity,* ed 5, St Louis, 2002, Mosby.)

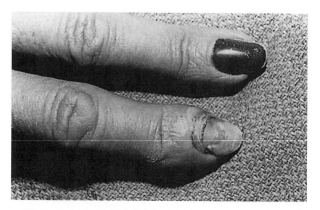

FIGURE 20-4 Chronic paronychia. (From Mackin EJ, Callahan AD, Skirven TM et al, editors: *Rehabilitation of the hand and upper extremity,* ed 5, St Louis, 2002, Mosby.)

CLINICAL *Pearl*

Paronychia is the most common hand infection. It may be acute or chronic.

With acute paronychia, the bacteria may be introduced by a hangnail, an ingrown nail, a tooth (e.g., cuticle or nail biting), or a manicure instrument. Erythema, swelling, and pain are noticeable at the base of the fingernail (Fig. 20-3). In children, paronychia is associated with finger sucking.[8]

Chronic paronychia is more common in people whose hands are frequently exposed to water.[1] This form is much more difficult to resolve than the acute type. Middle-aged women are affected most often, and individuals with diabetes are more susceptible to them (Fig. 20-4).

Artificial and acrylic nails contribute to fungal infections of the nail bed.[4,9] If a client with chronic paronychia uses artificial or acrylic nails, advise her to discontinue using them and explain the reason for this.

Eponychia

Eponychia differs from paronychia in that the infection involves the entire eponychium, along with one lateral fold. In eponychia, pus usually collects near the **lunula,** the white arch visible at the base of some fingernails.[4]

Felon

The finger pulp is divided into small compartments by septa. A **felon** is a deep infection of the finger pad involv-

ing these tiny compartments. Felons are very painful. A puncture wound or open injury usually precipitates the condition, and the thumb and index finger are most often involved. With these infections, pus is under pressure in a small, closed space; consequently, the area is marked by redness and an intense, throbbing pain. Felons have developed after repeated finger-sticks for blood tests.[8]

If a felon is left untreated, the abscess can extend toward the phalanx, leading to **osteomyelitis** (inflammation of bone and marrow) or **osteitis** (inflammation of bone). Felons also can cause skin necrosis and possible obliteration of digital vessels. Pyogenic arthritis of the distal interphalangeal (DIP) joint is another possible adverse effect.[4]

Subepidermal Abscess

Subepidermal abscesses are caused by *S. aureus* (Fig. 20-5). They occur on the volar digital pads between flexor creases or in the palm. If left treated, these infections can worsen, leading to involvement of the flexor sheath or deep compartment in the palm.[1]

Flexor Sheath Infection

Flexor sheath infections are also called **pyogenic flexor tenosynovitis** or **purulent flexor tenosynovitis.** *These are among the most destructive hand infections.* Pyogenic flexor tenosynovitis affects the index, middle, and ring fingers more often than the thumb and small finger. The mechanism typically is a puncture wound over the flexor crease at the metacarpophalangeal (MCP) or interphalangeal (IP) joint, where the skin is very close to the flexor sheath. Because flexor sheaths are poorly vascularized and richly synovial, they are an enticing environment for bacterial growth.[4,8]

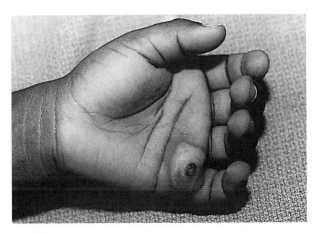

FIGURE 20-5 Subepidermal abscess in the palm of the hand. (From Mackin EJ, Callahan AD, Skirven TM et al, editors: *Rehabilitation of the hand and upper extremity*, ed 5, St Louis, 2002, Mosby.)

Flexor sheath infections may lead to permanent scarring and adhesions with reduced flexor glide, resulting in serious limitations of movement. Tendon necrosis also may occur, with outright destruction of the flexor sheath and progression of the infection.[1]

CLINICAL *Pearl*

Flexor tenosynovitis is recognized by the presence of **Kanavel's cardinal signs**: (1) slight digital flexion, (2) uniform volar swelling of the involved digit, (3) tenderness along the tendon sheath, and (4) pain with passive extension of the involved digit.[1,2,8]

Fascial Space Infection

Pus may develop in any of five fascial spaces, specifically (1) the dorsal subcutaneous space; (2) the dorsal subaponeurotic space; (3) the hypothenar space; (4) the thenar space; and (5) midpalmar space. Surgical drainage usually is performed for fascial space infections.[1]

COMMON MECHANISMS OF INJURY AND INFECTION

Human Bite

Human saliva is full of bacteria. Hand wounds can become contaminated with human saliva by several means: a fist striking the mouth, a bite, a toothpick or dental instrument, or nail biting. A wound caused by a fist striking the mouth is called a **fight bite** or **clenched-fist injury.** As the name implies, this type of injury typically occurs during a fight, and the client often does not seek prompt medical attention because the wound may

be small and appear unimportant. The injury often is seen in the dorsal third, fourth, or fifth metacarpal area, where the skin is supple and thin. The MCP joints are vulnerable areas that offer minimal protection of ligaments and cartilage. By the time the client seeks medical attention, advanced infection may be present.[1,4,8,10]

Animal Bite

All animal bites should be treated promptly and followed closely by medical personnel. Dog bites are more common than cat bites. Because dogs have powerful jaws, their bites tend to be crushing and superficial. Cats' teeth are sharper, therefore cat bites tend to look like punctures; these bites are quite likely to result in an infection.[2]

Some spider bites also can be very serious. With a spider bite, the victim may develop a rash over the torso, arms, and legs, as well as muscle and joint pain, chills, fever, enlarged lymph nodes, headaches, nausea, and vomiting. Remind clients that it is best to seek medical attention if they are in doubt about a bite. Bringing the remains of the spider (even if smashed) to the medical facility can be helpful.

Bite wounds are not sutured immediately because animal bites can quickly cause cellulitis and lymphangitis. Surgical closure, when needed, is postponed until all evidence of infection has resolved.[4]

Intravenous Drug Abuse

Infection can occur in drug users at sites of attempted venous access. The infection may manifest as a subcutaneous abscess, or it may involve joint spaces, flexor sheaths, or fascial spaces. Compliance problems related to drug use may complicate the medical management of these clients.[1]

Mycobacteria

Mycobacterial infections can be difficult to diagnose. When the hand is involved, *Mycobacterium marinum* is the most common cause of these infections. The injury usually is a puncture wound or skin abrasion the client incurs while working with a fish tank or while at a beach, lake, or pool. The infection manifests as a localized tenosynovitis or a chronic skin ulceration.[1] Infectious disease specialists may be involved in identifying the organism and managing the medical regimen.

Viruses

Herpetic whitlow is seen often among dental and medical personnel. It appears as one or more vesicles in the finger pad area. The client may report a history of herpes simplex infection on other parts of the body. The degree of pain reported exceeds the physical finding, and edema and erythema are present. The small, clear vesicles of herpetic whitlow may coalesce, and consequently the condition may be confused with a pyogenic bacterial infection. Medical management of herpetic whitlow involves allowing the virus to run its course. Incision and drainage are not performed because they may result in the development of a bacterial infection.[1,8]

TIMELINES AND HEALING

Time lines and healing for hand infections vary, depending on the client's medical status, the structures involved, and the extent of injury. Compartment release sometimes is required, and more severe cases may result in amputation. Delayed healing may be seen with deep wounds, secondary surgeries, or grafting.

NONOPERATIVE TREATMENT

Prompt wound care helps prevent hand infections. Clients initially may consider an injury a trivial problem and may not seek medical attention.[1] Always remind your clients: *when in doubt, it is safest to consult a medical expert early on.*

CLINICAL *Pearl*

If both infection and acute inflammation are present, the involved area should be immobilized to help prevent the spread of the infection and to reduce pain and edema. The area should be immobilized in a position that prevents deformity or stiffness, such as the **safe position (intrinsic plus position),** with the wrist in slight extension, the MCPs in flexion, and the IPs in extension.

With acute paronychia, early nonoperative treatment consists of medical management with systemic oral antibiotics, warm soaks, and resting the digit. If an abscess forms, surgical drainage is performed. Chronic paronychia is more difficult to treat. In these cases, antimicrobial agents, topical steroids, or antifungal agents may be administered over a prolonged period. A client with chronic paronychia should avoid exposing the hand to moist environments, especially water that contains irritants.[4]

Felons that are not treated within 48 hours usually require surgical drainage. Timely communication with the physician's office is important if the hand therapist

is the first person to recognize early signs of a possible felon. Pyogenic flexor tenosynovitis is best treated within 24 to 48 hours of onset. In this early period, conservative medical management includes administration of antibiotics, immobilization and elevation of the hand and wrist, and observation. If conservative care is sufficient, improvements should be noted within 2 days.

Keep in mind that as a hand therapist, it is not your job to diagnose any of the conditions discussed in this chapter. Instead, describe the clinical appearance to the physician's staff and let them do the diagnosing.

OPERATIVE TREATMENT

Therapy after surgery for a hand infection may include wound care, protective splinting, edema control as needed, and instruction in range of motion (ROM) exercises, depending on the structures involved. Less serious infections and those involving only a distal digit (e.g., paronychia) frequently do not require subsequent hand therapy.

When acute paronychia requires surgery, the nail plate may need to be partly or completely removed, depending on the accumulation of pus beneath the nail. Surgery for chronic paronychia may involve a procedure called *eponychial marsupialization,* in which an elliptic portion of skin in the proximal nail fold is removed.[1]

Felons are treated by surgical drainage, and subepidermal abscesses usually resolve with incision and drainage. Pyogenic flexor tenosynovitis is treated surgically by drainage, which is performed quickly if the condition was not treated initially within 48 hours or if conservative care does not result in resolution within 2 days.

More complicated conditions are most likely to be referred for hand therapy. The postoperative management of these clients must be individualized according to the structures involved and the client's needs.

Questions to Ask the Physician

- *What structures were involved in the infection?*
- *What precautions or guidelines are needed for active range of motion (AROM)?*
- *What are the wound care guidelines?*
- *Do you want the client to do home dressing changes?*
- *Is splinting desired? If so, what structures should be immobilized and in what position? Should the wrist be included in the splint?*

What to Say to Clients

If Infection is Suspected

"Check your hand for redness, swelling, heat, and pain. Call your doctor's office if you develop a fever, if you feel sick, or if you suspect your symptoms are worsening. Identifying these signs early can make a big difference in the speed of your recovery, therefore careful monitoring at home is extremely important."

Postoperative Clients

"It is very important always to keep your hand elevated above your heart so as to minimize swelling. Swelling leads to stiffness and pain, and managing swelling early promotes faster healing. It also makes it easier for you to recover function in the hand."

EVALUATION TIPS

- Do not cause unnecessary pain by evaluating ROM if infection is suspected. Defer any parts of the evaluation that are painful or that may later turn out to have been contraindicated.
- Before evaluating passive range of motion (PROM), find out whether it is contraindicated.
- If infection is suspected, describe and measure the symptomatic area (e.g., mark the erythematous portion) so that you can check for changes on the client's next visit.
- Check dressings for drainage and note the quality of the wound and the drainage (see Evaluation, Chapter 5).
- Watch for and document skin maceration.
- Monitor and document redness around sites of pins or other fixation devices. Pin tract infections can lead to osteomyelitis or osteitis. Instruct the client in pin site care according to the physician's preferences.

DIAGNOSIS-SPECIFIC INFORMATION THAT AFFECTS CLINICAL REASONING

When the therapist suspects that an infection is present, deciding how much supervision the client needs can be difficult. You also may not be sure when you should contact the physician's office. Try to determine the client's ability to monitor and manage the situation. If you feel you should contact the physician's office, try to do this while the client is with you in therapy.

Precaution. *It is better to have it documented that the physician's office was called than to wish later that this had been done.*

Make sure you give the client written instructions about calling the physician's office if symptoms persist or worsen. If the client cannot participate fully (perhaps because of cognitive or behavioral reasons), recommend

more therapy visits so that you can monitor the situation closely.

Wound care guidelines, including whether the area can be gotten wet, are determined by the physician. Reinforce these guidelines and explain that *getting an infected area wet can worsen the infection*. If the client lives in a hot climate, be extra careful to check for maceration caused by perspiration and to adjust the dressing guidelines as appropriate.

TIPS FROM THE FIELD
Splinting

Splinting is determined by the structures involved. Discuss splinting options with both the physician and the client and offer more than one choice if possible. If a client has digital stiffness after a metacarpal fracture but then develops flexor tenosynovitis, immobilization for the tenosynovitis will lead to greater stiffness of the hand. However, the tenosynovitis may be causing such pain that immobilization is necessary at least temporarily.

Wound Care

Practice wound care in therapy. If the client has someone to help perform dressing changes, include that person in therapy and practice together. Provide written instructions. When possible, provide sample dressings so that the client is more likely to buy the correct materials. Instruct the client not to change the dressing process unless advised to do so by the therapist or the physician's office.

Client Expectations

Clients may have a difficult time appreciating the complexity of their infection. Explain the implications but try to emphasize the positive aspects. Explain that managing the infection now will lead to less swelling and scarring, with quicker medical clearance to resume exercises.

Precautions and Concerns

- *Watch for redness, swelling, heat, and pain. Instruct clients also to check for these signs at home if they are performing dressing changes.*
- *Instruct clients to take their temperature and to notify the physician's office if they develop a fever.*
- *If the client is not complying with dressing guidelines (e.g., getting dressings wet or dirty), document this in the record.*

The Role of Therapy Assistants

- Reinforcing instructions regarding signs of inflammation
- Performing dressing changes
- Instructing the client and family in dressing changes and practicing these together
- Providing home instruction in wound care
- Assisting in wound inspection
- Modifying and refurbishing splints
- Performing exercises as supervised by the therapist
- Promoting maximal function with modifications for activities of daily living as appropriate
- Reinforcing precautions for wound care and dressings

CASE *Studies*

CASE 20-1

C.R., a female client, was bitten by a dog she was caring for in preparation for its adoption from the pound. She had multiple bites on the dominant left hand. The hand became infected, and she was hospitalized for intravenous antibiotic treatment.

After discharge from the hospital, C.R. was seen by a hand surgeon, who diagnosed her as having possible partial lacerations of the left extensor indicis proprius (EIP) and extensor pollicis longus (EPL) tendons. The hand surgeon indicated that she did not need surgical exploration at that time and that management through therapy was advised.

C.R.'s hand was very stiff and swollen. She lacked composite flexion of all digits. She had tightness of the index MCP joint with limitation of MCP passive flexion, but she also had an extensor lag at the MCP. Her thumb lacked composite flexion and also had an IP extensor lag. Bite scars were becoming hypertrophic in several sites and were adherent over the index MCP.

C.R. made good progress with manual edema mobilization (MEM), splinting, and exercise. The therapist monitored for signs of recurrent infection throughout her care. Because she had EPL involvement, a static splint supported her thumb in composite extension. Because she had EIP involvement, the same hand-based splint also provided index MCP extension. The therapist monitored the MCP joint tightness and corrected this condition with exercises for MCP flexion while observing for and preventing worsening of the MCP extensor lag. Extrinsic extensor tightness of the index and thumb resolved with exercise, and the therapist made sure not to create extensor lags by over-exercising flexion. Scar manage-

ment, psychologic support to help C.R. deal with her new fear of dogs, and incorporating home repair chores (her goal for recovery) into her exercises all helped the client improve. C.R. made excellent progress and was discharged from therapy with no edema, no extensor lags, full composite flexion of all digits, and signs of scar maturation in progress. All function was restored, although the hand scars bothered her cosmetically. C.R.'s case provides an example of the complicated sequelae that can be associated with hand infections.

CASE 20-2

B.F., an adult male construction worker, suffered a crushing injury at work. The dominant right index proximal phalanx was fractured, requiring percutaneous pin fixation, and the index flexor digitorum profundus (FDP) tendon was lacerated, requiring surgical repair. B.F. frequently came to therapy with filthy dressings and with evidence of dirt seeping inside his dressings to his wounds. The pin site was erythematous and painful. The physician prescribed treatment with oral antibiotics, and the physician and therapist instructed the client to keep the dressings dry and clean.

One day B.F. arrived for therapy with no dressings; instead he wore a waterproof Band-Aid that he had kept in place for about 48 hours. This Band-Aid was difficult to remove because of its strong adhesive. Underneath, the incision site was dehiscent and extremely macerated. The wound was deep and producing a serous discharge.

B.F.'s physician was called, and he was seen by the physician assistant that day. He was reinstructed in the proper use of dressings and was monitored closely until wound healing eventually occurred. The delay in wound healing caused a delay in medical clearance to initiate protected ROM. At discharge the client had stiffness of the index finger, which might have been less prevalent if his recovery had not been compromised.

CASE 20-3

H.W., a male client, sustained a fight bite of the left hand and a fracture of the left small finger metacarpal. Because he did not think his injury was serious, he did not promptly seek medical attention. He described himself as having "a problem with anger."

The fracture was treated with percutaneous pin fixation. Intravenous antibiotics were prescribed, and the client was not medically cleared to work at his job in heavy construction. The inability to work resulted in financial hardships for him, and he had limited insurance coverage for hand therapy. He was visibly frustrated by all of this and occasionally became agitated and angry in hand therapy.

H.W. thought that if he exercised aggressively, he would recover his hand function more quickly. Also, he was not accustomed to taking advice from females. H.W. painted his house without dressing protection. He overexerted with exercises and exceeded the tissue tolerances of his hand, despite the therapist's many attempts to explain that this would only slow his progress and could exacerbate the infection.

At discharge, the infection had cleared and ROM was adequate to allow H.W. to resume work tasks. However, he had residual MCP joint tightness that limited flexion, MCP extensor lag, and lack of full composite small finger flexion. The therapist recommended continued therapy, but he declined.

References

1. Nathan R, Taras JS: Common infections in the hand. In Mackin EJ, Callahan AD, Skirven TM et al, editors: *Rehabilitation of the hand and upper extremity*, ed 5, St Louis, 2002, Mosby.

2. Daniels JM, Zook EG, Lynch JM: Hand and wrist injuries. Part II. Emergent evaluation, *Am Fam Phys* 69:1949-1956, 2004.

3. Thomas CL: *Taber's Cyclopedic Medical Dictionary*, ed 13, Philadelphia, 1977, FA Davis.

4. Neviaser RJ: Acute infections. In Green DP, Hotchkiss RN, Pederson WC, editors: *Green's operative hand surgery*, ed 4, Philadelphia, 1999, Churchill Livingstone.

5. Wang QC, Johnson BA: Fingertip injuries, *Am Fam Phys* 63:1961-1966, 2001.

6. Zook EG: Anatomy and physiology of the perionychium, *Hand Clin* 18:553-559, 2002.

7. Zook EG, Brown RE: The perionychium. In Green DP, Hotchkiss RN, Pederson WC, editors: *Green's operative hand surgery*, ed 4, Philadelphia, 1999, Churchill Livingstone.

8. Clark DC: Common acute hand infections, *Am Fam Phys* 68:2167-2176, 2003.

9. Brown RE: Acute nail bed injuries, *Hand Clin* 18:561-575, 2002.

10. Chang M-C, Huang Y-L, Lo W-H: Infectious complications associated with toothpick injuries of the hand, *J Hand Surg* 28A:327-331, 2003.

21

Ganglion Cysts and Other Common Tumors of the Hand and Wrist

CYNTHIA COOPER

Basal cell carcinoma

Bowler's thumb

Carpometacarpal boss

Cutaneous fibrous histiocytomas

Dermatofibromas

Dorsal retinacular ganglion

Dorsal wrist ganglion

Enchondromas

Epidermal inclusion cyst

Fibrolipoma

Ganglion cyst

Giant cell tumors (xanthomas)

Glomus body

Glomus tumor

Hemangioma

Lipomas

Localized nodular tenosynovitis

Localized pigmented villonodular synovitis

Lymphangioma

Malignant melanoma

Mucous cyst

Neurilemomas

Neurofibromas

Occult dorsal carpal ganglion

Pulsatile

Pyogenic granuloma

Sarcomas

Schwannomas

Squamous cell carcinoma

Tendon sheath fibromas

Vascular tumor

Verruca vulgaris

Volar retinacular ganglion

Volar wrist ganglion

Xanthoma

GANGLION CYSTS

Ganglion cysts are the most common soft tissue tumors of the hand and wrist. They account for 50% to 70% of the masses found in this location. The onset of these cysts may be sudden or slow, and they can resolve spontaneously.

DIAGNOSIS AND PATHOLOGY

A **ganglion cyst** arises from the synovial lining of either a joint or a tendon sheath. The cyst usually is attached to the tendon, the tendon sheath, or the joint capsule. The etiology of ganglion cysts is unknown, although synovial herniation, mucoid degeneration, and trauma have been mentioned in the literature.[1] Women have more ganglions than men. The cysts appear most often in the second through fourth decades of life, but they can develop at any age, and pediatric cases are not rare.[1,2]

ANATOMIC SITES

The most common site of a ganglion cyst is the dorsal radial wrist (Fig. 21-1). A **dorsal wrist ganglion** usually originates in the area of the scapholunate ligament. A ganglion cyst may invade bone; this happens most often in the scapholunate area, but involvement of the capitate also has been reported.[1] Differential diagnoses for wrist ganglion cysts include lipomas, extensor tenosynovitis, and other tumors.[1]

The **volar wrist ganglion** is the second most common ganglion of the hand and wrist. During surgery, this type of ganglion sometimes is found to be much more extensive than expected. Volar wrist ganglions develop over the scaphoid tubercle (arising from the scaphotrapezial joint) or over the distal edge of the radius (arising from the radiocarpal joint) (Fig. 21-2). Branches of the radial artery may be intertwined with the cyst.[2]

The **volar retinacular ganglion** is the third most common ganglion cyst. This ganglion arises from the A1 pulley of the flexor tendon sheath of a digit. Volar retinacular ganglions are small, measuring about 3 to 8 mm. The cyst is a tender, firm, palpable mass that forms under the metacarpophalangeal (MCP) flexion crease, close to the digital nerve (Fig. 21-3).

A ganglion that is attached to the first extensor compartment is called a **dorsal retinacular ganglion.** A client

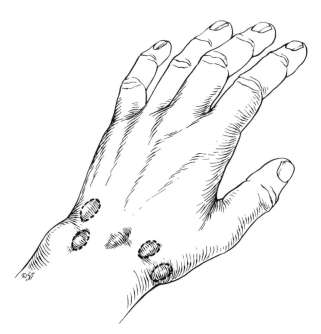

FIGURE 21-1 Sites where dorsal wrist ganglions may occur. The most common site is over the scapholunate ligament. (From Athanasian EA: Bone and soft tissue tumors. In Green DP, Hotchkiss R, Pedersen W et al, editors: *Green's operative hand surgery*, ed 5, Philadelphia, 2005, Churchill Livingstone.)

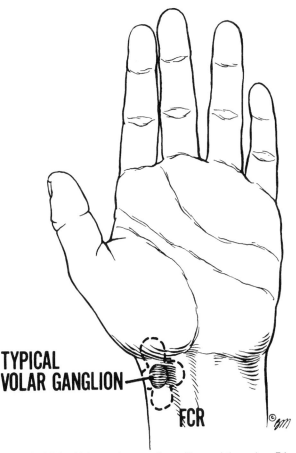

TYPICAL VOLAR GANGLION

FCR

FIGURE 21-2 Volar wrist ganglion. (From Athanasian EA: Bone and soft tissue tumors. In Green DP, Hotchkiss R, Pedersen W et al, editors: *Green's operative hand surgery*, ed 5, Philadelphia, 2005, Churchill Livingstone.)

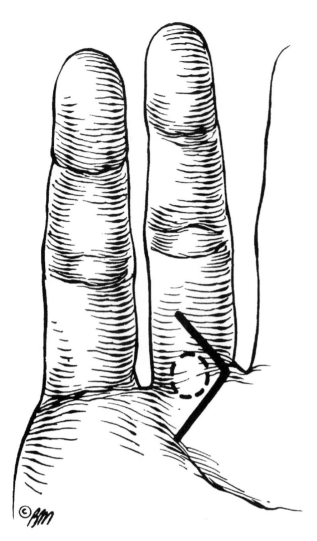

FIGURE 21-3 Volar retinacular ganglion. (From Athanasian EA: Bone and soft tissue tumors. In Green DP, Hotchkiss R, Pedersen W et al, editors: *Green's operative hand surgery*, ed 5, Philadelphia, 2005, Churchill Livingstone.)

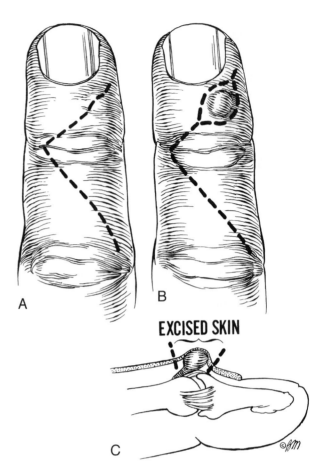

EXCISED SKIN

FIGURE 21-4 Mucous cyst. (From Athanasian EA: Bone and soft tissue tumors. In Green DP, Hotchkiss R, Pedersen W et al, editors: *Green's operative hand surgery*, ed 5, Philadelphia, 2005, Churchill Livingstone.)

with this type of ganglion usually has symptoms of de Quervain's tenosynovitis.[2]

An **occult dorsal carpal ganglion** is small and difficult to palpate, which differentiates it from a dorsal wrist ganglion. This type of ganglion may be overlooked during an examination; palpating with the wrist in extreme volar flexion can be helpful for detecting these cysts. Occult dorsal carpal ganglions usually are disproportionately painful and may be the cause of undiagnosed wrist pain. Differential diagnoses for an occult dorsal carpal ganglion include scapholunate ligament sprain and carpal instability. A thorough medical examination is important, because other conditions, as well as the ganglion, may be present.[2]

A **mucous cyst** is associated with degenerative arthritis of the small joints of the hand. The distal interpha-langeal (DIP) joint is the most common site. Clients who have these cysts usually are 50 to 70 years of age. Longitudinal nail grooving may be an early clinical sign of a mucous cyst. The cyst typically measures 3 to 5 mm and is situated between the dorsal DIP joint crease and the eponychium, to one side of the extensor tendon (Fig. 21-4). A differential diagnosis for a mucous cyst is Heberden's node (see Chapter 17).[2]

The ganglions described previously account for 90% of ganglion cysts found in the hand. The remaining 10% occur at other sites. A **carpometacarpal boss** is an osteoarthritic spur at the base of the second or third carpometacarpal (CMC) joint (or both). A boss is more evident as a prominent, firm, bony, tender mass when the wrist is flexed. Bosses occur more often in women than in men, usually between 30 and 40 years of age. They can be quite painful but may also be asymptomatic, and they may be confused with a dorsal wrist ganglion.[2] A dorsal proximal interphalangeal (PIP) joint ganglion is similar to the more common mucous cyst at the distal interphalangeal (DIP) joint. PIP joint ganglions are small and tender and may impede joint mobility. Ganglions also may develop within or on extensor tendons, typically over the metacarpals. These ganglions move proximally with digital extension, and they are associated with pain and snapping of the tendon during finger motion. Differential diagnoses include carpal boss and dorsal wrist ganglion. Ganglion cysts of the perionychium are closely associated with osteoarthritis of the DIP joint. Like a mucous cyst, a ganglion of the perionychium may cause a groove, ridge, or split in the fingernail.[3]

TIMELINES AND HEALING

Individuals vary in the amount of time it takes them to seek medical attention for a ganglion cyst. Some clients are bothered by the appearance of the cyst; others see their physician because the cyst is painful or they fear they may have a more serious tumor.

NONOPERATIVE TREATMENT

Conservative treatment of ganglion cysts at the wrist includes splinting and aspiration of the cyst, along with reassurance of the client that the mass is not malignant. Success has been reported with conservative care, even if multiple aspirations are necessary.[1,2] Many physicians recommend delaying surgery because of the postoperative complications of pain and stiffness. Scarring is also a concern for some clients.[1,2]

For mucous cysts, aspiration with or without injection of a steroid can be curative, but the recurrence rate exceeds 50%. The advantages of conservative treatment are that it can be performed conveniently in the physician's office and it is less invasive.[4] For volar retinacular ganglion cysts, needle rupture may eliminate the need for surgery, but this technique is not used often because possible injury of the radial artery is a concern. Aspiration is not performed if the ganglion cyst is located in a place where aspiration could injure a digital nerve.[1]

OPERATIVE TREATMENT

Decisions about surgery are not easy to make. Ganglion cysts frequently recur after surgical treatment, and recurrence is more likely if the ganglion was not completely excised. Other problems include persistent pain, stiffness, scarring, and nerve involvement.[1,2]

Surgery is recommended when a ganglion cyst is symptomatic (e.g., it causes nerve compression). Some authors suggest excising the joint capsule to prevent recurrence of a ganglion cyst at the wrist.[1] However, others have noted scaphoid rotary subluxation in association with this procedure.[1]

A bulky dressing is applied after surgery for a dorsal wrist ganglion. The client should keep the hand elevated and should perform proximal and also digital active range of motion (AROM) exercises. A smaller dressing is applied and wrist AROM is started after about 5 days. Wrist volar flexion exercises are important, because this motion may be limited initially. Sutures remain for about 2 weeks after surgery, and therapy continues until full range of motion (ROM) is achieved.[2] Static progressive splinting can be helpful if recovery of wrist ROM is difficult.

Therapy after surgery for a volar wrist ganglion is similar to that for a dorsal wrist ganglion. Wrist AROM exercises usually are started within the first 2 weeks, but the physician decides the course of therapy according to the client's needs.

For mucous cysts, simple excision is a less invasive option, but it is associated with a 28% recurrence rate. More extensive surgery involves complete excision of the stalk of the cyst, along with joint arthrotomy, capsulectomy, and excision of arthritic osteophytes. If the skin over the ganglion is thin or fragile, skin grafting may be required. The opposite side of the digit also is explored during surgery so that any occult cysts or hypertrophied synovial tissue can be detected and removed.[2] Complications of complete excision include nail deformity, persistent pain and swelling, and stiffness.[4] Some clients are concerned about finger cosmesis after surgery.

Questions to Ask the Physician

- *What structures were involved?*
- *If the ganglion was at the wrist: Is wrist stability a concern?*
- *What are the medical expectations for recovery of ROM?*
- *When is AROM to be initiated?*
- *What precautions are required (e.g., no PROM)?*
- *Are special guidelines necessary for wound care?*
- *Is a splint recommended? If so, in what position?*

What to Say to Clients

If Some Stiffness Is Expected after Surgery

"Your doctor has indicated that you may have some residual wrist stiffness. The priority here is to achieve a pain-free, stable wrist with movement that allows you to perform all your activities comfortably. It's important not to be aggressive or to push yourself when exercising. Avoid pain and focus more on the quality of your exercises so that they are done gently. This will prevent undesirable stress on your wrist while it heals."

EVALUATION TIPS

- Make decisions according to the situation. Defer circumferential measurements or volumetric measurements if a healing wound is present.
- Take special care to perform the initial ROM evaluation gently. These clients can be reluctant to move and may be concerned that ROM will disrupt healing. Do not measure PROM if this is contraindicated.

DIAGNOSIS-SPECIFIC INFORMATION THAT AFFECTS CLINICAL REASONING

If wrist stability is a concern, to not perform PROM exercises and make sure you have medical clearance before upgrading the program. If your client wants to try to recover wrist ROM quickly, explain that the clinical priority is pain-free stability, which is more important than maximal ROM at the risk of pain and instability. If necessary, remind the client often of this fact.

TIPS FROM THE FIELD

Splinting

Think about the purpose of splinting and make decisions accordingly. If appropriate and when permitted by the physician, use of a static progressive splint may be helpful for recovering wrist flexion after excision of a dorsal wrist ganglion.

A protective splint may be ordered for mucous cysts at the DIP. Try to promote maximum airflow over the area of the dorsal incision. Also try to avoid placing straps directly over the incision. This small splint may need to be taped in place at night time so that it is not dislodged during sleep. Instruct the client in PIP AROM of the involved digit and, when appropriate, perform isolated DIP blocking exercises of the uninvolved digits to prevent the development of a quadriga effect.

Client Expectations

The key to clinical success is a client with realistic expectations who accepts the possibilities of scarring and some stiffness. Spend as much time as necessary to educate the client about realistic clinical expectations. If a client seems overly concerned with measurable ROM gains that are inappropriate, focus on function. Monitor for signs of overexercising and keep explaining to the client that the quickest way to recover ROM is to work according to tissue tolerances. As necessary, remind clients that overexercising leads to stiffness and actually slows their progress; these can be difficult lessons for clients to learn.

Precautions and Concerns

- *Monitor wound healing and avoid exercises that disturb this.*
- *Following excision of ganglions at the wrist, emphasize proximal and digital ROM and explain that this will help overall recovery of wrist ROM.*
- *Keep balancing the concepts of pain-free stability with client desires to recover maximum ROM.*
- *Clients with mucous cysts often have DJD of the DIP joints of other digits. If this is the case, use caution with DIP AROM and encourage only pain-free DIP exercises of those digits.*

The Role of the Therapy Assistant

- Monitoring wound status
- Changing dressings and instructing the client in home dressing procedures
- Checking and modifying splints
- Performing exercises and upgrading the home exercise program as supervised by the therapist
- Instructing the client in modifications of activities of daily living to promote maximum function during the recovery of motion

OTHER COMMON TUMORS

Most soft tissue tumors of the forearm and hand are benign. Tumors can arise from fat, blood vessels, lymph vessels, nerves, skin, or bone.

DIAGNOSIS AND PATHOLOGY

Most hand tumors are painless; the exceptions are glomus tumors and tumors that put pressure on a nerve. A calcified tumor tends to appear more like an infection than a tumor. An excisional biopsy usually is performed if the soft tissue is solid. A tumor that varies in size is likely to be a ganglion cyst. A tumor that grows rapidly may raise suspicion of a malignancy, as does an excised tumor that quickly recurs.[1]

Types of Tumors

Giant cell tumors (xanthomas) are the most common solid tumors of the hand. Other names for this tumor are **localized nodular tenosynovitis** and **localized pigmented villonodular synovitis.** Giant cell tumors are grayish brown with yellow patches.[1] Despite their various names, giant cell tumors do not tend to be located at a tendon sheath and they do not exclusively contain giant cells.[5]

Lipomas, a common type of tumor composed of mature fat cells, are characterized by their soft consistency on palpation. Lipomas can arise anywhere fatty tissue exists, but they most often develop in the deep palmar space of the hand. Lipomas normally are asymptomatic and grow slowly; if symptoms develop, the cause usually is nerve compression. A lipoma that has a connective tissue component is called a **fibrolipoma.**[1]

Vascular tumors usually are congenital in origin. Failure of embryonic differentiation results in a **hemangioma** (a benign tumor of dilated blood vessels), a **lymphangioma** (a tumor of lymphatic vessels), or a congenital arteriovenous fistula. These tumors tend to enlarge slowly after birth and may become symptomatic. Diagnosis is facilitated by the reddish blue or blue color of the tumor. Some vascular tumors are **pulsatile** (i.e., they have a pulse). Vascular tumors that are not congenital are aneurysms, arteriovenous fistulas, pyogenic granulomas, or glomus tumors.

A **pyogenic granuloma** appears as a red mass that bleeds easily. It is categorized as a vascular tumor because it has abundant capillary granulation. This lesion is believed to occur after a traumatic injury that also involved an infection.[1]

A **glomus tumor** arises from either the neuromyoarterial apparatus or the **glomus body,** an arteriovenous anastomosis in the skin that functions as a thermoregulator. Glomus tumors tend to occur subungually (beneath the nail) and in distal finger pads. They cause cold sensitivity, lancing pain, and tenderness. Over time, glomus tumors can lead to erosion of bone.[1]

An **epidermal inclusion cyst** develops after an injury in which a segment of keratinizing epithelium is forced into subcutaneous tissue, where it produces keratin and becomes a tumor. These cysts occur most often in men 30 to 40 years of age, and the most common site is the distal phalanx of the left thumb and long finger.[5]

Nerve tumors are rare. The two most common types are **neurilemomas** (also called **schwannomas**) and **neurofibromas.** These tumor types differ histologically, although both are benign. Neurilemomas usually can be excised without damaging nerve fibers, whereas neurofibromas generally cannot be excised without destruction of nerve tissue. Neurilemomas arise from the Schwann's cells that surround nerve fibers. They tend to be found on the flexor forearm or hand in clients 40 to 60 years of age, and they may be misdiagnosed as ganglion cysts.[5]

Bowler's thumb is a fibrous enlargement of the nerve caused by repeated trauma of the thumb against the bowling ball. **Tendon sheath fibromas** are painless, solid tumors that grow slowly. Histologically, these tumors show no giant cells.

Epithelial tumors include **verruca vulgaris,** the common wart, which is benign and is caused by the human papillomavirus. Trauma may precede the development of warts, which are spread by contact. **Dermatofibromas,** also called **cutaneous fibrous histiocytomas,** are epithelial tumors composed of fibroblastic cells and some scattered histiocytes.[1]

Enchondromas, the most common primary bone tumors of hand bones, are benign, cartilaginous lesions. They account for 90% of hand bone tumors. Approximately 35% of these tumors occur in the hand. The most common location is the proximal phalanx, then the metacarpal, then the middle phalanx. Enchondromas do not normally develop in the carpus, although such cases have been reported.[5] An enchondroma may manifest as an area of localized, painless swelling, or it may be diagnosed after a pathologic fracture caused by minor trauma.[5]

Malignant epithelial tumors are associated with sun exposure, and the incidence of these tumors is on the rise.[1] The three types of malignant epithelial tumors are **basal cell carcinoma,** which is not common in the hand; **squamous cell carcinoma,** which can be fatal; and **malignant melanoma,** which arises from the melanocytes of the epidermis.[1]

Sarcomas are cancers that arise from muscle, vessels, fat, and fibrous tissue. They rarely develop in the forearm or hand. Sarcomas are categorized by their cell origin (e.g., fibrosarcoma and synovial sarcoma), and they can metastasize.[1,5]

TIMELINES AND HEALING

Timelines and healing for tumors vary, depending on the clinical situation. A complex case may involve a history of radiation therapy, resulting in poor tissue quality and slower healing. Each case must be discussed individually with the physician.

NONOPERATIVE TREATMENT

- Many *hemangiomas* resolve spontaneously, therefore delaying treatment is the customary practice for those that appear soon after birth.
- *Warts* are treated nonsurgically (e.g., with cauterization or cryotherapy).

OPERATIVE TREATMENT

- *Giant cell tumors* tend to be well encapsulated and usually can be excised completely. Recurrence rates of up to 10% have been reported.[1]
- Large *lipomas* can be difficult to excise. The recurrence rate is reported to be low.[1]
- *Hemangiomas* can be painful. Surgery for a hemangioma of the hand can be complex, and problems with avascularity can develop after surgery. Precise

techniques and close follow-up are necessary. Surgery for a *lymphangioma* is similarly challenging in terms of separating normal and abnormal tissues, but it usually is less problematic with regard to distal avascularity.

- *Pyogenic granulomas* are excised.
- *Glomus tumors* are excised.
- *Inclusion cysts* are excised. Recurrence may be related to incomplete removal of all epithelial cells from the subcutaneous area.
- As noted previously, *neurilemomas* usually can be excised without damage to nerve fibers. Because *neurofibromas* arise within the fasciculi of nerves, they tend to be more difficult to remove completely. Neurofibromas can occur as a solitary lesion or as several lesions, as is seen in von Recklinghausen's disease. Postoperative neurologic deficits are not uncommon with neurofibromas.[5]
- *Tendon sheath fibromas* are more difficult to excise than giant cell tumors, and surgery may involve the neurovascular bundle.
- *Dermatofibromas* usually are excised for differential diagnosis and to rule out malignancy.
- Surgical treatment of *malignant tumors* depends on the clinical findings. Extensive surgery and reconstruction may be required, and tendon transfers may be performed. Nerve function may be affected.

Questions to Ask the Physician

- *What structures were involved?*
- *What are the guidelines for wound care?*
- *What are the precautions and guidelines for AROM?*
- *What types of splinting, if any, are desired?*

What to Say to Clients

All guidelines related to tumor surgery depend on the clinical details of the individual case. Offer the client reassurance about recovering function as appropriate. Clients frequently ask therapists whether they have seen this type of case before; answer honestly. Explain the clinical expectations according to the physician's instructions and the surgical reports.

EVALUATION TIPS

- Be gentle and supportive. Tumors are scary to clients. The client may have gone through a difficult emotional time worrying about malignancy and may also be dealing with the impact of serious findings. Some clients may be undergoing radiation treatment or chemotherapy concurrently with hand therapy. They may not feel well while in your clinic. Appointments may be difficult to schedule if a client is on a rigorous medical regimen.
- Prioritize wound healing.
- Try to avoid any aspect of evaluation that causes pain.

DIAGNOSIS-SPECIFIC INFORMATION THAT AFFECTS CLINICAL REASONING

Ask about the history of the situation. In some cases, clients have gone through weeks or months of testing before the condition was finally diagnosed. Their lives and activity levels may be consumed by this. Helping them restore some normalcy in their lives may be as important as the medical and clinical aspects of your intervention. Work to achieve the best possible rapport with these clients.

Learn what structures were involved and anticipate the associated functional implications. Even minimal residual stiffness of a small finger DIP joint can be extremely frustrating to some clients.

No two clients with tumors are alike, even if the diagnoses are the same. A golfer with minimal stiffness after excision of a tendon sheath fibroma may be devastated by his residual limitations, whereas a young woman with sarcoma may undergo multiple tendon transfers and be fully functional. These experiences can be challenging and rewarding, both personally and professionally.

TIPS FROM THE FIELD
Splinting

Try to make splints functional whenever possible. Also, when feasible, teach clients how to put on and take off the splint by themselves. In complicated cases, a dynamic splint may provide function and a static splint may be needed for resting involved structures.

Client Expectations

Promote realistic but hopeful expectations for a functional recovery with a return to previous activity levels. Work with both the family and the client to achieve this. Find out what activities are most important to the client and incorporate these into treatment as soon as possible.

Precautions and Concerns

- *Make sure you understand the medical picture.*
- *Monitor wounds for signs of infection or slowed healing.*
- *Work closely with the physician throughout the course of care.*

The Role of the Therapy Assistant

- Providing modifications of activities of daily living and adaptive devices to maximize client's ability to function
- Monitoring wound healing
- Changing dressings and instructing clients in home dressing guidelines
- Checking and modifying splints
- Practicing and reinforcing appropriate exercises as supervised by the therapist

CASE *Studies*

CASE 21-1

Ganglion Cyst

R.S., a 34-year-old, left-dominant single mother of two small children, underwent excision of a left dorsal wrist ganglion and was referred to therapy after surgery. She works two jobs, and she had difficulty making time for her therapy appointments because of her busy work and family schedule.

R.S. was extremely hesitant to move her wrist when AROM was started, although the incision site was clean and dry. Pain was not a problem, but she feared "tearing something inside." The surgeon expected her to recover full wrist flexion. After a few weeks of therapy, she had good wrist extension, normal digital function, and normal proximal ROM but only about 5 degrees of wrist flexion. Her program was upgraded, but she still did not make progress. With the physician's approval, a static progressive wrist flexion splint was recommended, but R.S. refused the splint. She stated that she did not want to have to rely on a splint to recover and that she was concerned about the cost. The therapist documented that the splint had been recommended and refused. After a few more weeks, the therapist persuaded R.S. to try the static progressive splint. The client loved it because it was comfortable to use and she saw immediate results. One month later she was discharged from therapy with normal wrist flexion and extension.

CASE 21-2

Fibrosarcoma

A.L., a 64-year-old female, had undergone seven previous surgeries and radiation therapy for fibrosarcoma of the dominant right forearm. With every surgery she had been prepared for the possibility of amputation. The tumor had recently recurred, and she again underwent excision, with radiation therapy and tendon transfers for wrist and MCP extension function of all digits.

Healing was significantly delayed after surgery; large areas of thick eschar took over 8 weeks to heal. Medically, A.L. was not a candidate for grafting or debridement. She had been scheduled for more radiation therapy, but this was not done because of the compromised healing.

Because of the delayed healing and poor circulation, the hand therapist had to be very conservative with A.L.'s program. During the day, the client used a dynamic MCP extension splint with a short arc of motion protocol; at night, she wore a static extension splint. Because she lived 2 hours from the clinic, she requested as independent a program as possible. She was seen weekly.

When healing finally occurred, A.L.'s program was upgraded to promote functional grasp and pinch while avoiding worsening extensor lags. She had only minimal wrist flexion because of scarring, but she had functional wrist extension. She had MCP extensor lags throughout, but she also had enough composite flexion to hold large-handled implements.

A.L. loved to crochet. Her favorite devices from hand therapy were the functional splints that enabled her to hold her crochet hook. She was realistic in her expectations throughout therapy, and she commented more than once that she was just happy to have kept her arm. She celebrated every functional task she was able to perform.

CASE 21-3

Glomus Tumor

P.G., a female executive, underwent excision of a recurrent glomus tumor of the dominant right small finger. Her finger had become extremely painful, and she had undergone months of diagnostic testing. She even had become dependent on narcotics for pain relief. P.G.'s pain persisted after surgery. She had excruciating cold intolerance, which led to guarded posturing and resultant hand stiffness. She developed complex regional pain syndrome (CRPS), and her dependency on narcotics continued. She lost her job because she was unable to work.

P.G. required months of hand therapy, along with a coordinated pain management program. Teamwork and close communication were essential in this case. Over time she improved clinically, and the CRPS resolved. Hand and wrist ROM were functional, but she remained extremely sensitive in the incision area of the right small finger. In addition to undergoing a complete rehabilitation program for CRPS, the client was instructed in many alternatives for protecting the distal small finger. She stated that she believed these measures had been quite helpful for managing her pain and facilitating improved function.

References

1. Bush DC: Soft tissue tumors of the forearm and hand. In Mackin EJ, Callahan AD, Skirven TM et al, editors: *Rehabilitation of the hand and upper extremity*, ed 5, St Louis, 2002, Mosby.
2. Angelides AC: Ganglions of the hand and wrist. In Green DP, Hotchkiss RN, Pederson WC, editors: *Green's operative hand surgery*, ed 4, Philadelphia, 1999, Churchill Livingstone.
3. Sommer N, Neumeister MW: Tumors of the perionychium, *Hand Clin* 18:673-689, 2002.
4. Rizzo M, Beckenbaugh RD: Treatment of mucous cysts of the fingers: review of 134 cases with minimum 2-year follow-up evaluation, *J Hand Surg* 28A:519-524, 2003.
5. Athanasian EA: Bone and soft tissue tumors. In Green DP, Hotchkiss RN, Pederson WC, editors: *Green's operative hand surgery*, ed 4, Philadelphia, 1999, Churchill Livingstone.

22

Traumatic Hand Injury Involving Multiple Structures

PAIGE E. KURTZ

Traumatic hand injuries can be both the most daunting and the most rewarding conditions that hand therapists treat. Deciding where to start with a new evaluation can be intimidating for a therapist; however, once therapy is underway, and throughout the rehabilitation process, participating in a client's recovery can be remarkable and rewarding, from initial evaluation to final status and good function.

The systems approach is the easiest way to evaluate traumatic and complex injuries. Consider each individual system involved; then, for each system, determine the stage of the injury and how it can best be treated in light of necessary precautions. This approach makes it much easier to prioritize and treat each system according to its stage. Systems that should be considered include the skin (wound/graft), tendons (flexors or extensors or both), nerves, blood vessels (veins and arteries), and bones (fractures, fusions, and joint surfaces). Pain and edema are additional considerations.

Plan ahead throughout the course of therapy. If future surgery is likely, incorporate that fact into the goals of therapy and treatment planning. For example, if tenolysis or tendon grafting is likely, maximize passive range of motion (PROM); if tendon transfer is expected, maximize the strength of potential donor muscles. During the process, continually educate your client about what may be coming next.

Most traumatic hand injuries involve many different structures and systems. The most extreme and complex injuries require a **replant;** that is, an amputated finger, hand, or arm is reattached surgically to re-establish viability and function. Not all traumatic hand injuries involve a replant or **revascularization** (a surgical procedure to repair severed arteries or veins to restore blood supply to a limb). However, the precautions and the decision-making and treatment processes are similar across the spectrum of these injuries.

CLINICAL *Pearl*

Keep in mind that the goal of rehabilitation after a traumatic injury is not to regain a completely normal hand, but rather to regain maximal function with minimal pain.

As soon as possible, determine the reasonable functional outcome, given the extent of the injury; keep in mind that a client can be functional with less than "normal" range of motion (ROM). At this point, work with your client to set reasonable goals and expectations for both of you.

Precaution. *Achieving a pain-free hand with functional prehension, grip, and grasp is better than pushing to gain a few more degrees of ROM while jeopardizing stability, possibly increasing pain and edema, and reducing the chance of long-term success.*

Clients' satisfaction with their outcome is related to their expectations, as explained by the surgeon before surgery and reinforced by the therapist after surgery.[1]

ANATOMY

Traumatic, multisystem injuries can involve many different structures from the surface of the skin through to the bone. Complex injuries, including replants and revascularizations, may occur at any level of the extremity, from the upper arm to the fingertips. To treat these injuries successfully, therapists must have a thorough working knowledge of the anatomy involved. They must know the locations and workings of veins and arteries; the steps of wound healing; the anatomy and healing processes of tendons, ligaments, and bone; and the biomechanics and interrelationships of these tissues and structures during functional movement.

The therapist first must understand the mechanics of a "normal" (i.e., uninjured) hand, because this provides the basis for maximizing the client's hand function after surgery. If you understand the implications of the injury and the surgery, you will be better able to set realistic goals and formulate a good treatment plan. Decision making is related to healing times and sequences and may depend on the surgery performed. Some structures may need to be protected while others must be moved; this can be difficult to manage. Treatment of the traumatic hand injury can become a balancing act, requiring you to determine which joints to move and which structures to protect, and when stability is more important than mobility. Some stress on healing structures is good because it stimulates healing, but too much stress can cause a loss of stability. How far to push the therapy depends on the ultimate goals and expectations and on the aggressiveness and skills of the physician and therapist.

The therapist must know what tissues were disrupted and to what extent, the effect of different types of injuries on different tissues, and what surgical procedures were performed to repair those tissues. The position of the hand at the time of injury may affect which structures

were injured and at which level (i.e., the anatomic location of injury). The therapist must take into account the effect of the injury on surrounding, uninjured structures and attend to those uninjured structures throughout the extremity (e.g., the shoulder or elbow) to prevent additional loss of function.

Anatomically, consider the functional implications of the anatomy and the injury. Moran and Berger[2] have described seven basic maneuvers that constitute basic hand function; these include three types of pinch and four types of grasp. These can be further categorized into two primary functional uses of the hand: pinch between the thumb and finger (or fingers) and grip. Pinch is affected by a radial side hand injury, which influences prehension and fine motor coordination. Grip is affected by an ulnar side hand injury, which diminishes composite grip and stability. Keep these functional movements in mind when planning treatment and devising exercises and activities.

CLINICAL *Pearl*

Finger flexors offer more function than extensors. However, in activities of daily living, wrist extension generally is more useful than wrist flexion. The importance of the thumb's contribution to overall hand function cannot be ignored, and maintaining a good web space and opposition is critical. It is imperative to work for a strong, stable wrist; without it, finger function and grip strength will be impaired. Also, regaining functional use of the hand is very difficult without functional sensibility.

DIAGNOSIS AND PATHOLOGY

Traumatic hand injuries can be caused by many types of force, from sharp lacerations to crush injuries. The mechanism of injury (e.g., tearing, crushing, cutting, or twisting forces) and the cleanliness of the wound are important pathologic factors. A closed crush injury may show little visible damage but may involve fractures or **ischemia** as a result of extensive damage to internal structures.

Primary treatment typically is performed in the emergency department, ideally with immediate referral to a hand specialist and replant team. The hand surgeon evaluates the injury with regard to what can and cannot be salvaged and restored to good function. Many systems and algorithms are available to aid problem solving and prioritization in the emergency department and operating room. Generally, the thumb, if salvageable, is always replanted as a priority. With multiple-digit amputations, the surgeon tries to replant as many as practical. Replants are nearly always attempted at any level in children.

BOX 22-1

Surgical Procedures Used to Treat Complex Hand Injuries

SKIN
- Skin may be sutured in primary repair.
- Graft or flap may be placed for wound coverage.
- Skin may be left open for secondary closure to allow further debridement and to prevent constriction over vascular structures.

TENDONS
- Flexors and extensors are repaired.
- Tendon grafts or transfers or tendon removal is performed in preparation for a future graft, often with insertion of a temporary spacer.

NERVES
- Nerves are repaired with or without grafting.

BLOOD VESSELS
- Veins and arteries are repaired with or without grafting.

BONE FIXATION
- Bone fixation is performed using bone grafts, fixators, wires, pins, plates, screws, or other devices.
- Joint arthroplasty implant may be inserted where joint surfaces cannot be repaired.
- Joint fusion is performed.

Incomplete amputations are also treated with maximum aggressiveness.[3] Box 22-1 lists surgical procedures used to treat complex hand injuries.

TIMELINES AND HEALING

Operative Treatment

Most or all involved structures are repaired surgically, depending on the timing of surgery and the extent of injury. The hand surgeon evaluates which structures can be repaired and which cannot be salvaged and therefore must be amputated. Irrigation and debridement are performed first to remove contaminants and nonviable tissue.

The order of repair generally begins with stabilization of the injury. Blood flow and fracture stabilization are most critical, and these guide the surgeon's planning. Typically, bony injuries are fixed first, using techniques that are expedient but that also allow early ROM. Bone shortening may be done to allow for easier end-to-end repair of other structures. This ultimately can affect biomechanics, possibly resulting in compromised ROM.

Tendon repairs often are performed next unless the vascular status is severely compromised. When both flexors and extensors are involved, the surgeon tries to restore balance between the two, giving priority to functional flexion. Vascular and nerve repairs are performed next, and then skin coverage is addressed.

The initial goal of the surgeon is to restore the framework that allows the client and therapist to work toward a good functional outcome with a reasonably strong structure, optimal skeletal alignment and joint mobility, vascular flow, and the potential for functional tendon balance and glide. If the injury is extremely complex, scar, tendon, and nerve grafts, joint contractures, and other deficits may be addressed by further surgeries.

Many of the involved systems may be in different stages of healing after surgery. For example, a finger fracture may have good stability because of stable internal fixation, but an overlying skin graft or infection may delay wound healing. The systems approach can be very helpful for such cases.

Prioritize the systems during the initial evaluation. There is no specific hierarchy of systems; however, without healing in some systems, no further healing occurs in any of the others. The general order of importance is as follows:

1. Surgical repairs in arteries and veins (critical for providing nutrients for healing and survival of the repaired structures)
2. Bone injury, ligament injury, and fracture fixation (ROM exercises require a stable support structure)
3. Flexor tendons over extensor tendons (functional use favors flexors, although balance should be maintained as much as possible)
4. Nerves and sensibility (nerve recovery is a slow process; nerve injuries tend to be protected when nearby blood vessels and tendons are protected)
5. Edema (must be controlled and minimized because it may contribute to stiffness and fibrosis)
6. Wound, scar, and soft tissue (prevent and minimize contractures)
7. Pain (if pain is not managed, clients cannot perform exercises)

The priorities early in therapy (0 to 3 weeks after surgery or later, the acute phase) are to manage and protect repairs, prevent joint stiffness in all uninvolved joints, control edema, manage the wound, manage pain,

BOX 22-2

Information Needed from the Physician

Therapists should make sure they obtain the following information from the client's physician or surgeon.

1. What do I need to hold (i.e., protect) and what can I move?
2. What was injured, at what (anatomic) level, and what was repaired?
3. What type of injury was this (i.e., crush, tear, blade/laceration, type of blade, clean or dirty injury)?
4. With surgical repairs:
   - What structures were repaired and how?
   - What is the quality of the repairs?
   - What is the strength of the repairs?
   - Is there tension on any repairs?
   - What is the tendon quality; what is the relationship of the repair site to the pulleys?
   - How strong is any fracture fixation? Is anything fused? How is joint mobility? Was bone shortening performed?
   - Are any skin graft or flap precautions required?
5. Are any tissues or ROM to be protected?
6. Are there any tissues with questionable viability that should be watched closely?
7. What are your anticipated time frames for progression?
8. Were any structures not repaired? What is the plan for them?
9. What are your expected outcome and goals?

educate the client, and provide psychosocial support. As the client progresses into the intermediate phase (3 to 6 weeks after surgery), therapy focuses more on increasing ROM of involved structures, managing scarring, continuing wound care and protection, and initiating functional use of the involved extremity. Later phases focus on maximizing ROM, endurance, strength, and function.

Questions to Ask the Physician

Whenever possible, obtain a copy of the operative report. Make sure you and the physician have the same understanding of treatment goals and expectations; do not hesitate to ask for clarification when needed (Box 22-2). Other important questions include the following:

- *What types of repairs were done, and how strong are the repairs?*
- *What is the most appropriate splinting position?*[4]

- *What limits and restrictions were created by the surgical procedures?*

Therapists spend considerable time developing a rapport with their clients, which means that clients sometimes are more likely to report problems and concerns to the therapist than to the physician. Also, therapists often are more likely to notice subtle changes that indicate potential problems.

CLINICAL *Pearl*

Do not be afraid to confer with the physician on any information that appears to be important regarding the client's status, complaints, or problems.

What to Say to Clients

About the Injury

Try to give clients perspective about their injury and realistic goals for the outcome. Teach them that a good outcome is about getting enough movement to use the hand for normal everyday tasks but will not necessarily mean "normal" ROM. Work to develop a partnership: "I'm the coach, but you have to do the practices. We will work together to get you the best use of your hand. If you do not do your exercises consistently at home, there is nothing we can do a few times a week here in therapy that will make up for it."

Discuss the ramifications of not complying with contraindications and precautions: "If you are not careful about doing the exercises as I show you or you do not wear your splint, it could mean your hand will not heal as it should. It could even mean you'll need another surgery to fix your hand again."

Clients come to rely on their therapists for information, and they often ask questions they are afraid to ask the physician. Do not hesitate to refer the client to the physician for questions you cannot answer.

Clients often are more compliant with therapy and achieve better outcomes when the underlying anatomy and the healing process are explained to them in common terms. Try to explain what the client is attempting to achieve with specific exercises, using terms the client can understand. Provide basic information on how the flexors and extensors work and explain that many of the muscles that move the fingers originate near the elbow. When possible, use models, pictures, or drawings to show specific anatomic features. Explain how the normal anatomy was affected by the injury and what outcome the client should expect. If future surgery is likely, make sure the client understands that and incorporate it into the goals of therapy.

About Splinting

The splint is a critical component of protection and stability with traumatic injuries of the hand. Clients must understand that the splint serves both protective and corrective functions; therefore it is essential that they wear it between exercises.

Help them understand the importance of the splint and why the hand is positioned a certain way: "This splint is important for protecting the injured structures in your hand so that they can heal correctly. If you take the splint off and move out of the position in which it holds your hand, some of the repairs may not be able to handle the stress of the new position."

About Exercises

Most clients are afraid to move any part of the hand immediately after surgery, especially if they feel pain or have swelling or open wounds, or if they can see pins sticking out of the hand. The therapist must stress the importance of movement despite these problems: "You will not hurt your hand if you do the exercises just as I showed you. If you do not do the exercises, getting good movement back will be more difficult. We cannot wait for the swelling to go away, the pins to come out, or the wound to heal before we start moving your fingers. By that time, your fingers will be really stiff, and it will hurt more to move them."

EVALUATION TIPS

- The initial evaluation may be mostly "hands off" because of the client's pain and fear and, often, the need to establish trust and rapport at this time. Before seeing the client, gather all information available on the type of injury and the treatment to this point, especially the operative reports. The initial evaluation may be a time to gain trust and establish ground rules, to do an overview assessment of the status of various systems, and to perform necessary aspects of therapy (e.g., wound care and splint fabrication).
- When you begin an evaluation, ask whether the client is a smoker or diabetic or has any other health problems. These can delay healing in all systems.
- Make sure to ask about support systems, including friends and family. Monitor clients' behavior toward the injured hand: Are they able to look at the hand, or do they treat it as if it belonged to someone else or as if they would like to get rid of it? To achieve a good outcome, the client must develop "ownership" of the injured hand and take some responsibility for recovery.

- Visually inspect the following:
  - Vascular status (check skin color)
  - Wound status (use wound color system: black, yellow, red) (see Chapter 5)
  - Finger stiffness (*at the initial evaluation, measure full active range of motion [AROM] and PROM only if essential*)
  - Edema (e.g., minimal, moderate, or severe)
- Check ROM at uninvolved joints (e.g., shoulder and elbow)

CLINICAL *Pearl*

At the initial evaluation, obtaining specific measurements is not as important as making a global assessment of the client's status.

See Chapters 5 and 8 for more detailed information.

DIAGNOSIS-SPECIFIC INFORMATION THAT AFFECTS CLINICAL REASONING

The following sections present a general discussion of the critical areas to evaluate for each system, precautions and contraindications, and healing guidelines and timelines. More detailed information on a specific system is available in the relevant chapter in this text.

Bone Injury: Fracture

With a complex injury, all surrounding and unaffected joints should be moved immediately, if possible, depending on the type and location of fracture and the type of fixation. Beginning ROM exercises as soon as the physician permits helps enhance fracture healing. During the evaluation, consider precautions, the type of fixation, and the expected stability of structures. The surgeon may have elected to shorten bony structures at the time of fixation. This may allow for a cleaner, more stable fixation, and it facilitates end-to-end repair of tendons, nerves, and blood vessels in the area; however, it also may greatly alter the mechanics of musculotendinous units in the arm and hand.

Surgical fixation may be achieved with pins and Kirschner wires (K-wires), joint implants, plates and screws, interosseous wiring, or even joint fusion (Fig. 22-1). An important goal of surgery is to achieve as much stability as possible, creating the framework for movement in rehabilitation.[5]

Precaution. *Avoid excess stress at the fracture or fusion site or pin site and watch for infection.*

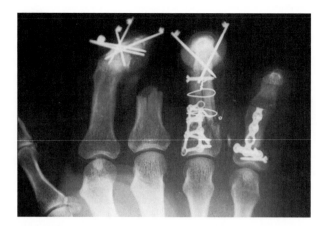

FIGURE 22-1 X-ray film showing amputation and internal fixation.

If revascularizations were done in conjunction with fracture fixation, the chance of delayed healing or nonunion is greater because of a decrease in the delivery of nutrients to the area.

Precaution. *A joint next to a fracture may need to be moved to begin ROM protocols. If this is the case, be aware of the location and type of fracture and the fixation and stability. Manually stabilize the bone during movement and do not torque across the fracture site.*

If the surgeon has established sufficient fracture fixation, ROM around a fracture site may be initiated immediately, starting from the midrange and progressing to full ROM as appropriate, observing precautions for tendons, nerves, and vascular structures.[6]

See Chapter 13 for further indications, contraindications, and typical timelines for healing.

Revascularization: Arteries and Veins

Revascularizations and replants often are categorized together as the most complex injuries because injury to an artery or vein (or both) with revascularization affects peripheral blood flow, which in turn affects the potential for survival of nearly every other structure in the hand. In complicated cases, surgeons may not repair both arteries into a digit; the digit therefore has decreased vascularity because of the repair and because it has only one functioning artery.[4,7] After surgery, these clients are placed in a "hot" (e.g., 75-80° F) room in the hospital to help increase peripheral circulation. Keep in mind that the decreased circulation after arterial repair affects the healing rate of the wound, tendon, and fracture in an extremity because of the decrease in peripheral circulation and delivery of nutrients to the area.

If possible, have the client exercise with the dressing off so that you can observe the vascular status. Ideally,

therapy should be performed in a comfortable, warm room, away from air conditioner vents. While working with the client, monitor the color, capillary refill, and temperature in the injured hand.

Precaution. *A dusky (grayish) finger or hand indicates severely diminished vascularity caused by arterial compromise; a purple color suggests venous congestion.*

Alert the referring physician if you note either a dusky or purple appearance.

A major precaution with revascularizations is to avoid anything that challenges the weakened peripheral vascular system. The client must not eat or drink anything vasoconstrictive, such as caffeine and chocolate. Smoking is prohibited because it causes severe vasoconstriction, reduces peripheral circulation, and affects the blood's ability to carry oxygen.[7] Compressive bandages (e.g., elastic stockinette, tape, or gloves) should not be used for 3 to 8 weeks, until the vascular status has stabilized. Monitor for compression caused by splint material and straps. Constantly check the color of the fingers with regard to capillary refill.

Another precaution to keep in mind is to avoid using cold treatments in the acute phase (3 to 6 weeks or longer after surgery). If the injury occurs during the winter, advise the client to keep the hand warm with a mitten, an oven mitt, or a scarf for both comfort and safety. Many experts recommend avoiding the use of a whirlpool, because it puts the hand in a dependent position; if a whirlpool is used, it must be run at neutral temperature.[4,8] Contrast baths should also be avoided, because they may cause vasospasm followed by vasoconstriction. Mild heat may be used 4 to 8 weeks after surgery, once vascularity has stabilized. However, keep in mind that the insensate hand does not have a warning system to let the client know when a substance is too hot; it also cannot dissipate heat as well (i.e., the tissue burns more easily). Although elevation is a good way to reduce edema, excessive elevation challenges the vascular system. The hand therefore should not be held significantly above the level of the heart, because this puts stress on the newly repaired arteries and can cause failure.[4]

Specific treatment considerations require positional protection of artery and vein repairs similar to that for flexor tendons (i.e., a splint with the wrist and fingers flexed, such as a flexor tendon dorsal protective splint), because neurovascular bundles generally are volarly located (see Chapter 16). If the bone was not shortened, the physician may need to use vein grafts to ensure adequate circulation without putting tension on the system. If tension is unavoidable, precautions must be observed, such as more flexed positioning in the splint and in therapy. If no other injuries or complications are involved, vascular structures can be moved soon after surgery. If tendon injuries or fractures occur in the same digit, follow the highest level of precautions to protect these structures appropriately.

Nerve Injury: Laceration and Repair

Like vascular injuries, nerve injuries often occur with flexor tendon injuries. In such cases, treat according to the appropriate flexor tendon protocol. Tension on the nerve guides decision making on protocols. As with tendon injuries, establishing early gliding is essential.

A nerve injury leaves part of the hand insensate. This is not a significant problem in the early phase of therapy, while the client is continually splinted. However, it becomes a concern when the client begins to perform activities of daily living (ADL) out of the splint.

Precaution. *The client must be taught to take care with ADL (e.g., heat, sharp objects); the eyes must be used as a sensory guide for the nerves. The therapist must cautiously use dynamic splinting and any other external compression, as well as heat and ice, because of the lack of a warning system for ischemia.*

A client with decreased sensibility may be unable to tell whether the temperature of a substance is excessively hot or cold.

A full sensibility evaluation is not necessary immediately after a traumatic hand injury. Because it takes some time for the repaired nerves to reinnervate an area, a cursory screening is practical at the initial evaluation to detect areas of sensory deficit. A full sensibility evaluation rarely is worthwhile earlier than 1 month after surgery. Follow-up re-evaluations should be performed approximately once a month thereafter, because nerves regrow slowly from the injury site to the distal fingertips.

After the client has regained protective sensation, begin sensory re-education to teach the brain to recognize signals from the peripheral nerves.[4] Start with constant pressure and moving touch. Begin with the client's eyes open and progress to eyes closed; vary between the involved and uninvolved side or area. Desensitization exercises should be performed for hypersensitivity.

CLINICAL *Pearl*

Remember that sensitivity to and intolerance of cold are common for up to 2 years after a nerve injury and sometimes longer.[7]

See Chapter 12 for more specific information.

Flexor and Extensor Tendons: Tendon Repair

Most hand therapists are familiar with the treatment of either flexor tendon injuries or extensor tendon injuries, but prioritizing becomes more difficult when the two must be treated at the same time. With a replant or if both flexors and extensors have been lacerated, priority almost always is given to the flexors over the extensors, because flexion is more important for function. However, the ideal is to maintain a normal balance between the two systems **(tenodesis).** A replanted hand or finger usually is splinted in a position similar to that for a flexor tendon injury, because the *safe position* is relatively balanced, slightly favoring the flexors and neurovascular bundles over the extensors. Gliding of involved structures should be increased as soon as possible so as to increase the delivery of nutrients, enhance healing, reduce edema, and reduce the potential for adhesions.

Treatment rules generally are the same as those for typical hand therapy protocols with regard to healing phases. Therapy after replantation should follow a version of the referring physician's preferred flexor tendon protocol, modified to protect the extensors. Generally, begin metacarpophalangeal (MCP) joint ROM, along with limited ROM of the proximal interphalangeal (PIP) and distal interphalangeal (DIP) joints, to prevent extensor lag and increase ROM via tenodesis. Major precautions are similar to those for flexor and extensor tendon protocols: protect against a full active fist or full extension of the fingers and avoid resistance until the structures have healed. If bone shortening was performed, the normal biomechanics of both the flexors and extensors will have been modified, therefore completely normal ROM is not a practical expectation.

For more specific information, guidelines, and protocols, see the description of early protective motion (EPM) later in this chapter; also see Chapter 16.

Edema

Increased edema causes increased resistance with AROM. This is a very important consideration in the introduction of early ROM for a complex traumatic injury. Long-standing, significant edema leads to increased fibrosis and scar formation. Edema can be evaluated by means of circumferential measurement, volumetric measurement (after wound closure), or visual, subjective assessment of the edema as minimal, moderate, or severe.

Treatment for edema begins with elevation of the hand to the level of the heart and not significantly higher. Excessive elevation challenges the damaged and repaired arterial system in the hand or arm.[8] It is important to avoid compression after revascularization until a stable, strong vascular flow has been re-established; this can take 6 to 8 weeks. AROM exercises can be performed as appropriate in the treatment protocol to create a pumping mechanism. Longstanding edema and the fibrosis that often occurs after a traumatic hand injury usually result in larger digits, and the client probably will have to have rings resized. To determine the most stable size, the client should wait 6 to 12 months after the last surgery to have jewelry resized.

Compression may be used after the vascular system has stabilized. Such devices and techniques include elastic bandages, compressive gloves, elastic stockinette, manual edema mobilization, or retrograde massage. See Chapter 3 for more specific management protocols.

Wound Healing and Scar Management

The presence of an open wound can change treatment priorities. Complex wounds often accompany complex injuries. Wound evaluation should include assessment and documentation of location, size, color (red/yellow/black), and drainage (type, color, and amount). Watch for signs of infection, which include redness that extends beyond the area of the wound, warmth, increased edema, increased pain, drainage, and unusual colors and odors.

Skin grafts must be treated with special care until they have stabilized. The precautions are similar to those for a typical wound, with special attention paid to avoiding friction and excessive compression over the graft site. Good nutrition is critical for wound healing, including an adequate intake of protein and vitamins. Encourage the client to discuss nutrition questions with the physician or other experts as appropriate.

Treat all wounds with care to avoid shear or mechanical stress from dressings and to prevent maceration while maintaining a moist wound bed.

Precaution. *Do not use cytotoxic chemicals, such as peroxide and povidone-iodine, on granulating wound tissue.*

Although agents such as povidone-iodine and peroxide are helpful for reducing contaminants in a wound, they also can affect the viability of new tissues.

In the early stages, wound care focuses on promoting healing and wound closure, preventing infection, and protecting healing structures.[8] In later stages, wound management involves efforts to modify and manage scarring through the use of scar massage, gel sheets, Otoform, elastomer, and so on. Therapy attempts to manage and control scarring while preventing future problems, such as the formation of adhesions and contractures. Keep in mind that scar heals all injured structures. Scar is essential for healing, but it must be managed to minimize adhesions, which limit tendon glide, and scar contractures, which occur as the scar matures. It is important to

control these two side effects of scarring because they limit ROM.

Scar tissue is different from normal skin tissue. It has less tensile strength and therefore may be more susceptible to abrasions and tearing. Scar tissue also sunburns easily and should be protected from sun exposure for approximately 6 months or until the scar is pale, soft, and supple. An easy way to protect scars on the hand is to cover them with a lip balm that has a high sun protection factor (SPF). The heavy, waxy balm stays on the scar, and the tube is portable and inexpensive.

See Chapters 1 and 19 for further information on wounds and scar management.

Pain

Pain affects the client's ability to deal with an injury and to follow a home exercise program. Pain is normal with a complex injury. However, when the pain is out of proportion to the injury for some time, a psychologic consultation may be beneficial.

Splinting

Appropriate splinting is important for supporting the injured hand, maintaining a position of balance, protecting the injured and repaired structures, and preventing future deformity. The splint typically used for a replant is similar to that for flexor tendon lacerations: a forearm-based dorsal block splint with the MCP joints in flexion and the interphalangeal (IP) joints in extension. The exact wrist position depends on the structures involved and the surgeon's preference.

CLINICAL *Pearl*

When fabricating a splint, consider the locations of pins, the vascular supply with regard to strapping and pressure areas, and tension on nerve or tendon repairs.

Prioritize the problems and splint for the most significant ones while maintaining a balance between the flexors and extensors.

Protocols for Mobilization

No true protocols exist for mobilization because injuries vary so widely. However, general guidelines are based on two approaches, delayed mobilization and early mobilization.

Delayed Mobilization

In some cases delaying mobilization is appropriate because it allows the initial inflammatory response to decline while structures heal in a balanced position. As a result, fewer precautions are necessary after the immobilization period. Delayed mobilization is ideal for young children or for any client who may not be fully cooperative.

For this technique, immobilize the hand in protected position (flexed wrist and finger, similar to the position used in a dorsal protective flexor tendon splint) and keep it wrapped in a bulky compressive dressing for 3 weeks. At 3 weeks after surgery, fit the client with a removable dorsal block splint (wrist flexion of 15 degrees, MCP flexed 50 to 70 degrees, and PIP/DIP joints fully extended to 0 degrees) and begin gentle AROM exercise of the replanted digit or digits, along with full AROM and PROM of uninvolved digits. At 4 weeks after surgery, add neuromuscular electrical stimulation (NMES) to assist with tendon glide. At 6 weeks, if the fracture is clinically healed, add dynamic splinting as needed. With medical clearance, initiate PROM in the replanted digit 6 weeks after surgery if fractures have healed sufficiently. Have the client begin using the hand for light ADL after 6 weeks, making sure precautions for the insensate parts of the hand are observed. Add strengthening exercises at 8 to 10 weeks after surgery after verifying fracture healing (Table 22-1).[10]

Early Mobilization

Early protective motion is a suggested replant treatment guideline that has been described in the hand therapy literature.[11,12] EPM is based on the premise that it allows for differential tendon glide and early movement while maintaining a balance between the flexors and extensors and minimizing the tension on repaired structures by means of tenodesis (in therapy this refers to mobilization

of one or more joints by using the tendinous connections that run past those joints and the relationship between flexors and extensors). Tenodesis is seen with the natural flexion of the fingers that occurs when the wrist is extended and the natural extension of the fingers that occurs when the wrist is flexed. This protocol can be used for digital or hand replants characterized by stable fixation and a clean injury.

Early Protective Motion I

The first treatment phase is EPM I. This phase begins 4 to 10 days after surgery (or 24 hours after discontinuation of anticoagulants), once viability of the replanted part has been established. Fit the client in a dorsal block splint with the wrist in neutral to slight flexion and the fingers in maximum practical MCP flexion and IP extension. The splint may be refitted as tolerated to increase MCP flexion and IP extension later in the program. Initiate clinical and home exercises at this time. Focus on using a gentle, passive tenodesis motion to proportionally move the MCPs, IPs, and wrist. Help the client passively extend the MCP and IP joints (naturally and with gentle assist) while the wrist is gently flexed (actively, if appropriate) (Fig. 22-2). Then help the client actively extend the wrist to neutral (with passive assist as needed) while you and gravity assist the fingers into MCP flexion (Fig. 22-3). Ideally, PIP and DIP extension are increased at the same time through viscoelastic forces in the hand. This movement must be proportional and balanced between flexors and extensors. The goal of EPM I is to establish gliding of the intrinsic and extrinsic flexors and extensors and the wrist and MCP joints to minimize stiffness while protecting involved structures.

Precaution. *EPM I should be modified if the MCPs are tight or severely limited by edema or joint stiffness, if bony fixation is not stable enough to tolerate ROM in nearby joints, or if related structures were repaired under tension.*

AROM should be performed regularly for all proximal joints throughout the day. Isometric exercises may be used to strengthen proximal musculature if the client is compliant; contralateral strengthening, by means of motor neuron retraining, may be used to minimize loss of strength.

Early Protective Motion II

The EPM protocol is advanced to passive EPM II 7 to 14 days after surgery, after a few days of EPM I movement. The goals of this phase are to reduce tendon adhesions, prevent PIP joint stiffness, provide differential tendon gliding, and improve tendon tensile strength. The client should continue EPM I while the intrinsic plus "table" and intrinsic minus "hook" exercises are added to the program to enhance differential gliding and gentle con-

TABLE 22-1

Delayed Mobilization Protocol for Replants

POSTOPERATIVE TIMELINE	EXERCISE OR INTERVENTION
0 to 3 weeks	No ROM
3 weeks	AROM of involved structures
	PROM of uninvolved structures
4 weeks	NMES
6 weeks	Dynamic splint
	PROM of involved structures
	Initiate use of hand for ADL
8 to 10 weeks	Strengthening exercises

ADL, Activities of daily living; *AROM,* active range of motion; *NMES,* neuromuscular electrical stimulation; *PROM,* passive range of motion; *ROM,* range of motion.

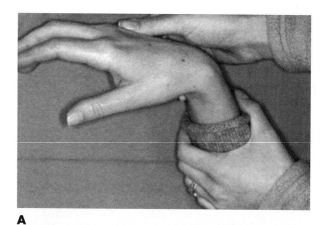

A

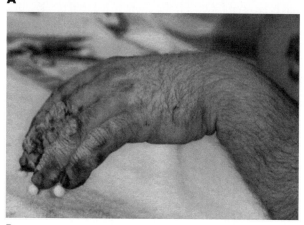

B

FIGURE 22-2   A and **B,** EPM I wrist flexion and MCP/IP extension.

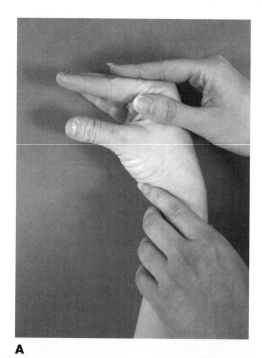

A

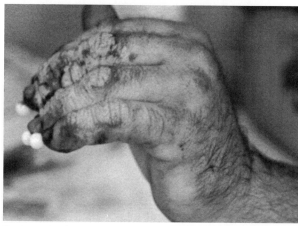

B

FIGURE 22-3   A and **B,** EPM I wrist extension with MCP flexion.

traction of the long flexors and extensors and intrinsics; the wrist remains neutral throughout the hook position. To create the hook position, passively extend the MCP joints and gently assist the PIP and DIP joints into slight flexion (Fig. 22-4).

Precaution. *Limit PIP flexion to less than 60 degrees until 4 to 6 weeks after surgery to protect the central slip. If resistance is felt, do not further progress ROM.*

From the hook position, move to the table position, using gravity to assist flexion of the MCP joints while assisting extension of the PIP and DIP joints into neutral (intrinsic plus) (Fig. 22-5). Interestingly, in the intrinsic plus position, the flexor digitorum superficialis (FDS) and flexor digitorum profundus (FDP) tendons are virtually inactive, because MCP flexion and PIP extension in this position are primarily achieved with the interossei and lumbricals. Therefore a strong contraction in this position should not overly stress the repairs to the long flexors or extensors.

Significant edema or extensor tendon damage will limit PIP joint ROM in this protocol.

CLINICAL *Pearl*

Slow, gentle movement helps reduce edema, gentle stress on healing tissues can help stimulate healing, and some gliding in the extensors can reduce extension-limiting adhesions. According to Silverman,[11,12] the hook to table movement is the most effective and safest movement that allows ROM at all three joints of the fingers, along with gliding of both long flexors (the FDS and the FDP) and all components of the dorsal mechanism and the extrinsic extensor (extensor digitorum communis [EDC]).

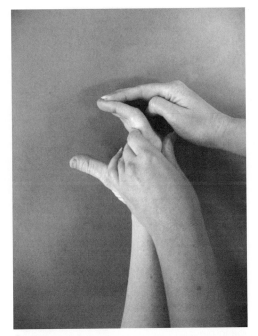

A

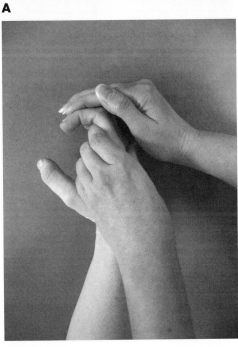

B

FIGURE 22-4 EPM II hook position.

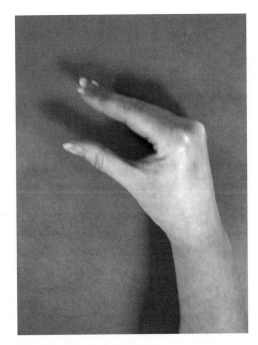

FIGURE 22-5 EPM II table position.

the intrinsic plus position. This upgrade allows initiation of active gliding in non–composite range, continuing use of tenodesis and relying on balance to move the intrinsic and extrinsic flexors and extensors without overstressing any system. Functional exercises may include picking up large beads and putting them into a container using modified prehension (Fig. 22-6).

At 4 weeks after surgery, the client may begin gradually to increase wrist extension past neutral with the digits loosely flexed, increasing overall tenodesis-related ROM. The client also should slowly progress toward full composite active flexion and extension at this time (depending on tightness).

Six weeks or later after surgery, add NMES as indicated for adhesions, gentle passive stretching, and more aggressive blocking exercises and upgrade functional exercises. Continue to progress with caution, given the likelihood that replanted or revascularized structures will heal more slowly than expected because of their less than optimal vascular and nutritional status. Introduce dynamic splinting as appropriate for stiffness, but in this area, also, keep in mind that circulation will be abnormal. Spread out pressure across as wide an area as possible with wide straps and cuffs and good splint contour and by keeping traction light.

If the physician has assessed and verified fracture consolidation, add pinch and grip strengthening as early as 8 weeks after surgery. Continue to upgrade the program, emphasizing reconditioning of the entire upper quadrant. Table 22-2 presents highlights of the timelines and interventions for EPM. (See Silverman and colleagues[11,12] and

Active EPM II is initiated 14 to 21 days after surgery. Progress to place and hold exercises by assisting the hand into the intrinsic minus hook position. Ask the client to hold the position with a gentle active contraction, then move the hand to the intrinsic plus table position and again ask for an active contraction. At this point, as appropriate and tolerated, add active gliding and isolated FDS gliding exercises and strengthen the interossei in

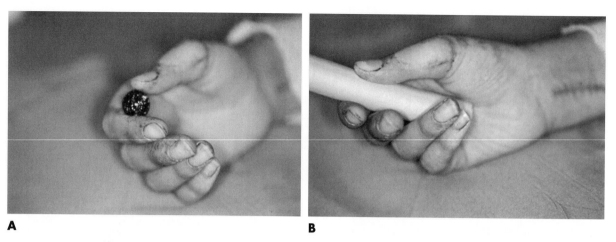

A   **B**

FIGURE 22-6   **A,** Functional prehension exercises. **B,** Functional grasp exercise.

TABLE 22-2

Highlights of Early Protective Motion (EPM) Protocol

POSTOPERATIVE TIMELINE	EXERCISE OR INTERVENTION
4 to 10 days	EPM I MCP extension with wrist flexion MCP flexion with wrist extension
7 to 14 days	EPM II passive Continue EPM I Passively move client's fingers between "table" MCP flexion with IP extension (intrinsic plus) and "hook" MCP extension with IP flexion (<60 degrees) (intrinsic minus)
14 to 21 days	EPM II active Continue EPM I and EPM II passive Place and hold hook and table positions Progress to active hook and table Isolated FDS tendon exercises Interossei strengthening (intrinsic plus) Light functional activities
28 days	Increase wrist extension to full with flexed fingers Progress to full active and passive finger ROM Begin gentle blocking exercises
6 weeks	NMES Passive stretching of involved structures Full nonresistive use for ADL (precautions for insensate hand) Dynamic splinting
8 weeks	Light strengthening exercises

ADL, Activities of daily living; *FDS,* flexor digitorum superficialis; *IP,* interphalangeal; *MCP,* metacarpophalangeal; *NMES,* neuromuscular electrical stimulation; *ROM,* range of motion.

Chan and LaStayo[4] for a more specific description of this protocol.)

Amputation

The hand surgeon generally makes every effort to salvage viable tissues in the hand. However, amputation is prefer-

able to spending time and energy trying to save a finger that ultimately would remain stiff, insensate, and non-functional. This is especially true if the stiff finger would interfere with the functioning of the remaining digits.[6]

From a therapy standpoint, amputations are simple to treat because relatively few precautions are required. The primary focus is on promoting uncomplicated wound healing and desensitizing sensitive tissues. Neuroma formation is a possibility, and this may be addressed through desensitization and use of a variety of gel sheeting products.

The most serious problem with amputations may be the psychologic effect on the client. Although a traumatic injury may result in a malformed hand, the loss of a digit often causes the greatest stress and concern. By emphasizing the positive effects of the amputation on overall functional recovery, the therapist can aid the client in coping with this loss. Functional or cosmetic prostheses may be helpful later, and showing the client pictures of these early on also can be helpful. If the client continues to greatly mourn the loss, referral to a psychiatric professional may be appropriate.

Secondary Procedures

Despite the hard work of both the client and the therapist, secondary procedures are common after therapy is completed and when a clinical plateau has been reached. During the last phase of therapy, as you head toward discharge, consider the remaining issues that may be addressed with a secondary surgery. Assess for and address tightness of the joint capsule, intrinsic and extrinsic tightness, tendon and scar adhesions, and scar contracture and plan ahead for future surgeries, which may include tenolysis, capsulectomy, joint contracture release, web space revision, tendon graft, and tendon transfers.[13] Maximizing PROM and strength is important before tenolysis. Work with the physician so that you understand the surgical procedures and objectives in advance; then, explain to the client the next surgery and the probable course of therapy so that you can help the person develop reasonable expectations.

Summary

Treatment of a traumatic hand injury requires simultaneous evaluation and management of many different types of injuries and the results of surgical procedures. An organized, logical systems approach allows you to assess each system individually and then prioritize the systems for treatment. Taking care to follow precautions is the guiding principle for treatment.

In traumatic hand injuries, the therapist can help produce noticeable improvements in appearance and function from initial evaluation to discharge. For this reason, treating these clients can be very rewarding.

Additional Thoughts on Diagnosis-Specific Information

- Determine which systems are involved, then prioritize them.

- Determine the stage of each system and decide how to treat this stage appropriately.
- Fracture fixation affects the appropriateness of early AROM and PROM.
- Healing varies with age, health, nutritional status, and smoking status. Vascular repairs can delay healing.
- Edema affects tendon glide by increasing resistance to movement, creating adhesions and fibrosis, and increasing pain.
- There is a fine line between being as aggressive as possible to improve the condition and being too aggressive. Some stress on healing systems encourages healing, but being too aggressive can lead to fracture nonunion or tendon rupture or other problems. The ideal is to move everything as early as possible without compromising the surgical repair. *Monitor tissue responses and adjust the therapeutic regimen accordingly if a flare reaction occurs.*
- Incorporate functional exercises into therapy as soon as possible. Clients who are medically cleared to perform AROM can work on picking up, holding, and turning objects in their hands or on passing items from hand to hand.

Precaution. *Respect pain; modify exercises for limitations.*

CLINICAL *Pearl*

Clients tend to respond better to short exercise sessions of fewer repetitions performed more often than to lengthy sessions performed infrequently.

- Work within a reasonable pain tolerance; ask clients to get to their end-range and then hold.
- Make therapy interesting, creative, functional, and purposeful.
- Consider functional outcomes: strength needs versus endurance needs for work and ADL.
- Strengthen every joint through the maximum available range.
- Strengthen proximal joints and the contralateral side as soon as possible after therapy.

See Chapter 4 for more information on strengthening.

Precautions and Concerns

Revascularizations (Arterial and Venous Flow)
- *Decreased circulation after arterial repair affects the rate of healing for wounds, tendons, and fractures because of*

the decrease in peripheral circulation and delivery of nutrients to the area. Typical protocol timelines generally must be extended by a few weeks.

- Keep the hand warm using a mitten, an oven mitt, or a scarf.
- In the early phase of healing, be very gentle when changing dressings; do not change them in cold, drafty areas.
- Emphasize to clients that they must not eat or drink anything vasoconstrictive, such as caffeine or chocolate. Smoking is prohibited.
- Do not use compressive bandages (elastic tape, gloves, sleeves) until vascular status has stabilized.
- Prevent compression from splint material and straps.
- Constantly monitor the color of the fingers with regard to capillary refill.
- Do not use cold treatments in the acute phase.
- Do not use a whirlpool, because it puts the hand in a dependent position.
- Do not use contrast baths, because they may cause vasospasm followed by vasoconstriction.
- Mild heat may be used once vascularity has stabilized. However, the insensate hand does not have a warning system to let the client know when a substance is too hot; also, it cannot dissipate heat as well (i.e., it burns more easily).
- Although elevation is a good way to reduce edema, excessive elevation challenges the vascular system; the hand should not be held significantly above the level of the heart.

Tendon Repairs

- Protect against a full active fist or full extension of the fingers.
- Avoid resistance from excessive co-contraction in early stages.
- Edema increases resistance during early ROM exercises; modify your approach if you encounter resistance.

Fractures

- Avoid excess stress at fracture, fusion, or pin sites while mobilizing a complex injury.
- If revascularization has been done in conjunction with fracture fixation, expect delayed healing or nonunion as a result of a decrease in the delivery of nutrients to the area.

Nerve Injury and Repair

- Nerve injuries leave part of the had insensate. Teach the client to use caution with ADL (i.e., avoid injury from exposure to heat or use of sharp objects).
- Use caution with dynamic splinting and any other external compression because of the lack of a warning system for ischemia.
- Also use heat and ice treatments cautiously.

- Remind the client that cold intolerance after a nerve injury is common for up to 2 years.

Incisions, Wounds, and Grafts

- Make sure that dressings do not exert shear or mechanical stress on healing wounds.
- Prevent maceration while maintaining a moist wound bed.
- Avoid using cytotoxic chemicals (e.g., peroxide, povidone-iodine) on granulating wound tissue.

The Role of the Therapy Assistant

In many cases, treatment of more complex injuries by nonspecialized therapists and assistants is neither appropriate nor ideal unless these professionals are closely supervised by the physician or a more experienced therapist or both (see Chapter 9 for more information).

CASE *Study*

M.H., a 15-year-old, right-hand dominant, male high school student sustained a complex laceration of his right hand while cutting a piece of wood with a saw blade during shop class. Because he was cutting wood, the wound was relatively clean. However, because the saw blade was an old one, it did a moderate amount of tearing damage. The following injuries were noted:

- Thumb: Amputation at the MCP joint
- Index finger: Laceration of FDS and FDP, radial and ulnar neurovascular bundles
- Middle finger: FDS and FDP laceration, open fracture of the metacarpal neck, lacerations of the radial and ulnar digital arteries and veins in the digit (radial digital nerve [RDN], ulnar digital nerve [UDN], radial digital artery [RDA], and ulnar digital artery [UDA])
- Ring finger: Laceration of FDS and FDP, RDN, UDN, UDA
- Small finger: Extensor tendon laceration

The following procedures were performed:

- Thumb: Replant with MCP arthrodesis, vein graft, flexor pollicis longus (FPL) tendon repair, extensor repair, nerve repair, artery repair
- Index finger (IF): Revascularization, repair of common digital artery to ulnar digital artery, FDS/FDP repair in zone II, repair of RDN/UDN
- Middle finger (MF): Debridement of metacarpal head and neck (intraarticular fracture), volar plate

repair, repair of common digital artery to ulnar digital artery, FDS/FDP repair in zone II, nerve repair
- Ring finger (RF): RDN/UDN repair, FDS repair in zone II, excision of FDP, insertion of Hunter rod
- Small finger (SF): Debridement, repair of 50% extensor laceration just proximal to PIP joint

M.H. had his first outpatient appointment with the hand surgeon 6 days after surgery. The physician changed his dressing, and he was referred for a splint and hand therapy. The splint order stated: "Orthoplast to tips, thumb spica, wrist 10 degrees' flexion, MCPs at 90 degrees in digits." The therapy referral requested "modified Duran protocol, no movement of thumb, ignore ext in SF (only partial injury)."

At his first hand therapy visit, M.H.'s hand was rebandaged with the lightest possible dressing, and he was fitted with a dorsal protective splint with slight wrist flexion and maximum reasonable MCP flexion. The thumb was positioned in midabduction for protection in a safe position and to minimize the potential for web space contracture (Fig. 22-7).

Although this had the elements of a complex injury, problem solving using the systems approach highlighted some exceptions worth considering in the treatment planning.

- The replant injury occurred in the thumb. Because of the importance of this digit, the surgeon opted for a delayed mobilization protocol to protect the revascularization and fusion. Also, because the thumb is relatively independent, it could be considered and treated separately from the others. While the thumb was primarily immobilized, tenodesis exercises to the fingers would have some effect on thumb gliding.
- Most of the tendon injuries occurred in the flexors, therefore they could be treated as simple tendon lacerations with revascularization and nerve repair. According to the surgeon's orders, the small finger extensor tendon injury was not treated as a precaution, and this led to implementation of a modified version of the Duran protocol.
- Precautions for revascularization were followed throughout therapy for the vascular repairs.
- The fracture at the thumb MCP joint was fused and was treated therapeutically as a fusion. The fracture at the middle finger MCP joint did not significantly affect any protocols.

INITIAL EVALUATION

At the initial evaluation, the following findings were noted:

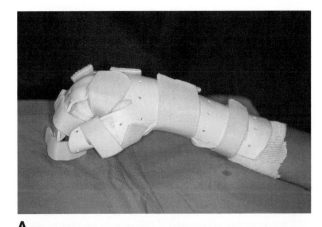

A

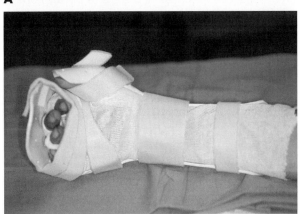

B

FIGURE 22-7 A and **B,** Dorsal protective splint with slight wrist flexion and maximum reasonable MCP flexion. The thumb is positioned in midabduction.

- Pain: 3 to 5 on a scale of 1 to 10 (3-5/10)
- Edema: Moderate in digits and palm
- Sensibility: NT (not tested), anticipated loss secondary to nerve injuries
- Wounds: Slight serosanguineous drainage
- ROM: Passive flexion to within 1 inch of palm; extension of MF, RF, SF to splint; IF has 30-degree flexion contracture at PIP; ROM to thumb not attempted

The therapist kept the initial evaluation brief and cursory to get a good overview of the situation.

THERAPY GOALS

Short-Term Goals

1. Protect injury and surgical repair through splinting and education
2. Increase passive flexion to the palm
3. Promote wound healing and closure

4. Initiate scar management program to minimize scarring and adhesions to maximize potential ROM

Long-Term Goals

1. Increase PROM of fingers to within normal limits (WNL) for potential AROM and function
2. Increase AROM of IF, MF, and SF to greater than 60% of normal limits
3. Client to use hand in more than 50% of ADL

In cases in which the therapist does not know specifically what to expect in terms of outcome, the easiest course is to predict a basic level of function and ROM. PROM must be maximized if there is to be any hope of regaining full AROM and to obtain the best results after secondary surgery.

HOME PROGRAM

Both the client and his mother were educated extensively about the surgical procedures performed, the expectations of surgery, and the necessity of a second surgery for replacement of the Silastic rod with an active tendon graft. They also were taught how to perform wound care, dressing changes, and ROM exercises. They were given the following initial home program.

Every other hour:

- Push the big knuckles down all together, hold 5 seconds each (passive MCP flexion).
- Push the big knuckle down, push the fingertip in, on each finger, one at a time; hold 5 seconds each; do 3 to 5 times per finger (passive composite flexion).
- Push the big knuckles in as far as able, straighten fingers (one at a time), relax, repeat 5 times (passive MCP flexion with active IP extension; enhances long flexor glide and intrinsic action).

Note that the home exercise program (HEP) was written in common terms that the client and his mother would understand.

At the client's second visit for therapy, tenodesis was added. The client was taught to combine wrist extension with a passive fist and then to flex the wrist and allow the fingers to extend naturally. The therapist was hopeful that some minimal gliding would occur in the thumb tendons without disrupting the healing and fusion there (Fig. 22-8).

THREE TO FOUR WEEKS AFTER SURGERY

At approximately 3 weeks after surgery, the physician gave approval to begin performance of a place and hold

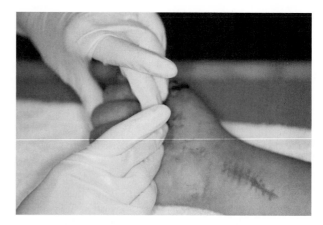

FIGURE 22-8 Early PROM at second postoperative visit.

fist to try to mitigate the heavy scarring that was forming. Heavy scarring that limits ROM suggests that the client is forming good scarring to heal the wounds and that the protocol may be progressed more rapidly. Whirlpool treatment was added, at a neutral temperature (approximately 94° F) and with the hand in a neutral position, to clean the wound and help manage pain, which had increased slightly with the upgrades in therapeutic exercises. Transcutaneous electrical nerve stimulation (TENS) was also tried for pain management but was not helpful. About 4 weeks after surgery, active finger flexion and extension exercises and blocked finger flexion exercises were added.

The physician was consulted about beginning thumb AROM. He approved initiation of IP blocking exercises with the still-healing MCP fusion protected, as well as abduction/adduction exercises. Because active finger and thumb ROM were now safe and acceptable, M.H. began to use his hand for light prehension exercises in the clinic and at home. He was not yet allowed to use the hand for ADL because of the concern that he might overdo it, especially with the thumb. He began functional prehension, picking up beads and grasping a foam tube (see Figures 22-8 and 22-9). Because scarring was becoming more of a problem, scar massage was increased at the volar MCP scars. M.H. was an exception to the typical delays in healing after a replant or revascularization because he was young and still growing. His body was able to produce new tissue, especially scar tissue, faster than most adults. His program therefore could be speeded up when it became apparent that scar formation was becoming an issue.

FIVE TO SIX WEEKS AFTER SURGERY

Five weeks after surgery, M.H.'s ROM evaluation showed that active MCP flexion was WNL, PIP flexion averaged about 55 to 60 degrees, and DIP flexion was about 17

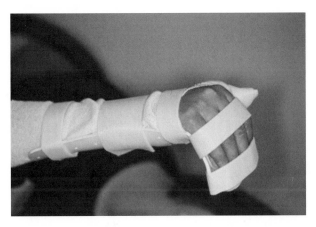

FIGURE 22-9 At 6 weeks after surgery, the dorsal block splint was converted to a volar design with a thumb web stretch.

degrees. MCP extension lag averaged −15 degrees, but the PIPs of the index, middle, and ring fingers were very limited in extension, at about −45 degrees. The client had full passive flexion of all fingers. The thumb web space showed tightness in both radial abduction (35 degrees) and palmar abduction (27 degrees), and he had only 10 degrees of thumb IP flexion. He had very good wrist ROM with wrist extension at 55 degrees and flexion to 73 degrees. Sensibility was functional with diminished protective sensation; the Semmes-Weinstein evaluation showed the thumb, IF, MF, and RF at 4.31 and the SF at 3.61.

A note was sent to the physician at this time stating that M.H. was "adherent, but gaining ROM" and that the web scar/contracture were a concern. The physician was asked when thumb PROM would be permitted, whether ultrasound treatment could be used for the scars, and whether the tolerable stretch for full passive extension of the fingers could be increased. The physician approved discontinuation of the protective splint, recommended splinting to try to increase the thumb web space, and approved ultrasound treatment for the scars. He allowed extension splinting "as per normal protocol." He told the therapist, "I doubt he'll get much thumb IP motion, but it's OK to begin PROM." Discontinuing protective splinting at 5 weeks after surgery is a bit unusual, but this young client apparently was forming a significant amount of scar and healing more rapidly than a full grown adult with the same injury. Sensibility, although diminished, was sufficient to protect him from additional injury and to allow use of the hand functionally in light ADL.

Changes in therapy included conversion of the dorsal block splint to a volar design with Otoform to scar for PIP extension. A thumb web stretch also was built into the splint (Fig. 22-9). M.H. began writing practice using a foam pen grip; he also practiced picking up marbles and

in-hand manipulation skills. Moist heat was added at 6 weeks after surgery, and ultrasound treatment with extension stretch was added to increase passive extension of the fingers.

SEVEN WEEKS AFTER SURGERY

At 7 weeks after surgery, the home program consisted of the following:

- Web spacer splint with Otoform, 4 hours a day and at night
- AROM and PROM exercises, including blocking, opposition, place and hold, and wrist ROM, 10 repetitions, 4 to 6 times a day
- Scar massage
- Light to moderate use of the hand for ADL, including writing and eating (Fig. 22-10)

In the clinic M.H. continued with moist heat, ultrasound treatment of scars, and one-on-one ROM exercises with emphasis on blocking. Mildly resistive activities were initiated, including use of a gripper with light tension (Fig. 22-11). The client used it in the normal position, gripping with the fingers, and also reversed it in his hand to pull down with the thumb. Putty rolling was done to stretch the fingers and elicit cocontraction of the finger and wrist flexors and extensors. The client also continued to practice writing and picking up pegs and marbles.

EIGHT WEEKS AFTER SURGERY

At 8 weeks after surgery, a baseline grip evaluation was performed. The right grip strength average was 10 lb and the left was 43 lb. The physician approved gentle strengthening, including the addition of putty exercises to the HEP, including gripping, pinching, and rolling. One of M.H.'s goals was to be able to carry a bucket of water or feed so that he could return to his summer job working on a farm. He therefore began a graded program of picking up and carrying weights in the clinic and at home, with the goal of working up to 20 lb. A Baltimore Therapeutic Equipment (BTE) work simulator was added in the clinic to help improve strength and endurance. By 12 weeks after surgery, the client primarily was performing a home program with upgrades for strengthening.

FOUR TO SIX MONTHS AFTER SURGERY

M.H.'s final evaluation was done approximately 4 months after surgery. Referring to his injured right hand, he said, "I can do anything with it" and demonstrated lifting a 20 lb weight. Grip strength in the right hand had increased to 42 lb. The findings at this evaluation are shown in the following box:

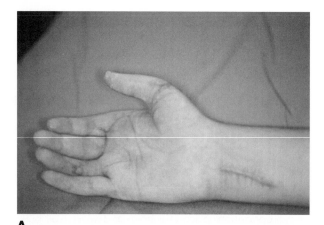

A

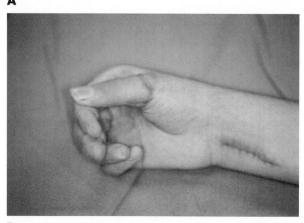

B

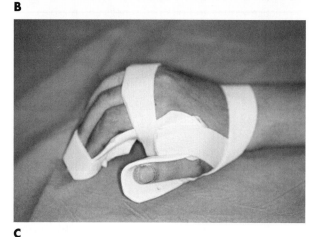

C

FIGURE 22-10   A to **C,** At 7 weeks after surgery, the client's home program consisted of ROM exercises. He also started using a web spacer splint.

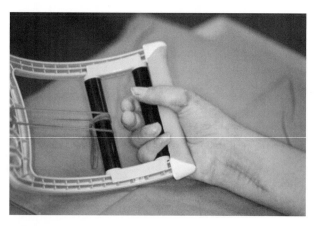

FIGURE 22-11 Client using a gripper at 7 weeks after surgery.

Measurements at Four Months after Surgery

ROM	THUMB	INDEX FINGER	MIDDLE FINGER	RING FINGER	SMALL FINGER
MCP		0/88	0/100	0/105	0/95
PIP		−40/95	0/80	0/77	0/95
DIP		0/20	0/15	0/0	0/82
Semmes-Weinstein test	3.22	3.22	3.22	2.83	2.83

	RIGHT HAND	LEFT HAND
Grip strength	42 lb	59 lb
Lateral pinch	14 lb	17 lb
Three-jaw pinch	14 lb	18 lb

M.H. returned to the surgeon 6 months after surgery. He had decided that he did not want a tendon graft to the FDP of the ring finger; he felt that he was functional, and he did not want to go through rehabilitation again. At this time several other surgical procedures were performed, including release of a thumb web space contracture (by **Z**-plasty); release of a volar skin contracture on the index finger (**Z**-plasty); and removal of the Hunter rod in the ring finger, which left the client with a *superficialis finger* (i.e., he had no flexion force at the DIP, which meant he could end up with a boutonniere deformity).

M.H. returned to therapy 9 days after surgery, and a splint was fabricated to maintain the web space and hold the index finger in full extension. He had minimal pain (0-2/10) and edema. Index finger extension was −30 degrees, radial abduction was 65 degrees, and palmar abduction was 60 degrees. The client was instructed in wound care and in full ROM exercises with emphasis on index finger PIP extension blocking and web space stretching. Because he was already familiar with therapy, he was seen only once a week for program and splint modifications and upgrades, which included the addition of strengthening exercises and a gel sheet.

M.H. was seen for the last time in therapy 6 weeks after surgery. He reported full functional use of the hand in all ADL and was prepared to return to his summer job soon thereafter. The final outcome measurements for this client are shown in the following box:

Final Measurements

ROM	INDEX FINGER	MIDDLE FINGER	RING FINGER	SMALL FINGER
MCP	0/90	0/99	0/95	0/90
PIP	−20/95	0/85	0/88	0/95
DIP	0/24	0/22	0/0	0/82

Grip strength   Right hand: 44 lb   Left hand: 62 lb
Thumb radial abduction: 60 degrees
Thumb palmar abduction: 60 degrees

References

1. Wilhelmi BJ, Lee WP, Pagensteert GI et al: Replantation in the mutilated hand, *Hand Clin* 19:89-120, 2003.
2. Moran SL, Berger RA: Biomechanics and hand trauma: what you need, *Hand Clin* 19:17-131, 2003.
3. Eddington LV: Replantation. In Clark G, Wilgis EFS, Aiello B et al, editors: *Hand rehabilitation: a practical guide*, ed 2, New York, 1998, Churchill Livingstone.
4. Chan SW, LaStayo P: Hand therapy management following mutilating hand injuries, *Hand Clin* 19:133-148, 2003.
5. Huish SB, Hartigan BJ, Stern PJ: Combined injuries of the hand. In Mackin EJ, Callahan AD, Skirven TM et al, editors: *Rehabilitation of the hand and upper extremity*, ed 5, St Louis, 2002, Mosby.
6. Freeland AE, Lineaweaver WC, Lindley SG: Fracture fixation in the mutilated hand, *Hand Clin* 19:51-61, 2003.
7. Jones NF, Chang J, Kashani P: The surgical and rehabilitative aspects of replantation and revascularization of the hand. In Mackin EJ, Callahan AD, Skirven TM et al, editors: *Rehabilitation of the hand and upper extremity*, ed 5, St Louis, 2002, Mosby.
8. Pettengill KS: Therapist's management of the complex injury. In Mackin EJ, Callahan AD, Skirven TM et al, editors: *Rehabilitation of the hand and upper extremity*, ed 5, St Louis, 2002, Mosby.
9. Sherman R, Pederson WC, LaVia AC: Replantation. In Berger RA, Weiss AP, editors: *Hand surgery*, vol 2, Philadelphia, 2004, Lippincott, Williams & Wilkins.
10. Cannon NM: *Diagnosis and treatment manual for physicians and therapists*, ed 3, Indianapolis, 1991, Hand Rehabilitation Center of Indiana.
11. Silverman PM, Willette-Green V, Petrilli J: Early protected motion in digital revascularization and replantation, *J Hand Ther* 2: 84-101, 1989.
12. Silverman PM, Gordon L: Early motion after replantation, *Hand Clin* 12:97-107, 1996.
13. Neumeister MW, Brown RE: Mutilating hand injuries: principles and management, *Hand Clin* 19:1-15, 2003.

23

Preventing and Treating Stiffness

BARBARA HAINES AND CYNTHIA COOPER

The transition from a flexible hand to a stiff hand involves the same elements that are present during the acute phase of hand injury: pain, immobilization, and scar formation. With efforts at prevention, residual stiffness may be minimized or even averted. Prevention requires awareness of the anatomic structures at risk and anticipation of the problems these structures may develop. Yet, even with appropriate early intervention, residual limitations may develop. Persistent hand stiffness can result in serious functional limitations, such as inability to make a tight fist.

ETIOLOGY

Most clients with hand injuries have pain, are immobilized, and form scar tissue; it is impressive, therefore, that they do not all develop serious restrictions. The degree of residual stiffness reflects the severity of the injury and pain and the duration of immobilization. Other factors that influence stiffness are age, general health, and tissue characteristics that affect scar formation or fibrotic responses. The presence of edema significantly worsens the outlook.

NONOPERATIVE TREATMENT

Range of motion (ROM) may be within functional limits (WFL) the first 1 or 2 days after injury, but an increase in collagen production, which contributes to stiffness, appears by day 4 or 5.[1] Elevation and early motion can control the formation of scar tissue and influence the orientation of the collagen so as to align, maintain, and restore appropriate gliding of tissues.[2]

Precaution. *Monitor ROM closely after an injury; stiffness can develop easily.*

Edema is the primary culprit after the injury itself. Edema causes vasodilation and impairs outflow, and these responses increase scar production and stiffness.[3] Techniques that can minimize edema include elevation, external compression, movement, and manual edema mobilization (MEM).[4] (See Chapter 3 for information on MEM.)

Pain can interfere with the client's efforts to prevent stiffness in the hand. When pain is controlled, the client is able to tolerate early ROM and edema reduction techniques. Pain can be managed by several treatment methods in addition to medication. High-voltage galvanic stimulation (HVGS) or transcutaneous electrical nerve stimulation (TENS), or both, can help relieve pain, allowing the clients to participate successfully in rehabilitation.[5]

When active motion is not medically permitted and edema is present, preventing the development of contractures in the hand is critical. The injured hand tends to rest in its weakest kinesiologic pattern.[6] Edema accumulates in the available space on the dorsal aspect of the hand, leading to a **position of deformity** (i.e., wrist in flexion, metacarpophalangeal joints [MCPs] in extension, interphalangeal joints [IPs] in flexion, and thumb in adduction). Splints can prevent contractures by positioning the hand in the **safe position,** also called the **intrinsic plus position** (i.e., wrist in 20 to 30 degrees' extension, MCPs in 40 to 60 degrees' flexion, IPs in extension, and thumb in abduction/extension). However, despite these interventions, the client's hand still may develop stiffness.

OPERATIVE TREATMENT

Acute stiffness is more likely to have a soft end-feel (see discussion of end-feel later in the chapter). Longstanding stiffness is more likely to manifest as a hard end-feel in joints and is prone to tightness of the musculotendinous units. Surgery may be done (e.g., capsulotomy or tenolysis) if therapy cannot resolve all the limitations. It is very important to achieve maximum passive range of motion (PROM) of the involved structures before corrective surgery is performed.

Questions to Ask the Physician

- *Are any precautions required regarding resistive exercise or PROM?*
- *Is this patient a candidate for surgery? If so, what surgery is anticipated and when?*

What to Say to Clients

About Soft End-Feel

"You have stiffness that feels spongy. This is a good sign that with exercise and splinting, you may be able to gain more motion. It is important to achieve gentle stretching with exercise and splinting. Remember, the stretching must be pain free to be effective."

About Hard End-Feel

"Although you may want to apply more force than I have demonstrated with your splints, your tissue will remodel itself more effectively with a gentle, prolonged force, called low load, long duration. You'll know your tissue is being coaxed to remodel effectively when you can wear a stretching splint comfortably for at least 20 minutes. Pain after wearing the splint for less than 20 minutes causes tissues to rebound and stiffen again. You'll achieve more flexibility from this prolonged, gentler approach. We know it can be challenging to keep your splint tension light or gentle, but it is truly the best thing you can do to help your tissues elongate. Generally speaking, the more times a day you can wear these gentle stretching splints, the more you will successfully reorganize your stiff tissues."

EVALUATION TIPS

When evaluating a client after injury, do the following:

- Distinguish between joint tightness and musculotendinous tightness, between intrinsic tightness and extrinsic tightness, and between extrinsic flexor and extrinsic extensor tightness. Also, assess for decreased function of the flexor tendons of the digits.
- Document hard end-feel versus soft end-feel at specific joints; assess and document the end-feel at regular intervals.
- Compare active range of motion (AROM) to PROM and factor these findings into your treatment plan.

Joint Tightness

Joint tightness is determined by assessing the quality of the joint end-feel.[7] **End-feel** is the passive movement carried out from the point where resistance is first met to the final stop in the available ROM.

A normal end-feel, also called a **physiologic end-feel,** can vary from individual to individual, depending on the person's body type and build and the anatomy of the particular joint. End-feel is described as soft, firm, or hard. A soft end-feel results from **tissue approximation** (the point where tissue upon tissue blocks further motion) or stretching (e.g., the bulk of the bicep muscle blocks full elbow flexion). A firm end-feel is the result of capsular or ligament stretching (e.g., the end-range during MCP flexion and extension). A hard end-feel results when bones or cartilaginous structures meet (e.g., elbow extension is blocked by bone on bone). Manual PROM is not effective with a hard end-feel.[8]

A **pathologic end-feel** is an end-feel with a location or quality that is abnormal for the particular joint. A pathologic end-feel may be the result of intrinsic, extrinsic, or joint tightness.

Joint contractures (PROM limitation of a specific joint because of ligament or joint capsule restrictions) may develop as a result of immobilization or trauma to the bone or the surrounding soft tissue. Other contributing factors include edema and prolonged disuse. The surrounding joint capsule becomes restricted, leading to joint stiffness.[9] Joint contractures are confirmed when PROM is limited and is unchanged despite repositioning of proximal and distal joints.[8] To prevent joint contractures in the hand, position the MCPs in 70 to 90 degrees of flexion and the IPs in full extension; this position prevents stiffness by placing the joint ligaments on stretch.

Intrinsic Tightness

Intrinsic tightness involves the lumbricals and the interosseous muscles. To identify interosseous tightness, place the MCPs in full extension (in hyperextension if available). Intrinsic tightness is confirmed when less passive IP flexion occurs with MCP extension than with MCP flexion.[10] Intrinsic tightness frequently develops after metacarpal fractures and crush injuries to the palm. It also can occur if the hand is placed in an intrinsic plus splint for a prolonged period, because this position puts the intrinsics on slack, allowing them to tighten in a shortened position.

Intrinsic tightness can result in lack of full composite fisting and weakness in power grip. It also can reduce the agility of the hand. To prevent intrinsic tightness, pay close attention to the status of the intrinsics and promote normalization of their length through positions of MCP extension with IP flexion. Hook fisting is a good exercise for this problem, and this exercise position also promotes FDP glide.

Extrinsic Tightness

To identify **extrinsic flexor tightness** (limited excursion of the volar muscles and tendons that originate in the forearm), passively maintain the fingers and thumb in full extension while passively extending the wrist. With extrinsic flexor tightness, the fingers will draw into flexion as the wrist is extended. Long flexor tightness frequently is seen with a laceration or open fracture on the volar surface. The flexors may also manifest a lack of **differential gliding** (freedom of movement of the long flexors relative to each other) between the flexor digitorum profundus (FDP) and the flexor digitorum superficialis (FDS).[11] Studies have demonstrated that 11 mm of differential gliding is normal between the FDS and the FDP at the wrist.[12,13] Lack of differential flexor gliding contributes to limited composite fisting and reduced

finger agility. Therefore it is important to perform differential flexor tendon gliding exercises as early as medically appropriate.

Conversely, to identify **extrinsic extensor tightness** (limited excursion of the dorsal muscles and tendons that originate in the forearm), passively maintain the fingers flexed while passively flexing the wrist. As the wrist is flexed, the fingers will draw into extension. Extensor tightness significantly weakens the power grip because of the lack of MCP flexion.

Web Space Contractures

Web space deformity is a result of a decrease in ROM at the carpometacarpal (CMC) joint of the thumb. Thumb stiffness is very difficult to correct. As yet no norms have been established for thumb CMC abduction and adduction ROM, therefore the therapist should compare the client's injured hand to the uninjured hand. With longstanding stiffness, the deforming pattern of thumb tightness is CMC adduction and slight IP flexion. Static splinting can help prevent web space contractures.

Direct trauma to or laceration of the first web space or adjacent structures, median nerve damage, ischemia, and infection all can result in web space contractures. The accumulation of edema between the dorsal fascia can pull the thumb into adduction. Functionally the client is unable to grasp a cup or lay the hand flat on a surface. Limited opposition of the thumb to the index finger (i.e., lack of a pad-to-pad pinch) can result in diminished ability to perform precision pinching.

Wrist Stiffness

Wrist limitation can be the result of prolonged immobilization, altered bony alignment, or damage to ligaments. Limited wrist motion can affect hand function significantly. Positioning the wrist in extension allows optimum power for grasping, whereas positioning it in flexion is necessary for other functional tasks. Joint mobilization techniques can help the therapist determine and treat the restriction. To prevent wrist stiffness, initiate ROM as early as medically possible and incorporate exercises with tenodesis action if these are not contraindicated.

Observing Movement

It is helpful to assess the client's sequence of movement and to teach the person how to use effective isolated motions. First, observe the movement. Look for free, smooth motion. Ask the client to grasp an object and have the person repeat the movement several times. The movement sequence may reveal the limitations in the hand. Note whether the client flexes the wrist first to achieve extension of the fingers.[14] Are the fingers initiating extension at the MCPs or the IPs? As the client grasps an object, observe where flexion is initiated. Note whether the wrist first must be extended to allow initiation of MCP flexion, followed by flexion of the IPs.[15]

DIAGNOSIS-SPECIFIC INFORMATION THAT AFFECTS CLINICAL REASONING

CLINICAL *Pearl*

If AROM and PROM are equal, focus first on gaining PROM. If PROM is normal and AROM is limited, focus on assisted AROM (AAROM) and structure-specific isolated exercises to promote AROM. If PROM is not normal but is greater than AROM, focus on gaining both PROM and AROM. Place-and-hold exercises with resistance at end-range are helpful.

If the client has musculotendinous unit tightness, control the position of the upper extremity proximally so that your exercise or splint achieves the pull at the proper isolated area. For example, if the client has extrinsic extensor tightness that limits full fisting, place the MCPs in flexion and then exercise or splint for IP flexion. If the client has extrinsic flexor tightness that limits full digital extension, place the wrist and MCPs in extension and then exercise or splint the IPs in extension, controlling for the pull at the specific area that is tight. If tightness of the FDP is a factor and you are trying to achieve the extension pull at the proximal interphalangeal (PIP) joint, you may need to make a gutter splint for the distal interphalangeal (DIP) joint so that the entire length of the FDP is controlled with the stretch at the PIP. Otherwise, the PIP may extend more but the DIP may flex more, preventing lengthening of the FDP.

TIPS FROM THE FIELD

When a client has stiffness in multiple joints and musculotendinous units, prioritizing and knowing where to start can be a challenge. Begin your treatment with a detailed assessment (see Chapter 5). Identify and distinguish between intrinsic tightness, extrinsic tightness, joint limitation, and/or muscle weakness. Assess for restricted tendon gliding. Each of these problems has tissue-specific solutions for restoring functional motion. Clients often have a combination of problems. In such cases, try to encourage the most functional position that allows the hand to perform activities of daily living (ADL) or specific vocational tasks. Table 23-1 presents treatment highlights and splint options for these various aspects of stiffness.

A client with stiffness of multiple digits at first may have joint tightness. As the joint tightness is corrected, the client may demonstrate musculotendinous tightness, which the therapist could not detect until the joint tightness had improved. As stiffness improves, be prepared to identify new findings and to change your treatment focus accordingly. Resistive exercise, if not contraindicated, is helpful for problems related to tendon adherence.

Prioritizing Treatment

If wrist limitations exist in both flexion and extension, first focus on wrist extension over wrist flexion. Extensor muscles are weaker than flexors, therefore they usually need more attention. Achieving 20 to 40 degrees of wrist extension is important for positioning and stabilizing the hand and for allowing maximum power for grasping when the digits flex.

If the client has stiffness of both digital flexion and extension, prioritize digital flexion over extension. Begin with emphasis on flexion, maximizing joint motion. Instruct the client in exercises to isolate the FDP and FDS, because these are important for achieving the coordinated motions required for tasks such as typing or playing an instrument. Add exercises for composite flexion to lengthen the extrinsic extensors. Remember to assess frequently for intrinsic tightness. Interosseous tightness must be corrected for the client to achieve maximum digital flexion. Alternating digital flexion exercises with intrinsic stretching and splinting may be helpful.

Next, turn your attention to achieving digital extension. Encourage IP flexion with an MCP block exercise splint to facilitate a hook fist; this maximizes FDP gliding and also promotes lengthening of tight interossei.[12] An effective way to exercise the EDC is to grasp a dowel, maintaining IP flexion, and then to extend the MCPs. To encourage intrinsic function for IP extension, block the MCPs into full extension and move from a hook fist position into IP extension. Depending on the client's individual needs, the better course generally is to sacrifice full digital extension and achieve maximum digital flexion than to forfeit full fisting.

Functional tasks require less than 40 degrees of wrist flexion. The wrist flexors are stronger than the wrist extensors, and wrist flexion usually improves more readily. Supination usually is more difficult to achieve than pronation. Some splints can support forearm supination and wrist extension simultaneously.

After you have gained motion, it is very important to maintain that motion through active exercise and functional use. Home exercise for progressive strengthening helps in gaining end-ranges. Initial baseline grip testing determines the resistance the client can use for exercise. If the client can grip 30 lb or more, resistance

TABLE 23-1

Treatment Highlights and Splinting Options for Stiffness Problems

PROBLEM	TREATMENT HIGHLIGHTS	SPLINTING OPTIONS
Joint contracture	• Heat • Slow, prolonged stretch • Joint mobilization at varied ranges • Place and hold with gained ROM[16]	
Supination/pronation	• Joint mobilization at all three locations (proximal, midshaft, and distal radioulnar joint); focus on supination as soon as possible	• Roylan supination/pronation splint • Joint active system (static progressive splint, Fig. 23-1)
Wrist stiffness	• Passive stretch with joint mobilization at end of ROM; begin with extension	• Phoenix outrigger with MERiT system (flexion/extension) (Fig. 23-2)
MCP/IP joint stiffness	• Joint mobilization with soft tissue massage of ligaments in stretched position (usually, joint restriction limits extension and soft tissue restriction limits flexion)	• Modified joint jack • Serial casting[17] • Dropout splint for multiple digits (Fig. 23-3)
Intrinsic tightness	• Heat • Soft tissue mobilization • Slow, prolonged stretch • Hook fisting • Final flexion exercises	• MCPs blocked into extension with IP flexion splinting (use serial static progression) • Intrinsic stretch splint (Fig. 23-4) • Exercise splint (Fig. 23-5)
Extrinsic tightness	• Heat • Soft tissue mobilization • Slow, prolonged, *composite* stretch • Muscle re-education and strengthening at end of gained ROM	
Long flexor stiffness	• Wrist rocking position with soft tissue massage of flexors while in this stretch position	• Wrist in maximum extension with isolated digits in extension (Fig. 23-6)
Long extensor stiffness	• Elbow extension combined with wrist in full flexion, then MCP flexion added **or** fingers wrapped into flexion with self-adherent wrap (e.g., Coban) then add elbow straight with wrist in flexion	• Stabilize wrist in neutral and apply outrigger for 90-degree pull of MCPs into flexion, adding IP flexion (Figs. 23-7 to 23-9) • Casting motion to mobilize stiffness (CMMS)[18]; used for a chronically stiff hand that is unresponsive to traditional techniques; key component is muscle re-education movement patterns (Fig. 23-10)
Web space contracture	• Heat • Deep soft tissue mobilization into web space • Serial static stretch	• Serial progressive splinting of web space; often web space splinting can be combined with other types of splinting (e.g., composite extension splint at night with web stretch)
Weakness	• Functional use (use it, use it, use it!) • Place and hold at end-range (isometric hold) • Progressive resistance (continue to upgrade the resistance)	

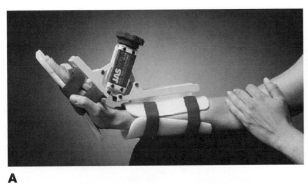

A

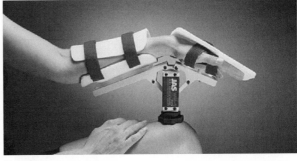

B

FIGURE 23-1 **A,** Joint Active System (JAS) static progressive splint for wrist extension. **B,** For wrist flexion.

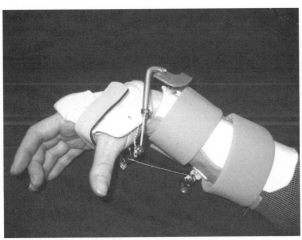

A

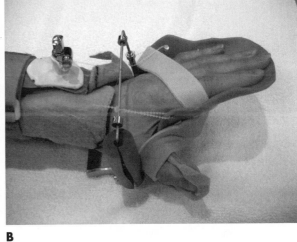

B

FIGURE 23-2 **A,** Phoenix outrigger with MERiT system for wrist flexion. **B,** For wrist extension.

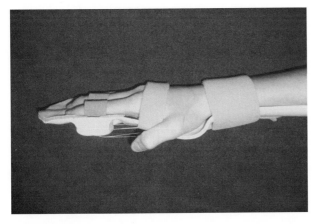

FIGURE 23-3 Dropout splint for multiple PIP joint contractures.

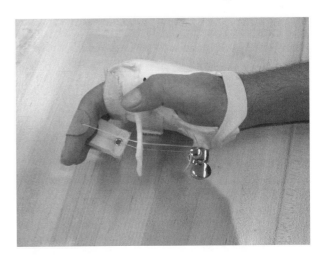

FIGURE 23-4 Intrinsic stretch splint for PIP joints.

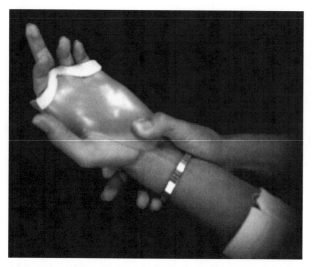

FIGURE 23-5 Exercise splint to isolate hook fisting and to stretch the intrinsics.

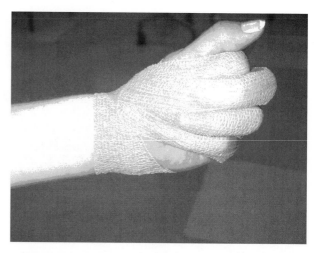

FIGURE 23-7 Flexion wrapping and paraffin dip. Be gentle with this technique and watch closely for signs of inflammation (e.g., pain, swelling, redness, worsening stiffness).

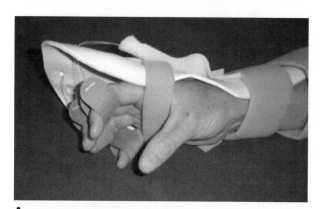

A

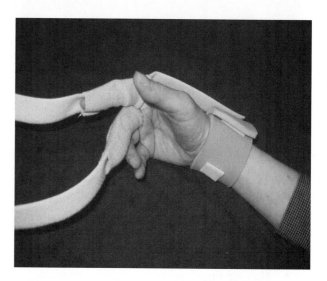

FIGURE 23-8 Gentle flexion strapping for composite splinting (initial steps).

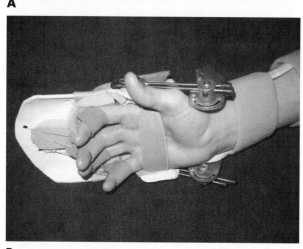

B

FIGURE 23-6 **A,** Static wrist splint with static progressive extension strapping of the digits to reduce tightness of the long flexors. **B,** Roylan serial static wrist hinge splint with static progressive extension of the digits.

greater than putty is needed to increase the power grasp. Graded grippers are effective for power grip strengthening, but watch closely for signs of inflammation.

Promoting Function

Some clients with stiff hands may not recover full functional hand use. Promote function with adaptive techniques and equipment according to the therapist's scope of practice. Clients who lack digital flexion (Fig. 23-6, 23-9) find the following items helpful:

- Foam built-up handles
- Grasping cuff (Fig. 23-11)

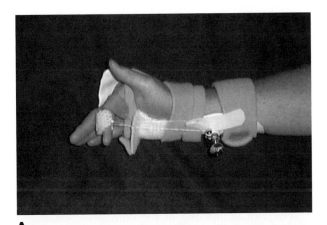

A

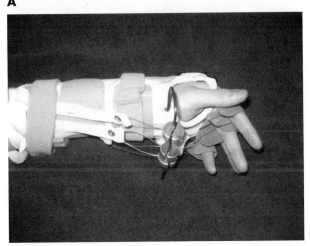

B

FIGURE 23-9 **A,** Composite flexion splinting with 90-degree pull at MCPs and strap to pull IPs into flexion; MERiT component has been added for static progressive splinting. **B,** MCP flexion splinting.

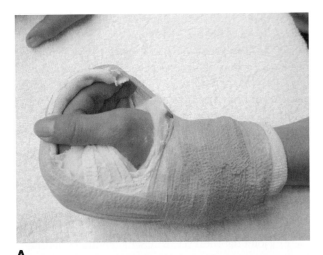

A

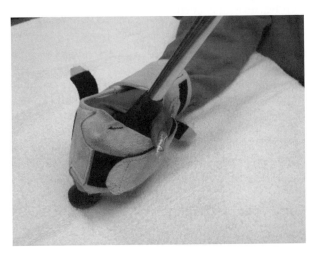

B

FIGURE 23-10 **A,** Casting for mobilization, maximal active flexion. **B,** Same cast with improved maximum flexion motion after 2 weeks of casting.

- Non-slip lining material attached to objects
- Senior grip modifications for golfers

SPLINTING TO TREAT STIFFNESS

AROM and PROM exercises often are not enough to overcome residual stiffness. Initiate splinting as soon as medically possible. With acute injury, splinting protects injured structures and helps minimize tissue tightness and deformity. With established stiffness, the goal of splinting is to reduce adhesions, lengthen tight tissues, and remodel and reorganize collagen.[19] Various types of splints can be used for stiffness. These include (1) functional splints, which can be used during daily activity; (2) exercise splints, which position the hand to isolate specific exercise motions (see Fig. 23-5); (3) night splints (typically serial static splints); and (4) intermittent day splints (dynamic or static progressive splints; see Figs. 23-6, 23-9).

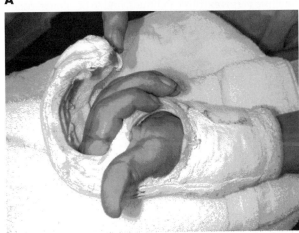

FIGURE 23-11 Grasping cuff.

Dynamic or static progressive splinting stimulates cells by keeping the tissues in a physical state of demand; the controlled stress allows collagen cells to sense the need to reorganize. This concept was beautifully explained by Paul Brand.[20] Brand states that the best way to lengthen tissues is to keep them in a constant state of mild tension through the use of low load, prolonged stretch using serial static forces. This type of stretch stimulates tissue growth in response to the stresses placed on the tissues.[21]

The principles of splinting are essential to the treatment of stiffness. Fundamental concepts of splinting are described in other chapters of this textbook. As mentioned previously, to correct longstanding stiffness, initiate splinting when the client has been medically cleared for PROM. Identify joint tightness versus musculotendinous tightness, intrinsic versus extrinsic tightness, and so on. Differentiate the types of end-feel for the various structures.

CLINICAL *Pearl*

Remember that splinting for isolated joint stiffness does not require immobilization of adjacent (proximal or distal) joints. However, splinting for tightness of a musculotendinous unit does require immobilization of adjacent joints.

Flexion Strapping

Fig. 23-8 shows examples of flexion strapping (flexion gloves are included in this category). This type of splinting or strapping does not control the exact site of stretch; rather, it achieves a generalized pull that may be effective in some cases, such as those with a soft-end feel. However, flexion strapping without proximal support may be ineffective at directing the gentle stretch to the area where it is actually needed. For this reason, splinting for longstanding stiffness frequently requires more exact positioning, including careful determination and control of proximal support.

Structure-Specific Splinting

Splinting should target the structures that are most limited. Tissues that are more restricted respond best to serial static lengthening. According to Brand,[20] "the use of splinting is only justified if the specific good will compensate the general harm and restrictions immobilization causes while splinting." (See Table 23-1 for an overview of a variety of tissue limitations and splinting options.)

Components of Splinting for the Stiff Hand

Base

- A circumferential base helps minimize distal migration.

- If the splint is forearm based, it should be three fourths the length of the forearm to allow more skin contact, which minimizes migration. The added length also provides a greater area for attachments.
- The use of a non-slip lining material on the strap or in the base may help minimize distal migration.
- Using D-ring straps helps provide a secure base and minimizes splint migration.
- Ample clearance at the distal palmar crease (DPC) is critical for improving MCP flexion.

Outriggers

- Frequent monitoring of the outrigger is crucial to ensure that traction is exerted at a 90-degree angle at each joint that is being corrected.
- Appropriate placement of the outriggers makes it easier for the client to wear the splint for the desired interval. Ideally, the client should be able to tell you where the pull is felt; this should be the specific structure you are trying to remodel.

Traction

- Serial static traction is the preferred method of lengthening soft tissue with a firm end-feel. This method allows for gentle, controlled lengthening of the tissue.
- Educate the client in the concept of low load, long duration splinting and allow the person to adjust the amount of force used. This improves wearing time and efficient use of the splint.
- The sling must distribute the pressure adequately to minimize discomfort. A more rigid sling should be used for a firm end-feel. For example, fabricate the sling from $1/16$ splint material rather than suede or leather.

Evaluating Your Splint

It is important to check the client and to analyze your splint to ensure the proper fit. Having the client stay and wear the splint for a while may be helpful, because it presents an objective demonstration of the results of your work. After making this observation, return to the client and critique the splint as if it were someone else's work. Check all the edges and look for any potential pressure areas. Ask the client to demonstrate how he or she puts on and takes off the splint and trouble-shoot any difficulties. Check skin tolerance, and look for pressure marks or areas that need refitting. Give the client written instructions regarding precautions and the wearing schedule. Clarify whether this or any other splint must be worn at night.

Precaution. *Give the client specific instructions for hygiene, skin care, and cleaning the splint. Caution the client not to allow pets to chew on the splint materials. If the splint has* small components, emphasize that these parts must not be left where small children might find them and put them in their mouths.

In some cases you may actually notice measurable ROM gains while assessing the splint for fit. Providing clients with goniometric findings reinforces the therapeutic regimen and helps promote good follow-through. Ideally, active exercises should be performed immediately after the splint is removed. This allows active stimulation of the remodeled tissue and reinforces the client's sense of functional improvement.

Splint Wearing Schedule

The wearing schedule depends on a number of factors, including how well the splint performs. If the splint is providing greater stretch than other exercises, I recommend that it be worn for 30 minutes or longer four to six times a day. The longer it is worn, the better it helps remodel tissues. Flexion splints usually are worn during the day, and extension splints are worn at night. It is important for the client to bring in the splint at every visit so that it can be reassessed and adjusted to accommodate ROM gains. As the client gains motion, the outriggers must be adjusted to ensure that the line of pull is correct. Depending on the tissues involved, the base also may need revising. Discontinue the splint when ROM has plateaued for 2 weeks. Thereafter, monitor ROM to make sure the gains are not lost. If motion is lost, have the client resume wearing the splint to recover and maintain motion.

Precautions and Concerns

- *Monitor tissue responses to exercise and splinting.*
- *Change the treatment regimen if pain is reported or if signs of flare occur.*

The Role of the Therapy Assistant

- Refurbishing splints and modifying them as determined by the therapist
- Reviewing instructions for the home program as identified by the therapist
- Modifications and adaptations for activities of daily living
- Reviewing skin inspection and tissue tolerances
- Reinforcing any precautions identified by therapists

CASE *Study*

V.C., a 48-year-old female, was involved in a motor vehicle accident. She was holding onto the steering wheel when the accident occurred, and the force of the impact

was transmitted to her forearms, resulting in an open midshaft fracture of the radius and ulna in the right forearm. V.C. underwent surgery at a local hospital, and the surgeon performed an open reduction and internal fixation (ORIF) of the radius and ulna. She was placed in a long arm cast after the surgery. The surgeon instructed her to "keep the arm elevated and to move the fingers." No formal therapy was ordered for the time she was in the cast, which was about 2 months; the client was referred for therapy after the cast was removed. Treatment was started 3 days after cast removal.

SUMMARY OF INITIAL EVALUATION

Observation: The client had moderate to mild edema throughout the right hand and digits. Her hand postured in the weakest kinesiologic position, with the wrist slightly flexed, the MCPs extended, the PIPs flexed, and the thumb adducted. The hand was very rigid in appearance, and the client was very guarded with any movement of her right limb. Prevention strategies of early motion and corrective night splinting while she was in the cast would have minimized digit restriction.

MEASUREMENTS

See Table 23-2.

PROBLEMS IDENTIFIED

- Limited AROM and PROM in all joints of the right forearm and hand; minimal stiffness at the elbow; shoulder is WFL.
- Moderate pain at end of passive motion
- Intrinsic tightness—soft end-feel
- Long flexor tightness with adhesion noted at volar midforearm at site of open fracture, limiting full wrist and digit extension—firm end-feel
- Significant scar adhesion at volar incision and injury site
- Inability to isolate FDP and FDS motions
- Moderate long extensor tightness, resulting in limited composite fisting
- Moderately limited thumb movement in all planes—firm end-feel
- Significant weakness for all functional uses of the right hand
- Inability to use right-dominant hand for any ADL
- Work restrictions limiting her to "paperwork only" (i.e., no lifting or forceful use) for current work restriction

After the therapist completed the evaluation, she explained to V.C. what she could expect over the 2 to 3 months of rehabilitation. She explained that initially V.C. should make slow, steady gains. She instructed her to be

TABLE 23-2

Case Study: Client's Initial Status

	ACTIVE ROM (DEGREES)	PASSIVE ROM (DEGREES)	COMMENTS
Supination	35	35	• Moderate pain at end of PROM and AROM
Pronation	50	50	• Moderate to severe adhesions at open fracture site, especially
Wrist extension	30	30	long flexors
Wrist flexion	25	30	• Limited isolation of FDS/FDP tendons
			• Grip: L: <5 lb R: 80 lb

	INDEX FINGER	MIDDLE FINGER	RING FINGER	LITTLE FINGER
MCP				
PIP	Only DPC measurements were taken at first visit.			45/
DIP				
DPC	7 cm	3.5 cm	4.7 cm	5 cm
Thumb abduction:	CMC: 30 degrees	MCP: 0/10	IP: 5/15	

sure to let the therapist know whether the treatment sessions were too vigorous, and she emphasized that a "no pain, no gain" approach was not helpful. Aggressive, painful therapy is detrimental and results in increased edema, stiffness, and scarring. The therapist informed the client that functional use would promote improvement over the following months and that at 6 to 9 months she probably would have maximal function in the injured hand.

TREATMENT

At V.C.'s initial visit the therapist performed only a general evaluation and took only a few detailed measurements (i.e., wrist movement and gross grasp, DPC crease measurements). In this initial interaction, the focus was on providing hands-on treatment with gentle soft tissue massage and on encouraging in the client a sense of confidence about the therapy process. Detailed objective measurements can be obtained by the third visit. After this first visit, the therapist requested all x-ray films and reports (including the operative report). She also asked the client's physician the following questions:

- Are any bony blocks present, especially with supination and pronation?
- Is there any damage to wrist ligaments that may result in pain and limited wrist motion?
- Is the fracture stable and able to tolerate unrestricted, pain-free ROM?

Treatment was initiated with the emphasis on regaining wrist extension. The therapist wrapped the fingers into comfortable flexion, dipped the hand in paraffin, and then applied a hot pack to the wrist and forearm. While the client received the heat treatment, the therapist

began gentle exercises of the hand to gain more finger flexion. Joint mobilizations were done throughout ROM to help gain wrist extension. Gentle scar massage was provided at the volar scar site; ultrasound treatment also was used for the volar scar. During the ultrasound treatment, the hand was placed in composite extension. This was combined with a contract-relax motion with gentle stretch. Scar retraction massage also was performed. Treatment was continued with AROM and place and hold exercises to provide muscle re-education. This sequence is used to gain motion at restricted joints and in movement patterns throughout the limb.

The client had minimal pain; however, if pain had occurred, the therapist could have tried HVGS to reduce it, allowing increased motion.[5] To maximize end ROM, special attention was paid to differential tendon gliding for the FDP and FDS and to isolated intrinsic stretch.

V.C. was given an exercise splint to isolate the hook fist pattern. (A trial use of electrical stimulation can be helpful if a client has significant weakness with flexor tendon pull-through. A home unit is provided if increased pull-through is noted with the stimulation.)

As the motion progressed and when V.C. was medically cleared for resistive exercise, strengthening tasks were continued, including the Baltimore Therapeutic Equipment (BTE) work simulator and functional job stimulation tasks (see Table 23-1).

V.C.'s home exercise program included the following elements:

- Edema control using a glove with the tips cut out; MEM
- Placement of a silicone gel sheet on scars at night

TABLE 23-3

Case Study: Client's Final Status

	ACTIVE ROM (DEGREES)	PASSIVE ROM (DEGREES)	COMMENTS
Supination	70	75	• Residual tightness of long flexors with composite reaching
Pronation	65	65	• Weakness with fisting
Wrist extension	40	50	• Minimal pain, stiffness
Wrist flexion	40	45	• Grip: L: 45 lb

	INDEX FINGER	MIDDLE FINGER	RING FINGER	LITTLE FINGER
MCP	0/90	0/90	0/85	0/80
PIP	WNL	WNL	WNL	15/WNL
DIP	0/70	WNL	0/70	0/60
DPC	1.5 cm	0.5 cm	1 cm	2.5 cm
Thumb abduction:	CMC: 55 degrees	MCP: 0/40	IP: 0/65	

- Differential tendon gliding with emphasis on hook fisting
- Gentle passive stretch exercise, including wrist rocking, with emphasis on isolation of the extensor carpi radialis brevis (ECRB) and tenodesis positions
- Strengthening, including putty and grippers
- Splinting (alternating composite flexion, extension, and intrinsic stretching)
- Joint jack for the small finger PIP joint

Table 23-3 shows V.C.'s final measurements.

References

1. Madden JW: Wound healing: the biological basis of hand surgery, *Clin Plast Surg* 3:3-11, 1976.
2. Cyr L, Ross R: How controlled stress affects healing tissue, *J Hand Ther* 11:125-130, 1998.
3. Casley-Smith JR, Casley-Smith JR: *High-protein oedemas and the benzo-pyrones*, Philadelphia, 1986, JB Lippincott.
4. Artzberger S: Edema control: new perspectives, *Phys Disabil Special Interest Section Quarterly* 20:1-3, March 1997.
5. Bettany JA, Fish DR, Mendel FC: Influences of high voltage pulsed direct current on edema formation following impact injury, *Phys Ther* 70:219-224, 1990.
6. Lister G: *The hand: diagnosis and indications*, ed 2, London, 1984, Churchill Livingstone.
7. Kaltenborn FM: Mobilization of the extremity joints: examination and basic treatment techniques, Olaf Norlis Bokhandel, Universitetsgaten, Oslo, 1980.
8. Colditz JC: Therapist's management of the stiff hand. In Mackin EJ, Callahan AD, Skirven TM et al, editors: *Rehabilitation of the hand and upper extremity*, St Louis, 2002, Mosby.
9. Frank C, Akeson WH, Woo SL et al: Physiology and therapeutic value of passive joint motion, *Clin Orthop* 185:113, 1984.
10. Bunnell S: *Surgery of the hand*, ed 2, Philadelphia, 1948, JB Lippincott.
11. Wehbe MA, Hunter JM: Flexor tendon gliding in the hand. II. Differential gliding, *J Hand Surg (Am)* 10:575-579, 1986.
12. Urbaniak JR, Cahill JD, Mortenson RA: Tendon suturing methods: analysis of tensile strengths. In American Academy of Orthopaedic Surgeons: *Symposium on tendon surgery in the hand*, St Louis, 1975, Mosby.
13. Schuind F, Garcia-Elias M, Cooney WP et al: Flexor tendon forces: in vivo measurements, *J Hand Surg (Am)* 17:291-298, 1992.
14. Long C: Intrinsic-extrinsic muscle control of the fingers: electromyographic studies, *J Bone Joint Surg (Am)* 50:973-984, 1968.
15. Arbuckle JD, McGrouther DA: Measurement of the arc of digital flexion and joint movement ranges, *J Hand Surg* 20B:836-840, 1995.
16. Stanley B: Therapeutic exercise: maintaining and restoring mobility in the hand, Chapter 7, *Concepts in hand rehabilitation*, Philadelphia, 1992, FA Davis.
17. Bell JA: Plaster cylinder casting for contractures of the interphalangeal joints. In Hunter JM et al, editors: *Rehabilitation of the hand: surgery and therapy*, ed 2, St Louis, 1990, Mosby.
18. Colditz JC: Plaster of Paris: the forgotten hand splinting material, *J Hand Ther* 15(2):144-157, 2002.
19. Brand PW, Hollister AM: *Clinical mechanics of the hand*, ed 3, St Louis, 1999, Mosby.
20. Brand PW: The forces of dynamic splinting: ten questions before applying a dynamic splint to the hand. In Hunter JM et al, editors: *Rehabilitation of the hand*, ed 2, St Louis, 1984, Mosby.
21. Bonutti PM et al: Static progressive stretch to establish elbow range of motion, *Clin Orthop* 303:128-134, 1994.

24

Dupuytren's Disease

CORNELIA VON LERSNER BENSON

Cords

Dehiscence

Dermofasciectomy

Diathesis

Fasciectomy

Fasciotomy

Limited (selective) fasciectomy

Nodule

Palmar aponeurosis

Peyronie's disease

Dupuytren's disease is a fairly common problem seen by hand surgeons and therapists. References to a condition characterized by an inward curling of the ring and small fingers are found as early as the twelfth century. In 1777, John Hunter, a British surgeon, accurately described the disease as a contracture of the palmar fascia. In the nineteenth century, the French provided the first extensive medical documentation of the condition, describing the characteristic flexion contractures of the fingers with dry, hard, stiff flexor tendons and palmar tissue. The disease was named after a French surgeon, Baron Guillaume de Dupuytren, who in 1831 performed the first fasciotomy (the removal of pathologic palmar fascia).[1] Much of the early history of the disease quite naturally centers on the attempts to determine the cause of the condition and the progression of the identifiable "palmar lumps" and on their treatment. Even today, the etiology of Dupuytren's disease is unknown, but a number of substantial theories have developed based on research findings and a modern understanding of cellular biology.

Dupuytren theorized that the disease arose from "microtrauma" caused by manual labor and intrinsic injury. However, this theory later was questioned when bilateral contractures were reported and similar clinical findings were seen in "upper class" clients who performed little or no manual labor.[2] Genetic and racial influences obviously needed to be investigated. This etiologic association gained popularity in the early 1900s, when the condition also became known as *Viking disease*, because it seemed to occur most often in regions that had been invaded by the Vikings. These areas included the western European coast, Poland, and the Ukraine. Currently the disease is most prevalent in Scandinavia and Great Britain.[2] Another interesting fact is that the disease is unknown in non-Caucasian races, even though these other populations make equal use of their hands; this seems to debunk the theory that overuse and trauma are the sole causes of the condition.

None of the available research conclusively links Dupuytren's contracture to hand dominance. However, the concept of microtrauma as a factor in the development of the disease has regained support. Manual laborers with small calluses in their palms often found that when they were promoted or retired and no longer performed manual labor, these early, unrecognized Dupuytren's contractures progressed rapidly.[2] Such cases seem to indicate that in individuals with an inherited **diathesis** (a bodily condition that predisposes a person to a particular disease), maximum manual labor keeps the hand in a state of physiologic normalcy, but when this level of use stops, the disease frequently progresses.[2]

Researcher John Hueston was the first to identify clients with an increased diathesis for the disease other then heredity.[2] He found that epilepsy, infection with the human immunodeficiency virus (HIV), alcoholism, and diabetes mellitus were closely related to the development of Dupuytren's disease. All these ailments are associated with the presence of oxygen free radicals and peripheral ischemia, and they are discussed later in the chapter in the context of treatment decision making. Manual work and hand injuries have a lesser implication in the cause of Dupuytren's disease than diathesis, but all these factors are considered in the decision-making process for surgical intervention and subsequent therapy.[3]

DIAGNOSIS AND PATHOLOGY

The typical client with Dupuytren's disease is a man in his 50s or older who notices a thickening or lump in his palm along the distal palmar crease at the axis of the ring finger. This **nodule** is the primary pathologic manifestation of Dupuytren's contracture, and it usually is the first sign the client sees. Later, **cords** arise, which are longitudinal manifestations of the thickening and contracting palmar fascia. Next, bands develop that extend longitudinally in the palm both proximally and distally into the finger. These pathologic cords and bands progress, causing shortening of and increased tension in the normal longitudinal fascial bands, called the **palmar aponeurosis.**[4]

In the early stages, Dupuytren's nodules may be confused with cysts, trigger finger, ganglions, and foreign bodies. However, Dupuytren's nodules usually are centered in the distal palmar crease or at the base of the thumb and extend proximally into the finger. They also are associated with pitting over the nodule or mass, fatty knuckle pads, disease in the opposite hand, **Peyronie's disease** (the formation of dense fibrous tissue on the penis), and a strong diathesis. As the disease progresses, it draws the fingers into a flexed position (Fig. 24-1).

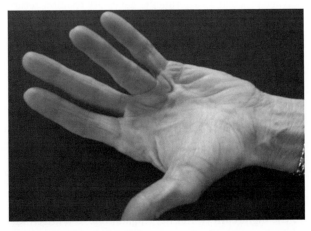

FIGURE 24-1 Early Dupuytren's disease; the ring finger is drawn into a flexed position at the MCP joint.

Women who develop Dupuytren's disease usually do so at an older age (in the 60s), and the progression of symptoms is less severe.

OPERATIVE TREATMENT

Indications for Surgery

Dupuytren's disease is a benign yet progressive process. Needle fasciotomy has been attempted, but the recurrence rate with this technique is greater than 50%. Radiation, enzymatic fasciotomy, and traction techniques also have been attempted, with limited or no success.

> **CLINICAL** *Pearl*
>
> Conservative nonsurgical treatment of Dupuytren's disease has been attempted but with little success. Currently, no effective, nonoperative treatment is available for the condition.[5]

The most successful treatment is surgical excision of the diseased palmar fascia. Indications for the surgery depend on the level of severity, whether joint contractures are involved, and the extent of functional disruption. The surgeon asks the client the following questions, and together they weigh the need for surgical intervention:

- Do you have a family history of Dupuytren's disease?
- How rapidly has this been progressing in your hand?
- Are you noticing the same condition in your feet or are there signs of Peyronie's disease?
- What is your biggest primary complaint and functional restriction?

A nodule alone, without contracture, is not an indication for surgery, and the client often just needs reassurance that the "lump" is not malignant. The most frequent functional complaints associated with the disease are difficulty putting the involved hand in a pocket and embarrassment about the curled fingers when shaking hands and waving. Flexion contractures greater than 30 degrees at the metacarpophalangeal (MCP) joint make using the hand difficult. This degree of flexion contracture is the indicator for surgery; lesser contractures are difficult to improve because of postoperative scar tissue.

Precaution. *Proximal interphalangeal joint (PIP) flexion contractures are more serious and more difficult to correct surgi-*

cally than MCP joint contractures, particularly with longstanding disease.

It is important that therapists make sure their clients have realistic expectations about finger function after surgery. Rarely is a finger completely corrected, particularly with multijoint involvement or contractures that have been present for years. Thumb contractures are not uncommon, and in severe cases Dupuytren's disease can limit the ability to extend and abduct the thumb. Clients with this condition often complain of having difficulty grasping large objects and using keyboards and computers. Again, the severity of contraction and of functional impairment determine the need for surgical intervention.

Precaution. *You may be asked to help explain to your client that repair involving late surgery or severe contractures may be only partly successful and may result in a poorly functioning digit.*

Surgical Techniques

Several techniques have been developed for surgical treatment of the skin and management of the fascia in Dupuytren's disease. The surgeon's preference and the severity of the disease dictate the procedure used. The four preferred types of fasciectomy for managing the diseased fascia are fasciotomy, regional or radical fasciectomy, limited selective fasciectomy, and dermofasciectomy.

Fasciotomy is the least complicated procedure. It most often is indicated when the disease does not involve PIP contractures. A local anesthetic is administered, and the surgeon works through an incision (often called a *blind stab*) between the skin and the fascial bands to divide the diseased fascia. This puts the surgeon at a visual disadvantage, because much of the procedure is performed without full tissue exposure. Colville[6] found that fasciotomy is most effective in older clients with MCP contractures. The technique has been modified so that a Z-plasty can be performed over the contracture band; in the modified procedure, the skin is opened in triangular flaps and the underlying cords and neurovascular bundles are exposed (Fig. 24-2). This modification also accommodates skin loss resulting from long-term palmar contracture.

Fasciectomy is the excision of fascia and palmar aponeurosis. Radical, or total, fasciectomy removes all fascia and palmar aponeurosis, both diseased and possibly diseased tissue. Fasciectomy most often is indicated for cases in which several fascial structures cause PIP contracture. However, the technique has fallen out of favor because the surgery is extensive and is associated with a high complication rate.

Limited (selective) fasciectomy is the surgical excision of only currently diseased tissue. It is most often used

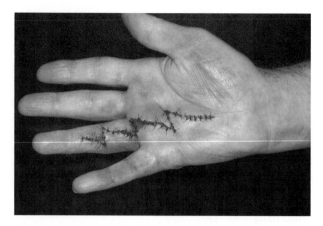

FIGURE 24-2 Postoperative view of an incision made during surgical treatment of Dupuytren's disease. The procedure involved a single finger fasciotomy using Z-plasty exposure.

with palm involvement only, particularly of the ulnar-side digits. Secondary operations to treat disease recurrence are more likely with this procedure, particularly in a client with a strong diathesis.

Dermofasciectomy involves the removal of both the diseased tissue and the overlying skin. The gap then is covered with a skin graft, or part of the wound is left open to heal by secondary intention. This is the McCash open palm technique, named after the surgeon who developed the procedure. McCash believed that an open palm wound had advantages over a skin graft; specifically, it acted as an open drain, preventing the formation of a hematoma, and it allowed for immediate range of motion (ROM) exercise.[7] This assertion later was substantiated by studies in which the total active motion of clients who had had closed surgery was compared with that of clients who had had open palm surgery.[7]

Amputation may be necessary in extreme cases of soft tissue loss or with severe, longstanding disease and contracture. Although controversial and extreme, this salvage procedure sometimes is necessary to allow return of function in a previously useless hand.

Complications

The incidence of complications arising from surgical treatment of Dupuytren's disease has declined in recent years because of advances in surgical and rehabilitative techniques and a better understanding of the tissue healing process. Complications occur in approximately 20% of Dupuytren's surgeries, most often in cases involving severe, extensive preoperative deformity and disease. Complications include infection, skin loss, hematoma, **dehiscence** (separation of the edges of the wound), injury of the digital artery and nerve, gangrene of a finger, loss of flexion, and complex regional pain syndrome (CRPS) (Fig. 24-3).

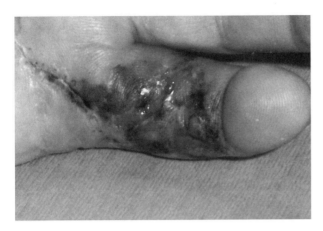

FIGURE 24-3 Incision showing dehiscence, skin necrosis, and infection, which are postoperative complications of surgery for Dupuytren's disease.

The complications can be divided into two categories: operative complications (infection, hematoma) and physiologic disturbances (CRPS, tissue loss, hypertrophic scarring, dehiscence, and loss of motion).[5] The therapist must monitor and manage physiologic contributions to these processes. Hand therapy techniques can minimize inflammatory cellular responses associated with the surgery and maximize tissue nutrition and oxygenation during rehabilitation.

Preoperative Evaluation Tips

Preoperative evaluations, although not often performed, are very helpful. By assessing your client's objective and functional status before surgery, you can eliminate the potential for some problems after surgery. Also, you can obtain a baseline measurement of the client's physical status, allowing for later measurement of outcome success and satisfaction (Box 24-1). In addition, preoperative evaluations are an excellent opportunity to educate clients about their postoperative course of care.

Perhaps the most useful component of the preoperative visit is the therapist's discussion with the client about the person's expectations, understanding of the postoperative course, and current functional limitations. Clients who are well informed about the course of their surgery and rehabilitation are more likely to comply with therapy and to express satisfaction with the outcome than are clients who later are surprised by the extent of the surgery or the commitment to therapy that recovery requires.

What to Say to Clients

- *Do you understand the progressive nature of Dupuytren's disease?*
- *Would you like me to review it with you?*

BOX 24-1

Steps in the Preoperative Evaluation

- Begin by obtaining active and passive joint measurements and volumetric measures.
- Perform a sensibility evaluation that includes Semmes-Weinstein monofilament testing and static two-point discrimination.
- Record grip and pinch strength when motion is sufficient for grasping the dynamometer and pinch gauges.
- Test the vascular integrity of the digits by performing Allen's test (see Chapter 5).
- Observe the sweating patterns in the client's hands. The client may have sensitive sympathetic (autonomic) nervous system function and may have sweaty palms if nervous during evaluation. *This is an important observation. It should be discussed with clients, particularly those undergoing radical surgery, because autonomic sensitivity puts an individual at greater risk for postoperative complex regional pain syndrome (CRPS).*
- Check for indicators of possible postoperative complications (e.g., increased pain, decrease in motion, dusky coloring on incisional borders). Many complications are predictable, and early detection can help minimize or prevent them.
- Initiate an outcome questionnaire appropriate to your profession or scope of practice, such as the Canadian Occupational Performance Measure (COPM) for occupational therapists or the Disabilities of the Arm, Shoulder and Hand (DASH). These questionnaires are used later to measure surgical and therapeutic success and function (see Chapter 6).

- *Did the doctor discuss the extent of your surgery? Do you still have questions?*
- *Are you aware that this surgery will require you to participate in hand therapy several times a week for several weeks?*
- *Do you notice that your palms sweat easily?*
- *Do you smoke or drink alcohol regularly?*
- *Would you like to see a photograph or sketch of the splint you will be wearing after surgery?*
- *What things are difficult for you to do now that you hope to be able to do better after surgery?*
- *What goals do you have for the surgery?*

"It is important for you to understand your role in avoiding possible complications after surgery. The operation will allow you to better straighten your finger, but after surgery you will need to wear a splint during the day to be sure that this straightening is maintained. You also will need to attend therapy two or three times a week so that the therapist can help you exercise, regain the use of your hand, and care for your incision. Complying with this program is critical for making the most of the surgery."

"If you smoke or drink alcohol regularly, it is important that you avoid these habits after surgery to improve the blood supply and delivery of nutrients to your hand and the healing tissue. Research has shown that better tissue nutrition and less trauma help Dupuytren's clients heal better and with fewer complications."

It may be helpful to show clients a photograph or sketch of the splint they will wear after surgery.

POSTOPERATIVE TREATMENT

Individualized treatment planning is critical for clients who have undergone surgery for Dupuytren's disease. The plan of care must reflect the nature and extent of the surgery and of the client's functional deficits and goals. Good communication with the surgeon makes this process much easier.

Early Phase: 24 Hours to 4 Days

A primary requirement is to maintain the surgical gains achieved in the operating room. Also, avoiding tension and mechanical stress on the neurovasculature and incision are critical to allowing better delivery of nutrients to the tissues.

Various approaches to splinting have been described and researched. A dorsal or volar splint can be fabricated that includes both the affected digits and neighboring digits. A dorsally based splint puts less pressure on the surgical site (thereby preventing compromised nutrition) while maintaining the extended finger position. It also allows clients to control their progress in digital extension up to the splint hood. Volar-based splints are thought to increase intentional pressure on the surgical site, allowing management of the scar (Fig. 24-4).[8] The referring physician may make this determination, or you may choose the type of splint based on your personal and clinical preferences.

Diagnosis-Specific Information That Affects Clinical Reasoning

The exact resting angle of the splint is based on the surgical disruption of the neurovasculature, the previous degree of contracture, and any tissue color and temperature changes that occur during splint fabrication. If the digit had a mild contracture, if the PIPs were not involved, and if no sensory changes were noted before or after surgery, the wrist can be splinted in neutral position with the MCPs in 0 to 20 degrees of flexion for the first days

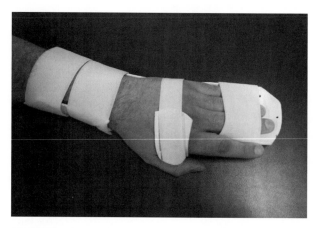

FIGURE 24-4 Volar-based wrist and hand splint with the wrist and MCPs in neutral position.

after surgery if the tissue responses are good. Good tissue response is evidenced by client comfort and by the absence of color, sensory, or temperature changes.

Precaution. *If the involved digit develops a dusky (gray) color or becomes ischemic, immediately reduce the degree of extension and eliminate any source of pressure or vascular compromise from dressings or splints.*

Ultimately the fingers and thumb, when involved, should be positioned in the greatest amount of safe extension the tissue can tolerate to maintain the gains achieved surgically.[7] You can fabricate the splint in full MCP and PIP extension and allow your clients gently to self-progress the finger position between therapy visits through increased strap tension. The splint is worn at night and periodically during the day between exercise sessions or according to surgeon's preference, when this information is available (Fig. 24-4).

With a longstanding or more complicated contracture treated with an extensive fasciectomy, all tension should be eliminated at the wound site for the first 2 weeks. These clients benefit from temporary MCP positioning at 40 degrees with the wrist in neutral position to avoid local hypoxia or further tissue stress (see Figure 24-5).[9] Research has shown that splinting the MCPs in slight flexion for the first 2 to 3 weeks of wound healing to relieve tension on the wound does not result in any loss of ROM in digital extension.[10] The splint is worn at night and periodically during the day; it is removed for bathing and dressing, wound care, and gentle exercise. This wearing schedule is monitored to ensure that it achieves the established goal: maintaining the digital extension achieved in the operating room. In both of these types of splints (see Figs. 24-4 and 24-5), position the interphalangeal (IP) joints during these early postoperative days in as neutral position as the client's tissues can tolerate.

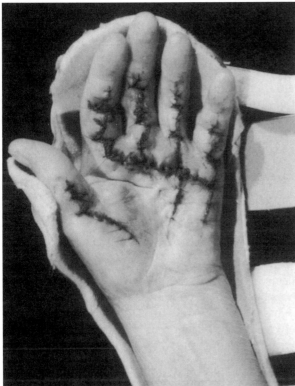

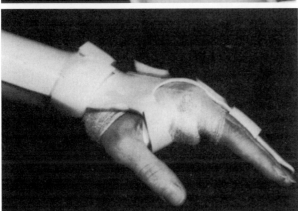

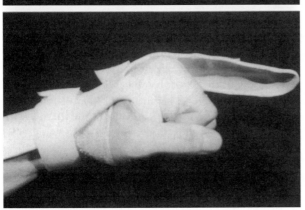

FIGURE 24-5 Dorsal static protective splint used immediately after surgery; this type of splint allows active flexion but limits full extension. (From Evans RB, Dell P, Fiolkowski P et al: A clinical report of the effect of mechanical stress on functional results after fasciectomy for Dupuytren's contracture, *J Hand Ther* 15:331-339, 2002.)

Precautions and Concerns

- *The client's fingers should remain warm and pink during splint wear.*
- *The client should not have any significant increase in pain while wearing the postoperative splint.*
- *The client should not have any sensory changes during splint wear.*
- *If the client is losing extension between therapy visits, the wearing time for the splint must be increased.*
- *If the client is having difficulty with active motion, the splint should be removed more often during the day.*

Wound Care

It is best to receive specific wound care guidelines from the surgeon. The surgeons with whom I work recommend the following:

- If the wound has not undergone skin grafting and if the palm stitches are intact, gently begin cleansing the wound with mild soap and water by the third postoperative day.
- The wound may continue to drain in the first days after surgery. Changing the dressing will be easier and less disturbing to the new tissue if a nonadherent gauze or dressing (e.g., an Adaptic contact layer) is used between the skin and the gauze wrap. *Use only one layer of the nonadherent gauze; use of more than one layer can contribute to maceration.*
- Dressings should be changed daily. This gives both the therapist and the client regular opportunities to inspect the wound for signs of infection, drainage, hematoma, and vascular changes.

Precaution. *Clients who have had a skin graft or flap procedure will have a thick, soft bolus dressing, which should not be disturbed. Do not remove this dressing for 5 to 7 days or until the surgeon has re-evaluated the client.*

By this time the graft has grown into the wound bed; you must be meticulous and delicate in changing the dressing to preserve this cell growth. Most grafts require a moist environment to prevent desiccation of the tissue, therefore a wet-to-dry dressing or antibacterial ointment should be applied unless otherwise specified by the surgeon.

Precaution. *Remember, it is always best to have specific dressing orders from the surgeon.*

- If ordered by the surgeon, a mild whirlpool treatment (96° to 98° F [35° to 37° C]) can be used to help restore tissue elasticity and to cleanse the wound in clients who have undergone the open palm technique.

Precaution. *Do not add cytotoxic chemicals, such as povidone-iodine (Betadine), to the whirlpool.*

Edema Control

Swelling is normal in the inflammatory phase of wound healing, but controlling swelling reduces fibrosis. Gross edema in the area around the wound reduces the blood supply and oxygen delivery to the wound, thereby interfering with healing by reducing the proliferation of granulation tissue.[11] As with many postoperative clients, management of edema after surgery for Dupuytren's disease includes elevation of the limb, light compressive dressings or self-adherent wrap (e.g., Coban), and gentle, controlled motion. The client should have little pain.

Precaution. *If severe pain develops during the first few days and the client reports needing a higher dosage of pain medication, inspect the wound and immediately refer the client back to the surgeon.*

If a hematoma has developed, the client may need additional surgery[11]; this is determined by the hand surgeon. Assess hand color and temperature changes frequently. *When vascularity is compromised, compression and cool compresses are contraindicated.*

CLINICAL *Pearl*

An edematous wound environment helps sustain and perpetuate a chronic inflammatory state, which is associated with excessive scarring.

Exercise

Gentle active digital flexion exercises usually can be started 3 days after surgery, depending on the status of the wound. When beginning this program, avoid extension greater than the limits of the splint and also avoid aggressive blocking exercises.

Precaution. *Early forced extension can cause vascular compromise, which can lead to loss of the digit.*

Active flexion and tendon gliding exercises of the digits and the thumb, if involved, should be performed every 2 to 3 hours within 3 to 4 days after surgery, if the tissues tolerate this regimen. Isolated exercises for the PIPs and the distal interphalangeal (DIP) joints are included in the home program. In the clinic, gentle flexion place and hold exercises can be initiated and progressed according to the tissue responses to therapy. Be sure to monitor tissue responses and take care to avoid stressors that provoke a flare reaction (e.g., increased swelling and pain).

Clinical Reasoning Considerations in Progressing Exercises

- How severely was the hand impaired before surgery?
- How quickly does the digit (or digits) lose flexion or extension with extended splint wear?
- Is the client compliant and cooperative?
- Is the exercise provoking an inflammatory response?

If a skin graft was placed, defer active motion until the surgeon has inspected the graft for viability and has authorized gentle exercise. Then, gentle active flexion, tendon gliding, and place and hold exercises are appropriate.

If the open palm technique or dermofasciectomy was performed, early motion often can be started on the first postoperative day. However, you must prepare the client for the appearance of the large, open wound in the palm. Unless you address this early, the client probably will be very alarmed and hesitant to exercise with such a wound. Having the hand surgeon also discuss this with the client can be helpful.

What to Say to Clients

About the Splinting Schedule

"You will need to wear your splint at night when you sleep and for most of the day to make sure your fingers stay as straight as the surgeon had them in the operating room. However, we don't want your fingers to get so stiff from splinting that it becomes difficult for you to make a fist. That means that during the day, you need to be sure to determine whether your hand needs more or less time in the extension position. If you find it hard to make a fist every 2 to 3 hours, after four or five attempts, leave the splint off for a while, let your hand rest in a relaxed position, and perform your exercises occasionally to make another fist. Conversely, if straightening your hand to fit the splint as it is today becomes harder and harder, make sure that you wear the splint often and that you are providing gentle extension stretch to the tissue without causing pain or discoloration of your fingers."

Provide written instruction with this program to ensure compliance.

About the Open Palm Technique

"You are going to have an opening in your palm that is allowing extra fluids and some blood to drain. This also helps new cells grow into the space. Do not be afraid to move your hand while your wound is still open. It will actually make moving less painful and allow you to move earlier."

Suggest including a spouse or close friend to provide support and to reduce fear and anxiety.

Postoperative Weeks 2 to 3

Splinting

After the first 2 to 3 weeks, the splint program requires frequent adjustments for proper fit and wearing times are modified. If the splint was positioned with less than full MCP extension to reduce tissue stress in the early phase, you can begin upgrading extension at 2 to 3 weeks after surgery. Make serial adjustments gradually and monitor closely for signs of tissue anoxia and other adverse effects, such as tissue color change or pain.

Tips for Clinical Reasoning about Progression of the Splint Position

* Does the finger change color within 10 minutes of adjustment of the splint position?
* At visits later in the week, does the client complain of increased pain or burning in the hand at rest or with use?
* Are the borders of the wound gray or white?

Precaution. *Gray or white wound borders indicate a compromised blood supply, which affects wound healing.*

* Is the palm red, inflamed, or painful?
* Does the wound show any sign of dehiscence?
* Is moving the fingers significantly more difficult during the day after splint wear?

If such negative effects occur, continue MCP flexion blocking to protect the hand for 2 more weeks. However, the client may tolerate PIP extension splints at this time. If the PIP was contracted before surgery, the central slip may be attenuated and the volar plate and oblique retinacular ligament may be tight after surgery.[12] For these cases, construct a volar trough splint for the proximal and middle phalanges and leave the distal phalanx free. Use soft strapping to provide a gentle extension stretch at the PIP joint, and encourage the client to move the DIP into flexion periodically. This small gutter splint can

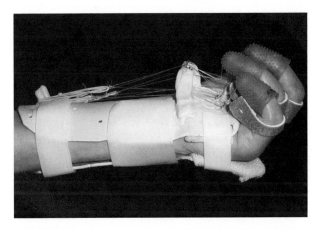

FIGURE 24-6 This composite flexion splint can be used after 2 to 3 weeks of therapy if flexion limitations require dynamic splinting. *The therapist must monitor the condition closely to prevent loss of extension ROM.*

be worn within the protective postoperative splint. Serial casting or static progressive splinting may be necessary if the PIP contracture is firmer or does not improve with use of the gutter splint.

Dynamic flexion splinting is rarely needed for Dupuytren's clients who are closely monitored. However, if you note significant loss of passive flexion, begin early composite dynamic flexion splinting to prevent joint contractures, shortening of the extrinsic flexors, and further loss of motion (Fig. 24-6). Dynamic flexion splints should be used according to the principles of low load, long duration splinting. Pain should not increase with this splinting program (see Chapter 23).

Wound Care and Scar Management

The stitches are removed approximately 2 weeks after surgery if the incision is well healed. Occasionally the surgeon leaves a single stitch in place for a longer period if the skin is under tension or slow to heal, such as at the volar MCP crease. *Clients with diabetes or other medical problems also may heal more slowly.* Minimizing tension and stretching along the incision line helps reduce heavy scarring and hypertrophy. If a stitch remains in place (and the surgeon recommends it), continue soaks and cleansing with mild soap and water. Heat or fluidotherapy can be used to improve tissue extensibility when the wound is fully closed and the graft is secure and mature enough to tolerate it. *Take care not to burn this fragile tissue.* Using silicone gel sheets or silicone-polymer pressure inserts (e.g., elastomer) over the incision may aid scar remodeling and minimize or prevent hypertrophy[13]; this is most important for primarily closed incisions. The gel sheets or inserts can be worn at night inside the splint and intermittently during the day (Fig. 24-7). Begin scar

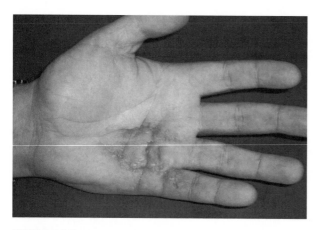

FIGURE 24-7   Three weeks after surgery, a thick, hypertrophic scar has developed. The scar should be treated with ultrasound, gentle massage, and silicone gel sheets.

massages daily in the home program and in the clinic to aid scar remodeling and desensitization.

Precaution. *Do not perform aggressive massage that irritates the scar or surrounding tissue; this can increase thickening of the scar.*

Treatments

Iontophoresis with saline has been shown to minimize excessive scar formation and can be used at 3 weeks after surgery in Dupuytren's clients. Saline seems to work as a sclerosing agent when delivered with iontophoretic current. The saline (1.5 ml in 2.5% aqueous solution) is delivered via the cathode.[14]

Continuous-wave ultrasound therapy also can be used in this phase. Because this treatment enhances soft tissue mobility and reduces stiffness, it is used to increase tissue temperature and precondition the hand before massage, stretching, or exercises.

Exercise

At 2 to 3 weeks, include active blocking exercises in both the daily home exercise program and the therapy session to maximize differential tendon gliding. In the clinic, use one hand to stabilize the more proximal joints and the other hand as a target to improve the client's tendon pull-through. Teach the client to perform a similar technique at home by stabilizing the more proximal joint (see Chapter 1).

What to Say to Clients

"I'm going to help you with your exercises so that you can learn to help individual tendons and muscles work independently. I'm going to hold the base of your finger still, and while I do, I want you to bend the tip until you touch my other finger. I'm using my finger as a target to encourage you to make a strong effort."

Adjust the position of your target finger as necessary and avoid causing any pain.

Precaution. *Pay close attention to signs of a flare reaction and inflammation after exercise.*

By working closely with the physician, you can aid medical decision making on when medicines such as Neurontin or Medrol or nonsteroidal antiinflammatory drugs (NSAID) should be used to reduce inflammation and interrupt the cycle of pain. If you note signs of a flare reaction, increase the frequency of therapy and implement treatment strategies for as outlined in the chapter on pain syndromes (see Chapter 18).

Postoperative Weeks 3 to 6

Splinting

If full extension is limited, fabricate a serial static splint to be worn during sleep for gentle, prolonged stretch. Adjust the splint and monitor progress and digit changes regularly in follow-up therapy visits. Combine this composite splinting program with individual PIP splints or serial casting for residual contractures. Differentiate joint tightness, intrinsic tightness, and extrinsic tightness and determine splint choices and positions accordingly.

Scar Management

If hypertrophic scars develop, continue to use silicone gel sheets for 12 hours daily, along with ultrasound therapy and deep massage combined with progressive desensitization. Iontophoresis with dexamethasone (if that medication is not contraindicated) can be used if the incision is painful or burning.

Exercise

Emphasize differential tendon gliding in this phase, as well as blocking exercises and oblique retinacular ligament stretch of DIP flexion with PIP extension. Initiate strengthening and light simulated job activities while observing the clinical response.

Precaution. *Avoid excessive repetition of exercises and monitor for signs of carpal tunnel syndrome.*

Postoperative Week 8 and Later

Progress the exercise program to strengthening and work simulation. These upgrades may include putty exercise, the BTE Work Simulator, tool use, and lifting and carrying to tolerance. The client should continue to wear the splint and gel sheet or silicone insert at night. Explain that the client also should monitor extension changes for 3 to 6 months after surgery.

The Role of the Therapy Assistant

- Providing preoperative client education
- Assisting with splint fabrication and modifications
- Assisting with wound care
- Managing edema
- Instructing the client in the home program, splint application, and precautions
- Providing family instruction and support training
- Teaching the client and family modifications for activities of daily living
- Monitoring for symptom flares during therapy sessions

CASE *Study*

B.L. is a 61-year-old, right-hand dominant machinist of Scandinavian descent. The only significant findings in his past medical history are that he is diabetic and a social drinker. He has no memory of a serious injury to his right upper extremity, but in the last year he has noticed that he has lost the ability to straighten the ring and small fingers of his right hand, and this seems to be getting worse. He remembers his father having something similar, but the condition was never addressed by a physician. B.L. states that the contracture "annoys" him, because although he can still use tools, he can no longer straighten his fingers enough to get his wallet out of his pocket. He also hesitates to greet people with a handshake because he cannot clear his palm of his last two fingers. He consulted a hand surgeon, and they decided that surgery was necessary because of the level of contracture and the progression of these changes.

EVALUATION

The physician worked closely with the hand therapy staff in the same building and requested a preoperative evaluation. The findings were as follows:

AROM	Right ring finger:	Right small finger:
	MCP: 47-95 degrees	MCP: 51-98 degrees
	PIP: 0-110 degrees	PIP: 19-108 degrees
	DIP: 0-55 degrees	DIP: 0-60 degrees
Grip and pinch (Jamar Dynamometer, rung position II)	Right hand: 89 lb	Left hand: 112 lb
Volumetric measurements	Right hand: 572 ml	Left hand: 566 ml
Sensation		
Von Frey monofilament testing for light touch sensation	3.22 bilaterally to volar fingertips	
Two-point discrimination	5 mm or normal bilateral fingertips	

Special tests
- Normal result on Allen's test for vascular function.
- No significant sweating in the palm during testing.
- Canadian Occupational Performance Measure (COPM): In functional performance measure, client noted five functions significantly impaired by his injured hand: putting his hand in his pocket, waving, using a keyboard, carrying, and grasping a large pipe wrench at work.

SURGICAL PROCEDURE

The physician performed a McCash open palm procedure to resect the diseased tissue that caused the contracture at the MCPs. An additional dissection was needed to release the PIP of the small finger and to remove diseased bands (Fig. 24-8). The palmar wound was left open to heal by secondary intention, with **Z**-plasty closure into the small finger; the sutures were to be removed in 2 weeks. The client's hand was covered in a wet-to-dry dressing over the palm and a bulky gauze wrap, and he was instructed to return to the physician's office in 2 days.

TWO DAYS AFTER SURGERY

The physician referred the client back to the hand therapist and prescribed whirlpool treatments, ROM exercise, edema control, and splinting. Although the client had no sympathetic signs before surgery, a dorsal extension splint was provided that allowed 30 degrees of MCP flexion the first 1 to 2 weeks; this prevented compromised delivery of nutrients to the tissue and wound bed, as well as anoxia. The PIPs were placed in extension to the hood of the splint. AROM exercises were initiated immediately, with 10 repetitions of gentle flexion to the palm every 2 to 3 hours and extension to the splint's

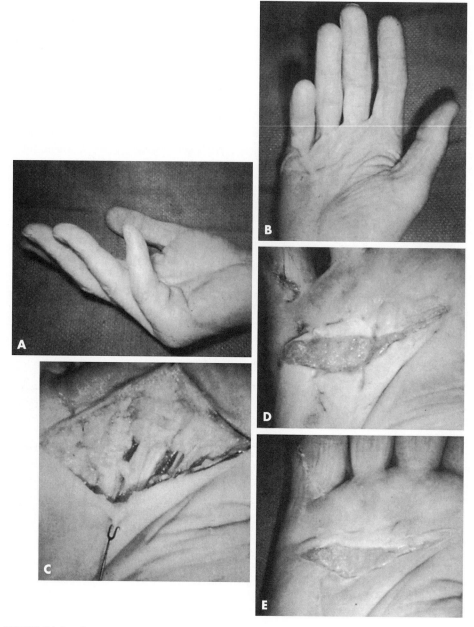

FIGURE 24-8   Open palm technique for resecting diseased tissue. (From Schneider LH: The open palm technique, *Hand Clin* 7:724-725, 1991.)

limits. Active flexion to the distal palmar crease was limited, measuring 2.5 cm in the ring finger and 2.8 cm in the small finger. Wound care included a cool whirlpool treatment (95° F [35° C]) during his clinic visits and daily dressing changes of wet-to-dry dressings at home. Edema management included elevation and AROM. The client was seen for therapy three times a week; at each visit he was given a sterile whirlpool treatment followed by elevation and exercises for AROM, tendon gliding, and gentle passive flexion stretch within tolerance.

ELEVEN DAYS AFTER SURGERY

B.L. had no adverse responses to splinting, the granulation bed around his palmar wound was good, and he was ready to have the PIP stitches removed. He was able to make a full active fist but struggled to maintain extension. His splint was modified at 2 weeks to increase the MCP position to 0 (neutral); the tissue reaction was watched closely, and B.L.'s wearing schedule was monitored.

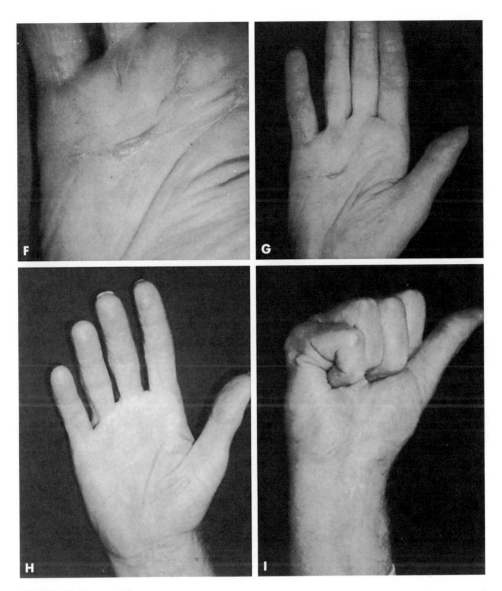

FIGURE 24-8 cont'd

TWO WEEKS AFTER SURGERY

With his splint adjusted and his stitches removed, B.L. demonstrated good extension and flexion at the MCPs and limited discomfort with exercise and splinting. Edema was minimal, but the limitations in PIP extension continued. More isolated exercise was given to the PIPs, and the client was given a gutter splint to wear at night with mild tension into PIP extension. This was to be followed by blocking exercise in the morning after removal of the splint. The palmar wound had not yet fully closed, and B.L. was instructed to keep it moist and clean.

THREE AND ONE-HALF WEEKS AFTER SURGERY

The palmar wound was closed, and PIP extension was resolved. The client's only complaint concerned the dense wound and palmar hypersensitivity. A daily desensitization program was added, along with ultrasound treatments in the clinic. B.L. also was given a silicone gel sheet for use at night. His splinting time was reduced to 2 hours in the morning, 2 hours in the evening, and nightwear, and he was monitored closely for changes in ROM. The therapist incorporated hand activities, including manipulating money, using the computer keyboard, and grasping and releasing large objects, to address the client's preoperative functional goals.

FIVE WEEKS AFTER SURGERY

B.L. began gentle strengthening exercises and lightly resistive tool grasp, along with desensitization.

TWELVE WEEKS AFTER SURGERY

The client returned to his job as a machinist. He was delighted with his outcome.

References

1. Elliot D: The early history of contracture of the palmar fascia. Part 3. The controversy in Paris and the spread of surgical treatment of the disease throughout Europe, *J Hand Surg* 14:25-31, 1989.
2. Hueston JT, Seyfer A: Some medicolegal aspects of Dupuytren's contracture, *Hand Clin* 7:759-763, 1991.
3. McFarlane R, MacDermid J: *Dupuytren's disease: rehabilitation of the hand and upper extremity,* St Louis, 2002, Mosby.
4. Luck JV: Dupuytren's contracture: a new concept of pathogenesis correlated with surgical management, *J Bone Joint Surg* 41A:635-664, 1959.
5. Hurst L et al: Dupuytren's disease: In Clayton A, Peimer MD, editors: *Surgery of the hand and upper extremity,* New York, 1996, McGraw-Hill.
6. Colville J: Dupuytren's contracture: the role of fasciectomy, *Hand Clin* 15:162-166, 1983.
7. Chick L, Lister GD: Surgical alternatives in Dupuytren's contracture, *Hand Clin* 7:715-719, 1991.
8. Mullins PA: Postsurgical rehabilitation of Dupuytren's disease, *Hand Clin* 15:167-174, 1999.
9. Evans RB: Dupuytren's Contracture, ASHT Scientific Session 2002, September 19-22, Ottawa, Canada.
10. Evans RB, Dell P, Fiolkowski P et al: A clinical report of the effect of mechanical stress on functional results after fasciectomy for Dupuytren's contracture, *J Hand Ther* 15:331-339, 2002.
11. Evans RB, McAuliffe JA: Wound classification and management: rehabilitation of the hand and upper extremity, St Louis, 2002, Mosby.
12. Smith P, Breed C: Central slip attenuation in Dupuytren's contracture: a cause for persistent flexion of the proximal interphalangeal joint, *J Hand Surg* 19A:840-843, 1994.
13. Ohmori S: Effectiveness of Silastic sheet coverage in the treatment of scar keloid, *Aesthet Plast Surg* 12:95-99, 1998.
14. Michlovitz S: Ultrasound and selected physical agent modalities in upper extremity rehabilitation. In Mackin EJ, Callahan AD, Skirven TM et al, editors: *Rehabilitation of the hand and upper extremity,* ed 5, St Louis, 2002, Mosby.

25

Upper Extremity Problems in Clients with Central Nervous System Dysfunction

MICHELLE ABRAMS

Hand therapists may be asked to treat clients with upper extremity problems resulting from neurologic impairment, or they may see a client with an orthopedic diagnosis who also happens to have a neurologic disorder. As an example in the first case, a physician refers a client to hand therapy in order to reduce a contracture caused by **rigidity** from **Parkinson's disease.** As an example in the second case, a physician refers a client who has carpal tunnel syndrome because of overuse of the unaffected arm years after that client sustained a stroke. In both of these cases the hand therapist must be able to incorporate treatment techniques appropriate to the neurologic impairment. This chapter addresses commonly encountered neurologic disorders that affect the upper extremities. This chapter is not meant to be all-inclusive but instead to provide an overview of commonly seen diagnoses. These diagnoses are **postpolio syndrome,** stroke, **multiple sclerosis,** Parkinson's disease, and **essential tremor.** The resource list at the end of this chapter offers additional information specific to these diagnoses for clients and therapists.

POSTPOLIO SYNDROME

From 1875 to the 1950s, **poliomyelitis** vastly affected the population of the United States. Discovery of an immunization in the early 1950s put a virtual halt to the spread of this epidemic in nations with access to the vaccine. More than 50 years after the implementation of the vaccine, health care professionals are treating these clients for problems that manifest later in life.

Diagnosis and Pathology

Poliomyelitis, more commonly referred to as "polio," is caused by a virus that attacks the motor neurons of the anterior horn cells of the spinal cord, resulting in varied symptoms ranging from minor muscle weakness to complete paralysis.[1] Sensation is not involved.

The diagnosis of postpolio syndrome (PPS) is based on a history of poliomyelitis and complaints of a random pattern of increased muscle weakness that does not follow a nerve root or peripheral nerve distribution. Additional symptoms may include severe fatigue; muscle pain, cramping, or **fasciculations** (muscle twitch); joint pain; sleep apnea; intolerance to cold; and depression.[2] Arm pain occurs in approximately 64% of persons with PPS and generally is associated with the overuse of muscles compromised by the use of mobility aids such as wheelchairs or crutches.[3] A higher prevalence of mild osteoarthritis occurs in the hands and wrists in the PPS population than in normal individuals for the same age group.[4]

Timelines

Onset of PPS occurs approximately 30 to 40 years after having polio. Muscle weakness, a common symptom, is caused by overuse of the muscles that originally were affected. Clients may fear that this weakness is a return of the polio virus, and it is important to clarify and reassure them about this distinction. Clients may be referred to hand therapy because of muscle weakness, joint and muscle pain, and decreased functional hand use.

No drug or surgical treatment is known to reverse the effects of PPS. The role of the hand therapist is to preserve strength, reduce the risks of overuse syndromes, assess for beneficial adaptive equipment, instruct the client in energy conservation and joint protection, and provide custom splinting to support weak muscles, minimize pain, and increase functional hand use.

Nonoperative Treatment

Exercise

Precaution. *It has not been determined whether exercise in clients with PPS is beneficial or harmful.[5] The motor unit or muscle is susceptible to overuse by nature of the disease. Therefore strenuous exercise that exceeds joint and/or muscle tolerance may exacerbate PPS.*

Therapy should focus on increasing aerobic capacity, strength, and activity tolerance.[6] Persons with PPS should not exercise to the point of fatigue. They should use only light resistance that is less than their maximum ability. The goal of exercise is to increase endurance and avoid injury or overuse.

Agre et al.[5] examined the effects of a combination dynamic and isometric 12-week home exercise program in clients with PPS. The weight used for the dynamic portion of the exercises was determined by the rate of perceived exertion of the subject. Weights were selected that were perceived as "somewhat hard" during the trials but were categorized by the subject as less than "very, very hard" after 3 sets of 12 repetitions. Subjects significantly increased muscle strength, work performance, and activity tolerance without adverse effects to the muscles or motor units.

In a similar study, clients with PPS were asked to participate in a low-intensity, alternate-day exercise program.[7] This study revealed no deleterious effects on the motor unit or muscle, nor did it find any positive trend in muscle physiology. These authors theorized that the low-intensity nature of their exercise program did not challenge the motor unit sufficiently to cause measurable positive changes in the muscle fibers.

Upper extremity exercises should be performed with weights and repetitions that provide a comfortable and submaximal challenge for the client. The hand therapist routinely should complete manual muscle tests on clients who participate in nonfatiguing resistance exercises to ensure that the exercise regimen is not causing weakness because of overuse.

Activities of Daily Living

Other nonoperative treatment includes instruction in lifestyle changes such as proper body mechanics and use of adaptive equipment to reduce stress on the joints of the upper extremity. Appropriate adaptive equipment may include built-up handles for eating utensils and self-care items for reduced grip strength, as well as reachers and sock aids to assist with limited mobility. Custom splinting may increase functional hand use. For example, a dynamic wrist extension splint enhances natural tenodesis grasp, and a metacarpophalangeal extension-blocking splint reduces hyperextension of the metacarpophalangeal joints associated with intrinsic weakness of the hand. Solutions such as these can improve grip and pinch function.

Modalities

Widar and Ahlstrom[8] determined that joint pain in the upper extremity of clients with PPS is worse in the evening and is exacerbated by physical strain and climatic factors such as cold temperatures and rain. The hand therapist should emphasize night splinting, rest, and the cautious use of heat, which can reduce pain.[8] *The client should avoid ice.*

Operative Treatment

No operative intervention is known to reverse the effects of PPS, but some clients undergo orthopedic surgery to correct joint, tendinous, or muscular deformities that are a result of the syndrome. Wheelchair-dependent clients or crutch users may have rotator cuff injuries because of overuse and may benefit from arthroscopic debridement to improve function and relieve shoulder pain. If there is paralysis or weakness of the opponens pollicis, functional opposition can be restored by tendon transfer. Tendon transfers also are done to improve function of the wrist extensors, maximizing tenodesis for grasp function.[1]

Questions to Ask the Physician

- *Is there evidence of a rotator cuff tear or a ligamentous injury?*
- *Is this client a candidate for corrective surgery to improve function and/or reduce pain?*

What to Say to Clients

About the Diagnosis

"Postpolio syndrome is caused by the overuse of muscles that were affected by the polio virus in the past. This diagnosis requires that we take care not to aggravate the symptoms further."

About the Pain

"A common aftereffect of postpolio syndrome is upper limb pain. The use of mobility aids such as wheelchairs or crutches can increase arm pain. Interestingly, this pain more often involves the upper extremity that was not affected originally by the polio process. Overuse syndromes of unaffected limbs can lead to much of the functional limitations seen with postpolio syndrome. It is helpful to minimize pain by performing gentle exercise, practicing joint protection principles, and possibly splinting in order to maintain functional arm use."

About Concurrent Osteoarthritis

"If you have lower extremity weakness, you are more prone to overuse your arms. This can result in osteoarthritis in your hands and wrists. Hand splinting might be beneficial but might interfere with your use of canes or crutches. We need to work together to find a good balance that includes protecting your joints and using the adaptive equipment that you need."

About Energy Conservation Techniques/Joint Protection Principles

"Try to avoid reaching whenever possible. Bring objects close to your body when lifting or moving items. This helps you to avoid strain on your shoulders and elbows. Keep your wrists in a neutral position whenever possible during activities such as typing and knitting." Discuss joint protection principles in terms of activities of daily living (ADL) and work.

About Splinting

"Splinting can be used to protect your arm or to increase function. The splint helps keep your arm in a position that will rest the joint and reduce pain. Certain kinds of splints also help enhance your grip to make holding on to items easier."

About Exercises

"Perform exercises that increase aerobic capacity, isometric strengthening, and endurance. Avoid heavy resistance or pushing beyond comfort because this may lead to other problems, such as tennis elbow or rotator cuff tears." You may need to reinforce this continually until the client verbalizes and demonstrates an understanding of how to perform exercises safely.

Evaluation Tips

- A comprehensive client history is the most important part of the evaluation. Key questions include the number of years since the initial onset of the polio-virus, the muscles/limbs affected by the virus, and the muscles/limbs that are symptomatic.
- Note the current use of mobility aides and adaptive equipment for ambulation and ADL function.
- Use the Canadian Occupational Performance Measure (if appropriate to your professional scope of practice) to achieve a client-centered treatment plan.
- Note the client's pain level at its worst and at its least throughout the day and night.

Precaution. *Avoid strenuous manual muscle tests or grip/pinch testing if this causes an increase in pain.*

Diagnosis-Specific Information That Affects Clinical Reasoning

PPS is the reemergence of a disease process that was thought to be resolved.[9] Profound psychological symptoms may accompany the syndrome. Incorporate individually meaningful activities, and try to address the stresses that accompany the role changes in this population.

Polio survivors have attained educational and socioeconomic levels higher than those of the general population.[2] Their motivation for success is also evident in their quest for rehabilitation when the disease process re-emerges. Therapists should balance intense motivation with education to avoid overdoing it.

Tips from the Field

- Postoperative hand therapy for the PPS client should follow physician guidelines for the specific operation but may need to be modified to be gentler and more conservative. Do not overstress the involved joints or muscles.
- Always work with the client to balance joint protection with functional ability. Splinting might be beneficial, but clients may not comply with the splint-wearing schedule if the splint interferes with the use of mobility aids or completion of work tasks.
- Convey that you understand how hard the client had to work to recover his or her function following the original illness. Explain that with PPS now, working as hard as before is injurious. Rather, by protecting the muscles and joints, the client can perserve function.

- Find individually appropriate ways to change clients' behaviors of ignoring their pain. Consider an activity log. Look at pacing, schedule changes, and lifestyle modifications to get more rest throughout the day.

Precautions and Concerns

- *Continually monitor the client's rate of perceived exertion during exercise, and do not exceed safe and productive levels of exercise.*
- *Avoid painful exercise.*

CEREBRAL VASCULAR ACCIDENT

Cerebral vascular accident (CVA), or stroke, is the most common neurologic disease in adulthood, newly affecting more than 750,000 persons in the United States each year.[10] Two thirds of stroke survivors have residual neurologic deficits that impede function. A CVA can have devastating effects on occupation and ADL independence. Hand therapy has tremendous potential for restoring function, but a good therapist must address all aspects of the deficits, including cognitive, perceptual, and sensory losses, in order to maximize optimal recovery.

Diagnosis and Pathology

Strokes are categorized as **ischemic** or **hemorrhagic.** An ischemic stroke is caused by blockage of cerebral blood flow. A hemorrhagic stroke is caused by bleeding into the brain. Physicians use magnetic resonance imaging or a computed tomography scan to diagnose the extent of damage and area affected by the stroke. These tools may be helpful in predicting the recovery of function.

The most common stroke involves the middle cerebral artery.[11] Ischemia of the middle cerebral artery results in contralateral **hemiplegia** (full or partial paralysis of one side of the body)/**hemiparesis** (muscular weakness or partial paralysis restricted to one side of the body), sensory deficits, contralateral **homonymous hemianopsia** (loss of visual field in the corresponding right or left half of each eye), and **aphasia** (a language disorder resulting from a neurologic impairment that can affect auditory comprehension and/or oral expression). Box 25-1 lists typical perceptual and cognitive characteristics associated with right versus left hemispheric CVA. This population has unilateral impairments in motor control or possibly complete loss of function in one arm. Stroke causes loss of cortical regulation of normal subcortical responses and results in patterned **synergistic movements** and abnormal reflexes such as upper extremity **hypertonicity** (the muscle constantly is tensed because of increased tone) or **flaccidity** (muscles lack tone).[12] Synergistic movements

BOX 25-1

Perceptual and Cognitive Deficits Typical with Cerebral Vascular Accident

RIGHT HEMISPHERIC CEREBRAL VASCULAR ACCIDENT WITH LEFT HEMIPARESIS/HEMIPLEGIA

Deficits may occur in the following:
Hand-eye coordination
Spatial relationships
Figure-ground discrimination
Form constancy
Visual neglect
Emotional lability
Poor judgment
Denial of disability
Body image; not recognizing own body parts
Retaining information
Problem-solving ability
Attention span

LEFT HEMISPHERIC CEREBRAL VASCULAR ACCIDENT WITH RIGHT HEMIPARESIS/HEMIPLEGIA

Deficits may occur in the following:
Motor apraxia
Initiation and termination of tasks
Sequencing and problem solving
Poor frustration tolerance
Language skills—aphasia
Processing delays
Verbal and motor perseveration
Compulsive behavior; poor judgment
Severe distractibility

CLINICAL *Pearl*

Clients with complete limb paralysis typically recover voluntary movement in the order of flexion of the shoulder, followed by flexion of the elbow, wrist, and fingers, and supination of the forearm. Clients recover simultaneous flexion and extension of all fingers before being able selectively to activate individual digits.[12]

Visual neglect and sensory deficits of the affected side limit recovery of motor function and ADL independence because the client is less likely to attend to or initiate activities with the involved extremity.[13] Cuing clients to attend visually to their affected side during active movement and functional activities enhances healing and improves function.

General Guidelines when Evaluating Clients with Cerebral Vascular Accident

Sensory testing in clients with upper motor neuron deficits (e.g., CVA) differs from sensory testing in clients with lower motor neuron deficits (e.g., peripheral neuropathy). With CVA, the goal of sensory testing is not to identify the level of innervation as in peripheral neuropathies, but rather to assess the presence or absence of the sensation that typically is controlled cortically.

Proprioception is the awareness of joint position in space. Clients with deficits in proprioception are at risk for injury to the affected arm and also have difficulty applying the appropriate amount of pressure to hold on to items such as styrofoam cups or eggs without breaking them. They often may be unaware of having their small finger caught on the lip of a table or in the arm of their wheelchair. They do not understand why their arm will not move where they want because they do not recognize or sense that their finger is caught. Visual cuing, verbal direction, and weight-bearing activities can assist in improving function with deficits in proprioception. To assess proprioception during the evaluation, prevent tactile input to the volar or dorsal surface of the client's arm or hand. Instead, hold only the lateral aspects of the arm and move each joint in flexion or extension with the client's vision occluded. The client indicates whether the body part is moving "up" or "down" to correspond with flexion or extension.

In addition to proprioception, sensory evaluation should include assessment of two-point discrimination at the fingertips with points being less than 1 cm apart. If deficits exist in this area, the client will be dramatically less likely to initiate activities with his or her hemiplegic

are gross patterns of movement in flexion or extension that occur as a result of interruption in cortical control. All muscles involved are neurologically linked, and when one of these movements occurs, movement in some or all of the other linked muscle groups occurs simultaneously. These patterns of movement can be nonfunctional, for instance, when a client attempts to reach and grab an object, because a flexor synergy causes flexion of the digits and elbow at the same time. The desired movement would be for the elbow to extend while the digits flex.

Timelines and Healing

The most significant spontaneous neurologic recovery from stroke occurs within the first 2 months.[12] Many health care professionals believe that neurologic recovery can continue to occur for up to 1 year and even longer following the onset of symptoms.

arm.[12] Include visual perceptual testing as well in the evaluation. If a formal or standardized visual-perceptual assessment is not available in the clinic, a gross assessment may include having the client read a paragraph from a magazine out loud or identify all of the M's, for example, on a sheet of paper filled with different letters. Ask the client to draw a clock or a person in order to identify visual neglect and/or body schema deficits. Successful completion of these tasks indicates that the client does not have significant visual neglect or deficits in spatial orientation.

Test posture or tone by assessing the reaction of a muscle to a quick stretch. Tone typically is described as "none," "minimal," "moderate," or "severe." Include these classifications in the evaluation so that the tone can be reassessed in response to treatment modalities or prolonged stretching through splinting.

Nonoperative Treatment

Addressing Tone and Pain
Dependent edema and soft tissue contractures can be minimized by proper extremity positioning. An arm trough or lap tray for the wheelchair-dependent client provides the affected shoulder with support to reduce **subluxation** (partial dislocation of a joint), helps to reduce edema in the hand, and minimizes possibility of upper extremity injury by the arm being caught in the wheel of the chair or bumped against walls or doorways. The occasional use of a sling can assist with shoulder subluxation and minimize pain and dependent edema during ambulation.

CLINICAL *Pearl*

Minimization of sling use when one is not ambulating is imperative in order to maximize functional arm use during activities.

Clients often experience pain with abnormal tone, whether they have **hypotonicity** (lack of tone) or hypertonicity. Therapists can use kinesiotaping to inhibit hypertonicity, to minimize shoulder subluxation caused by the flaccidity or hypotonicity of the rotator cuff musculature, or to reduce dependent edema. Instruction in kinesiotaping is available through continuing education courses.

Research is lacking to support any sustained effects of functional electric stimulation on upper extremity function. However, functional electric stimulation of the extensor digitorum communis may be useful clinically to help a client practice grasp and release tasks. This may be most beneficial to a client who has functional grasp

but cannot perform active release. A therapist also can use functional electric stimulation to decrease tone by stimulating the antagonistic muscle (e.g., stimulating the triceps in order to reduce biceps tone).

Activities of Daily Living/Motor Control
Learned nonuse occurs as the client no longer uses the affected arm in activity. Although it is important to teach clients one-handed techniques to regain ADL independence, it is equally important to encourage use of the affected arm as much as possible. Doing so facilitates **neuroplasticity** (the ability of the brain to recover structurally and/or functionally after injury). Because simultaneous finger flexion and extension return before individual digit isolation, the client should focus on using the affected hand for a gross grasp assist or stabilizing hand in functional activities before trying in-hand manipulation and fine motor control. An example would be stabilizing a lotion bottle with the affected hand while taking off the cap with the unaffected hand. By capitalizing on increased flexion tone in the hand, the client can squeeze lotion with the hemiparetic hand onto the unaffected arm and then, possibly with hand-over-hand assistance, can rub the lotion in by using gross movements of the shoulder and elbow. Other examples of appropriate functional activities include buttoning clothes and cutting food, which can be simulated by small object in-hand manipulation and using putty of graded resistances.

Motor control also can be improved through graded fine motor coordination activities. Examples include pegboards (graded large to small), handwriting or tracing tasks, and picking out small objects from a bowl of rice or beans. Practice and upgrading of activities may lead to improved motor control.

Traditional constraint-induced therapy restricts the client from using the unaffected arm for 90% of waking hours for 14 days. Page et al.[14] report that a modified constraint-induced therapy program might be an effective treatment method to improve arm function in clients with learned nonuse. Clients receive 6 hours of continuous therapy training for 10 days. The modified treatment includes 30 minutes of activity during therapy with the unaffected arm restrained so the affected arm is forced to achieve the goals of the selected task. The therapist can devise a home exercise program using a constraint-induced approach during ADL. The unaffected hand can be restrained easily by holding a tennis ball and then placing a sock or stockinette over that arm. This comfortable position prohibits the use of the unaffected arm.

Range of Motion/Exercise
Performance of daily range of motion of the affected arm is important in order to maintain joint mobility and to

prevent contractures. Teach clients and/or caregivers self-range of motion or passive range of motion exercises early in the rehabilitation process. Because a quick movement will trigger increased tone, teach them to perform passive range of motion exercises in a slow manner. Instruct the client how actively to assist with the range of motion exercises as much as possible. If a caregiver is not present, teach the client self-range of motion exercises with emphasis on how to move the affected arm safely.

Bilateral asymmetric movement is thought to increase cortical reorganization and thereby improve function. Initiate repetitive bilateral arm exercises such as pulleys, an upper arm bike, or pushing and pulling activities of the arms such as simulating use of poles in cross-country skiing. If a client cannot grasp the equipment with the hemiparetic arm, the therapist should secure the client's hand carefully with a strap. A study by Whitall et al.[10] showed that bilateral arm training with rhythmic auditory cuing improved motor function in the hemiparetic arm of stroke clients.

Splinting
Splinting can be used to reduce tone or **spasticity** and to improve function.

Precaution. *Use more rigid thermoplastic material when combating increased tone or spasticity, but instruct the client and/or caregiver to check for pressure areas, especially on the fingertips, because increased flexor tone will cause the fingers to curl and can create skin problems.*

Apply padding along the volar aspect of the fingers and provide well-fitted broad straps along the dorsum of the hand to distribute pressure over a greater surface area. It can be difficult to fabricate a splint for a client with increased tone. It helps to have another therapist, an assistant, or a family member present to assist in positioning the arm or hand.

CLINICAL *Pearl*

When fabricating an elbow extension splint, position the arm in shoulder abduction to reduce biceps tone. In forming a hand- or forearm-based antispasticity resting hand splint, hold the thumb in abduction to help reduce digital flexor tone.

If there is weakness of the wrist extensors, use a semirigid or rigid wrist cock-up splint to achieve a more functional position.

Sensory Reeducation
A client with sensory loss is at risk of injury to the affected extremity. If protective sensation and pain sen-

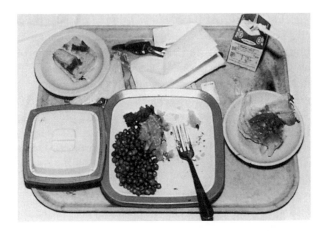

FIGURE 25-1 Clients with homonymous hemianopsia, or visual neglect, frequently ignore one side of their environment, including the food on the left side of their tray. They must be trained to compensate for this visual-perceptual deficit. (Waters RL, Wilson DJ, Gowland C: Rehabilitation of the upper extremity after stroke. In Hunter JM, Mackin EJ, Callahan AD, editors: *Rehabilitation of the hand: surgery and therapy*, St Louis, 1995, Mosby.)

sibility are absent, instruct the client visually to observe the position of the arm often to avoid possible injury. Advise the client to test bath water temperature and the heat or sharpness of an item with the unaffected extremity. In addition to compensatory strategies for safety, initiate sensory reeducation in an effort to improve sensibility. Refer to the chapter on nerve injury for more on sensory reeducation.

Visual-Perceptual Retraining
Visual neglect is defined as a client's inability to perceive entire regions of space contralateral to the brain lesions (Fig. 25-1). Neglect is more common and severe following strokes in the right hemisphere. Therapists should instruct clients, their families, and caregivers in ways to compensate for this perceptual loss. These include verbal cuing of clients to turn their heads toward their affected side to promote their ability to notice and localize items in their environment. Have clients use the affected arm to reach for objects placed outside their visual field. This stimulates enhanced motor function of the arm and also helps retrain attention to the environment and depth perception. Creating scavenger hunts within the clinic is a fun way to stimulate clients' ability to scan their environment.

Operative Treatment

Flexor tendon lengthening for mild spasticity or contracture can improve extensor strength and increase active range of motion in the wrist, thumb, or fingers.[12] Following this surgery, the hand and wrist are immobilized for about 3 weeks, and then comprehensive hand therapy is initiated, including functional electric stimulation of wrist and finger extensors and gentle passive range of motion to the wrist and finger flexors. Treatment progresses to include active exercises and functional activities that incorporate wrist and finger extension along with full grasp of the hand.

In a client with a nonfunctional contracted hand, surgery can correct severe wrist and finger deformities by flexor lengthening procedures. In these instances, the goal of surgery is to correct deformities that cause pain or impede hygiene, not to improve upper extremity function.

Questions to Ask the Physician

- *Is this client a surgical candidate for flexor tendon lengthening?*
- *Is this client currently on a medication regimen to reduce spasticity?*

What to Say to Clients

About the Diagnosis

"Often following strokes, your emotions will shift rapidly, and you might find yourself crying more than before. This is a normal occurrence and is related directly to what happened in your brain. Our job is to help you focus on your strengths and to regain your maximum level of independence."

About Positioning/Splinting

"Splinting can be used to help protect your arm or increase your arm and hand function. By using a hard plastic material, we can prevent joint tightness and keep the muscles balanced for best use in the future if you start to regain active movement in your hand."

About Exercise

"Quick movements in your arm will just increase the sense of tightness. It is important to do your exercises in slow, controlled movements so that your muscles can relax and get a good stretch."

About Functional Activities

"Every day, try to use your affected arm in some way. Pay attention to it, because the more you attempt to use it, the more likely you are to see positive changes."

Evaluation Tips

- Evaluate the client's motivation, muscle function, motor control, cognition, sensation, and visual-

perceptual skills in order to achieve a comprehensive evaluation.
- Avoid unnecessary distractions, interruptions, or stimuli.
- Monitor the client's level of fatigue and frustration. Complete the various portions of the evaluation in several sessions, if needed.
- Emphasize function when able. Clients may achieve a higher level of success, and the therapist can assess a client's ability more accurately during a functional activity as opposed to rote exercise or isolated movements.

Diagnosis-Specific Information That Affects Clinical Reasoning

When the client exhibits sensory and/or cognitive deficits, he or she may not be able to complete the exercises or self-range of motion in a safe way. Include caregivers when appropriate during exercises and range of motion activities.

Because it is common for a client to demonstrate **lability** (shifts in emotional state) and frustration following CVA, it is important to choose activities that will not elicit extensive frustration. Try to provide an adequate challenge to highlight strengths and gently point out areas of weakness that therapy can address. A client who is not motivated and is frustrated easily will not benefit from modified constraint-induced therapy.

When treating clients who are more than 1-year post-CVA, focus treatment on normalizing tone, preventing muscle and joint contractures, and instructing in one-handed techniques to improve functional independence. Make these decisions based on the client's current physical, cognitive, and visual-perceptual deficits.

Tips from the Field

- Treatment principles for clients with neurologic disorders differ from those for clients with orthopedic disorders. When treating an orthopedic client, it is important to gain good proximal strength before working on distal functioning. In contrast to this, when treating a neurologic client who has sustained a stroke, allowing patterned or synergistic movements proximally sometimes can aid in recovering distal functioning. It is always important to focus on function and compensatory strategies to increase ADL independence.
- Refer to your clients as "stroke survivors," not "stroke victims." Teach this concept to family members and caregivers. Explore avenues for members of the family to vent that do not embarrass or offend the client. An example of this would be a family member who

describes the client as a burden on the family in the presence of the client.

- Carpal tunnel syndrome resulting from overuse is common in the client's unaffected arm following a stroke.[15] Always work with the client to balance joint protection with functional ability. Splinting and rest might be beneficial but should not interfere with using mobility aids or completing basic ADL. Symptom management, prevention, and early intervention related to carpal tunnel syndrome are important in clients who have had CVAs.
- It may be helpful to keep an activity log of tasks completed with the affected arm throughout the day. This record identifies gains to the client and reinforces the benefits of the client's efforts, thereby reducing learned nonuse.

Precautions and Concerns

- *Applying moist heat to the affected extremity can reduce tone briefly and promote increased range of motion, but use caution and check the skin vigilantly if the client has any sensory losses.*
- *Postoperative hand therapy for the stroke survivor should follow physician guidelines for the specific operation.*

MULTIPLE SCLEROSIS

After trauma and arthritis, multiple sclerosis (MS) is the third leading cause of disability in adults 20 to 50 years of age.[16] Because of the nature of the disease, its implications on function vary tremendously and can include cognitive, motor, and sensory disturbances. Whether treating the physical effects of MS or working with a client with MS who sustained a wrist fracture, a therapist must always assume that the disease process will influence the progression and outcome of therapy.

Diagnosis and Pathology

MS is a chronic and typically progressive **demyelinating** (disrupting the myelin sheath that surrounds and insulates the axon of some nerves) disease of the central nervous system. Plaque or scar tissue develops on the myelin sheath of nerve fibers, which results in partial, complete, or intermittent blocks of nerve conduction. As nerve conduction is impaired and inflammation occurs, neurologic dysfunction ensues. The symptoms of MS depend on the location of the plaque or affected nerve fibers (Box 25-2). Clients often present to therapy with generalized fatigue, decreased ADL independence, and weakness or spasticity in the upper extremities.

The cause of MS is unknown at this time. Physicians diagnose MS by a review of the client's history, laboratory

BOX 25-2

Summary of Common Signs and Symptoms of Multiple Sclerosis

MOTOR SYMPTOMS
Spasticity and reflex spasms
Weakness
Contractures
Gait disturbance
Fatigue
Cerebellar and bulbar symptoms
Resultant swallowing/respiratory difficulties
Nystagmus
Intention tremor

SENSORY SYMPTOMS
Numbness
Pain (most often of musculoskeletal origin)
Paresthesia
Dysesthesia
Distortion of superficial sensation

VISUAL SYMPTOMS
Diminished activity
Double vision
Scotoma
Ocular pain

BLADDER/BOWEL SYMPTOMS
Urgency
Frequency
Incontinence
Urinary retention
Constipation

SEXUAL SYMPTOMS
Impotence
Diminished genital sensation
Diminished genital lubrication

COGNITIVE AND EMOTIONAL SYMPTOMS
Depression
Lability
Disorders of judgment
Agnosia
Memory disturbance
Diminished conceptual thinking
Decreased attention and concentration
Dysphasia

(From Frankel D: Multiple sclerosis. In Umphred DA, editor: *Neurological rehabilitation*, St Louis, 2001, Mosby.)

studies, and neurologic examination.[16] Diagnostic tests include cerebrospinal fluid analysis, nerve conduction studies, and brain imaging such as magnetic resonance imaging or computed tomography scans.

Timelines and Healing

Multiple sclerosis presents in three different patterns: (1) the classic pattern characterized by exacerbations and remissions; (2) a progressive pattern with a slow or fast worsening of symptoms without remissions; and (3) a combination of the two that includes exacerbations and remissions at the onset of the diagnosis but gradually becomes a disease of progressive decline.[17] The course of the disease is unpredictable, and the prognosis varies dramatically among individuals. No cures or operative treatment exists to eliminate the disease. The primary goal of medical treatment is to minimize the severity, amount, and length of exacerbations in order to improve function.

Nonoperative Treatment

Addressing Pain and Spasticity

CLINICAL *Pearl*

Sixty-five percent of clients with MS experience clinically significant pain.[18]

Spasticity and deconditioning that result from MS contribute to **dysesthesias** (sensory impairment) in the limbs, joint pain, and musculoskeletal pain. In therapy, address spasticity through splinting, positioning, stretching, and gentle range of motion exercises. Encourage clients to ask their physicians about pharmacologic agents that may inhibit tone or spasticity in the upper extremities as appropriate. Be careful to word this discussion in a way that does not exceed your scope of practice and does not sound like you are prescribing or suggesting medication to the client. Instruct the client in proper body mechanics to avoid overstressing joints and causing more musculoskeletal pain.

Modalities

Clients with MS typically are intolerant of heat.[16] A client with heat sensitivity experiences augmented signs and symptoms of MS with increases in core temperature and climatic temperature. A fever, environmental conditions, or excessive physical activity can lead to increased temperature.

Precaution. *Therapists should avoid using modalities such as moist hot packs or fluidotherapy. They also should emphasize the importance of rest and should avoid excessive physical exertion that will exacerbate symptoms during treatment.*

In contrast, cooling the client has produced favorable results. Persons with MS commonly use cooling techniques such as immersion in cold water, cold showers, ice packs, iced drinks, and the use of a liquid cooling garment.[19] In studies, most subjects with MS reported that 30 minutes of cooling resulted in less fatigue and increased motor control, with beneficial effects lasting from 1 to 4 hours. Therefore, it is advisable to include cold or ice modalities in therapy to increase function and enhance participation in conditioning exercises or ADL retraining.

Activities of Daily Living

Principles of treatment for clients with MS are similar to those for clients with PPS. Therapy includes instruction in lifestyle changes such as the use of proper body mechanics, energy conservation techniques, and adaptive equipment to compensate for weakened musculature and to reduce stress on the joints of the upper extremities. Adaptive equipment may include built-up handles for eating utensils and self-care items for reduced grip strength, as well as reachers and sock aids to compensate for limited mobility. See the PPS section in this chapter for information on splinting to enhance ADL function. For clients who experience hand tremors as a result of MS, try weighted utensils for self-feeding and wrist weights during ADL tasks. More suggestions for compensation of tremors can be found in the sections on Parkinson's disease and essential tremor later in this chapter.

Because clients with MS often have impaired sensation, incorporate compensatory strategies as described in the section on CVA. Sensory reeducation also may be effective in increasing sensory awareness.

Range of Motion/Exercise

Clients with MS can have weakness in the upper extremities caused by demyelination of the upper motor neurons, fatigue, disuse, or spasticity in the antagonistic musculature. Although exercise will not thwart the disease process, it does improve the overall health in the individual and buffers psychological, social, and physical problems associated with inactivity[17] (Fig. 25-2).

Therapeutic exercise can strengthen musculature affected by disuse, increase strength in nonaffected muscles to assist with compensation, and combat the spasticity of antagonistic muscles. Stress the importance of rest breaks throughout the exercise program to avoid fatigue. Instruct the client to complete exercises at sub-

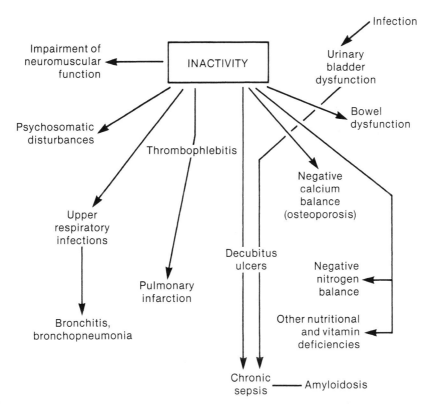

FIGURE 25-2 Inactivity chart. (From Bauer H: *A manual on multiple sclerosis,* London, 1997, International Federation of Multiple Sclerosis Societies.)

maximal resistance with frequent repetition in order to avoid overuse.

Questions to Ask the Physician

- *Is this client currently on a medication regimen targeted at reducing spasticity?*

What to Say to Clients

About the Diagnosis

"MS can be a frustrating disease because it tends to be unpredictable. It is important to find time to do the things that make you happy and relieve stress. Let's work together to see if we can identify ways for you to be able to do these things, even when your symptoms are aggravated."

About Positioning/Splinting

"Splinting can be used to reduce the pain in your arm or to increase function. The splint also can compensate for weaker muscles by holding your hand or wrist in a certain position that gives your fingers the best possible grip strength."

About Fatigue and Environmental Conditions

"It will take you twice as long to recover if you allow yourself to get to the point of complete exhaustion. Pace yourself. If you spread out your daily activities instead of condensing them all into the morning, you'll have more energy throughout the entire day. Also, it is important to know that heat could make your symptoms worse. Try to stay in air-conditioned areas and avoid hot showers."

About Exercise

"Although exercise isn't going to cure MS, it can give you more energy and strengthen your muscles. Listen to your body and respect the pain or fatigue. Do not overdo it or you could be risking additional pain or injuries. Yoga and exercise classes also have been shown to help with fatigue."[20]

About Activities of Daily Living

"Prioritize where you want to spend your energy. Delegate tasks you do not really enjoy so that you can save your energy for the things you do enjoy."

Evaluation Tips

- Activity tolerance and functional strength may vary during different times of day and in response to medications. Learn when the client feels he or she has the most energy during the day, and schedule therapy sessions at those times.

- Goal setting should be client-centered. Address different goals for exacerbation versus remission phases. Even if clients have hand function when in remission, instruct them in the use of adaptive equipment when their hand use may be impaired during exacerbations.

Diagnosis-Specific Information That Affects Clinical Reasoning

Commonly occurring cognitive deficits include impaired abstraction and problem solving, poor visual-spatial skills, delayed information processing, memory problems, and decreased attention.[16,21] Although clients with MS tend to have delayed information processing, they typically perform the tasks well as long as they are given additional time to process the information. Consider the client's abilities to follow through with treatment plans and to follow multistep instructions when communicating with these clients. Involve the family and caregivers as appropriate.

MS differs from insults such as a complete spinal cord injury or stroke because of its progressive nature. Clients and the health care team must acknowledge the symptoms as waxing and waning. Therapists consistently should reevaluate treatment plans and address the changing needs of the clients. They also should consider the psychological effects of depression and despair that can coincide with a progressive disease such as MS.

Tips from the Field

- Clients often rely on spasticity in their lower extremities to assist in functional transfers. By treating this spasticity, clients may experience increased weakness in their legs with resulting reduction in functional mobility. Help clients become aware of the functional benefits and the possible disadvantages of treatments for lower extremity spasticity.
- Stretching should be performed to decrease spasticity before initiating therapeutic exercise. This helps increase flexibility, increases circulation, and may help avoid possible injury.
- Clients with MS often find it easier to warm up with proximal exercises such as shoulder and trunk exercises before attempting activities requiring hand strength or fine motor coordination. Activities should progress from proximal to distal.

Precautions and Concerns

- *Avoid heat modalities in treatment, and recognize that excessive physical activity can raise the client's core temperature.*
- *Prioritize pacing with therapeutic exercise.*

PARKINSON'S DISEASE

James Parkinson first described the symptoms of Parkinson's disease as "the shaking palsy" in 1817. Today, Parkinson's disease is considered one of the most common movement disorders in the United States, affecting approximately 1% of the general population and up to 10% of the population over 65 years of age.[22] Parkinson's disease is a progressively debilitating disease that often eventually results in complete loss of ADL independence. In Parkinson's disease, the characteristic tremor is a **resting tremor** that tends to abate with functional or intentional hand use. The symptoms of Parkinson's disease affect functional hand use, mobility, and cognition (Table 25-1). Whether a physician refers a client with Parkinson's disease to therapy for instruction in the use of adaptive equipment to increase ADL independence or because of an unrelated injury, the therapist must factor in the symptoms of the neurologic disorder to the treatment.

Diagnosis and Pathology

Parkinson's disease is a chronic, progressive, degenerative disease caused by the loss of dopamine-producing neurons in the substantia nigra of the brainstem and the presence of Lewy bodies.[23,24] The lack of dopamine results in the reduced ability of the brain to coordinate and control movement and balance. Physicians typically diagnose Parkinson's disease by observing two of three cardinal motor signs (tremor, rigidity [stiffness], and **bradykinesia** [slowness]) and noting a positive and consistent response to L-dopa, a medicine used to increase levels of dopamine in the brain. Currently, brain imaging studies and laboratory tests to assist physicians in diagnosing Parkinson's disease do not exist.

Timelines and Healing

Many believe that Parkinson's disease results from a combination of genetic and environmental factors.[23] Pharmacologic agents normalize the dopamine activity in the brain and reduce the symptoms of Parkinson's disease. Over time, these medications become less effective and can have side effects such as nausea and vomiting, hypotension, and arrhythmias in high dosages; therefore, clients must be closely medically managed.

Signs and symptoms of Parkinson's disease usually begin unilaterally, but eventually they affect bilateral limbs and the trunk. Other early signs include lack of arm swing during ambulation and **micrographia** (small, illegible handwriting).[16] In Parkinson's disease, the bradykinesia and rigidity can impair functional mobility, ADL independence, and safety more so than the **postural tremors,** or resting tremors. With attempts at goal-directed movements, the tremors dissipate slightly. Over

TABLE 25-1

Summary of Common Signs and Symptoms of Parkinson's Disease

CLINICAL SIGNS AND SYMPTOMS	COMMON CLIENT COMPLAINTS
Resting/postural tremor	Tremor; shaking
Bradykinesia (slowness of movement)	Slowed movements when completing bathing, dressing, and general activities
Rigidity	Stiffness; aching muscle pain
Hypokinesia (small-amplitude movement)	Trouble rolling in bed; difficulty standing up from a chair
Loss of postural reflexes	Falling often; poor balance; tripping
Sudden "freezing" of movement during activity	Difficulty following through with activities of daily living
Festinating (shuffling) gait/decreased arm swing in ambulation	Trouble walking
Dementia	Memory loss; depression
Autonomic dysfunction (slowed gastrointestinal motility, urinary retention, orthostatic hypotension)	Loss of bowel or bladder control; light-headedness with positional changes
Dysphagia/dysarthria	Difficulty swallowing; speaking rapidly or whispering
Masked facial expressions	Family members report lack of smiling or showing emotions
Flexed posture	Stooped posture; feeling "hunchbacked"
Micrographia (small handwriting)	Change in handwriting

time as the Parkinson's disease progresses, clients experience other symptoms involving bowel and bladder function, orthostatic hypotension, postural instability, and **dysphagia** (difficulty swallowing). Late-stage dementia occurs in approximately one third of all clients with Parkinson's disease. Medications and physical rehabilitation address the symptoms of Parkinson's disease, but there is currently no cure for this disease.

Nonoperative Treatment

Addressing Tremor

Physiologically, tremor is the involuntary oscillation of a body part resulting from contractions of the antagonistic muscles.[25] In Parkinson's disease, these tremors typically are noticed during times of inactivity, disappear during sleep, and improve with intention or goal-directed movements. Emotional state, motor activity, and general health can modulate tremor. Because the tremor worsens with anxiety or stress, it is helpful to teach the client relaxation and self-stabilization techniques.

Although not scientifically proven, clients with tremor have noticed that the use of distal wrist weights (cuffs) may reduce symptoms during functional activities or at rest. Most rehabilitation supply companies sell weighted utensils, such as forks and spoons, and weighted holders for toothbrushes, pens, and razors. Some clients find these beneficial. Other adaptive devices are button hooks, zipper pulls, sock aids, and elastic shoelaces. Plate guards and nonslip placemats can make self-feeding easier when one hand is nonfunctional because of the tremor or **dyskinesias** (involuntary movements).

Besides strategies such as weighted implements, clients with tremors also may need to modify tasks. For example, if clients cannot complete bill-paying tasks, they may find it easier to pay their bills online or over the phone.

Addressing Rigidity

Rigidity, or resistance to movement, is caused by the constant contraction of the antagonist muscle groups. **"Cogwheeling,"** common in clients with Parkinson's disease, is identified by jerky movements and is considered rigidity superimposed on tremor.[23] *Rigidity often is associated with musculoskeletal pain.* These clients respond well to heat modalities, stretching, and gentle range of motion exercises. If there are muscle contractures, try splinting the upper extremity in an antispasticity splint using thermoplastic material, or try a static progressive splint that applies a low-intensity stretch against the contraction of the antagonist muscle group. Instruct the client to check skin integrity often because the tremor may lead to skin problems or breakdown.

Addressing Bradykinesia

Bradykinesia is a slowing of spontaneous and automatic movement that limits initiation of tasks or modification of an action once it has begun. Research has shown that a single auditory cue can help clients with Parkinson's disease to produce faster and more forceful movements.[26] Instruct clients to give themselves single auditory cues during ADL and with functional mobility. The rhythmic nature of counting out loud and singing also helps clients with Parkinson's disease move in a smoother or more coordinated fashion. Teach clients with Parkinson's disease to count their steps when walking, rising from a toilet seat, or reaching for an item.

A book by John Argue[27] explains how automatic movement no longer exists in the client with Parkinson's disease. For this reason, each coordinated movement must be broken down into single steps with auditory cues. Argue's book provides exercises that use this technique to promote flexibility and mobility.

Exercise

Weakness and deconditioning in clients with Parkinson's disease can be caused by inactivity and by physiological changes in muscle efficiency that occur because of altered central innervation.[16] Research on strengthening the lower extremity in clients with mild to moderate Parkinson's disease shows enhanced muscle strength at the same rate of normal subjects of similar age.[28]

Operative Treatment

Deep brain stimulation (DBS) is an alternative to ablative surgery of the structures in the brain that cause the symptoms of Parkinson's disease. High-frequency electric stimulation of specific brain targets can mimic the effect of a lesion without the need for destroying brain tissue.[29] In DBS, an electrode is implanted into the target area within the brain and is connected to a battery source usually located in the client's chest area. The stimulator settings can be adjusted easily postoperatively to increase efficacy or reduce adverse reactions. DBS, in principle, is reversible and does not preclude the use of possible future therapies for Parkinson's disease.

Placement of the DBS in the subthalamic nucleus or internal pallidum produces a beneficial effect for the more global symptoms of Parkinson's disease such as bradykinesia or rigidity. In an attempt to abolish tremor in mild cases of Parkinson's disease, the DBS is placed in the thalamus. These surgeries can be performed for bilateral or unilateral symptoms. The DBS is placed contralateral to the side of the affected limb.

Questions to Ask the Physician

- *Is this client a candidate for deep brain stimulation?*
- *Are there any clinical signs related to medication tolerance that you would like us to monitor?*

What to Say to Clients

About the Diagnosis

"The symptoms of Parkinson's disease can have a significant impact on your function and enjoyment, such as eating out at restaurants, going to the theater, or garden-

ing. It is important to try to find strategies to help you continue to participate in activities you like to do. One strategy is to maximize the best or most functional times of your day and to prioritize your daily routines with this in mind."

About Positioning/Splinting

"By positioning your arm in a splint, you may get to relax the muscles that are working as part of the tremor. By relaxing these muscles, your quality of movement may improve."

About Exercise

"It is possible to get stronger despite the diagnosis of Parkinson's disease. Many times, individuals with Parkinson's disease get weaker just because they don't use their affected arm anymore. By exercising, you may gain strength, increase your energy level, and feel healthier in general."

About Functional Activities

"The most important thing that therapy can do for you is help you regain or maximize your sense of independence. By using adaptive equipment or modifying the way that you do activities, you may be able to participate better in day-to-day activities."

Evaluation Tips

- Use the Canadian Occupational Performance Measure to determine client-centered goals if this is appropriate to your profession's scope of practice. Clients respond favorably to a positive emotional state with minimizing of stress. Therapy that is client-centered is most successful.
- Find out if your clients have an "on" or "off" time of the day. Typically, symptoms worsen just before the next dose of medication; this is considered an off time. Consider this in your evaluation and treatment planning. Working with clients may be easier from a functional standpoint while they are on, but they also may benefit from treatments that mimic real-life occurrences during their off stage. An example of this is practicing bed mobility while they are off.
- Perform cognitive screening as appropriate, possibly at on and off times.
- Include family members or caregivers in home exercise programs for clients with Parkinson's disease who appear to have cognitive deficits.

Diagnosis-Specific Information That Affects Clinical Reasoning

Clinical depression is reported in nearly 50% of all clients with Parkinson's disease compared with 7% of the general population.[22] Clients with Parkinson's disease might be more reluctant to participate in social gatherings because of their symptoms. Identify goals that address broader issues of quality of life. When the client demonstrates cognitive deficits, modify instructions accordingly.

Tips from the Field

- Clients with Parkinson's disease often have masked facial expressions. Do not assume that they lack emotions. Being less expressive makes it more difficult to monitor pain during range of motion or stretching activities. Therefore it is important to talk with your clients to confirm that they are comfortable with the treatment.
- During treatment and when performing ADL, encourage the client to bring activities as close to their body as possible. Using their proximal musculature can help to stabilize their distal extremities and may reduce tremors.

Precautions and Concerns

- *Mood changes or depression are associated with Parkinson's disease. Report these signs to the referring physician because they may be treatable.*
- *Shaving or other activities with sharp instruments such as using scissors or knives may be dangerous if motor control is compromised.*

ESSENTIAL TREMOR

Essential tremor (ET) is characterized by postural and **intention tremors** (rhythmic shaking that occurs in the course of a purposeful movement), typically affecting the hands or the head. ET is worsened by stress. ET is the most common movement disorder, affecting 1 million to 3 million persons in the United States.[30] In ET the characteristic tremor occurs with intentional use of the extremity and tends to be quiet at rest. ET also is called **action tremor.** As in the case of Parkinson's disease, this disease is slowly progressive, but the symptoms are limited to tremor and generally do not affect mobility. ET does not alter cognition. Clients with ET typically are spared of complete loss of independence, but their upper extremity function can be dramatically affected, with serious social ramifications.

Diagnosis and Pathology

The cause of ET is unknown. ET may be sporadic or it may be familial.[30] In the familial form, an autosomal dominant gene exists, and the tremors typically present early in the client's life. As the clients age, the tremors typically worsen. In the sporadic form the incidence of ET increases with age and does not discriminate regarding race or sex.

Timelines and Healing

ET has only one clinical manifestation—tremor. Unfortunately, this sole symptom also can lead to psychological and social impairments, resulting in embarrassment often associated with the tremor. The tremor of ET does not always respond satisfactorily to the current available drug therapy. Also, some clients do not like the side effects of these medications. Some believe that beta-blockers temporarily reduce tremors and control elevated heart rates that often occur as the client goes on a social outing or is in a more stressful situation. In approximately 50% of the clients, diminished tremor occurs for about an hour following ingestion of small amounts of alcohol. In contrast to the tremor of Parkinson's disease, the tremor in ET gets worse with attempts at activities such as writing, eating, drinking a glass of water, or dialing a phone. Stimulants such as caffeine and nicotine also may worsen tremor temporarily. ET generally is considered a slowly progressive disorder, with the advancement of the disease process defined by an increase in the tremor amplitude or an extension of the tremor to previously unaffected body parts. Increased mortality is not associated with the diagnosis of ET.[25] As in the case of Parkinson's disease, a cure does not exist currently for ET, but operative treatment such as DBS reduces the symptoms and is discussed later in this chapter.

Nonoperative Treatment

Addressing Tremor

As stated previously, tremor is the involuntary oscillation of a body part caused by contractions of the antagonistic muscles.[25] With ET, tremors worsen with intention or voluntary movement, and emotional state, motor activity, and general health can modulate tremor. With ET the tremor worsens as the arc of motion is increased.

As for the client with Parkinson's disease, teach the client with ET to implement relaxation techniques to help minimize symptoms because tremors worsen with stress. Try having the clients use distal wrist weights (cuffs) to reduce symptoms during functional activities. (See the previous section on Parkinson's disease.) In addition, stabilizing the upper extremity proximally and repositioning the task to minimize the amount of motion at each joint can be helpful. Long-handled devices help reduce the arc of movement needed in some tasks (e.g., a long-handled eating utensil).

Addressing Social Isolation

Clients with ET experience embarrassment because of their tremor, which leads to social isolation. Cooper et al.[30] demonstrated that briefly cooling the affected limb in clients with ET quieted their tremor and improved their functional hand use. In a subsequent prospective randomized crossover trial, these researchers[31] found that the benefits of cooling lasted up to 60 minutes. This may be an effective technique for clients to use before social outings. Clients with ET are typically aware of the times of day and the types of activities that augment symptoms. Reinforce the benefits of planning community or social activities during optimal times of the day and include activities that minimize tremor. As an example of activities that minimize tremor, a client could suggest going to a movie or hiking as opposed to playing miniature golf.

Persons with ET may use new technology to their advantage. They can swipe bank cards for automatic withdrawal of funds instead of having to write out checks with a shaky hand. Most computers have a setting to control the rate at which the keyboard and mouse respond to movement. By decreasing the sensitivity of the keyboard and mouse, the client with tremor will have more control at the computer.

Operative Treatment

DBS is an alternative to ablative surgery of the structures in the brain that cause the symptoms of ET. The rationale for its use is the same as for Parkinson's disease. In cases of ET, the DBS is placed in the thalamus. Researchers show that DBS is an effective form of treatment, with thalamic DBS for ET having a success rate of approximately 90% in dramatically reducing tremor.[25] As for Parkinson's disease, DBS can be completed for bilateral or unilateral symptoms, and it is placed in the brain contralateral to the affected limb.

Questions to Ask the Physician

- *Is this client a candidate for deep brain stimulation?*
- *Are there any clinical signs related to medication tolerance that you would like us to monitor?*

What to Say to Clients

About the Diagnosis

"The symptoms of essential tremor can have a significant impact on your function and enjoyment, such as eating out at restaurants, going to the theater, or gardening. It is important to try to find strategies to help you continue to participate in activities you like to do. One strategy is to maximize the best or most functional times of your day and to prioritize your daily routines with this in mind."

About Functional Activities

"The most important thing that therapy can do for you is help you regain or maximize your sense of independence. By using adaptive equipment or modifying the way that you do activities, you may be able to participate better in day-to-day activities."

Evaluation Tips

- Use the Canadian Occupational Performance Measure if appropriate to your professional scope of practice to determine client-centered goals. As with Parkinson's disease, clients' symptoms respond favorably to a positive emotional state with less stress. This can be achieved through purposeful and goal-directed activities.
- Complete the evaluation in a private area away from other clients, so that the client is not uncomfortable during the assessment of the tremor.

Diagnosis-Specific Information That Affects Clinical Reasoning

Clients with ET are often younger and may be in the prime of their careers. They may be fearful from having seen their parents experience the same symptoms. Treatment focuses on improving function by strategizing upper extremity positions, proximal support, and consideration of cooling techniques.

Tips from the Field

- During treatment and when performing ADL, encourage clients to bring activities as close to their bodies as possible. Using their proximal musculature can help to stabilize their distal extremities and may reduce tremors.
- Long-handled devices promote function in clients with ET by reducing the arc of motion needed for the task. Because action tremor worsens as the arc of motion increases, using longer-handled tools can be helpful.
- Instruct clients in the following tips to assist with tremor:
  - Place a napkin between the cup and saucer to avoid rattling.
  - Use auto dial on a cell phone or have the operator place the call.
  - Avoid soup, spaghetti, and other difficult foods while at restaurants, or ask for the food to be served in a tall mug to allow for more time with

contact between the spoon and the side of the mug before placing it in your mouth.
- Use straws with liquid foods.

Precautions and Concerns

- *Mood changes or depression are associated with ET. Report these signs to the referring physician because they may be treatable.*
- *Shaving or other activities with sharp instruments such as using scissors or knives may be dangerous if motor control is compromised.*

CASE *Studies*

CASE 25-1: CEREBRAL VASCULAR ACCIDENT

A man who sustained a stroke in 1994 with right-sided involvement presents to the clinic for treatment of repetitive strain injury in the left arm. He has no functional use of his right arm, ambulates with a cane, and is independent in ADL by using modified or one-sided techniques. He complains of numbness and tingling in his first three digits on his left hand and soreness at the left lateral epicondyle and extensor wad.

Because the client has had a stroke in the past, the therapist includes a brief cognitive and visual-perceptual screening in the initial evaluation to assist in appropriate treatment planning. The therapist does not focus treatment on trying to regain function in his right arm but rather addresses overuse of the left arm.

Unlike the client with postpolio syndrome (see the section in this chapter), it is unrealistic to advise the client to minimize use of his left arm. Without his arm, he is unable to maintain independence. Therefore therapy involves symptom management of carpal tunnel syndrome and lateral epicondylitis with instruction in proper body mechanics to minimize further strain on the upper extremity.

CASE 25-2: CEREBRAL VASCULAR ACCIDENT

A 34-year-old woman sustained a stroke and presents to the clinic with left hemiparesis. She has always been right-hand dominant, so she does not initiate tasks with her affected left hand. She has good emerging movements in her affected arm, but her learned nonuse is limiting her chances for recovery.

By participating in modified constraint-induced therapy during treatment and over gradually extended periods of the day, she understands that there are tasks that she can complete with her left hand. By the end of the first week of therapy, she is using her left hand to operate the television remote control, to push her glasses to the bridge of her nose, and to turn the pages of her favorite magazine. She documents her activities in which she uses her left hand daily, which allows her to visualize and appreciate the objective gains that she is making in functional arm use.

CASE 25-3: PARKINSON'S DISEASE

A client with Parkinson's disease has been seen in therapy for 2 weeks when the therapist and family begin to note changes in the client's affect. She has become increasingly frustrated and no longer seems motivated to participate in exercises and activities of daily living.

The therapist advises the client and family to discuss these mood changes with the physician. In the meantime, the therapist reassesses the client's personal goals and makes attempts to create new goals that may elevate the client's mood. The client reveals that she misses working in her garden. Therapy works on planting small potted flowers with the use of wrist weights, nonslip padding to stabilize the potted plant on the table, and weighted gardening tools.

The client is now aware of modified gardening activities that she can complete successfully, and she appreciates the therapist's recommendation to seek medical attention for her recent mood change.

CASE 25-4: ESSENTIAL TREMOR

A doctor refers a client to hand therapy for extensor digitorum communis repair of his index finger. The therapist notices that the client has tremors in his hand when he attempts to complete active range of motion and therapeutic putty exercises. In talking to the client, the client reveals that he has essential tremor and that using that hand has been difficult for several years. The therapist takes this opportunity to instruct the client in the use of various adaptive equipment and modified activities to minimize the symptoms and improve functional hand use. The client dons a distal wrist weight on the affected arm during active range of motion and strengthening activities and makes sure to bring the work surface as close to his body as possible to allow the proximal musculature to help stabilize the tremor.

Resource List

- American Parkinson Disease Association
- American Stroke Association
- International Essential Tremor Foundation
- National Institute of Neurological Disorders and Stroke
- National Multiple Sclerosis Society
- National Parkinson Foundation

- *Parkinson's Disease and the Art of Moving* by John Argue (ISBN: 1-57224-183-7)
- Unified Parkinson Disease Rating Scale

References

1. Keenan MAE, Waters RL: Heterotopic ossification. In Skinner HB, editor: *Current diagnosis & treatment in orthopedics*, New York, 2003, Lange Medical Books.
2. Chasens ER, Umlauf MG: Post-polio syndrome, *Am J Nurs* 100(12):60-65, 2000.
3. Koh ESC, Williams AJ, Povlsen B: Upper-limb pain in long-term poliomyelitis, *QJM* 95:389-395, 2002.
4. Werner RA, Waring W, Maynard F: Osteoarthritis of the hand and wrist in the post poliomyelitis population, *Arch Phys Med Rehabil* 73:1069-1072, 1992.
5. Agre JC, Rodriquez AA, Franke TM: Strength, endurance, and work capacity after muscle strengthening exercise in postpolio subjects, *Arch Phys Med Rehabil* 78:681-686, 1997.
6. Salcido R: Rehabilitation of the post-polio client, *Topics in Geriatric Rehabilitation* 15(3):95-98, 2000.
7. Agre JC, Rodriquez AA, Franke TM et al: Low-intensity, alternate-day exercise improves muscle performance without apparent adverse affect in postpolio clients, *Am J Phys Med Rehabil* 75(1):50-58, 1996.
8. Widar M, Ahlstrom G: Experiences and consequences of pain in persons with post-polio syndrome, *J Adv Nurs* 28(3):606-613, 1998.
9. Jubelt B, Agre JC: Characteristics and management of postpolio syndrome, *JAMA* 284(4):412-414, 2000.
10. Whitall J, McCombe Waller S, Silver KH et al: Repetitive bilateral arm training with rhythmic auditory cueing improves motor function in chronic hemiparetic stroke, *Stroke* 31(10):2390-2395, 2000.
11. Pedretti LW, Smith JA, Pendleton HM: Cerebral vascular accident. In Pedretti LW, editor: *Occupational therapy: practice skills for physical dysfunction*, St Louis, 1996, Mosby.
12. Waters RL, Wilson DJ, Gowland C: Rehabilitation of the upper extremity after stroke. In Hunter JM, Mackin EJ, Callahan AD, editors: *Rehabilitation of the hand: surgery and therapy*, St Louis, 1995, Mosby.
13. Kalra L, Perez I, Gupta S et al: The influence of visual neglect on stroke rehabilitation, *Stroke* 28(7):1386-1391, 1997.
14. Page SJ, Sisto SA, Levine P: Modified constraint-induced therapy in chronic stroke, *Am J Phys Med Rehabil* 81(11):870-875, 2002.
15. Sato Y, Kaji M, Tsuru T et al: Carpal tunnel syndrome involving unaffected limbs of stroke clients, *Stroke* 30(2):414-418, 1999.
16. Orsini JA, Dombovy ML: Multiple sclerosis and Parkinson's disease rehabilitation. In Lazar RB, editor: *Principles of neurologic rehabilitation*, San Francisco, 1998, McGraw-Hill.
17. Frankel D: Multiple sclerosis. In Umphred DA, editor: *Neurological rehabilitation*, St Louis, 1995, Mosby.
18. Kerns RD, Kassirer M, Otis J: Pain in multiple sclerosis: a biopsychosocial perspective, *J Rehabil Res Dev* 39(2):225-232, 2002.
19. Ku Y-TE, Montgomery LD, Lee HC et al: Physiologic and functional responses of MS patients to body cooling, *Am J Phys Med Rehabil* 79(5):427-434, 2000.
20. Oken BS, Kishiyama S, Zajdel D et al: Randomized controlled trial of yoga and exercise in multiple sclerosis, *Neurology* 62(11):2058-2064, 2004.
21. Demaree HA, DeLuca J, Gaudino EA et al: Speed of information processing as a key deficit in multiple sclerosis: implications for rehabilitation, *J Neurol Neurosurg Psychiatry* 67:661-663, 1999.
22. Abudi S, Bar-Tal Y, Ziv L et al: Parkinson's disease symptoms: patients' perceptions, *J Adv Nurs* 25(1):54-59, 1997.
23. Goldsmith C: Parkinson's disease, *Am J Nurs* 99(2):46-47, 1999.
24. Paulson HL, Stern MB: Clinical manifestations of Parkinson's disease. In Watts RL, Koller WC, editors: *Movement disorders: neurologic principles & practice*, San Francisco, 2004, McGraw-Hill.
25. Cersosimo MG, Koller WC: Essential tremor. In Watts RL, Koller WC, editors: *Movement disorders: neurologic principles & practice*, San Francisco, 2004, McGraw-Hill.
26. Ma H-I, Trombly CA, Tickle-Degnen L et al: Effect of one single auditory cue on movement kinematics in patients with Parkinson's disease, *Am J Phys Med Rehabil* 83(7):530-536, 2004.
27. Argue J: *Parkinson's disease and the art of moving*, Oakland, Calif, 2000, New Harbinger Publications.
28. Scandalis TA et al: Resistance training and gait function in clients with Parkinson's disease, *Am J Phys Med Rehabil* 80(1):38-43, 2001.
29. Volkmann J: Deep brain stimulation for the treatment of Parkinson's disease, *J Clin Neurophysiol* 21(1):6-17, 2004.
30. Cooper C et al: The effect of temperature on hand function in clients with tremor, *J Hand Ther* 13:276-288, 2000.
31. Cooper C, Evidente VGH, Hentz JG, Bernstein SC: Randomized crossover trial of cool temperature immersion treatment to improve hand function in patients with essential tremor. Paper presented at the American Society of Hand Therapists annual meeting, Charlotte, North Carolina, October 2004.

26

Pediatric Hand Therapy

LYNN BASSINI AND MUKUND PATEL

KEY TERMS

Amyoplasia

Arthrogryposis multiplex congenita

Athetosis

Avulsion injury

Axonotmesis

Camptodactyly

Cerebral palsy

Clinodactyly

Compartment syndrome

Complex tasks

Congenital clasped thumb

Crush syndrome

Delta phalanx

Distal arthrogryposis

Epiphyseal distraction (chondrodiastasis)

Epiphysis

Epitendinous suture

Fasciotomies

Flaccidity

Grasp

Hemiplegia

Hypoplasia

Kirner's deformity

Longitudinal radial ray deficiency

Malunion

Manipulation

Neuropraxia

Neurotmesis

Paresthesia

Physis

Pincer (pinch) grasp

Pinch

Play skills

Pollicization

Prehension

Quadriga effect

Quadriplegia

Radial club hand

Rupture of the brachial plexus

Simple tasks

Spasticity

Tenodesis effect

Volkmann's angle

Volkmann's Passive Muscle Stretch Test

Windblown hand

In pediatric hand therapy, it is critical to understand a child's growth and development, to apply sharp observation skills, to perform ongoing evaluation, and to use treatment protocols that are scientific and creative. Early intervention provides therapeutic and educational intervention designed to treat and educate children and their parents during the critical stages of development. With early intervention, development can be enhanced, modified, or accelerated to prevent or lessen the effects of disabling conditions. This chapter addresses pediatric hand therapy topics that therapists and students are most likely to encounter. At times there may be contradictory instructions from different surgeons for a given problem. This chapter provides solutions that may help in such instances.

We have divided this chapter into two sections: general principles of pediatric hand therapy and common pediatric hand conditions.

GENERAL PRINCIPLES OF PEDIATRIC HAND THERAPY

GROWTH AND DEVELOPMENT

A child brings into this world a unique personality, unpredictable growth, and a genetic blueprint. Each child is influenced by his or her environment and nurturing influences. For a child to develop a skill, the musculoskeletal, neurologic, and cognitive functions must be intact and integrated. If the child has an atypical posture caused by failure of one of these, this posture will become permanent through repetitive practice. Efforts to develop normal movements then may be unsuccessful because atypical patterns have been established. If the hand does not perform a variety of movements, it will develop muscle imbalance and contractures. Timely therapy and surgery prevent the sequela of abnormal postures.

Certain definitions help one to evaluate the child's performance and select the appropriate treatment plan (Box 26-1).

BOX 26-1

Definitions

Grasp occurs between the fingers and the palm.
Pinch is between any finger and the thumb.
Prehension is grasp or pinch (flexion) and release (extension).
Manipulation requires combinations of movements consisting of grasp, pinch, and prehension.
Play skills require hand, upper extremity, body, and lower extremity coordination.

Grasp progresses from reflex grasp to purposeful grasp, from proximal to distal, and from ulnar to radial hand. Grasp progresses from mass movements to individualized finger movements and from hand grasp to finger **pinch.** Purposeful grasp develops between 4 and 12 months. Crude grasp begins in the proximal palm. Fine grasp develops in the distal palm. Key pinch develops first proximally and later distally. Pulp pinch begins in the proximal pulp. Tip **pincer (pinch) grasp** then develops in the distal pulp. Grasp, pinch, **manipulation,** and **play skills** develop in that sequence. Hand dominance develops between the age of 36 and 48 months (Table 26-1; Fig. 26-1).

Manipulation Skills

Hand function does not develop in isolation. Hand function is the result of neurologic development, physiologic maturation, and functional development of learned patterns of movement and motor control. The evolution of the cortical mechanisms in human beings enables the hand to reach its high levels of skill. The ability to perform such fine finger movements depends on the motor and sensory cortices. As the child plays with his or her hands, the sensory input is assimilated continuously and guides movements such as sustaining grasp around a peg or tying shoelaces. Tactile perception integrates the information from sensory end-organs including the proprioceptors to achieve coordinated movements in which agonist and antagonist muscles work in a smooth pattern. The three types of manipulative hand movements are the following[1]:

1. Finger to palm: moving a coin from the fingers to the palm
2. Palm to finger: moving a coin from palm to fingers
3. Rotation: simple and complex. Simple is a 90-degree rolling of an object between fingers, as in unscrewing a cap of a bottle. Complex involves a 180-degree rolling motion of an object between fingers, as in turning a pencil to the eraser side. A key factor in hand manipulation is the ability simultaneously to integrate stability and mobility. One object must be moved around in the hand while another object is stabilized, usually in the ulnar digits. A combination of fine movements constitutes a functional task, such as picking up a paper clip and securing it to a paper.

Table 26-2 describes growth and development of manipulative motions.

Play Occupations

The development of play occupations integrates the skills of pinch, grasp, and manipulation to produce purposeful

TABLE 26-1

Development of Grasp

AGE	DESCRIPTION OF GROWTH AND DEVELOPMENT
Birth to 4 months	Basic reflexes are mediated by the brainstem and spinal cord mechanism. Infant thrusts arms and legs in space while supine.
3 months	Movements for ambulation begin. Body turns from side to side. Eyes follow moving object facing midline. While supine, infant swings at an object held at 1 foot from face.
4 months (Fig. 26-1, A)	Reflexive grasp: object held between the hand and body. While supine, hands come together intentionally to meet in midline or at the mouth.
5 months (Fig. 26-1, B)	Proximal palmar grasp with mass finger flexion of digits 2, 3, 4, and 5 against the proximal palm. Elbows extend, reach for objects and grasp. Grasp is sweeping with no specific thumb and finger movement. Balance still is developing, and body follows direction of reach, using vision to direct movement.
6 months (Fig. 26-1, C)	Midpalmar grasp with fingers flexing simultaneously to hold an object in midpalm. Infant begins to sit independently. Learning progresses rapidly, and hands become free to develop.
7 months (Fig. 26-1, D)	Radial palmar grasp: index and middle fingers flex around object. Thumb pushes object into radial palm. Crawling begins.
8 months (Fig. 26-1, E)	Raking grasp: fingers, hand, and arm move as one unit and "rake" object into palm. Radial fingers flex more than ulnar fingers.
9 months (Fig. 26-1, F)	Radial digital grasp: thumb opposes object against radial two fingers. Object is held between the proximal finger joints and the thumb. Key pinch or scissor grasp is apparent. Object is secured between the adducted thumb and the radial side of the flexed index finger.
10 months (Fig. 26-1, G)	Thumb tip to finger tip. Pincer (pinch) grasp.
12 months (Fig. 26-1, H)	Thumb tip to finger tip pinch. Neat pincer (pinch) grasp.

TABLE 26-2

Development of Manipulation

AGE	DEVELOPMENT OF MANIPULATION
Birth to 6 months	Manipulation is absent or not defined.
7 months	Crude raking: Child holds an object between finger pads and thumb pad.
8 months	Child maintains fingers in flexion while thumb grasps against the index. Intrinsic muscles are not functioning. Child has no effective fine control of metacarpophalangeal joint flexion and interphalangeal joint extension (no intrinsic-plus)
9-12 months	Child refines thumb pad to finger pad pinch. Movement is enhanced by slight supination of forearm and wrist extension.
12-18 months	Intrinsic function begins, and metacarpophalangeal joint flexion becomes effective. Manipulation progresses from clumsy ulnar to delicate (precision) radial side. Child can use utensils as long as physical and mental capabilities allow problem solving.
18-36 months and beyond	Lateral pinch, all grasps, and manipulation continue to be mastered.

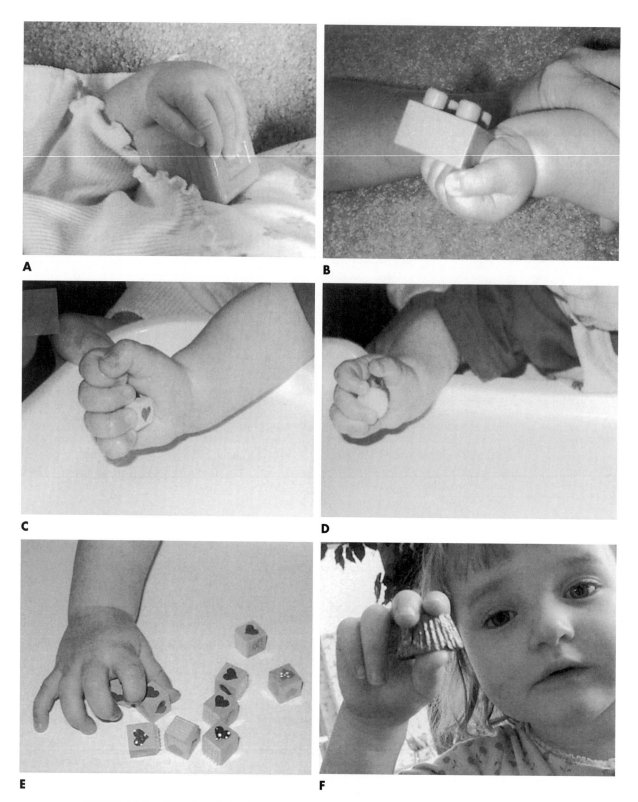

FIGURE 26-1 Growth and development. **A,** At 4 months—reflexive grasp with object held between the hand and body. **B,** At 5 months—proximal palmar grasp with mass finger flexion of digits 2, 3, 4, and 5 against the proximal palm. **C,** At 6 months—midpalmar grasp with fingers flexing simultaneously to hold an object in midpalm. **D,** At 7 months—radial palmar grasp with index and middle fingers flexed around object. Thumb pushes object into radial palm. **E,** At 8 months—raking grasp in which fingers, hand, and arm move as one unit and rake object into palm. Radial fingers flex more than ulnar fingers. **F,** At 9 months—radial digital grasp in which thumb opposes object against radial two fingers. Object is held between the proximal finger joints and the thumb.

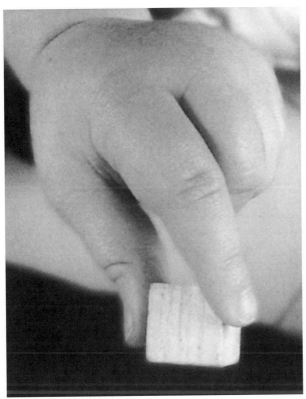

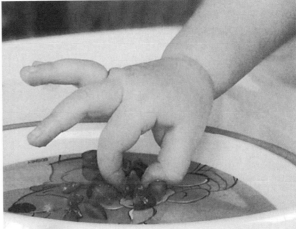

H

FIGURE 26-1 cont'd G, At 10 months—thumb pulp to finger pulp pinch. Pincer (pinch) grasp. **H,** At 12 months—thumb tip to finger tip pinch. Neat pincer (pinch) grasp. (From Edwards SJ, Buckland DJ, McCoy-Powlen JD: *Developmental functional hand grasps,* Thorofare, NJ, 2002, Slack.)

movement. In our view, tasks may be simple or complex. **Simple tasks** involve minimal variability of movement. An example of this is eating, which involves similar and repetitive patterns of movements to manipulate the utensils. **Complex tasks** involve unpredictable patterns of movement in time and space. They require greater demands on the child to adapt, such as throwing and catching a ball. In complex tasks the movements vary each time the task is performed, and the child must have a repertoire of skills to adjust to the varying demands of the activity. Table 26-3 describes growth and development of play skills.

The hand cannot perform successfully without a stable base. The stabilization of the trunk maintains postures against gravity and allows the body to move through space in a smooth and coordinated way, ensuring efficient placement of the arm. The control of stability and mobility of the arm and hand is needed for precise digital grasp. The hand simultaneously requires eye-hand coordination to determine appropriate arm and hand placement. Hand function is part of this complicated synergistic process.

CLINICAL *Pearl*

When one is evaluating a child's hand function, it is crucial to look at proximal parts of the extremity and the trunk.

The development of hand function depends on socioeconomic and cultural environmental influences, cognitive ability, and the sensory and musculoskeletal integrity of the child. Normal variations in the development of grasp, pinch, **prehension,** manipulation, and play skills may occur. The quality of movement can range from clumsy to artistic in different children of the same age. The intellectual cortical development also may vary between children of the same age. Some children excel in some skills but not in others within the same age group. Certain motor skills may be advanced or lagging but still may be within the normal limits for an age group. If a child is referred for clumsy or awkward

TABLE 26-3

Development of Play Occupations

AGE IN MONTHS	DEVELOPMENT OF PLAY OCCUPATIONS
Birth to 6 months	Child reaches for object, uses palmar grasp, moves the object from hand to mouth and from hand to hand and can play with hands at midline.
6-12 months	Child mouths toys, bangs objects to make noise, waves toys in the air, releases toys in container, rolls a ball, grasps small objects with finger tips, points to toys with index finger, and crudely uses tools. Simple tasks include minimal variability of movement and similar and repetitive patterns of movement, as in eating.
12-18 months	Child scribbles with a crayon, holds two toys in one or both hands, releases toys in container, and uses two hands, one to hold and one to manipulate.
	Reconstructive surgery is addressed. The size of the hand is large enough for surgical manipulation. From 6 to 12 months the child begins to develop his or her own immunologic defenses. From 12 months onward, the child's own immunity has maximized, and chances of infection are least.
	Complex tasks begin to develop: unpredictable patterns of movement in time and space. Movements vary each time. The child must have a repertoire of skills to adjust, as in throwing and catching a ball.
18-24 months	Child completes a five-piece puzzle, builds a tower, draws a line or circle, strings beads, uses simple tools such as a toy hammer, and turns pages.
	Neuromuscular development proceeds proximal to distal. Gradually the elbow, wrist, and finally the metacarpophalangeal joint become the mobile part, and the shoulder stabilizes the arm (simple to complex tasks).
24-36 months	Child snips with scissors, traces and colors, lines up objects, holds crayon accurately, and plays with toys that have moving parts (complex tasks continue to be mastered).
36-48 months	Hand dominance is developing. In a small percentage of children, hand dominance is not defined until age 9. An attempt at forcing dominance may hinder development. Development of bilateral hand function is essential for hand skills.

motor skills, observe the child over a period of time. Teach the parents the activities and function consistent with the child's age. The child may catch up or may need additional help in certain areas.

The motor functions in the hand are static or dynamic. Static functions include grasp and pinch. Dynamic functions include prehension, manipulation, and play occupations. Grasp and pinch require fingers and palm. Manipulation requires the ability to grasp or pinch in combination with prehension (grasp and release) and coordinated wrist, elbow, shoulder, and body movements.

COMPONENTS OF PEDIATRIC HAND THERAPY

This chapter provides basic information and strategies for a therapist to build a successful therapeutic relationship with the best outcomes possible. The main components of hand therapy in the pediatric population are assisting physicians with the medical plan, evaluation, treatment, and parent and child education.

Assisting the Physician in Carrying out the Medical Plan

The ideal, but not always the most practical, arrangement is for the therapist to be by the side of the physician. Being present with the hand surgeon during the initial consultation allows for clear understanding of the problems and the medical plan to follow. One's presence with the physician aids in deciphering a doctor's prescription. Communication with the physician regarding the status of the child's condition is an ongoing process.

Evaluation

The evaluation process continues at every visit. More often than not, limited information is obtained from only one session. The child may be fearful, fussy, or in pain. It may take several sessions until sufficient information is gathered.

Children's amazing ability to heal and adapt requires that the evaluation and treatment program be monitored and adjusted constantly. Once a thorough understanding of the child's condition and communication between the parties involved have been established, evaluate the child as follows:

1. Observe and document the child's problems. Ask the child to grasp a toy if evaluating the status of a flexor tendon. Hand him or her a small block in the palm to see if the child is able to pull the thumb out of the palm. Then offer the block on the radial side of the hand and see if the child can extend the thumb further. Finally, hold the child's palm against the table and see whether the child can retroposition the thumb. The activity needs to represent the movement that you are evaluating accurately and must be appropriate for the child's age.
2. Request and review the medical prescription, operative report, or other available information.
3. Evaluate the severity of pain and grade it if possible with a visual analog scale or descriptive language (e.g., mild, moderate, or severe).
4. Check the condition of the hand for swelling, color, scar, wound, and infection.
5. Analyze cognition, sensation, range of motion, strength, general coordination, and eye-hand coordination.
6. Perform specific tests using necessary tools (goniometer, dynamometer): Wrinkle Test, and standardized developmental tests such as Peabody, Bayley Test, Bruininks-Oseretsky Test of Motor Proficiency, Erhardt Test, and HELP Checklist.

Treatment

Treatment Plan

Precaution. *Be careful to follow the medical prescription and the surgeon's protocol.*

Identify the problems that are appropriate to treat. Identify the child's development and functional level, and select the therapeutic methods and tools. Development of short-term and long-term goals is crucial. The short-term goals may be from session to session. They may be as simple and important as keeping the cast dry and intact or improving the range of motion for an affected finger. Review your goals during each session and change them as new situations arise.

CLINICAL *Pearl*

Be sure to praise accomplishments, keep eye contact, pay attention to detail, move slowly, and be consistent but flexible.

Splinting and Casting

Splinting is an important component in the care of the child's hand. Splinting skills are acquired over time. Fabrication of a successful splint on a child who may not be cooperative is a challenge. The splint must meet the objectives set forth and also must be accepted and tolerated by the child and the family.

Keep in mind the strengths that the child may have. Try not to take function away, even temporarily, if possible. One must observe and evaluate the child carefully before using any splinting. One must weigh the advantages of splinting. If the problem is mild and the child has a major developmental and sensory deficit, the splint may only add to the confusion.

Precaution. *Either do not splint or be extremely cautious when there is poor sensation, vulnerable skin, or a nonverbal child. Do not use any small pieces in your splinting that potentially can be pulled off and swallowed.*

Splinting is performed for the following reasons:

- To increase function (Fig. 26-2)
- To prevent deformity (see Fig. 26-12 on the CD)
- To correct deformity (Fig. 26-3)
- To protect healing
- To restrict motion
- To allow for tissue growth and remodeling

The materials, components, and straps available have varied qualities that one must consider carefully. A lighter neoprene may be useful when only mild stiffness or increased tone is the problem. A thicker plastic may be used over neoprene when greater support is required. A light and flexible plastic is appropriate for the newborn or very young child. However, the therapist can use the material with which he or she feels more skillful. In general, the splint should be as light as possible, easy to put on, yet not easy to pull off by the child. The splint should not have too many movable components or small pieces, and whenever possible, the therapist should make it fun. This can be achieved through color, stickers, and a positive outlook or even a nickname, such as the "ballerina glove" or "your cool mitt."

Prefabricated splints are difficult to match perfectly with the problem. One size fits few. They may be soft and look pretty, but they are often ineffective.

Precaution. *A splint that does not fit well or does not position the digit in the desired location actually may interfere with the development of the child.*

A poor splint adds to the confusion and becomes a negative variable to the development of play occupations. *Above all, do no harm.*

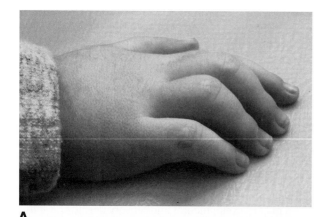

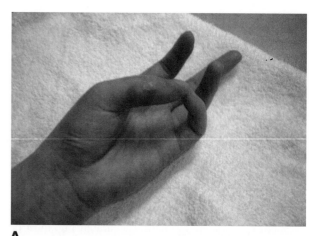

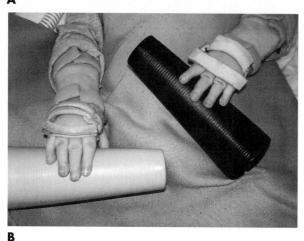

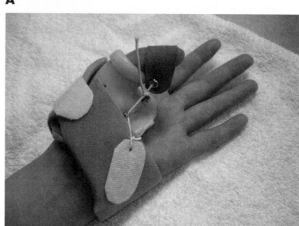

FIGURE 26-2 **A,** Metacarpophalangeal joints are in extension and proximal interphalangeal joints are in flexion because of intrinsic weakness in a 4-year-old child with familial neuromuscular disease. **B,** Forearm-based splint holds wrist in extension. Extension blocking bar positions the metacarpophalangeal joints in flexion allowing proximal interphalangeal joints to extend. This converts intrinsic-minus hand into intrinsic-plus hand.

FIGURE 26-3 **A,** Interphalangeal joint is stiff in extension after reconstruction of radial collateral ligament following excision of radial component of duplicate thumb. **B,** Hand-based dynamic splint is used to block metacarpophalangeal joint and gently flex interphalangeal joint with a looper. The elastic band is threaded through a pulley on the radial side of the palm, and the force is adjusted with Velcro as needed.

Splinting Schedule

One schedule does not fit all children. Some conditions may require full-time immobilization, such as in tendon repair. Other conditions may require a night resting and stretching splint and a day functional splint, such as in Erb's palsy and burns. Monitor tolerance and skin sensitivity, and teach parents to do the same. Children with daytime increased tone may not have increased tone during sleep, so you may need to rely on the parents' information or schedule a nighttime appointment. If a child is sick, tired, or hungry, it may be difficult to assess the comfort of the splint. Instruct the parents to keep a log of the wearing schedule. Splinting and casting are only a part of the total rehabilitation program.

Casting Principles

The plaster cast technique for remodeling and mobilization holds the joint or muscle tendon in the position of maximum resting length for a given time.

Precaution. *The splint and cast must be removed immediately when the fingers turn blue or white, when there is skin breakdown, or when the child appears in distress.*

This position over time induces actual tissue growth, not just stretch. Repeated casting lengthens tissue and ultimately decreases joint and soft tissue stiffness. Encourage exercise between casting sessions to maintain active range of motion. The cast can be removed once or twice per week for the finger to be exercised for 15 or 20 minutes, followed by recasting if necessary. The remodeling process requires enough time in the cast to promote regrowth of tissue.

BIOMECHANICS

CLINICAL *Pearl*

Application of a small but constant force has been shown to be more effective in remodeling (lengthening) tissue than intermittent application of large forces.

The selection of the most appropriate splint and its forces often involves trial and error rather than a scientific method. That is why constant reevaluation and vigilance are needed to achieve the safest and most effective force and splint application. We do know, however, that the pressure exerted on the skin should not exceed capillary pressure, which averages 30 to 35 mm Hg, or ischemia may result. According to Weeks and Wray,[2] an average person can tolerate 6 oz of force for up to 4 hours, or less force, for a longer period. This further alerts us against splinting an anesthetic hand or a more fragile pediatric skin. Brand and Hollister[3] state that in a short application of less than 2 hours, ischemia should not be a factor. They also warn of small tolerable stresses, applied repetitively, which can lead to shearing of tissues over time.

The force required to move a slightly stiff joint is small and simply may require positioning of the digit in the desired position. However, a force required to remodel a more contracted joint may vary between 100 to 300 g of force.

Precaution. *The force used by the therapist to position the finger "gently" into an improved position should not cause tissue blanching and damage.*

Always monitor the child's comfort and skin color.

CLINICAL *Pearl*

Rapid growth of the hand in a child mandates frequent changes or adjustments of casts or splints.

Hand length doubles during the first 2 years of life. Each hand deformity is unique and needs creative splinting or casting. Casting a child successfully is fun but challenging. Casting has potential for serious complications. These are related to tight cast, rapid cast wear and tear, broken cast, and loose pieces that curiously find a way into a mouth, nose, or ear.

BOX 26-2

Guidelines on When to Splint, Cast, or Monitor

When to cast rather than splint:

1. If a flexion contracture is greater than 20 degrees at interphalangeal joints
2. If the lateral deformity (radial or ulnar deviation) is greater than 20 degrees at interphalangeal joints
3. Serially to correct radial deformity as in a radial club hand
4. When therapy or splinting alone are not reducing a contracture

Do not cast if:

1. There is skin irritation or a rash.
2. Parents are unreliable in keeping appointments.
3. Contracture or deformity is mild (less than 20 degrees) and can be treated with splinting or hand therapy.
4. Other developmental or cognitive problems are greater than the physical limitation and actually may interfere with the child's overall performance.
5. Sensation is compromised because of nerve or brain injury.

Box 26-2 presents key indications, considerations, techniques, precautions, and tips on casting.

THERAPY STRATEGIES

Select a therapy program that works with the parents' lifestyle and routine. Ask the parents to ascertain a realistic amount of therapy/play time that they actually can follow. Often, other family members need to be involved. A daily log of time spent and clear exercise and picture handouts are important to avoid confusion and to maximize the benefits of splinting and stretching time. Make the parents accountable for it. Draw a "therapy contract" if necessary that delineates the parents' responsibilities.

Box 26-3 contains key strategies that the therapists can incorporate into their bag of skills. The objective is to keep it short, simple, and useful.

Parent and Child Education

Parents can make or break a favorable outcome. Parents often tend to focus on the child's abnormalities. Luckily, children focus on their normalities. Try to be optimistic but always realistic. Show concern and care, but always stay professional. Be available to parents and follow through on tasks, such as calling the doctor, getting

BOX 26-3

Key Strategies

STRATEGIES FOR IMPROVING RANGE OF MOTION
- Therapy program should match the client's age.
- Set specific times aside to exercise, such as bath time and feeding time.
- Incorporate range of motion into daily activities; make it fun.
- Develop a routine.
- Start with a few repetitions, 3 to 5 minutes per activity.
- Keep activity in front of the child; distract the child's other hand with a toy.
- "Hand hold" should be gentle during active-assisted or passive movements.
- Check for proper positioning of the hand and the rest of the body.
- Perform an activity analysis to make sure that the movements desired are taking place.
- Look out for unnecessary shoulder and elbow movements during fine motor activities done by wrist, hand, and fingers.

STRATEGIES FOR IMPROVING MUSCLE STRENGTH
- Check with the physician to see whether the child is ready to begin strengthening, as in tendon repair or fracture management.
- Move from range of motion to resistive function.
- Introduce heavier objects gradually.
- Introduce resistive activities such as putty, velcro, stickers, magnets, push-down buttons, and pull-apart blocks.
- Increase the time spent performing an activity, and keep track of the time.
- Maintain activities within pain tolerance.
- Strengthen the desired muscles.
- Prevent imbalance patterns that arise because of muscle weakness, as in thumb-in-palm deformity or spasticity in cerebral palsy.

STRATEGIES FOR IMPROVING DEXTERITY
- Activity selection is defined by chronologic or functional age.
- Define the child's intrinsic problem.

- Grade activities and toys from simple to complex.
- Allow the child enough repetitions over time to master the skills.
- Interject a simpler task to provide an experience of success while performing a series of complex tasks.
- Use functional activities, such as buttoning, lacing, and tying.
- Address stability of proximal joints to enhance dexterity of distal joints.

STRATEGIES FOR IMPROVING SENSATION
- Increase sensory experiences by providing a variety of textures, sizes, shapes, and weights.
- Allow enough time for exploration and play.
- Perform two-handed activities with vision and with vision occluded so that the child can relearn and become aware of the diminished sensation.
- If heat is used, make sure the medium is warm, not hot, and check the temperature often.
- During play, make sure the child is not pressing too hard so as to get sensory feedback and cause skin irritation.
- Train the child to use vision to compensate for sensory loss.

STRATEGIES FOR REDUCING HYPERSENSITIVITY
- Explain the activity to the child beforehand.
- Introduce tactile activities slowly.
- Begin with brief moments of touch.
- Mother may need to touch the objects first to allow the child to develop trust.
- Watch the child's face to determine sensory response.
- Begin with familiar objects—smooth, soft objects before coarse objects.
- Increase time of exposure gradually.
- Vibration is fun.
- Incorporate the sensory experience with play.
- Warmth is usually pleasurable, and play in a warm bubble bath can be fun.

equipment, and providing them with written literature. From the beginning, try to build a trusting relationship. Tell the parents that if the child is not able to do the exercises or wear the splint, they should communicate this to the therapist. The usefulness of the splint then can be assessed accurately, and the exercise program can be adjusted.

All parents hope for a normal child. The realization that there is a birth defect or injury is often earth-

shattering. Parents are with the child for longer periods and provide important information that leads to better care. Information such as position during sleep, neglect of an extremity or digit during play, wrist and hand postures that may not seem normal to them or equal between hands, and children biting at their fingers are just a few examples of important parental input.

Parents are dealing with their anxiety and expectations, and they often experience feelings of guilt over their child's problem. Make parents your partners in therapy by giving them responsibilities. For parents simply to bring the child to the office is not sufficient. They need to be accountable for the splint or cast and exercise program. This will make them feel that they truly are helping their child and thereby will help reduce some of their confusion and anxiety.

What to Say to Clients

The therapist must be physically gentle with the child and cautious with words. The therapist needs to praise parents for their work and to teach them when they are not following directions. For example, "You are doing very well with the exercises at home, but the baby feels a little stiff in this direction." Demonstrate the exercises several times and have the parents feel the stiffness. "I would like you to do it a bit slower, count to ten each time, and support the baby's chest with your other hand." Perform the exercise on the baby while holding onto the parent's hand, and guide them until they can do it independently. Ask the parents whether the technique is clear and whether they are comfortable with the new instructions. Record the instructions for the parents. You may have to draw a picture to make it more clear.

COMMON PEDIATRIC HAND CONDITIONS

CONGENITAL DEFORMITIES

The congenital anomalies of the hand and upper extremity are described in alphabetical order for ease of retrieval.

Embryology

Congenital anomalies affect 1% to 2% of neonates, and approximately 10% of neonates have upper extremity abnormalities.[4] Congenital limb anomalies are second only to congenital heart disease in the incidence of birth malformations. Most anomalies occur spontaneously or are inherited.[5] Limb bud formation begins approximately 4 weeks after gestation and is complete by 8 weeks. The majority of limb anomalies occur within this time of rapid and fragile limb development. Constriction bands occur from ninth week of gestation to birth.

The limb bud is first visualized at 26 days after fertilization when the embryo is about 4 mm in length from crown to rump. The bud rapidly develops through 47 days of life until the embryo length is close to 20 mm. At 52 to 53 days after gestation when the embryo is between 22 and 24 mm of length, the fingers are entirely separate.[6] Joint formation follows, and proper joint development

requires intact neuromuscular activity and joint motion for modeling. Eight weeks after fertilization, embryogenesis is complete and all limb structures are present.[7] The majority of upper extremity congenital anomalies occur during this 4 to 8 week period of rapid and fragile limb development. Fetal development continues between 8 and 36 weeks, during which time joints develop as a result of muscle contraction. Lack of muscle contraction during this time for unknown reasons leads to stiff joints as seen in arthrogryposis.

CLINICAL *Pearl*

The majority of congenital anomalies affect the finger, hand, and wrist. Deformities of the forearm, elbow, and shoulder are less frequent but are equally important.

Classification

Swanson's classification[8] of congenital anomalies of the upper extremity has been used by the American Society for Surgery of the Hand, American Association for Hand Surgery, and International Federation of Societies for Surgery of the Hand, but when a child presents to the hand surgeon or therapist, Flatt's classification[9] by clinical site is practical. Swanson's classification explains embryologic basis of deformities and is divided into seven types as shown in Box 26-4.[8]

The following are commonly encountered congenital deformities of the hand and upper extremity that benefit from hand therapy. All possible conditions are not included.

Arthrogryposis

Arthrogryposis, so named by Rocher in 1913, now generally is known as **arthrogryposis multiplex congenita.** Arthrogryposis is a congenital neuromuscular disease that presents as a syndrome of nonprogressive joint contractures at birth.[10] Multiple forms occur that vary in presentation, severity, and number of joints involved.[11] Hand deformity is a common manifestation in the arthrogrypotic child. The majority of the hand deformities consist of two types: one is a thumb-in-palm deformity with the fingers in intrinsic-plus position, and another type is flexion contractures of the fingers at the interphalangeal joints.

Diagnosis and Pathology

Arthrogryposis may be generalized or localized to the distal extremity (**distal arthrogryposis;** Fig. 26-4, *A*). In both types, there is arthrofibrosis of the joints and weakness or wasting of muscles.

BOX 26-4

Swanson's Classification of Congenital Hand Anomalies

I. FAILURE OF DIFFERENTIATION
Syndactyly: fibrous, osseous, complex
Synostosis: radioulnar synostosis

2. DUPLICATION
Preaxial   Thumb duplication
Central   Digits 2, 3, 4
Postaxial   Little finger; supernumery fifth finger

3. OVERGROWTH
Macrodactyly

4. FAILURE OF FORMATION
Transverse arrest   Below-elbow amputation
Longitudinal arrest Radial, ulnar, central deficits
Intersegmental   Phocomelia

5. UNDERGROWTH
Hypoplastic thumb
Brachydactyly

6. CONGENITAL CONSTRICTION BAND
Occurs between 8 and 36 weeks of gestation

7. GENERALIZED ANOMALIES AND SYNDROMES
Madelung's deformity: failure of volar growth
    plate of distal end of radius
Costello syndrome/nail-patella syndrome

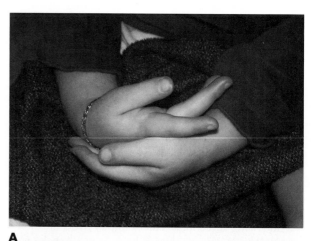

A

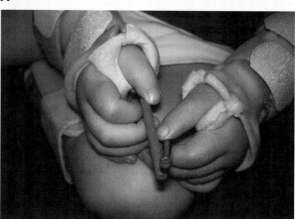

B

FIGURE 26-4   A, Child with distal arthrogryposis has wrist flexion and digital extension posture. **B,** The splints extend the wrist, allowing digital flexion and improving hand function.

Amyoplasia (classic arthrogryposis) is the most common form and is characterized by symmetric positioning of the limbs. Amyoplasia occurs sporadically.[10] The upper extremities posture with shoulder adduction and internal rotation, elbow extension, forearm pronation, wrist flexion, and hand ulnar deviation. The digits are postured in flexion and are stiff. The contracted clasped thumb is a common finding in arthrogryposis and creates functional difficulties.[4] Additional clinical features are waxy skin devoid of skin creases, considerable muscle wasting, and a paucity of subcutaneous tissue.

The joint contractures result from lack of motion during fetal life. Embryologic defects that lead to lack of fetal limb movement may be related to muscle abnormalities, nerve anomalies, or vascular insufficiency. The precise cause remains unknown.

Nonoperative Treatment

The treatment of arthrogryposis is individualized to each child's needs. Upper extremity treatment goals include achieving independent function. Adaptive equipment is helpful in maximizing independence.[7]

Precaution. *The mainstays of early treatment are frequent passive movement of all involved joints and judicious use of splints.*

A static splint helps to position the wrist in extension and facilitates finger flexion for improved function (Fig. 26-4, B). Static progressive splinting creates a low load and prolonged stretch and may be helpful for diminishing contractures. An increase in passive motion is beneficial for function and enhances the outcome of surgical reconstruction. Smith and Drennan[12] demonstrated that passive stretching, serial casting, and splinting are most efficacious in correcting wrist contractures of distal arthrogryposis.

Operative Treatment

Surgery usually is recommended before school age (4 or 5 years of age) to minimize compensatory movements and maximize mainstream school function. Goal of postoperative hand therapy is to maintain joint motion achieved during surgery and to prevent further contractures after the wounds have healed.

Questions to Ask the Physician

Nonoperative Treatment

- *How often should parents and I apply passive range of motion to the joints?*
- *How many hours a day should the child be splinted?*
- *How long may the finger, wrist, or elbow be left without a splint?*

Operative Treatment

- *What procedures were done? (Ask for an operative report.)*
- *What range of motion does the doctor expect the child to achieve?*
- *Are there any precautions?*

What to Say to Clients

About the Deformity

"Without treatment, deformity will not improve."

About Splinting

"The child should wear the splints daily, during the day and night."

About Exercises

"Move the joints through maximum range as tolerated by the child. Exercises need to be performed several times a day."

Evaluation Tips

Explore activities of daily living needs to improve independence. Measure range of motion of finger joints with wrist in extension and flexion to differentiate between **tenodesis effect** and joint contracture.

Diagnosis-Specific Information That Affects Clinical Reasoning

Child and parent compliance is critical to achieve expected goals.

Treatment Recommendations

Use a team approach between the family, physician, speech therapist, physical therapist, and teachers. A daily program consisting of stretching, active range of motion, and strengthening is carried out. The goal is to achieve independent function. Watch how the child plays, and outline the abnormal postures that may lead to contractures. Splint appropriate joints to enhance function and prevent contractures.

CLINICAL *Pearl*

Exercises, splinting, and adaptive equipment are the hallmark of treatment.

Precautions and Concerns

- *If the child appears uncomfortable during splint wear, adjust or remove the splint.*
- *If the skin becomes red, swollen, or broken down, discontinue splinting.*

The Role of the Therapy Assistant

Supervise the child's home and office splint and exercise and play programs as developed by therapist.

Camptodactyly

Camptodactyly is a painless flexion contracture of the proximal interphalangeal (PIP) joint that is usually progressive.[5] The fifth finger most commonly is involved. Table 26-4 describes the three types of camptodactyly.

Diagnosis and Pathology

Camptodactyly is rare and occurs in less than 1% of the population. Camptodactyly occurs without intraarticular or periarticular PIP joint swelling. The metacarpophalangeal (MCP) and distal interphalangeal (DIP) joints are not affected, although compensatory deformities may develop. Most cases of camptodactyly are sporadic. However, camptodactyly can be inherited and is considered an autosomal dominant trait with variable expressivity and incomplete penetrance. Most cases are mild and asymptomatic and probably do not warrant treatment. Camptodactyly is bilateral in approximately two thirds of the cases, although the degree of contracture is usually not symmetric. Camptodactyly may affect radial fingers, although the incidence decreases toward the radial side of the hand.

Almost every structure about the PIP joint has been implicated. These include skin, collateral ligaments, volar plate, flexor and extensor tendons, intrinsic muscles, retinacular ligaments, bones and joints, flexor tendons, and intrinsic muscles (lumbricals and/or interossei).

Camptodactyly is diagnosed when there is a finger deformity in the flexion extension plane at the PIP joint. If there is a fixed bone or joint deformity, splinting or casting will not correct the contracture. One must confirm this finding with radiographs before initiating treatment.

TABLE 26-4

Classification of Camptodactyly

TYPE	OCCURRENCE	CHARACTERISTICS
I	Infant or congenital	Isolated finding and usually limited to the fifth finger
II	Preadolescence or acquired	Often does not improve spontaneously; may progress to a severe flexion deformity
III	Associated with a variety of syndromes	Usually involves multiple digits of both extremities

Timelines and Healing

Prolonged and continuous splinting and casting are necessary until the correction is satisfactory to the child and the parents. Complete discontinuation of the splint should be delayed until skeletal maturity because the deformity may progress.[13-15]

Nonoperative Treatment

Conservative treatment is the mainstay for mild camptodactyly of 30 degrees or less of contracture. The child and family should be instructed to undergo splinting or serial casting or should accept the deformity. Static splinting at night is recommended to prevent progression after acceptable improvement with casting. A preliminary period of nonoperative treatment is almost always attempted to decrease any fixed flexion deformity.[14,16,17] Formal therapy usually is required and includes stretching, splinting (static and dynamic), and serial casting.

In infants, the cast or splint must be forearm-based to fit adequately and to decrease the chances of removal. The recommended duration of splint wear per day varies among investigators.[14,15,17] Hori et al.[14] used full-time dynamic splinting for "a few months," followed by 8 hours per day after correction was achieved. Miura et al.[15] requested full-time splint wear but accepted 12 hours per day in young children. Benson et al.[16] encouraged 15 to 18 hours of splint wear per day in the young infant and 10 to 12 hours per day as the child grew. Irrespective of the initial splinting regimen, part-time splinting needs to be continued for a long time.

Conservative treatment with passive stretching, splinting, and casting results in decrease in the amount of PIP joint contracture.[14,15,17] Formal therapy, a compliant child, and prolonged diligent splinting are prerequisites. Superior results are obtained in a motivated child with a mild deformity.[17] Hori et al.[14] reported on 24 clients (34 fingers) with small finger camptodactyly who were treated with a splinting regimen. The average follow-up time was almost 4 years. Twenty fingers had "almost" full extension, nine had improved, three were unchanged, and two were worse. The average flexion contracture improved from 40 to 10 degrees after treatment. Benson

et al.[16] treated 22 clients (59 digits) with a therapy program and reported their results at a mean follow-up of 33 months. Type I camptodactyly (13 clients or 24 PIP joints) improved from a 23-degree flexion contracture to 4 degrees shy of full extension. Type II camptodactyly (4 clients or 5 PIP joints) were relatively noncompliant with therapy and achieved minimal correction. Type III camptodactyly (30 PIP joints in 5 clients) possessed a varied amount of deformity. Twelve of these 30 PIP joints lacked at least 15 degrees of extension and improved to almost full extension.

Operative Treatment

When deformity is severe and the child's desire for correction is great, surgery is done to address the underlying pathologic anatomy: skin, collateral ligaments, volar plate, flexor and extensor tendons, intrinsic muscles, retinacular ligaments, bones and joints, and intrinsic muscles (lumbricals and/or interossei).

Questions to Ask the Physician

- *How long should the finger be casted?*
- *When may I switch to splinting?*
- *How long may the finger be left without cast or splint?*

What to Say to Clients

About the Deformity

"Your deformity cannot be corrected quickly. Casting and splinting will be necessary for months or years. The final correction may not be complete. You may choose to undergo surgery if the final correction is not satisfactory to you. The deformity is mostly cosmetic, and function of the hand tends to be satisfactory."

About Splinting

"We will start with serial casting to stretch the deformity slowly. Once the deformity is reduced to mild degree (less than thirty degrees of proximal interphalangeal joint contracture), a static splint will be applied. This may be worn day and night as much as possible. The splint may be removed for hygiene and play. Older children will need a dynamic splint such as a reverse knuckle bender during daytime and static splinting during nighttime. We recommend splinting only for children who show enthusiasm for correction of proximal interphalangeal joint. Do not wet the cast. Cover the arm in plastic bag while cleaning the body. If cast becomes wet accidentally, come in for a new cast. If the finger tip is blue or pale, remove the cast and come in for a new cast."

About Exercises

"Between casting and splinting sessions, the proximal interphalangeal joint and hand may be used for playing and exercises."

Evaluation Tips

- Measure PIP joint range of motion with the wrist in extension and flexion. If the range of motion of the PIP joint changes, the flexor digitorum superficialis is short and is the cause of flexion deformity.
- Determine whether the deformity is cosmetic or functional.

Tips from the Field

Use the cast and splinting only in compliant children. The cast should be changed once or twice a week.

Precautions and Concerns

- *If there is pain, remove cast immediately by soaking the hand in warm water.*
- *If the color of the finger tip is pale, purple, or blue, remove the cast immediately by soaking the hand in warm water.*
- *Keep the cast dry at all times to prevent skin maceration.*
- *If a regular appointment for cast change cannot be kept, notify your therapist and remove the cast.*

The Role of the Therapy Assistant

This technique is for therapists with advanced training in hand therapy. Therapy assistants must be trained by an experienced hand therapist before attempting to cast a finger.

Treatment Recommendations

We strongly recommend casting over splinting. Casting is the mainstay of treatment in our practice because the cast is more secure and remains in the desired position. We use cast for deformities of 30 degrees. As correction is obtained to less than 30 degrees, we switch to splinting. In between casting or splinting sessions, encourage the child to play using the affected finger.

Clinodactyly

Clinodactyly is not a diagnosis. The term means deformity of the finger in a medial or lateral plane. Clinodactyly is a complaint a client makes and a finding on physical examination. Diagnosis is made once the cause of deformity is identified.

Diagnosis and Pathology

The four common causes of clinodactyly are inherited deformity in the small finger, **delta phalanx** in the thumb, clinodactyly as a part of rare syndromes, and posttraumatic deformity in any finger.

Clinodactyly presents most commonly as an isolated radial inclination of the *small finger,* because of the middle phalanx adopting a triangular[18] or trapezoidal shape. This form of clinodactyly is inherited as an autosomal dominant trait and is often bilateral. Expression of the trait is variable, with males more likely to express the phenotype. In Australia, a delta middle phalanx–producing clinodactyly of the little finger is the most common deformity. Isolated, severe clinodactyly may occur in the neonate or infant, although most occur later as the angulation becomes more obvious with growth. The reason for presentation is usually cosmetic because compensatory abduction of the small finger prevents substantial interference with flexion.

Clinodactyly of the thumb occurs because of an extra triangular phalanx between the proximal and distal phalanx. Jones[19] suggested the term *delta phalanx* for this triangular bone, and this term is in general use. In the hand of a child with Apert's syndrome, the thumb may have a delta phalanx and may present as clinodactyly.

Clinodactyly also is seen as part of many syndromes and complex hand anomalies. The asymmetric development of secondary ossification centers in phalanges produces this anomaly.

Posttraumatic clinodactyly is the most common deformity of fingers in children following articular fractures. It was present in 19% of finger fractures in children.[20] When deformity or deviation is greater than 10 degrees, overlapping of the fingers in flexion may occur and may require treatment.

Clinodactyly is diagnosed when the finger deformity is in medial-lateral plane. No deformity occurs in the flexion-extension plane.

Timelines and Healing

Unless treated, the angle of deformity does not change.

Nonoperative Treatment

The splinting of clinodactyly has no support in the literature. Kozin[7] categorically considers splinting clinodactyly pointless. If the **epiphysis** is open, we use

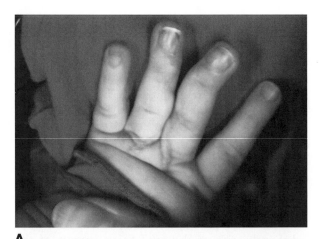

A

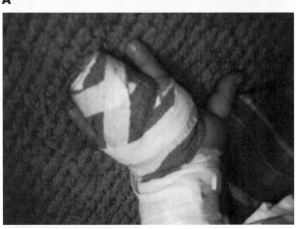

B

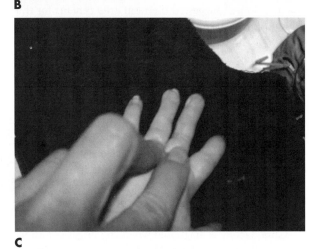

C

FIGURE 26-5 A, Clinodactyly in a child after syndactyly release. **B,** Serial casting was done twice a week for 6 months. **C,** The distal interphalangeal joint deformity has improved.

serial casting in the same manner as Ilizarov's method of gradual **epiphyseal distraction (chondrodiastasis).** We have seen correction in four children with serial casting. We currently are investigating this method (Fig. 26-5).

Operative Treatment

Correction of a bent phalanx requires an osteotomy to realign the digit. Resection of the longitudinal epiphyseal bracket may be done to balance longitudinal growth potential of the shortened side of the digit. The extra phalanx in thumb clinodactyly is resected to restore length and alignment of the digit.

Questions to Ask the Physician

- *Should I attempt casting of this deformity?*
- *How long should the finger be casted before surgery is considered?*

What to Say to Clients

About the Deformity

"Your deformity cannot be corrected without surgery. Casting and splinting are controversial and may be necessary for months or years. The final correction may not be complete. You may choose to undergo surgery if the final correction is not satisfactory to you. The deformity is mostly cosmetic, and function of the hand tends to be satisfactory."

About Casting and Splinting

"We will start with serial casting to stretch the deformity slowly. Once the deformity is reduced to mild degree (less than 30 degrees of proximal interphalangeal joint contracture), a static splint will be applied. This may be worn day and night as much as possible. The splint may be removed for hygiene and play. We recommend splinting only for children who show enthusiasm for correction of the deformity. Do not get the cast wet. Cover the arm in plastic bag to bathe the baby. If the cast becomes wet accidentally, come in for a new cast. If the finger tip is blue or pale, remove the cast and come in for a new cast."

About Exercises

"Between casting and splinting sessions, the finger and hand may be used for playing and exercises."

Evaluation Tips

Measure the angular deformity by tracing the finger on a paper, by hand printing, or by taking radiographs once every 3 months. Record the range of motion of the PIP joint and DIP joint.

Tips from the Field

Use the cast and splinting only in compliant children. The cast should be changed once or twice a week.

Precautions and Concerns

- *Precautions and concerns are the same as for camptodactyly.*

The Role of the Therapy Assistant

This technique is for therapists with advanced training in hand therapy. Therapy assistants must be trained by an experienced hand therapist before attempting to cast a finger.

Kirner's Deformity

Diagnosis and Pathology
Kirner's deformity is a specific skeletal deformity characterized by progressive palmar and radial curvature of the distal phalanx of the small finger.[21] The presence of dorsovolar curvature distinguishes Kirner's deformity from clinodactyly of the small finger. The curvature is progressive and painless, bilateral and symmetric. The deformity may be inherited as an autosomal dominant trait. The deformity occurs sporadically in at least half of the cases. Kirner's deformity typically develops in late childhood or adolescence. The child may have some discomfort associated with this stage. Joint motion at the DIP joint is preserved. Kirner's deformity has been seen in cases of Cornelia de Lange's syndrome, Silver's syndrome, Turner's syndrome, and Down syndrome.

The differential diagnosis includes traumatic injury to the **physis** (growth plate) or physeal injury caused by burns or frostbite.

Timelines and Healing
The deformity is progressive if left untreated. Prolonged and continuous splinting and casting are necessary until the correction is satisfactory to the child and the parents. Complete discontinuation of the splint should be delayed until skeletal maturity.[13-15]

Nonoperative Treatment
Some investigators have reported prolonged serial splinting useful in correcting the deformity if applied in the early stages and before completion of growth. Freiberg and Forrest reported successful correction with prolonged splinting.[21a] According to Kozin,[7] splinting can be attempted in the immature child, and it needs to be monitored rigorously to be effective. Our choice of treatment is casting the finger.

In infants, the cast or splint must be forearm-based to fit adequately and to decrease the chances of removal. Irrespective of the initial casting, part-time splinting needs to be continued for a long time.

Operative Treatment
Once the epiphysis is closed and the deformity is established, multiple osteotomies with Kirschner wire stabilization may improve the appearance. Corrective surgery is deferred until the child is able to participate in the decision-making process because surgery is performed to improve appearance rather than function.

Questions to Ask the Physician

- *How long should the finger be casted?*
- *When may I switch to splinting?*
- *How long may the finger be left without cast or splint?*
- *When should the splinting or casting be terminated in favor of surgery?*

What to Say to Clients

About the Deformity
"Your deformity cannot be corrected quickly. Casting and splinting will be necessary for months or years. The final correction may not be complete. You may choose to undergo surgery if the final correction is not satisfactory to you. The deformity is mostly cosmetic, and function of the hand tends to be satisfactory."

About Casting and Splinting
"We will start with serial casting to stretch the deformity slowly. Do not get the cast wet. Cover the arm in plastic bag while cleaning the body. If the cast becomes wet accidentally, come in for a new cast. If the finger tip is blue or pale, remove the cast and come in for a new cast. Once the deformity is mild, a static night splint is recommended."

About Exercises
"Between casting and splinting sessions, the hand may be used for playing and exercises."

Evaluation Tips
- Measure the angular deformity by tracing the finger on a paper, by hand printing, or by radiographs once every 3 months.
- Record the range of motion of the PIP joint and DIP joint.

Tips from the Field
Use the cast and splinting only in compliant children. The cast should be changed once or twice a week.

Precautions and Concerns

- *If there is pain, remove the cast immediately by soaking the hand in warm water.*

- *If the color of the finger tip is pale, purple, or blue, remove the cast immediately by soaking the hand in warm water.*
- *Keep the cast dry at all times to prevent skin maceration.*
- *If your regular appointment for cast change cannot be kept, notify your therapist and remove the cast.*

Treatment Recommendations

Cast the fingers with deformity greater than 20 to 30 degrees and allow motion between casting sessions. We recommend splinting for deformities less than 20 to 30 degrees. Surgery is reserved for clients who insist on correction of deformity and after they reach maturity.

Congenital Clasped Thumb (Thumb-in-Palm Deformity)

Congenital clasped thumb refers to a spectrum of thumb anomalies that range from mild deficiencies of the thumb extensor mechanism to severe abnormalities of the extrinsic and intrinsic muscles, web space, and soft tissue and joint contractures. A persistent flexed adducted thumb variously has been called congenital clasped thumb,[22] thumb-in-palm deformity, or flexion adduction deformity of the thumb. When associated with ulnar deviation of the fingers at the MCP joints, the condition is called **windblown hand.** Congenital clasped-thumb deformity may manifest as part of a more generalized disorder, but it is more prevalent as a sporadic finding rather than as part of a generalized disorder. A separate category of clients are those with spastic adduction deformity of the thumb resulting from brain damage, as in **cerebral palsy.**

Weckesser et al.[23] classified congenital clasped thumbs into four groups. Group I consists of isolated clasped thumb. Group II consists of flexion contracture of the fingers. Group III consists of flexion contracture of the thumb. Group IV is a miscellaneous category.

Diagnosis and Pathology

The characteristic posture of thumb-in-palm deformity is flexion of the MCP joint and adduction of the first metacarpal. This causes the thumb to lie across the palm. In the newborn, it is normal for the thumb to be clutched intermittently in the palm, and it is only by the third month of life that the infant begins to incorporate thumb movement into grasp. For this reason, the diagnoses of thumb-in-palm deformity may be made only after the third month of life. In some cases the interphalangeal joint is flexed because of the absence or **hypoplasia** of the extensor pollicis longus tendon. In the spastic thumb-in-palm, the associated features of cerebral palsy should make the diagnosis apparent.

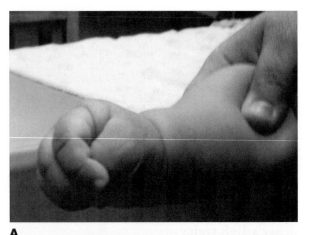

A

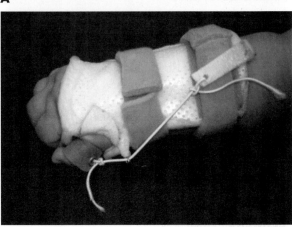

B

FIGURE 26-6 A, Eight-month-old infant has only thumb-in-palm deformity. **B,** Dynamic thumb abduction assist splint pulls thumb out of the palm, prevents contracture, and allows unimpeded digital grasp.

A practical classification of clasped thumb has been proposed by Mih[22] and by McCarroll.[23a] A type I clasped thumb is usually supple, with absence of or hypoplasia of the extensor mechanism. A type II clasped thumb is complex with additional findings of joint contracture, collateral ligament abnormality, first web space contracture, and thenar muscle abnormality. A type III clasped thumb is associated with arthrogryposis or its related syndromes. In this case the extensor mechanism may be deficient or normal.

Nonoperative Treatment

Children with congenital clasped-thumb deformity, especially those under 2 years of age, respond well to splinting of the thumb (static or dynamic) in a position of extension and abduction. In nearly all children, splinting should be tried for at least 3 months and possibly for 6 months or longer (Fig. 26-6).

Tsuyuguchi et al.[24] reported on 43 clients with 75 clasped thumbs. Forty-two thumbs were treated with splinting alone, 16 were treated with surgery, and 17 were observed. Those without soft tissue contracture did well with splinting in 19 hands. Initial treatment of the type I clasped thumb includes splinting of the affected joints in extension. The goal is to prevent additional attenuation of the hypoplastic extensor mechanism and to allow hypertrophy over time. Full-time splinting for 2 to 6 months has been shown to be effective. Miura et al.[15] reported on 96 hands in 66 clients who underwent splint application. Seventy percent of children who were splinted within 12 months of birth obtained good results. In contrast, only 21% of children older than 1 year had success after splinting. None of the children older than 2 years of age had a successful outcome.

Operative Treatment

Surgery is warranted in situations in which splinting has failed or if the child is older than 2 years of age. The degree of impairment, however, must be considered during formulation of a treatment plan. Mild MCP joint extension lag does not hinder hand function and does not always require treatment. Frequently, adolescents are seen with a mild clasped thumb that has never been treated, and they report no problems.

CLINICAL *Pearl*

Considerable lack of thumb extension that interferes with grasp warrants treatment.

Any associated thumb MCP joint or thumb-index web space contracture requires surgical treatment. Initially, serial casting or splinting may be tried to stretch the taut skin and correct the contracture. Correction of the residual contracture must be incorporated into the surgical planning. In the Weckesser et al.[23] study, surgery in group II clients with arthrogryposis multiplex congenital produced less satisfactory results.

Questions to Ask the Physician

Nonoperative Treatment

- How long during the day and night should I splint the hand?
- For how long will I continue splinting before surgery?

Operative Treatment

- What structures were reconstructed? (Ask for an operative report.)

- What is the therapy protocol following surgery?
- What are the precautions?

What to Say to Clients

About the Deformity

"If the deformity is not addressed, it will not get better. Very mild deformity may respond to play therapy; moderate deformities may require splinting and therapy; severe deformities require preoperative therapy, surgery, and postoperative therapy."

About Splinting

"Your child may need splinting during play and during the night. In moderate to severe deformity, casting and dynamic splinting may be used."

About Exercises

"Exercises will be used in all cases of severity."

Evaluation Tips

- Check if the deformity can be passively corrected. (Check MCP joint and interphalangeal joint active and passive flexion and extension.)
- Observe the child play and note the active movements and lack of movements.
- Check for the effects of tenodesis by flexing and extending the wrist and noting thumb flexion and extension.

Tips from the Field

A satisfactory result depends on compliance of the child and the parents.

Treatment Recommendations

For type I cases, we recommend a static splint with the wrist in extension and the thumb in opposition and abduction. The splinting program is supplemented with strengthening activities with and without the splint. For type II cases, we use a night immobilization splint to position the thumb-in-palmar abduction. During the day, we use a mobilization splint with or without a dynamic component. The program is supplemented with strengthening activities. Type III cases are treated as in type II with the addition of serial casting. The treatment is needed for longer periods during the day and over time. Partnership with parents is our principle precept.

The Role of the Therapy Assistant

Supervise clients' home and splint programs as developed by therapist.

Radial Club Hand

The term **radial club hand** has been used widely and has been accepted to describe congenital **longitudinal radial ray deficiency,** a hand that is radially deviated at the distal forearm in the shape of a golf club.

Diagnosis and Pathology

Radial deficiency is a spectrum of malformations affecting the structures of the radial side of the forearm (radius, radial carpus, and thumb), including hypoplasia (undergrowth) of the bones and joints, muscles and tendons, ligaments, nerves, and blood vessels. Radial deficiency is bilateral in 50% of cases. The majority of cases are sporadic. Radial deficiency is associated with Holt-Oram syndrome, thrombocytopenia, and Fanconi's anemia. Modified Bayne's classification is useful in diagnosis and treatment. Table 26-5 describes Bayne's classification.[25]

The goal of radial ray deficiency management is to correct the deformity, to improve the function of the hand and upper extremity, and when possible to improve the cosmetic appearance. Three treatment options are available: no treatment, manipulation and stretching with plaster casts and splinting, and surgical correction. Treatment indications vary with the severity of the deformity and the age of the child.

Nonoperative Treatment

Children with type 0, 1, or mild type 2 radial deficiencies may require only stretching, exercises, and splinting or serial casting. A tight webspace is stretched and casted. The ulnar collateral ligament of the MCP joint is often insufficient.

Precaution. *It is important not to worsen joint laxity with splinting and casting.*

Operative Treatment

When considerable radial deviation is present, tendon transfers and soft tissue releases are indicated. Kozin[7] prefers serial casting for preoperative soft tissue stretching and starts this shortly after birth. The wrist is stretched as close to neutral as possible, and a long-arm cast is applied. The cast is changed weekly with further correction each time. If the wrist can be stretched to neutral, a custom-fabricated long-arm splint is applied. The parents are instructed to continue stretching the wrist several times each day until centralization is performed.[4]

Questions to Ask the Physician

All Clients

- What are the skeletal and soft tissue deficits present in the hand, wrist, forearm, and elbow? (Ask for x-ray films and magnetic resonance imaging findings.)
- What other organ deficiencies are present?
- What are the functional deficits and goals of treatment?

Nonoperative Clients

- How long should I cast the child's wrist?

Operative Clients

- What structures were reconstructed? Skin, collateral ligaments, tendon transfer?
- If **pollicization** was done, what soft tissue and bone procedures were done? What was the stability of the carpometacarpal and metacarpophalangeal joints before and after the surgery?
- What is the postoperative protocol?
- What are the precautions?

TABLE 26-5

Modified Bayne's Classification of Radial Longitudinal Deficiency

TYPE	THUMB	CARPUS	DISTAL RADIUS	PROXIMAL RADIUS
0	Hypoplastic or absent	Absence, hypoplasia, or coalition	Normal	Normal, radioulnar synostosis, or congenital dislocation of the radial head
1	Hypoplastic or absent	Absence, hypoplasia, or coalition	>2 mm shorter than ulna	Normal, radioulnar synostosis, or congenital dislocation of the radial head
2	Hypoplastic or absent	Absence, hypoplasia, or coalition	Hypoplasia	Hypoplasia
3	Hypoplastic or absent	Absence, hypoplasia, or coalition	Physis absent	Variable hypoplasia
4	Hypoplastic or absent	Absence, hypoplasia, or coalition	Absent	Absent

Modified from Bayne LG, Klug MS: Long-term review of the surgical treatment of radial deficiencies, *J Hand Surg (Am)* 12:169-179, 1987. In James MA, Bednar M: Deformities of the wrist and forearm. In Green et al: *Green's operative hand surgery,* ed 5, Philadelphia, 2005, Churchill-Livingstone.

What to Say to Clients

About the Condition

"If both wrists and thumbs need surgery, the first procedure is done at six months of age, so that all the procedures can be adequately spaced and completed by eighteen months of age or thereafter."

About Splinting

"If the condition is unilateral, surgery may be postponed until the age of one year. The deformity is corrected with serial casting and splinting during this time."

About Exercises

"Exercises are done to strengthen the upper extremity and to incorporate both hands for function."

Evaluation Tips

- Check the mobility of index finger joints before pollicization.
- Check stability of the ulnar collateral ligament of the MCP joint.
- Check whether the carpometacarpal joint is present or absent.
- Record the angulation of the radial clubbing at every visit.

Tips from the Field

An index finger that is stiff before pollicization will result in a stable thumb for gross grasp. A mobile index finger will result in a stable thumb that can participate in pinch activities. After surgery, develop a proper pinching pattern between the pollicized thumb and the adjacent finger. Prevent scissoring of the remaining fingers.

Precautions and Concerns

- *Prevent further laxity of the ulnar collateral ligament of the MCP joint when you cast the thumb to improve web space.*
- *Do not allow the cast to get wet.*

Treatment Recommendations

Start serial casting of the wrist as soon as possible, using a forearm-based splint or cast. Casting can begin as early as the child is born. Cast the wrist once or twice a week. When the cast is removed, engage the child in age-appropriate activities, and provide gentle passive motion. Supplement the cast with a removable plastic splint in case the cast comes off or is removed by the parents. Once the hand is aligned with the forearm, the surgeon can balance the wrist surgically with added ease. Retrain the pollicized thumb as soon as possible.

The Role of the Therapy Assistant

The assistant helps the therapist in reinforcing the home and office exercise program.

BIRTH INJURIES

Cerebral Palsy

Cerebral palsy is a birth injury of the brain that causes irreversible upper neuron disorder characterized by an increase of muscle tone **(spasticity)**, tendon jerks, and hyperexcitability of the stretch reflex. This results in weakness, lack of smooth movement, joint contractures, decreased functional ability, pain, and possible nerve compression.

Diagnosis and Pathology

The upper motor neuron causes hyperexcitability of flexor group of muscles when the effect of lower motor neuron is neutralized. The infant or child may have motor, sensory, and cognitive deficits that span from **flaccidity** to spasticity to **athetosis.** Deficits may involve one extremity, one side of the body **(hemiplegia),** or both sides of the body **(quadriplegia).** Sensibility of the affected part usually is diminished, and the intelligence of the child is variable.

Evaluation Tips

- The typical posture of the extremity is shoulder internal rotation, elbow flexion, forearm pronation, wrist flexion, fingers in flexion, and thumb positioned in the palm. The evaluation includes the following deficits:
  - Motor deficit: volitional activity, spasticity, and resulting joint contractures because they determine treatment plan. Evaluate active range of motion, activities of daily living, strength, and dexterity.
  - Sensory deficit: determines splint application and surgical outcome. Evaluate sensation in every child. Sensation is a predictor of functional ability of the extremity. In a cognitively impaired child, it is difficult to assess the sensibility of the affected part.
- Cognitive ability is important to evaluate because treatment outcome is compromised in children with diminished intelligence and communicative skills.
- Hand function may be graded as described in Table 26-6.

Timelines and Healing

The neurologic status is static, but resulting joint contractures are progressive. New problems arise as the child

TABLE 26-6

Functional Grading of the Hand by Green and Banks, Modified by Samilson and Morris[9,22]

GRADE	DESCRIPTION
Poor	Use of hand as paper weight
	Poor or absent grasp and release
	Poor control
Fair	Use of hand as a helping hand
	No ability to use hand in dressing
	Moderate grasp and release
	Fair control
Good	Use of hand to help in dressing, eating, and general activities
	Effectual grasp and release
	Good control
Excellent	Good use of the hand in dressing and eating
	Effectual grasp and release
	Excellent control

grows. Deterioration of function occurs when joint contractures are allowed to progress in severe cases. Contractures possibly can be prevented in mild cases.

Nonoperative Treatment

Treatment goals are to prevent deformity, expand function, enhance hygiene, and improve appearance.

Splinting, if applied properly and consistently, may prevent and reduce contractures, facilitate movement, inhibit spasticity, lessen pain, and improve function (Fig. 26-7). With the addition of new chemical agents to reduce spasticity, splint usage has become more realistic.

One must keep in mind that proper positioning of the extremity is necessary. For example, splints designed to keep fingers in extension also must include wrist extension. Otherwise, a compensatory and predictable pattern of deformity will occur. The extrinsic tendons of the fingers cross the wrist as well.

Prolonged and gradual mobilization splinting of the wrist and fingers of a spastic hand over time may achieve a more functional position. However, if not maintained, the deformity gradually returns.

CLINICAL *Pearl*

Splinting the spastic upper extremity is a challenge even to the hand therapist with experience.

Furthermore, the neurophysiologic effects of splinting have not been studied and tested fully. We do not use the prefabricated splints in our practice. The Snook "spasticity reduction splint" was studied by McPherson[26] and was found to have an immediate and marked reduction of tone. This splint positions the wrist in 30 degrees of extension, finger MCP joints in abduction and 45 degrees of flexion, interphalangeal joints in extension, and thumb in abduction. We fabricate splints according to the needs of each child. These include a resting splint at night to stretch the elbow, wrist, fingers, and thumb comfortably into functional position. We use day splints to enhance function by extending the wrist and positioning the thumb out of the palm. The thumb position must allow it to oppose the index and middle fingers.

Operative Treatment

CLINICAL *Pearl*

Surgery is most beneficial in children who are less affected and have mild to moderate spasticity. Surgery is least helpful in children with severe involvement, uncontrollable spasticity, and athetosis.

Surgery is reparative and not curative. The goal of surgery is to rebalance the extremity. A combination of joint stabilization procedures, tendon lengthening techniques, and tendon transfers are used. Transfer of the flexor carpi ulnaris to the extensor carpi radialis is a common procedure and is used to reduce wrist flexion deformity.[27] Once the wrist is placed in extension, passive digital extension is impaired (tenodesis effect). Lengthening of the finger flexor muscles allows the hand to release objects. For thumb-in-palm deformity, augmentation of thumb extension and abduction may be achieved by rerouting the extensor pollicis longus tendon and by releasing spastic intrinsic muscles (thenar muscles and adductor pollicis).

Questions to Ask the Physician

- *What are the results of electromyography, if performed? Request an electromyography report.*
- *What surgical procedures were performed? Request an operative report.*
- *What is the protocol for tendon transfer, tendon lengthening, and joint stabilization?*
- *What precautions are necessary during therapy?*

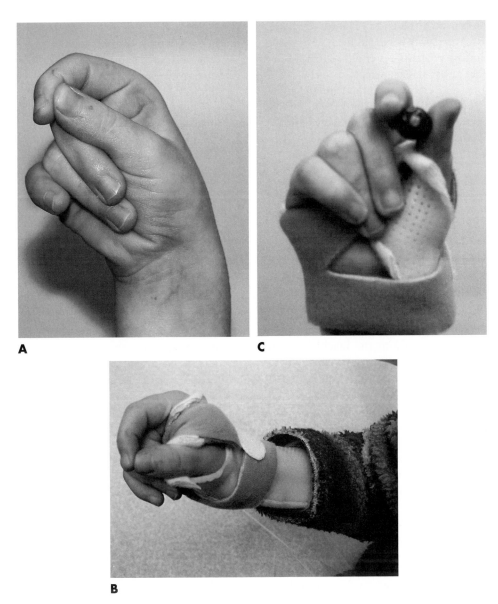

A

C

B

FIGURE 26-7   A, This child with cerebral palsy has ulnar deviation of the wrist and inability to perform pulp or tip pinch. **B,** Splint has corrected ulnar deviation of the wrist and facilitates pulp to pulp pinch. **C,** Splint facilitates flexion if interphalangeal joint of the thumb and allows for a neat pincer grasp.

What to Say to Clients

About the Condition

"Treatment will improve but not restore function. Treatment needs to be continued until the child grows up and beyond."

About Splinting

"Without splinting, joint deformities will occur or increase, and function will deteriorate."

About Exercises

"Exercises are performed to maintain joint mobility and improve muscle balance."

Tips from the Field

Compliance from the child and parents ultimately determines the outcome.

Precautions and Concerns

- *Assess sensibility of the affected part and cognitive deficit of the child before applying splints or casts. The pressure sore threshold is decreased with these two problems.*

Treatment Recommendations

Fabricate a splint for the spastic hand because each child has different degrees of spasticity, contracture, skin tolerance, cooperation, and cognitive ability. To maintain a working relationship with the child's family, physician, and other treating therapists is crucial in order to have an effective splinting program. After all, splints do not treat spasticity but rather manage symptoms such as contracture, abnormal movement, pain, and limited function. Splinting is only one component in the management of a child with cerebral palsy; other components include stretching, active range of motion, and the use of adaptive equipment.

The Role of the Therapy Assistant

Therapy assistants can help in stretching the spastic muscles. They also can monitor the exercise program set up by the therapist.

Obstetric Brachial Plexus Palsy

The infant with obstetric brachial plexus palsy is born with paralysis of proximal or distal muscles of the upper extremity resulting from injury to the brachial plexus during delivery. Sensory loss is always variable. These infants have varying degrees of rupture (Sunderland II to IV), and their ultimate neuromuscular recovery from spontaneous recovery and tendon transfers still has not been compared with their recovery with microsurgery and tendon transfers.[28]

Obstetric brachial plexus injury has a reported incidence between 0.38 to 1.56 per 1000 live births. Perinatal risk factors include large-for-gestational-age infants (macrosomia), prolonged labor, multiparous pregnancies, previous deliveries resulting in obstetric brachial plexus palsy, breech delivery, vacuum or forceps usage, and difficult deliveries.

Without question, the role and timing of microsurgery are the most controversial issues in the care of these infants. No controversy exists about the prognosis of avulsion injuries, they do not recover. The controversy hinges on prognosis and treatment of **rupture of the brachial plexus.** The difference in outcome between non-microsurgical treatment with later tendon transfers and early microsurgical treatment has not been determined definitively. In either case, the role of therapist is paramount to maintain the mobility of the shoulder, elbow, wrist, and fingers in wake of muscle reinnervation. With our current state of knowledge, therapists play an undeniable role in the care of infants with obstetric brachial plexus palsy, whether parents elect only therapy followed by tendon transfers or therapy followed by microsurgery and more therapy.

Anatomy and Pathology
The brachial plexus receives contributions contiguously from the fifth cervical (C5) to the first thoracic (T1)

ventral spinal nerve roots. The brachial plexus innervates every muscle in the upper limb.

One has three anatomic considerations in determining the severity of the injury:

- Anatomic site of the injury: The location of injury may be at the root level or peripheral to root level in the plexus. The root level injury involves avulsion of the nerve roots from the spinal cord within the foramina of the vertebra and is called **avulsion injury.** There is motor loss (anterior motor root avulsion) and sensory loss (posterior sensory root avulsion). The posterior root has the cell body of the sensory nerves in its ganglion, and the injury is often termed *preganglionic.* Electric sensory function is intact, although clinically the sensation is lost as the root is avulsed from the spinal cord proximal to the ganglion. An injury distal to the roots (is extraforaminal and postganglionic) and may affect the trunks, divisions, cords, and/or branches of the plexus. Complete disruption along these segments is termed a *rupture* and results in motor and sensory loss. Avulsion injuries are irreparable and are treated with nerve transfers. Ruptures along the brachial plexus can be repaired by excision of neuromas and interposition of nerve grafts. Many brachial plexus injuries are found to have avulsions and ruptures at surgical exposure. Fortunately, these severe avulsion or rupture injuries are in the minority and have been cited as between 8% and 25% of all brachial plexus birth palsies.
- The nerve injury may be a **neuropraxia** (Seddon 1), **axonotmesis** (Seddon 2), or **neurotmesis** (Seddon 3) in order of severity. Avulsion and rupture injuries are neurotmesis. Nerve rupture may be incomplete or complete (neurotmesis).
- The injury may be a stretch or traction injury of the nerve with intact neurons (neuropraxia) or intraneural rupture of neurons (axonotmesis). Eighty percent of all obstetric brachial plexus palsies are of this type and recover spontaneously, incompletely, or completely.

Diagnosis
Diagnosis is made predominantly by physical examination. Recovery is dynamic, and there is an evolution to the clinical examination over the first few weeks and months of life. The most important aspect to the examination is to prognosticate recovery. Therefore serial examinations on a 1 to 3 month basis in infancy are critical to predict outcome and indications for surgical intervention.

Clinically, Narakas has categorized clinical continuum of palsy into four groups according to the severity of the motor deficit (Box 26-5).[29]

Categories of Obstetric Brachial Plexus Palsy

- *Group I:* The mildest clinical group, group I represents a classic Erb's palsy (C5-C6) with loss of shoulder abduction and external rotation, elbow flexion, and forearm supination. Wrist and digital movements are intact. Ninety percent of those in this group spontaneously recover fully. This is because the injury is not avulsion type and the target shoulder and elbow muscles are a shorter distance from the location of the injury.
- *Group II:* This group includes C7 along with C5 and C6 involvement. Wrist and digital extension are absent. The prognosis is poorer with C5 to C7 injury because the target muscles are located farther from the site of the injury. Obstetric brachial plexus palsy most commonly involves the upper trunk (C5-C6) with or without injury to C7. Group I and II compose approximately 80% of obstetric brachial plexus palsy.
- *Group III:* This group includes clients with flail extremity without Horner's syndrome. All roots of brachial plexus are injured without avulsion of nerve roots.
- *Group IV:* This group includes clients with flail extremity and Horner's syndrome (drooping eye lids, myosis, enopthalmos, and anhydrosis). Prognosis is poor because the nerve roots are avulsed. The entire plexus (C5 to C7) is injured. Group III and IV constitute approximately 20% of the obstetric brachial plexus palsy. An isolated Klumpke's paralysis (C8-T1) is rare, and the target muscles in the hand are located farthest from the injury, and thus prognosis is poor.

By assessing the function of several nerves that arise close to the ganglion, one often can determine by physical examination the level of the lesion. Specifically, the presence of Horner's syndrome (sympathetic chain); an elevated hemidiaphragm (phrenic nerve); winged scapula (long thoracic nerve); and the absence of rhomboid (dorsal scapular nerve), rotator cuff (suprascapular nerve), and latissimus dorsi (thoracodorsal nerve) function raise significant concern about a preganglionic lesion. Preganglionic lesions can be reconstructed only microsurgically by nerve transfers, most commonly with thoracic intercostal nerves or a branch of the spinal accessory nerve. Postganglionic ruptures have reconstructable proximal and distal nerve beyond the zone of neural injury. Thus a postganglionic injury is a peripheral nerve lesion that can be reconstructed with nerve grafts if necessary.

Defining and grading specific muscles in an infant is difficult. Gilbert and Tassin[30] modified Mallet's classification,[31] which assesses more global motor function of the upper trunk as opposed to isolated muscle testing. This system assesses global abduction, global external rotation, hand-to-mouth, hand-to-neck, and hand-to-spine activities on a score of 1 to 5, where 1 is no function, 5 is normal function, and grades 2 to 4 denote progressive strength. Clarke's "cookie test" is an important test in the recovery of biceps muscle when the infant can move a cookie to his or her mouth because Clarke advocates microsurgery as late as 9 months in those infants who fail the cookie test.[32] Microsurgical reconstruction at that relatively late time was of positive benefit. Thus microsurgery between 3 and 9 months of age has been found to be useful.

The radiographic studies may improve the quality of preoperative planning, but the final decision regarding the presence or absence of an avulsion injury still is made intraoperatively.

Neurophysiologic studies often underestimate the severity of injury and falsely provide optimism regarding recovery. At present, most microsurgeons ultimately rely on physical examination to assess recovery and to decide on timing of surgical interventions.

Timelines and Healing
The majority of brachial birth palsies are transient. Those infants who recover partial antigravity upper trunk muscle strength in the first 2 months of life should have a full and complete recovery over the first 1 to 2 years of life.

Infants who do not recover antigravity biceps strength by 5 to 6 months of life should have microsurgical reconstruction of the brachial plexus because successful surgery results in a better outcome than natural history alone.

Those infants with partial recovery of C5 to C7 antigravity strength during months 3 through 6 of life will have permanent, progressive limitations of motion and strength, as well as risk the development of joint contractures in the affected limb. At some point, these limitations cross the line from clinical observations to functional impairment with permanent consequences.

This is most evident about the shoulder where children with incomplete recovery almost universally develop an internally rotated, adducted shoulder. With the development of limited glenohumeral motion, a universal increase in compensatory scapulothoracic motion occurs. Parents notice the scapular winging. These clients can have functional limitations for above-shoulder, facial, and occipital region activities.

Nonoperative Treatment
Eighty percent of birth palsies with spontaneous recovery (complete or an incomplete) can be managed effectively

with physical and occupational therapy. If recovery is incomplete, secondary tendon transfers and osteotomies are done to improve their function. The role of the therapist begins early. Parents are anxious and confused. Engaging them in the hands-on process from the start allows them to feel that they are helping their child and making the condition better. The parents are the ideal therapists because the child feels the most comfort in their arms, and they are with the child throughout the day and night.

The therapist teaches the parents and monitors the child's progress. Carefully teach parents through demonstration, repetition, drawings, and clear verbal and written instructions. Repeat these regularly. Parents are often so distraught that they may not attend to or focus carefully on the teaching.

Initially, a gentle home program is begun at 7 to 10 days of life. This is followed by a formal occupational, physical, or hand therapy program with home supervision in infants who do not recover rapidly in the first month of life.

CLINICAL *Pearl*

Full glenohumeral range with scapular stabilization is the goal.

Abduction and external rotation splints have been used to improve or maintain range of motion. Compliance can be poor, and these splints may increase the risk of injury to the physis and developing joint. At present there are no data to guide the clinician on the indications and expected outcomes from shoulder abduction and external rotation splints, electric stimulation of muscles, and Botox (botulinum toxin) injections.

Precaution. *The failure to maintain full passive range of motion of the shoulder joint puts the child at risk for the development of glenohumeral deformity.*

The glenohumeral deformity progresses from normal (I) to posterior glenoid deformity (II), to humeral head subluxation and further glenoid dysplasia (III), to the development of a false glenoid (IV), to flattening of the glenoid and the humeral head (V). If the child fails to recover external rotation strength and motion, significant functional consequences occur. External rotation of the shoulder is necessary to achieve above-horizontal shoulder activity (i.e., reach the hand to the occiput and forehead). Scapulothoracic winging can compensate for limited glenohumeral motion in all planes except external rotation. In this circumstance, the scapula abuts the

posterior thorax. This leads to significant limitation of function because of the inability to place the hand appropriately in space for many activities. In addition, weakness about the shoulder further limits hand use away from the body. The child has difficulty placing and maintaining the hand at a desired location in space because of fatigue. The affected limb, therefore, most often will be used at the child's side or with support from furniture or the ipsilateral leg.

The primary aim of treatment is to maintain full passive shoulder rotation with full abduction of the glenohumeral and scapulothoracic joints. To achieve this, exercise both upper extremities together. Tell parents to take the child through range of motion as the child and they interact and play and also to schedule additional times such as before meals and during the bath. Two to 3 minutes of exercises are recommended.

Exercises need to be individualized. Movements that are not actively present must be maintained passively, and those that appear weak need to be resisted gently. For example, the shoulder must be adducted for medial and lateral rotation while making sure that the child is supported with a gentle yet secure hand. The inferior glenohumeral angle is maintained into adducted position by gently holding the scapula against the ribs when flexing or abducting the arm. The parents need to be reminded to exercise both upper extremities. Recommend that each exercise be repeated 2 to 5 times at each session. The number of sessions is individualized for each client.

Limitation of active supination is common in children with incomplete recovery of their brachial plexus birth palsy. When combined with an internal rotation contracture and external rotation weakness of the shoulder, this deficiency becomes more obvious. These children posture in pronation and raise their hands toward their mouth with considerable abduction and internal rotation with a neutral or pronated forearm. Correction of the shoulder problem improves the forearm motion because shoulder adduction, external rotation, and forearm supination are complementary motions. However, in the absence of full biceps strength, often some unresolved supination weakness is evident. Therapy, splints, and electric stimulation do not seem to resolve this problem. Surgery rarely is indicated for mild supination loss.

Fortunately, the majority of children with a brachial plexus birth palsy have an upper trunk lesion with near-normal recovery of the wrist and hand. The C8 and T1 nerve function often recovers without significant limitation. The C7 functional recovery may be incomplete with some limitation of wrist and finger extension, but frequently there is sufficient compensatory function by tenodesis strength that surgery is not indicated.

Operative Treatment and Therapy

The clinical data by Gilbert et al.[33] is classic for defining the timing of recovery of biceps antigravity function as an indicator of long-term outcome. The outcome with biceps recovery beyond 6 months was poor and served as the basis for microsurgical intervention. Subsequently, microsurgery was recommended for infants with no antigravity biceps recovery by 3 months of life.

As noted by Waters,[28] there are limits to the present information available for the clinician to make decisions regarding timing of microsurgical intervention and ultimate outcome of these clients versus natural history and tendon transfers. Within these limits, Waters presently cares for these infants in the following ways:

- Observe all infants with brachial plexus birth palsy who begin to have antigravity biceps muscle recovery in the first 3 months of life. Perform physical and occupational therapy until recovery is complete or plateaus to maintain a full range of motion of all joints of the upper limb, especially shoulder abduction and external rotation.
- If there is Horner's syndrome and failure of recovery of some antigravity biceps strength by 3 months, surgery is performed at that time. Nerve grafting is performed if there are any intact nerve roots. Nerve transfers are almost always necessary because of avulsion injuries and limited viable proximal nerve roots. Transfers of a branch of the spinal accessory nerve, T2 to T4 intercostal nerves, and anterior fascicles of the ulnar nerve (requires an intact C8-T1 root) are performed as appropriate.[13,31] The hand, wrist, elbow, and shoulder are prioritized in that order.
- If there is progressive recovery of wrist extension and finger extension without Horner's syndrome, Waters[28] waits for 5 to 6 months to determine whether some antigravity biceps function will return. If there is still no adequate return of biceps function by 5 to 6 months, surgery is performed at that time. Neuroma resection and nerve grafts or nerve transfers are performed based on intraoperative findings.
- All nonoperative clients are followed closely for the first 9 months of life to be certain recovery is progressive. In the rare instances of failure of biceps recovery to progress to sufficient antigravity strength by 9 months of life (i.e., a positive cookie test), microsurgery is performed.

In summary, final diagnosis of nerve avulsion and rupture is made at the time of surgical exploration. Excision of neuromas and interposition of nerve grafts for ruptures and nerve transfers for nerve root avusions are the mainstay of microsurgical reconstruction.

Postoperative immobilization is with a well-padded stockinette sling and swathe that binds the arm to the side. If there is any concern that neck motion will cause undue tension on the neural repairs, the neck is included in the immobilization. Arm immobilization is discontinued at 4 weeks. Shoulder and arm range of motion is initiated at this time to prevent contracture development. The parents are informed that improved function will not occur for 6 to 18 months. Therapy is of the essence during this time to maintain passive range of motion of the shoulder, elbow, wrist, and fingers in the wake of muscle reinnervation. Failure to observe progressive recovery of the biceps by 9 months is of concern. Reexploration and additional microsurgery may be indicated for the failure of biceps recovery by 9 to 12 months after surgery.

Questions to Ask the Physician

- *What studies were done to support preganglionic versus postganglionic lesion?*
- *When does the doctor plan to consider microsurgical reconstruction and why?*
- *What lesions were found at surgery that are different from clinical evaluation?*
- *What nerve grafts and transfers were done?*
- *What is the expected reinnervation time and of which muscles?*

What to Say to Clients

About the Injury

"Nerve root avulsion injuries occur inside the spinal canal and are not repairable, require nerve transfers, and do not always have favorable results. Nerve rupture injuries are repaired with removal of nerve scar and replacement with nerve grafts, and results may be better than waiting for recovery to occur on its own."

About Splinting

"Night splinting prevents contractures, and day splinting assists the child to position the wrist so that the child can grasp a toy and effectively use fingers. Watch skin for irritation."

About Exercises

"Passive, active-assisted, active, and gently resisted exercises are of essence to keep muscles, joints, ligaments, and nerves supple in wake of muscle reinnervation and recovery."

Evaluation Tips

- Always examine the opposite arm, because bilateral lesions occur in 2% of the cases.
- Evaluation of global function of the extremity than of individual muscles is easier in an infant.

- Watching the child play gives one information on abnormal posturing, muscle imbalance, joint contractures, neglect of extremity indicating sensory loss, and compensatory movements.

Tips from the Field

Separately mobilize glenohumeral motion from scapulothoracic motion. Mobilize both extremities together. Contracture of glenohumeral motion eventually leads to restricted scapulothoracic motion and scapular winging.

Precautions and Concerns

- *The primary concern is to maintain shoulder abduction and external rotation.*
- *Protect the flail and insensate extremity from injury. Do not let the extremity hang by the side of the body. Protect the extremity from being trapped under the body when the child turns over.*

Treatment Recommendations

Use facilitation techniques such as tapping, vibration, stroking, and touching over the muscles that you wish to stimulate. The children enjoy the sensations, and these in turn provide stimulus to move the joints. Do not use electric stimulation in children because they do not seem to tolerate it. Assist the child in the activities that he or she otherwise would not perform. Muscles that are not affected also need to be strengthened. Look at the balance and mobility of the neck, trunk, and upper and lower extremities. Use splinting to enhance function and prevent contractures. Parental involvement is the cornerstone of an effective approach.

The Role of the Therapy Assistant

The therapy assistant may help the therapist in carrying out range of motion exercises. The assistant may play with the child to facilitate involvement of the affected extremity.

ACQUIRED TRAUMA

Fractures

The hand is a child's instrument in the discovery of the world and thus becomes vulnerable.[34] Children's bones absorb higher energies of trauma before they fracture. The greater collagen-to-mineral ratio in a child's bone provides the elasticity and stretch qualities that adult bone no longer has. Growth presents an opportunity for a fracture to align itself over time. Certain injuries around

the physis have the potential for long-term morbidity if not treated correctly. The outcome is not apparent for many years.

CLINICAL *Pearl*

Of all fractures in children, 65% to 70% occur in the upper extremity.

Diagnosis and Pathology

Growth plate fractures were classified by Salter and Harris, and their classification is in general use (Fig. 26-8). The classification is useful in predicting prognosis of growth deformity. Salter-Harris fracture types III and IV have the worst prognosis. Angular deformity or shortening of the bone may occur because of cessation of growth in part or all of the physis.

Timelines and Healing

CLINICAL *Pearl*

Because of rapid healing and remodeling in the young, fractures heal in about half the time it takes for an adult.

Continued growth at the physes corrects residual angular deformity after the fracture heals. Rapid healing also may present the potential of a **malunion** or a deformity to occur if treatment is delayed. Frequent radiologic review after fracture manipulation is necessary in a child to prevent deformity.

Nonoperative Treatment

Therapy rarely is needed in children after fractures have healed. Children resume activities when pain subsides. This is their best therapy. However, the physician may refer a child for therapy after fracture treatment when severe soft tissue injuries are associated with the injury. The other indication for therapy in a child is an epihysial fracture with malalignment. Serial casting, dynamic splinting, or buddy taping to the adjacent finger helps to remodel the malalignment if the fracture is close to the physis. This is a nonoperative form of epiphyseal distraction (chondrodiastasis). In many ways, therapy for fractures in children is similar to adults. Assess pain, sensation, joint motion, strength, and function. Evaluate the need for splinting, casting, and compression bandages and establish an appropriate home program.

Type	Poland	Salter-Harris	Ogden

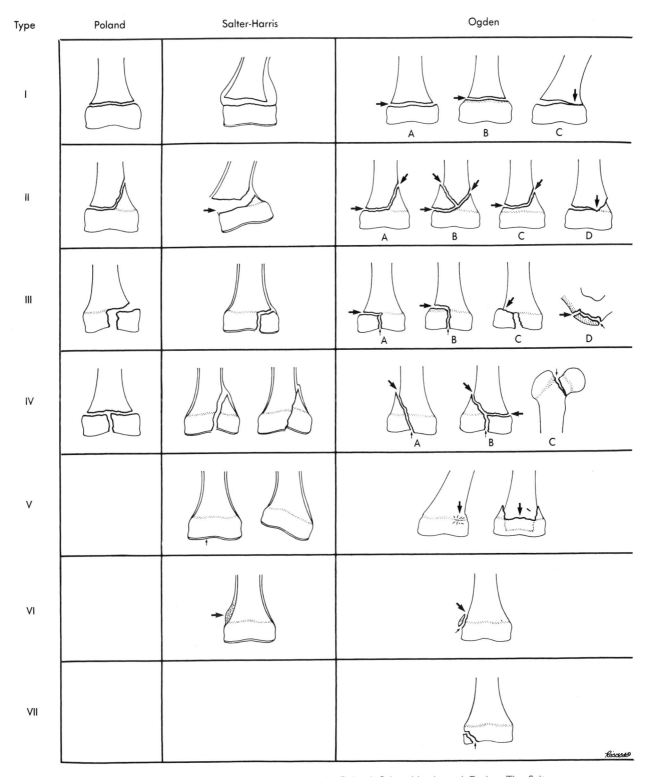

FIGURE 26-8 Classification of physeal injuries by Poland, Salter, Harris, and Ogden. The Salter-Harris classification of epiphyseal fractures includes six subtypes. *Type I,* Epiphysis is separated from metaphysis. *Type II,* Epiphysis is separated from metaphysis and a metaphyseal fragment is attached to epiphysis. *Type III,* Fracture line crosses only epiphysis. *Type IV,* Fracture line crosses metaphysis, physis, and epiphysis. *Type V,* Crushing injury of physis. *Type VI,* Rang added perichondrial ring injury that may cause the periphery of physis to close prematurely. (From Canale ST, editor: *Campbell's operative orthopaedics,* ed 10, St Louis, 2003, Mosby.)

Operative Treatment

One must know the location and stability of fracture and the method of fixation used by the surgeon. The stability of the fracture determines aggressiveness with which the adjacent joints may be mobilized. One also must address the treatment of the soft tissue injury.

What to Say to Clients

About the Injury

"Here is the diagram of your fracture. Note the growth plate (physis) at the end of the bone. It is here that the bone grows in length and circumference. Growth of bone helps to remodel the fracture alignment."

About Buddy Taping, Splinting, and Casting

"Buddy taping, dynamic splinting, and casting may help remodeling over an extended time."

About Exercises

"Exercises help to incorporate the injured finger, hand, or wrist into play activities."

Evaluation Tips

- Evaluate baseline pain, swelling, range of motion, and any malalignment while the child is at rest and during play activities.
- If a child has suspicious or multiple fractures, consider the possibility of abuse at home and notify the proper agencies.

Tips from the Field

Once communication has been established between the physician, child, and parents and a diagnosis has been made and discussed, consider the strongest splintage possible. Children are magicians when it comes to removing dressings and casts. Plenty of surgical adhesive tape and casting reinforcement are necessary to prevent the cast from being pulled off or destroyed.

CLINICAL *Pearl*

Above-elbow casts and splints are recommended for children because they are more difficult for them to remove.

State clear explanations and instructions, repeat them, and write them down. Educate the parents and the child in the care of the extremity while in the cast, including elevation techniques, protection of the healing fracture, and mobilization of joints once the cast is removed.

Precautions and Concerns

- *If a complication occurs or a cast is no longer secure, immediately communicate with the treating physician.*
- *When dealing with complications such as **compartment syndrome** and tendon ruptures, time is crucial. This quick communication process may allow for improved outcomes in many clients.*

Treatment Recommendations

Age, cognitive level, and fracture stability affect the therapeutic process. Keep the sessions short, fun, age-appropriate, and within pain tolerance. Establish clear goals in the treatment plan. If a child is hesitant to move because of pain, initiate the session with warm media such as water with bubble bath, fluidotherapy, paraffin, or warm compresses. Moving objects in a container with rice, taking out hidden surprises, and playing with familiar toys help the child to initiate needed joint movements. The therapist may need to fabricate splinting for night or day in order to protect or align healing tissues and to correct deformity. The child may not be ready to play sports or even squeeze putty, but the child needs to move joints actively to prevent stiffness. Many children do not need much therapy. Once the pain has subsided, they are allowed to play, and stiffness dissipates rather quickly. However, some children do become stiff because of a lengthy immobilization or a severe crushing injury. Children need individualized attention to restore joint motion and hand function.

CLINICAL *Pearl*

Interestingly, older children often need more therapy than younger ones.

The Role of the Therapy Assistant

An adult can cooperate, but a child often is crying and pulling away during splinting or casting. Therapy assistants can be helpful in distracting or amusing the child and can help the child maintain positions needed for splinting.

Flexor Tendon Injuries in Children

One out of 100 children cared for at a large pediatric referral center has a tendon laceration. Age, size, growth potential, and limited cooperation influence the clinical examination, surgical technique, and postoperative rehabilitation. Therapists need to have a clear understanding not only of the anatomy but also of the surgical procedure performed by the surgeon. The therapist needs to ask questions regarding the type of repair performed, its strength, and the presence of other affected structures.

Timelines and Healing

- Full immobilization is done for the first 4 weeks.
- Passive flexion and active extension are done under therapist's supervision as early as 2 weeks in exceptionally cooperative children and parents.
- Active flexion without loading is allowed after first 4 weeks of immobilization.
- Resisted flexion is delayed as much as possible. *We do not advocate sports activities in children until at least 4 months after repair. This also includes activities such as carrying heavy books.*

Nonoperative Treatment

Nonoperative treatment is indicated in unique situations of old avulsed or lacerated flexor digitorum profundus tendons in zones I or II. If the child has adapted to lack of DIP flexion, it is unreasonable to risk tendon adhesions or rupture by performing a tendon graft.

Operative Treatment and Therapy

The principles of tendon repair are similar in children and adults: minimal debridement of the tendon, gentle handling of tissues, minimal disturbance of the flexor tendon sheath and pulley system, use of a core suture for strength, and use of an **epitendinous suture** for easy gliding, reducing gap formation and for additional strength.

The postsurgical hand therapy in children is different from that used in adults. Following surgery, the child is placed in a cast for comfort and to protect the repair. In a young child, this cast may include the elbow. The elbow is flexed at 90 degrees and wrist at slight flexion, and the MCP joints are blocked in comfortable flexion. The child is protected with an above-the-elbow cast for 3 weeks and then is provided a below-the-elbow cast. The therapist peforms passive flexion as soon as prescribed by the surgeon. This may be as early as 1 week. Parents' cooperation dictates the degree of early passive mobilization. If there is any doubt about cooperation of the child or the parents, carry out a full 4 week immobilization. Otherwise, we like to start passive motion once the wound is healed, usually after 1 week. The child's hand remains immobilized when not in our office. We do not use dynamic traction or early active range of motion in a young child. Our philosophy is to protect the repair, the splint, and the child from using the hand. *When in doubt, protect.* Dealing with adhesions is preferred to repairing a ruptured tendon. We do not trust teenagers with an adult protocol, except in select cases.

Questions still remain regarding the functional outcome following flexor tendon repair in children. Only a few studies are available, and nothing has been written on extensor tendons in this age group. In a combined study of three hand surgery practices, 78 clients younger than 16 years who had sustained flexor tendon lacerations in zones I or II of 95 digits were studied by O'Connell et al.[35] in 1994. The average postrepair follow-up period was 24 months (range, 3 to 144 months). Client age was divided into three groups: birth to 5 years, 6 to 10 years, and 11 to 15 years. All profundus repairs in zone I returned excellent function. Isolated flexor digitorum profundus and combined flexor digitorum profundus and flexor digitorum superficialis repairs in zone II achieved comparable results when managed with an early passive motion program or following immobilization for 3 or 4 weeks.

Precaution. *Immobilization for longer than 4 weeks resulted in an appreciable deterioration of function.*

Digital motion following zone II flexor digitorum profundus and superficialis injuries treated with 4 weeks of immobilization or early motion was not significantly different in the three age groups studied. Digits with associated digital nerve and/or palmar plate lacerations fared less favorably compared with isolated tendon lacerations. In many digits, a modest improvement in digital motion was found when clients returned after several years of growth.

In a retrospective review performed at Mayo Clinic, Moran et al.[36] studied flexor tendon injuries that occurred in children less than 16 years of age between 1988 and 2002. Only lacerations occurring in zones I or II were evaluated. Tendon repairs were performed with a modified Kessler technique with an epitendinous repair for all zone II injuries and a Bunnell pull-through repair in cases of distal zone I injuries. Postoperative therapy consisted of total immobilization in 7 children and early controlled mobilization in 36 children. Return of total active motion (TAM) was evaluated with the Strickland and Glogovac method where the extension lag is subtracted from the sum of the flexion at the PIP and DIP joints. Overall, 43 clients were identified, ages 2 to 15 (mean age, 8.9 years). Seventy-three flexor tendons were injured. Twenty-three percent of tendons were injured in zone I, and 77% were injured in zone II. Eighty-five percent of injured tendons were repaired primarily within 72 hours; the remainder had delayed primary repairs (range, 4 days to 9 weeks). Postoperatively, 36 clients were treated with early controlled mobilization (Duran protocol), and 7 clients were treated with plaster immobilization for 3 weeks. Mean follow-up was 2 years (ranging from 6 months to 3 years). The TAM percentage was determined by dividing the range of motion by 175. Eighty-three percent had excellent or good results with a mean TAM of 79%. Mean TAM in zone I injuries was 87.5% and in zone II injuries was 70.8%. Complications occurred in 2 children with one tendon rupture (2%) and 1 child requiring tenolysis (2%). Previously reported rupture rates are 7% to 12%. The one case of rupture occurred in a 2-year-old who came out of her cast at 1 week postoperatively. Variables such as postoperative regimen and timing of surgery had no significant effect on the final result. Digits in which nerve or arterial repairs were performed showed some reduction in mean TAM compared with digits in which only tendon repairs were performed (mean TAM 72.3% versus mean TAM 85.4%, respectively). Also, no significant difference in outcome was found when children less than 6 years of age were compared with those ages 6 to 15. In conclusion, a satisfactory functional result can be expected after primary repair of flexor tendons in children. Though the numbers were small, there was no clear relationship between age, time elapsed from injury, or application of postoperative splint and overall TAM values. Complication rate was 5%. Though no significant outcome difference was seen between children less than 6 years of age, the physician should use plaster in those clients in whom rupture has the highest likelihood.

Questions to Ask the Physician

- *What structures other than flexor tendons [bone, joint, nerves, blood vessels, flexor tendon sheath] were repaired? (Request an operative report.)*
- *What protocol do you want me to follow? Immobilization or early passive flexion?*
- *Clarify precautions.*

What to Say to Clients

About the Injury

"Tendon injuries heal with difficulty because circulation to the tendons is poor. The hand will be in the cast, and the fingers should not be used for any activities. Even after four weeks of immobilization, it may take many months until the hand is strong enough for play activities."

About Splinting and Casting

"Children tend to destroy their casts or splints or pull them off. Parents must monitor the integrity of the cast frequently every day. The cast must remain dry at all times. The arm must be covered with a plastic bag during bathing or washing. Make sure the cast or splint is in the prescribed position and has not slipped."

About Exercises

"No exercises are expected of children at home. A restricted set of exercises will be prescribed after the cast or splint is removed at four weeks. No other exercises or activities are allowed until six weeks. Exercises will change with time. To prevent tendon rupture or adhesions, children and parents must not deviate from the prescribed instructions. All exercises will be done under the supervision of the therapist."

Evaluation Tips

- Monitor pain, wound healing, edema, and undue inflammation. *Notify the surgeon if there is excessive pain, edema, and inflammation or wound dehiscence.*
- Monitor the integrity and desired position of the cast or splint. Adjust the splint or cast as frequently as needed.
- If the child or parents do not follow instructions or miss appointments, alert the doctor.
- If you elect the passive flexion protocol, measure and monitor the range of motion of finger joints.

Tips from the Field

See the child as often as possible. Parents must be given written instructions on what the child can and cannot do. Review these instructions at every session. Ask the parents and child what activities they do at home with the affected extremity. Communicate with the physician frequently on the overall status of healing.

The child's compliance often dictates the result following flexor tendon repair. The child and parents must understand that flexing an unaffected finger may put undue stress on the repaired tendon of the adjacent finger because they share the same muscle in the forearm.

Precautions and Concerns

- *The child and parents must understand the **quadriga effect** of one finger motion on an adjacent finger. Flexing an unaffected finger may put undue stress on the repaired tendon of the adjacent finger because they share the same muscle belly in the forearm.*

Treatment Recommendations

Follow the immobilization protocol in the younger child and consider early mobilization in the older child as he or she approaches adult age in select cases. Immobilize the repair with an above-elbow splint. When prescribed by the surgeon, initiate a passive flexion protocol as early as 2 weeks after repair. This is done strictly under the experienced therapist's supervision. See the child as often as possible every week. From 4 to 6 weeks, the child is allowed active movement within a limited arc of motion, still protected in the splint. A pad in the palm restricts a full grip. At 6 weeks, full active mobility is allowed, but not until 16 weeks can the child participate in sports. During this period between 6 and 12 weeks, the child is allowed light play activities. The therapist also may fabricate an MCP blocking splint to promote movement at the PIP joint or use a buddy splint to encourage function of an adjacent digit. We do not immobilize repaired tendons after 4 weeks as advocated by O'Connell et al.[31] Improvement can continue beyond 12 to 18 months. Keeping the child and the parents involved with the therapy and splinting at home and at the office is a challenge. Because of children's amazing flexibility and ability to remodel, they rarely require tenolysis. Overly enthusiastic early mobilization may lead to a tendon rupture with its unpleasant sequela for the child, parents, surgeon, and therapist.

The Role of the Therapy Assistant

Therapy assistants help to enforce the selected protocol in the office and home.

Compartment Syndrome and Volkmann's Ischemic Contracture

Gulgonen[37] has reviewed the history, pathophysiology, diagnosis, and treatment of Volkmann's contractures in detail, and we present a concise version of his description. In his classic article, Richard von Volkmann[38] described the contracture and the ischemic condition that resulted from trauma, fractures, bandaging, and edema.

Diagnosis and Pathology

In the compartment syndrome, Volkmann's ischemic contracture, and **crush syndrome,** the primary pathologic event is increased compartment pressure within a confined space.[11] The duration and the severity of this increased pressure determine the progression of the disease to Volkmann's ischemic contracture. Displaced supracondylar humeral fractures, most common in children between 3 and 13 years of age, are a classic cause of Volkmann's ischemic contracture. Caouette-Laberge et al.[39] and Kline[6] have reported compartment syndrome in neonates from birth trauma. Other causes of compartment syndrome are prolonged direct pressure of collapsed buildings on crushed extremities; high doses of barbiturates, in which case all protective reflexes are lost and victims rest on a hand or arm for long periods; intraarterial barbiturate or propoxyphene injections; snake bites; hemophiliac bleeding; thermal and electric burns; overwork of the muscles; and intraoperative complications.

The diagnosis of compartment syndrome is primarily clinical and is based on symptoms and signs of muscle and nerve ischemia. The most important symptom is pain. Persistent, increasing pain, usually out of propor-

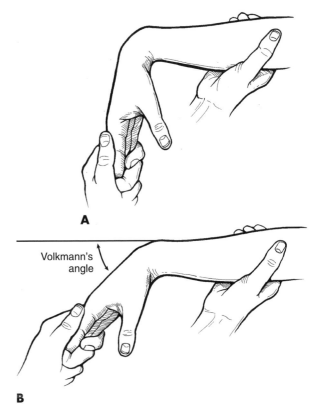

FIGURE 26-9 Volkmann's test for digital flexor tendon tightness and Volkmann's angle. **A,** The digits are held extended with the wrist flexed. **B,** The wrist is extended with the digits extended. With no flexor tendon tightness, full extension of the wrist is possible. Wrist extension to less than neutral (Volkmann's angle) grades severity of muscle contracture. (From Carlson MG: Cerebral palsy. In Green DP, Hotchkiss RN, Peterson WC, et al, editors: *Green's operative hand surgery,* ed 5, St Louis, 2005, Churchill Livingstone.)

tion to that expected from the existing injury, not decreased by immobilization, and increase in pain despite elevation of the limb and medications are the most typical findings. In children, profound anxiety in the presence of an increasing analgesic requirement has been found to be a reliable indicator of a compartment syndrome. **Paresthesia** indicates nerve ischemia. After 8 hours of total ischemia, irreversible changes in the nerve can be expected. In addition, the **Volkmann's Passive Muscle Stretch Test** (Fig. 26-9) and a sense of stony hardness during palpation of the proximal forearm are typical findings.

Treatment

When circulation in the muscles and nerves stops because of increased compartmental pressure, an irreversible condition arises unless this pressure is relieved within 6 to 8 hours. The muscle fibers can be lost irreversibly if a delay ensues. Only early diagnosis and treatment can prevent Volkmann's contractures.

Early treatment during the acute stage involves first the removal of external pressure if this exists. Any tight cast or bandage should be removed completely. Acute **fasciotomies** performed promptly and correctly help muscles to regain their normal function.

After release of acute compartment syndrome and before reconstructive surgery is commenced, hand therapy with passive stretching and dynamic splinting is done because limitation of muscle excursion by fibrosis gradually leads to loss of joint motion and subsequent ligament, capsule, and joint contracture. This early conservative therapy is an important part of the overall treatment. Children have considerable fear, pain, abnormal postures, decreased sensation, and poor function. All are challenges for even experienced therapists. Perform a careful assessment of the sensory and motor functions. Ongoing communication with the physician and parents is crucial. Warm not hot media, soft textures, and soft massage can be used to comfort the child. Desensitize the area, try to relax the extremity, and provide passive range of motion and gentle stretch. Encourage the child to participate in age-appropriate activities. Splinting at night provides a slow stretch and extends the wrist and fingers. Gradually adjust splints to decrease the contracture. Use a splint to position the wrist in extension and allow fingers to flex during the day. You may need to use serial casting and dynamic splints for rigid contractures. Use gloves and elastomer (silicone) to remodel scar tissue. This is all done before reconstructive efforts are started 3 to 4 months after the acute injury.

Untreated children and those with delayed decompression have established contracture of muscles and joints. Holden has divided the established contracture into two types: (1) contracture that is distal to or at the site of the injury and (2) contracture that is mild, moderate, or severe.[40]

In Holden type I contractures the injury to the vessels is located proximal to the fascial compartment. In Holden type I, mild type, the degeneration of the muscles is located in the deep flexor compartment, mainly as limited infarction of the profundus muscles. The clinical picture is characterized by flexion contracture of long and ring fingers and occasionally of the little and index fingers. In Holden type I, moderate type, also known as the "classic or typical type," the moderate muscular degeneration is in the deep flexor compartment, affecting the flexor digitorum profundus, flexor pollicis longus, and pronator teres, and there also may be partial involvement of the wrist flexor muscles and the flexor digitorum superficialis. The wrist is held in a flexed position, and the fingers show an intrinsic-minus deformity. Sensory disturbances are present in the area of the median and sometimes the ulnar nerves. Holden type I, severe type, results in muscular degeneration of all flexor muscles and pronators and partial or total involvement of the extensor muscles, and occasionally the intrinsics, with severe degrees of contracture. The median and ulnar nerves are involved. The forearm muscle mass has a firm, "woody" consistency. The deformation of the hand and fingers is usually in an intrinsic-minus position, characterized by hyperextension at the MCP joints and flexion at the interphalangeal joints.

Holden type II contracture is caused by direct trauma to the forearm, such as externally applied localized pressure, tight dressings, entrapment under heavy objects, local crush injuries, forearm fractures, or thermal injuries, with ischemia developing at the site of the injury. In Holden type II, mild type, the muscle injury is in the limited area of direct trauma, with the muscles being partially fibrotic. No interruption or entrapment of the nerves occurs. In Holden type II, moderate type, all the superficial and deep flexor muscles from the surface inward are involved. The extensor muscles may be involved as well. The median and ulnar nerves are involved. These localized nerve lesions can cause neuralgias, paresthesias, and sometimes dystrophic changes at the fingertips. Holden type II, severe types, usually are neglected cases beginning in childhood but may follow severe localized crush injury under collapsed weights in mass casualties. From the site of injury to distally, the whole extremity is usually atrophic and severely contracted with neural involvement. The fingers show a fixed intrinsic-minus deformity. In more distal injuries with overwhelming intrinsic contracture, an intrinsic-plus deformity may develop with adduction of the thumb and MCP flexion and interphalangeal extension contractures of the fingers.

The surgical procedures that are done in various stages determine postoperative hand therapy. Following is an outline of procedures done in different stages of severity:

- *Mild contracture:* Skin release, Z-plasty lengthening of tendons
- *Moderate contracture:* Resection of scarred muscles; Z-plasty tendon lengthening; in Holden type I, muscle slide; in Holden type II, tendon transfers according to individual situation; exploration and release of the median and ulnar nerves; possible soft tissue coverage
- *Severe contracture:* Innervated free muscle transfer for function and coverage; reconstruction of protective sensation (neurolysis or nerve grafting); in Holden type II, carpectomies or arthrodesis of the wrist and correction of intrinsic contractures

Questions to Ask the Physician

- *What muscles [superficial, deep] and nerves [median, ulnar, radial] were compressed and damaged [ischemic or infarcted] during decompression of compartment? During reconstruction of Volkmann's contracture?*
- *What procedures were done during decompression [decompression of which compartments, excision of muscle infarcts, decompression of nerves] and reconstruction [muscle slide, tendon release, tendon transfer, proximal row carpectomy, intrinsic contracture reconstruction, free muscle transfer, wrist fusion, nerve grafts]?*
- *What precautions are necessary during therapy?*
- *When should I start passive motion, active-assisted motion, and active and resisted motion?*

What to Say to Clients

About the Injury

With early decompression, say, "Your strength and sensation will recover with time and therapy." With delayed decompression, say, "Additional surgical procedures will improve function, but a prolonged period of therapy will be necessary before and after reconstructive procedures are done."

About Splinting

"Day functional splints and night stretching splints will be used. They will be modified as contractures decrease and function improves."

About Exercises

"Exercises will be performed in the therapy and at home. Precautions will be taken to perform them without worsening pain."

Evaluation Tips

Determine **Volkmann's angle** as a baseline to determine the severity of contracture and to determine improvement with therapy and surgery. Volkmann's angle is the angle of flexion that the wrist assumes when the fingers and wrist are extended maximally by the examiner (see Fig. 26-9).

Precautions and Concerns

- *Beware of sensory loss when splinting and exercising the wrist and fingers.*
- *Children with pain need motivational activities that are fun and done within their pain tolerance.*
- *Carefully monitor appointments because children and parents do not keep their appointments because of pain involved with therapy.*

Treatment Recommendations

Early management prevents development of contracture. Remove tight dressings, and contact the surgeon promptly and personally as soon as you suspect compartment syndrome. Follow the basic principles of splinting, stretching, and mobilization as outlined before. Select methods that relieve a child's discomfort such as warm, not hot, media (fluidotherapy, warm water); soft and soothing textures; and gentle massage. This helps to soothe the area, relax the muscles, and gain the child's trust. This allows you to initiate gentle stretch and active-assisted motion. Use night splints to stretch. Motivate and reward the child to use his or her hands during activities of daily living and play.

The Role of the Therapy Assistant

Supervise the child's home and office splint and exercise and play programs as developed by the therapist.

CASE *Studies*

CASE 26-I: ARTHROGRYPOSIS MULTIPLEX CONGENITA

A.A. was referred to therapy soon after birth with a diagnosis of arthrogryposis multiplex congenita. Most if not all joints of the body were affected with contractures. Joints were painful on passive range of motion. Shoulders were in adduction and internal rotation, elbows in extension, forearms in pronation, and wrists in flexion and ulnar deviation. Thumbs were positioned into the palm, and the fingers were partially flexed. A.A. was able to move his hands above his head but could not flex his elbows. Passive elbow flexion, forearm supination and wrist extension, and finger flexion and extension were restricted and painful.

Goals of treatment included increase in active and passive range of motion of all joints to facilitate development of sitting, crawling, and eventually standing and walking. The goals for improving hand function included facilitating grasp, pinch, prehension, manipulation, play, and activities of daily living skills. Wrist extension splints were used during the day to allow the fingers and thumb to flex and extend. Night splints were used gently to stretch the thumb out of the palm, extend the fingers, and align the wrist into extension and radial deviation as much as possible. During the day, the joints were mobilized almost hourly by the parents, family, volunteers, and therapists. All the stages of development were enhanced and integrated as the child grew. Parents complied with the maximum benefit of the child. The therapists and medical team regularly communicated with each other and with the parents. The splinting and therapy program was modified continuously as needed.

The child was able to sit, stand, and walk, but these milestones were delayed. At the time of this writing, the child is 5 years old and walks with leg braces. He walks up and down stairs holding on to the rails. He rides a bike, uses in-line skates, and even can do head stands. With trunk extended and shoulder externally rotated, he can compensate and flex the elbow enough to position his hands to reach the mouth, face, and head. The left hand has improved remarkably. He can extend, flex, and oppose the fingers and make a fist when the wrist is extended, nevertheless weakly. He does not have enough wrist extension strength to oppose fingers and to hold a pencil to write unless his wrist is supported in extension with a splint. On the right side, he still lacks forearm supination, wrist extension, and finger extension. The thumb pulls somewhat out of the palm and into opposition with the wrist splinted in extension. Dexterity has improved appropriate for his age, but muscle strength is lacking. He can work with screws and bolts but lacks strength to use a hole puncher. He can bring food to his mouth and pour milk but cannot quite cut meat and still needs assistance to dress and bathe.

The future plan is for A.A. to become independent at school. At home, we expect him to become independent in toilet activities. He requires assistance to put on and take off braces. Safety precautions are warranted in activities that may require greater strength and flexibility than he has. Ongoing treatment will continue until he reaches maturity and beyond.

CASE 26-2: RADIAL CLUB HAND

S.S. was referred to therapy by her orthopedic surgeon a few days after birth with a diagnosis of right radial club hand with a floating thumb (Fig. 26-10, *A*). She is a healthy child, born following a full-term pregnancy and cesarean section delivery. Her hand surgeon recommended that her hand be casted and splinted to correct the wrist deformity before pollicization planned at 1 year of age.

The goals in therapy were the following: to correct the wrist radial deformity through passive range of motion, corrective casting (Fig. 26-10, *B*), and splinting; to encourage active range of motion of the right upper extremity through reaching and play activities; to monitor and engage in fine motor skills as they develop; to strengthen weak muscles that are necessary for stability of her trunk and upper extremity; to encourage bilateral motor coordination; to reduce the pain in her hand; and to monitor appropriate milestones in development.

S.S. was seen in hand therapy 3 times per week in addition to following a home program of casting, splinting, range of motion, and play therapy. She has a loving and involved family. S.S. has thrived in this environment. By 4 months she began reaching out and swiping toys with her right arm in the cast. Although she preferred to use her left, by 6 months she no longer ignored her right side and incorporated both sides during play. She developed raking with her right hand digits and scissoring to grasp a toy between her index and third digit. Her thumb had no metacarpophalangeal joint and lay limp.

At 2 years (25 months) S.S. underwent pollicization. The prognosis for thumb function was good because she had a flexible index finger to pollicize. After an immobilization period of 5 weeks, S.S. was referred back to hand therapy. Initially, S.S. ignored her new thumb and was in discomfort when we touched her hand. During play, S.S. wanted to grasp toys as before surgery, between index and middle digits (scissoring; Fig. 26-10, *C*). Parents and grandparents participated in the retraining process, teaching her to use the thumb in opposition. Treatment included massage to the hypersensitive scar, gentle passive range of motion to thumb interphalangeal joint, and gentle positioning of the thumb in the opposition plane to encourage pincer development, fine motor coordination, and play skills with her "new" thumb.

S.S. is now $2^{1}/_{2}$ years old. Her thumb opposition continues to improve (Fig. 26-10, *D*). She is using her right thumb more but often but needs to be reminded especially when she is tired or "cranky." She throws and catches a ball and plays with pegs and puzzles appropriately. She still needs work in developing fine manipulative skills. The radial deformity of the wrist is now minimal. S.S. enjoys wearing a splint that corrects it and provides her with stability as she plays. She continues to attend therapy weekly. At age 3 she will no longer be eligible to participate in the Early Intervention Program. S.S. will be reevaluated by her hand surgeon and hand therapist to determine whether further hand therapy will be necessary. We are confident that S.S. will have very good use of her right hand. The cooperative family was crucial to successful rehabilitation. The left normal hand continues to be the dominant hand as is true in most clients with pollicizations.

CASE 26-3: BRACHIAL PLEXUS PALSY

H.F., a 4-month-old girl, was referred to hand therapy by her physician with a diagnosis of brachial plexus palsy. Her left upper extremity was significantly abnormal in posture. The active range of motion included partial shoulder flexion, internal rotation, and abduction. Significant limitation of shoulder active external rotation and abduction were apparent. Slight tightness of the scapulohumeral angle was evident. H.F. had no elbow, wrist, and hand active range of motion (Fig. 26-11, *A*). The finger flexor muscles were tight. No contractures were present.

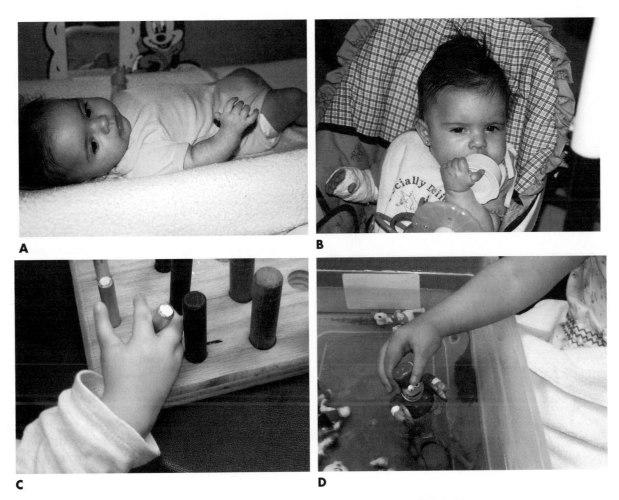

FIGURE 26-10   A, Newborn infant has radial club hand with a floating thumb (absent carpometacarpal and metacarpophalangeal joints). **B,** Serial casting is initiated as soon as possible to correct radial deviation of the wrist, 2 to 3 times a week. **C,** Pollicization was done at the age of 2 years. The wrist deformity is corrected to neutral, but because of muscle imbalance, removable splint is used several hours a day. Child is being trained to prevent scissoring of index and middle fingers as is carried over from before surgery. **D,** Child is trained to oppose new thumb with middle finger.

At 4 months of age the parents of this child were given a poor prognosis for spontaneous recovery because active elbow flexion was absent. The physician advised microsurgery between 5 and 6 months of age.

The therapist carefully reviewed all medical records and established communication with the mother, who was saddened and concerned. Evaluation consisted of clinical observation, musculoskeletal assessment, and the Peabody Developmental Motor Scales (PDMS-2) to provide a clearer picture of H.F.'s current level of function. It was clear that H.F. had significant delays in motor, sensory, and cortical awareness of her affected left extremity.

The treatment plan consisted of instructing the mother in performing exercises on the baby while prone, supine, and sitting with support. This included passive range of motion of the entire extremity, with special emphasis on shoulder abduction and external rotation. The mother was instructed in facilitation techniques to provide sensory and motor feedback using vibration, tapping, and stroking. The importance of allowing the child to play, explore, and reach out with the affected extremity was emphasized. Light rattles were placed on the baby's hand. Mom was asked to assist in shaking them. Appropriate handling techniques were reviewed and a schedule was determined for exercises and splinting.

The physician prescribed a day mobilization splint to position the wrist in extension and allow the digits to flex (Fig. 26-11, *B*) and a different night forearm immobilization splint to stretch the wrist and digits comfortably, especially the thumb (Fig. 26-11, *C*). We practiced the

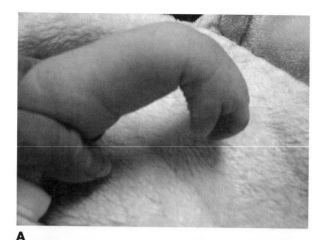

A

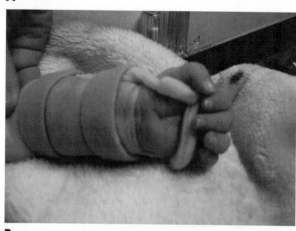

B

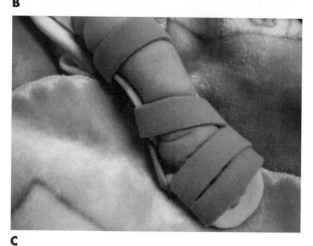

C

FIGURE 26-11 **A,** Four-month-old infant with obstetric brachial plexus injury at C4 to C7. Infant lacks wrist and digital extension. **B,** Wrist is extended with palmar bar, allowing fingers to flex; thumb is extended with a bar in the first web. **C,** Night splint gently stretches wrist, fingers, and thumb to prevent contractures.

exercises and splint application and gave written instructions to the mother.

Surgery was performed at the age of $7^1/_2$ months. The C5-C6 and C7 portions of the nerve trunk neuromas were resected and were grafted with sural nerves to reinnervate suprascapular nerve, musculocutaneous nerve, radial nerve, and axillary nerves. The extremity was immobilized in a sling and swathe with shoulder adducted and internally rotated for 6 weeks.

The infant was referred to hand therapy once the immobilization was discontinued. Therapy included passive ranging of the shoulder, elbow, wrist, and fingers through full range of motion. All exercises were performed with scapula stabilized in adduction. The passive stretches included glenohumeral abduction, external rotation in adduction, and external rotation in 90 degrees of shoulder abduction. Each stretch was held for 30 seconds. We instructed the mother to perform the same exercises at least 3 times a day, and reviewed the precautions mentioned before. We showed the mother how to support the flail extremity when she held her infant. The scars were sensitive and were to be massaged. We taught the mother how to do this. The finger and shoulder were tight 2 weeks after initiation of therapy, and these joints were stretched more often. Normal activities that were age-appropriate were started, including shaking a rattle, weight bearing on the floor, and holding a ball with two hands with mother's help. At the time of this writing, a resting splint was being used at night and a wrist extension splint was being used during the day. The future treatment depends on recovery of various muscles.

References

1. Elliott JM, Connolly KJ: A classification of manipulative hand movements, *Dev Med Child Neurol* 283-296, 1984.
2. Weeks PM, Wray RC: *The management of acute hand injuries: a biological approach,* St Louis, 1973, Mosby.
3. Brand PW, Hollister A: *Clinical mechanics of the hand,* ed 3, St Louis, 1999, Mosby.
4. Ezaki M: Treatment of the upper limb in the child with arthrogryposis, *Hand Clin* 16:703-711, 2000.
5. Smith R, Kaplan E: Camptodactyly and similar atraumatic flexion deformities of the proximal interphalangeal joints of the fingers: a study of thirty-one cases, *J Bone Joint Surg* 50A:1187-1203, 1968.
6. Kline S, Moore J: Neonatal compartment syndrome, *J Hand Surg* 17A:256-259, 1992.
7. Kozin SH: Upper-extremity congenital anomalies, *J Bone Joint Surg* 85A:1564-1576, 2003.
8. Swanson AB: A classification for congenital limb malformations, *J Hand Surg* 1A:8-22, 1976.
9. Flatt AE: *The care of congenital hand anomalies,* St Louis, 1994, Quality Medical Publishing.

10. Sells J, Jaffe K, Hall J: Amyoplasia, the most common type of arthrogryposis: the potential for good outcome, *Pediatrics* 97:225-232, 1997.

11. Hargens A, Mubarak S, Akeson W: Current concepts in the pathophysiology, evaluation and diagnosis of compartment syndrome, *Hand Clin* 14:371-383, 1998.

12. Smith DW, Drennan JC: Arthrogryposis wrist deformities: results of infantile serial casting, *J Pediatr Orthop* 22:44-47, 2002.

13. Flatt AE: Crooked fingers. In *The care of congenital hand anomalies*, St Louis, 1994, Quality Medical Publishing.

14. Hori M, Nakamura R, Inoue G et al: Nonoperative treatment of camptodactyly, *J Hand Surg* 12A:1061-1065, 1987.

15. Miura T, Nakamura R, Tamura Y: Long-standing extended dynamic splintage and release of an abnormal restraining structure in camptodactyly, *J Bone Joint Surg* 17B:665-672, 1992.

16. Benson LS, Waters PM, Kamil NI et al: Camptodactyly: classification and results of nonoperative treatment, *J Pediatr Orthop* 14:814-819, 1994.

17. Siegert J, Cooney W, Dobyns J: Management of simple camptodactyly, *J Hand Surg* 15B:181-189, 1990.

18. Wood V, Flatt A: Congenital triangular bones in the hand, *J Hand Surg* 2A:179-193, 1977.

19. Jones J: Delta phalanx, *J Bone Joint Surg* 46B:226-228, 1964.

20. Leclercq C, Korn W: Articular fractures of the fingers in children, *Hand Clinics: Pediatric Upper Extremity* 16:523-534, 2000.

21. Kirner J: Doppelseitige verkrummung des kleinfingergrundgliedes also selbstandiges krankheitsbild, *Fortschr Rontgenstr* 36:804-806, 1927.

21a. Frieberg A, Forrest C: Kirner's deformity: a review of the literature and case presentation, *J Hand Surg* 11A:28-32, 1986.

22. Mih A: Congenital clasped thumb, *Hand Clin* 14:77-84, 1988.

23. Weckesser EC, Reed JR, Heiple KG: Congenital clasped thumb (congenital flexion-adduction deformity of the thumb): a syndrome, not a specific entity, *J Bone Joint Surg* 50A:1417-1428, 1968.

23a. McCarroll HR, Jr: Congenital flexion deformities of the thumb, *Hand Clin* (3):567-575, 1985.

24. Tsuyuguchi Y, Masada K, Kawabata H et al: Congenital clasped thumb: a review of forty-three cases, *J Hand Surg* 10A:613-618, 1985.

25. Bayne LG, Klug MS: Long-term review of the surgical treatment of radial deficiencies, *J Hand Surg* 12A:169-179, 1987.

26. McPherson JJ: Objective evaluation of a splint designed to reduce hypertonicity, *Am J Occup Ther* 35(3):189-194, 1981.

27. Green WT, Banks HH: Flexor carpi ulnaris transplant and its use in cerebral palsy, *J Bone Joint Surg* 44A:1343-1352, 1962.

28. Waters PM: Pediatric brachial plexus palsy. In Green DP, Hotchkiss RN, Pederson WC et al, editors: *Green's operative hand surgery*, ed 5, Philadelphia, 2005, Churchill Livingstone.

29. Narakas AO: Injuries to the brachial plexus. In Bora FW, Jr, editor: *The pediatric upper extremity: diagnosis and management*, Philadelphia, 1986, WB Saunders.

30. Gilbert A, Tassin JL: Reparation chirurgicale du plexus brachial dans la paralysie obstetricale, *Chirurgie* 110:70, 1984.

31. Mallet J: Paralysie obstetricale du plexus brachial: Traitement des sequelle: Primaute du traitement de l'epaule: Method d'expression des resultants, *Rev Chir Orthop Reparatrice Appar Mot* 58 (suppl 1):166-168, 1972.

32. Clarke HM, Curtis CG: An approach to obstetrical brachial plexus injuries, *Hand Clin* 11:580-581, 1995.

33. Gilbert A, Hentz VR, Tassin JL: Brachial plexus reconstruction in obstetrical palsy: operative indications and post-operative results. In Urbaniek JR, editor: *Microsurgery for major limb reconstruction*, St Louis, 1987, Mosby.

34. Roberts A: Special considerations in children's fractures. In Gupta A, Simon KPJ, Scheker LR, editors: *The growing hand diagnosis and management of the upper extremity in children*, London, 2000, Mosby.

35. O'Connell SJ, Moore MM, Strickland JW et al: Results of zone I and zone II flexor tendon repairs in children, *J Hand Surg* 19:48-52, 1994.

36. Moran SL, Farahmand AE, Amadio P: Repair of zone one and zone two flexor tendon injuries in children. Paper presented at the American Association for Hand Surgery annual meeting, Conference Scientific Paper Session 2B: Tendon, Puerto Rico, 2005.

37. Gulgonen A: Compartment syndrome. In Green DP, Hotchkiss RN, Pederson WC et al, editors: *Green's operative hand surgery*, ed 5, Philadelphia, 2005, Churchill Livingstone.

38. Volkmann R: Die ischaemischen Muskellahmungen and Kontrakturen, *Zentralbl Chir* 8:801-803, 1881.

39. Caouette-Laberge L, Bortoluzzi P, Egerszegi E et al: Neonatal Volkmann's contracture of the forearm: a report of five cases, *Plast Reconstr Surg* 90:621-629, 1992.

40. Holden CEA: The pathology and prevention of Volkmann's ischemic contracture, *J Bone Joint Surg* 61(B):296-300, 1979.

27

Geriatric Hand Therapy*

CYNTHIA COOPER

". . . a child passes through the years into old age, but when exactly does he become 'old'; or if no such moment exists, then does the word have any meaning?"

From Mr. Mee by Andrew Crumey (New York, 2000, Picador)

The older population consists of persons who are at least 65 years of age. By 2010, 56 million Americans will be 60 years of age or older, and 6 million will be at least 85 years old.[1] In 1998, adults over the age of 65 accounted for 12.7% of the population. By the year 2030, adults over the age of 65 are projected to account for 20% of the U.S. population.[2] Persons who are older than 85 years of age make up the segment of our population that is growing most rapidly.[3]

A larger geriatric population will result in a greater proportion of geriatric hand therapy clients. Learning about the unique features of older clients will enable therapists to individualize effective treatment programs. Although accommodating their special needs may prolong the initial treatment, it can increase therapists' effectiveness, improve client compliance, and produce a more successful clinical outcome.[4]

Nonelderly caregivers have difficulty imagining what it is like to be elderly.[5] Six million elderly persons residing in the community (i.e., not in nursing homes or other assisted-care facilities) experience difficulty with at least one activity of personal care, and more than 7 million experience difficulty with at least one activity of home management.[1] Because we all stand a chance of someday being elderly, any improvements we make for older persons today may benefit us tomorrow.

This chapter explores the effects of aging on tissues and identifies changes associated with aging that may influence the appropriateness and effectiveness of hand therapy. The goals of this chapter are to sensitize hand therapists to the process of aging and to promote clinical efficacy with older clients.

AGEISM

Our societal values promote gerontophobia, or fear of aging, which in turn fosters age bias. Advertising media bombards us with unsubtle idealizations of youth and beauty that reinforce negative perceptions about aging and implicitly devalue older persons. Social distance and age segregation further compound the problem.

AGING AND BODY IMAGE

Cultural standards for female beauty are associated with youthful characteristics. Our media is glutted with young, thin women promoting products developed to defy chronologic age and to maintain a youthful appearance.[1] Having to cope with an external fixator, incisional scar-

---

*Adapted from Cooper C: The geriatric hand patient: special treatment considerations. In Mackin EJ, Callahan AD, Osterman AL et al, editors: *Hunter, Mackin & Callahan's rehabilitation of the hand and upper extremity*, ed 5, St Louis, 2002, Mosby.

ring, or deformity can complicate already existing issues of cosmesis in older clients.

ELDER ABUSE

By conservative estimate, approximately 500,000 persons experience elder abuse each year. Older persons who live with family are at greater risk, with women being more vulnerable than men to abuse that may be physical, financial, or psychological.[6]

Spiral fractures and transverse or oblique midshaft digital fractures might raise suspicion of physical abuse, whereas flexion or extension contractures may indicate physical neglect.[7] Victims may be afraid to report their abuse because of the fear of being placed in a nursing home.

BABY TALK

Stereotypes of elderly persons commonly include the notion of incompetence. This may contribute to the use of baby talk when communicating with older persons. Talking too loudly, using a higher pitch, and choosing words that normally are used with pets and babies also may occur.[8] The therapist should avoid these condescending dynamics; however, it can take awareness and practice to change these habits.

TIPS FROM THE FIELD

Be aware of your attitude toward elderly clients. One study of physical therapists found less aggressive goals associated with negative attitudes about aging. Underestimating clients' potentials based on their age could deprive them of opportunities to maximize their function and independence.[9]

Make special efforts to treat and connect with older clients as persons, not as numbers or ages. For instance, many older hand therapy clients obviously put time and thought into their appearance before coming to therapy. When appropriate, it can be effective genuinely to compliment older clients on their appearance.

TIMELINES AND HEALING: CHANGES ASSOCIATED WITH AGING

Skin, Soft Tissue, and Wound Healing Changes Associated with Aging

Age-related changes in skin predispose older persons to injury after even minimal trauma. Age also contributes to slower healing.[10,11] Changes include reduced dermal thickness and decreased contact of and adherence between the dermis and epidermis. Physiologic changes demonstrated in animal models include reduced cellular proliferation, altered wound metabolism, and altered remodeling of collagen. Such findings help explain the increased incidence of skin wounds in the elderly.[12,13]

Dryness and loss of skin turgor,[14] lower overall strength of incisional wounds, and higher dehiscence rates[11] occur with aging.[11,15] Skin tears among institutionalized elderly persons appear to occur most frequently in the forearm, with the hand, elbow, and arm being the next most frequent locations.[13]

Precaution. *The elderly can heal successfully, although age causes them to heal more slowly. Other concomitant medical conditions, such as vascular disease, steroid use, or cardiopulmonary disease, which are seen more often in older clients, also can slow the healing process.[11,12]*

Tips from the Field
Slight mechanical traumas that may occur with dressing removal, especially adhesive dressings, pose potentials for injury because of skin vulnerability associated with aging.[12] Splint edges may be more problematic as a result of the fragility of older skin.

Precaution. *Remove dressings with extreme care, and touch the client gently. Select soft, wide splint straps, and pad splint edges to minimize shearing forces on the skin. Provide conservative guidelines for checking the skin. Use extra care with routine clinical equipment such as treatment table edges or exercise equipment handles.*

Muscle Changes Associated with Aging

Muscle strength tends to be stable through age 50 years. It decreases by 15% per decade from age 50 to age 70 years and again by 30% from age 70 to age 80 years. By 80 years of age, persons have lost almost half of their motor neurons, motor units, muscle fibers, muscle strength, and muscle mass.[10,16] Hand atrophy associated with aging tends to affect the interosseous and thenar muscles.[17] Loss of muscle mass may explain the reduction of grip strength noted with aging. Changes in muscle fiber type and motoneuron abnormalities also occur.[18]

Immobilization itself has significant negative effects on skeletal muscle. Immobilization causes shortened muscle length with segmental necrosis at muscle fiber ends, with myofibril contracture. This may result in partial denervation[19] or may predispose the involved muscles to atrophy.[20] Interestingly, immobilization can even lead to changes in muscle fiber type.[21]

Tips from the Field
Decreased muscle strength results in reduced capacity for physical activity and may contribute to functional dependence. Because decreased muscle strength also may increase one's risk for injury,[10] use care in testing. On a

brighter note, a clinical study has demonstrated that the hand muscles of elderly subjects can be strengthened by a training program.[22]

Sensibility Changes Associated with Aging

Studies have demonstrated age-related changes in sensibility, including the touch/pressure threshold. The degree of deterioration of tactile sensitivity may vary among subjects. Interestingly, blind elderly subjects were found to have better sensitivity in a digit used for reading braille, but not at other sites. Individual differences may result from changes in circulation, thinning of receptors, or age-related disease or trauma.[23] Sensory changes may make it difficult to perform fine motor tasks such as manipulating splint straps or dynamic components.

Precaution. *Be extra cautious with guidelines for monitoring splint edges, strap tightness, or other possible pressure spots.*

Neuromuscular Changes Associated with Aging

Sensorimotor decline may be among the most apparent changes associated with aging. Motor function such as finger tapping, sensory perception, and central processing are slowed with age. Speed-based psychomotor skills reach their peak at approximately age 20 years and tend to decline thereafter.[17] Skills used infrequently are most affected by age.

Essential tremor is the most common movement disorder that manifests with intentional use of the extremity. Essential tremor also is called intention tremor or action tremor. The cause is unknown, but the incidence of essential tremor increases with age. Stress or emotional situations such as the stressful demands and unfamiliar surroundings of a busy hand clinic can exacerbate the severity of essential tremor.[24,25] A therapist may notice essential tremor as a client dons or doffs a splint.

Resting tremor typically is seen among clients with Parkinson's disease. Resting hand tremor is described as "pill-rolling." It lessens with hand activity. Like essential tremor, resting tremor also worsens with emotional stress.[24,25]

Tips from the Field

Because stress has negative effects on cognitive processing, motor tone, and movement quality, try to communicate with the older client in stress-relieving ways. Provide a calming environment, and try not to rush the client.

Persons with problems of motor tone may have an unsteady gait, which may further increase their risk of their falling.[26] Eliminate obstacles that could cause a fall and provide assistance with ambulation as appropriate.

Physiologic and Functional Changes Associated with Aging

Chronic degenerative disease has surpassed infectious disease as the major health threat in our nation.[27] Arthritis, hypertension, and hearing loss are the most prevalent chronic conditions of the elderly.[17]

Most persons who are 65 years of age or older have at least one chronic condition.[2,28] Fifty percent have neurologic problems, the most common cause of limited function in the elderly[17]; 49% have arthritis; 37% have hypertension; 32% have hearing impairments; 30% have heart disease; 17% have cataracts; 17% have sinusitis; 16% have orthopedic problems; 9% have visual impairment; 9% have diabetes[28]; and 8% have severe visual impairment.[15]

Hearing loss affects approximately 40% of persons older than 75 years of age and results in significant emotional and social problems, including communication barriers[29] that dramatically affect their quality of life.[30] Changes in temporal organization associated with aging can lead to interruption of the sleep-wake cycle and can be extremely problematic.[31]

CLINICAL *Pearl*

When treating a client whose hearing is impaired, sit directly facing the client to promote lip-reading. Speak clearly and slowly.[14]

Osteoarthritis is the most common arthritic condition occurring in older persons. Most older individuals demonstrate some radiographic changes indicative of osteoarthritis.[32] As many as 80% of persons older than 65 years of age may have significant pain that is caused by osteoarthritis.[33] Rheumatoid arthritis, a debilitating condition,[34] affects females 2 to 3 times more often than males, with frequency increasing for persons older than 65 years of age.[32] More than 90% of persons with rheumatoid arthritis have clinical involvement of the hands.[35]

Precaution. *Because arthritis can contribute to reduction in grip strength and fine motor skills, areas already affected by aging, splint application by the client may be doubly difficult in these situations.*

Osteoporosis causes more than 1 million fractures yearly and affects between one third and one half of all women who are menopausal. After the age of 50 years, a woman has a 40% chance of incurring an osteoporotic fracture at some time.[36]

Physical performance generally improves into the middle of the second decade and then decreases as persons age.[37] Capacity for physical work also decreases with age[38] as persons experience more chronic conditions that limit their activity level.[2] This decline in physiologic status limits function and raises the morbidity associated with chronic diseases.[39]

Mental impairment limits the self-sufficiency of 3.3 million elderly persons in the United States. Another 2.5 million older persons live alone despite their need for a caregiver.[28]

Tips from the Field

Older persons who maintain a physically active lifestyle demonstrate less functional decline than those who are not active.[37] Therefore, look for ways to sustain the activity levels of elderly hand therapy clients while they recover from upper extremity injuries.

The treatment space itself may pose problems. Doors should not be heavy to open, and doorways should be wide enough to accommodate wheelchairs. Waiting areas should be free of obstacles or types of carpets that may challenge ambulation with assistive devices. Such obstacles might even cause falls. Lighting should be good.[14]

Pain Associated with Aging

Pain is a common problem with profound effects on the quality of life and ability to function of the elderly population. Pain in the elderly can result in depression, limited socialization, disturbance of sleep, and problems with ambulation, all of which contribute to increased cost and use of health care services. Pain can result in deconditioning and poor gait, leading to falls, polypharmacy, greater cognitive dysfunction, and even malnutrition. Pain significantly can degrade the quality of life of residents in long-term care facilities.[33]

Musculoskeletal causes of pain, especially osteoarthritis, predominate.[33] Pain is associated with diseases accompanying aging, such as cancer and neuromuscular disorders.[40] From 25% to 50% of elderly persons in the community and 45% to 80% of residents in nursing homes suffer from significant pain.[41]

Older clients who want to please the caregiver may not report their pain, may have stoic attitudes about pain and aging, or may not feel permitted to express their pain.[40] They might hesitate to discuss their pain because of fear of diagnostic tests or possible medication-related side effects.[41]

Tips from the Field

Talk with your clients about pain, and instruct them to report any pain associated with their therapy.

Depression/Suicide Associated with Aging

The elderly population has the highest risk for suicide.[42] Depression is actually the most common functional disorder of the elderly,[43] affecting up to 25% of this population.[44] Signs of depression, which may be vague, include anorexia, apathy, fatigue, self-neglect, weight loss,[14] social withdrawal, sleep disturbance, decreased involvement in activities, and hopelessness.[44]

Physical disability is associated strongly with depressive disorders.[45] Because pain contributes to depression, hand therapy clients who are in pain therefore may be at heightened risk of experiencing depression.

I have been moved by the frequency with which older hand therapy clients reveal tearfully that they are grieving for a deceased spouse or recently have experienced some other loss. The clinical problem necessitating hand therapy may heighten their emotionality, their loneliness, or simply their need for a caring listener.

Tips from the Field

Because physical activity has associated psychological benefits,[44] make every effort to restore clients' preinjury levels of physical activity. Encourage regular physical exercise that is safe for clients.

Typical Cognitive Changes Associated with Aging

The typical declines in cognition associated with normal aging are usually minimal. Elderly persons who stay physically active may perform well on all cognitive measures beyond the age of 80.[17] Sensory stimulation and exercise are related positively to abilities in reasoning, cognition, reaction time, and working memory among the elderly.[46] Older persons who continue to participate in daily activity perform better on memory tasks and intelligence tests.[47] Interestingly, younger but less active persons may not perform as well as older active persons.[17]

Memory in normal aging tends to remain available for material that is relevant or has been well learned.[17] Older persons can retain memorized information as long as can younger persons. However, the time it takes to retrieve a memory may increase. In persons who stay active intellectually, memory may even improve.[48]

Neurologic changes expected with senescence are differentiated from those associated with disease. Older adults often complain about memory loss (typically associated with names), misplacing items, and forgetting conversations and everyday events. They may be slower to learn in new or unfamiliar situations or to process novel information. However, they may respond well to suggestions of adaptive strategies such as appointment books, calendars, lists, or reminder notes. Short-term memory may be more likely to deteriorate with age if the content seems irrelevant.[17]

Clinically Significant Cognitive Changes Associated with Aging

Alzheimer's disease is the most common cause of dementia. Aging itself is the highest indicator for developing Alzheimer's disease.[49] Cardiovascular accident is the second most common cause.[50]

Dementia of the Alzheimer's type is a neurodegenerative disorder that affects approximately 7% of the geriatric population.[51] Alzheimer's disease is reported to occur in 3% of persons who are 65 to 74 years of age, in 19% of persons who are 75 to 84 years of age, and in 47% of persons who are 85 years and older. Approximately 50% of 90-year-olds are clinically demented.[52,53] External factors that can accelerate the onset of dementia include nutrition, drugs, and cardiovascular disease.[52]

Because of medical advances on longevity, health care providers will be seeing greater numbers of older clients, more of whom may have dementia.[53] Growing numbers of older hand therapy clients means a greater chance of cognitive impairment among some of them.

With dementia, various intellectual processes are limited, resulting in interference with work or social function. The primary symptom of this syndrome is memory loss.[49] Anomia (difficulty with naming objects) is a typical early symptom of Alzheimer's disease.[46] Other symptoms of dementia include disturbances in orientation, abstraction ability, judgment, language, and constructional ability[49]; difficulty with composing, sending, receiving, and understanding a message[46]; psychomotor retardation[54]; sleep disturbances[31]; reduced appetite; social withdrawal; loss of libido; and decreased concentration.[54] Personality changes, which usually are not associated with normal aging,[17] occur with dementia.[49]

Most dementia cases are irreversible, but 20% to 30% are reversible if diagnosed early. Reversible cases may be caused by depression, medications, or nutritional or metabolic deficiencies.[50]

Tips from the Field
A person who has communication impairments still may be able to comprehend simple statements. Speak in grammatically correct, simple sentences, and convey only one piece of information with each sentence.[50] Avoid distractions and multiple stimuli.

A person who has difficulty with spatial relationships may not be able to apply a splint or its straps properly. This challenge is compounded with more complicated splint demands (Fig. 27-1).

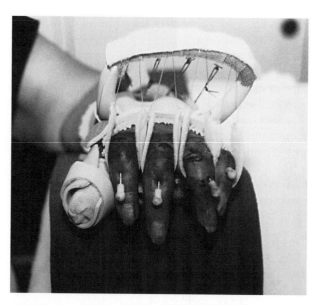

FIGURE 27-1 This postoperative dynamic splint for a 76-year-old patient with rheumatoid arthritis requires dexterity, coordination, and good judgment to be used properly. (Courtesy John L. Evarts.)

COMMUNICATING WITH OLDER HAND THERAPY CLIENTS

Therapists should make an extra effort to establish a good rapport with their older clients. Older clients may be slower in most of their behaviors,[55] which can be challenging to a busy therapist with a full schedule.[4] In addition, they may have difficulty ignoring irrelevant stimuli[56] such as dialog among therapists, ambient noise, and other interruptions. Try to help the client focus by eliminating distractions and by redirecting, talking, and touching. Instructions or demonstrations must not be overcomplicated. Humor is helpful but should be used with sensitivity and discretion.

The following suggestions may improve communication effectiveness with elderly persons[57]:

- Do not use baby talk. Do not call the client "sweetie" or "honey."
- Do not condescend. Remember that you are speaking to an adult.
- Do not shout. Shouting distorts speech perception and also may embarrass the client. Lower your voice, and face the client directly.
- Interact with the client directly. Include the person accompanying the client as appropriate but not to the exclusion of the client.
- Ask the client whether he or she can see well before assuming so.
- If the client can see well, use visual aids whenever possible.

- If the client has traditional learning and memory problems, focus on activities of daily living.
- Avoid interruptions.
- Remember that many older persons still can learn, grow, and develop.
- Express interest in the person. If the client is given an opportunity to tell about his or her life, you may find yourself fascinated by a remarkable or moving story.
- Be patient, or recruit another caregiver.

STRATEGIES FOR SUCCESS

- Schedule the treatment at the client's "good" time, which is frequently midmorning or early afternoon.[14]
- Provide extra time to treat elderly clients to accommodate the possibility of slower physical performance or slower cognitive processing.
- Try not to rush older clients. If you do, they actually may slow down.
- Eliminate or minimize interferences and ambient stimuli.
- Enhance learning by using physical practice with simultaneous verbalizing and written instructions.[58]
- Minimize dexterity demands.
- Simplify strap requirements on splints; permanently secure one end of each strap to the splint. Color-code the ends of straps (consider checking for color blindness); mark where straps should meet.
- Simplify overall numbers of splints, devices, exercises, or instructions.
- Physically acknowledge the client's presence. Therapeutic touch of a disoriented client may enhance his or her ability to focus on the task.

Questions to Ask the Physician

- *Does this client have concomitant medical problems?*
- *If the diagnosis is a fracture, what is the fracture status?*
- *If an elective surgery is planned and there are questions about the client's cognitive status, ask about performing a cognitive screening before deciding to schedule elective surgery.*
- *A splint may limit a person's ability to drive safely. Because there can be medical-legal issues of driving while wearing a hand splint, refer this difficult question to the physician.*

What to Say to Clients

"In some but not all circumstances, healing may be slower in an older client. This could be more likely to happen

if you have a history of steroid use or medical problems such as diabetes or vascular disease. Preventing or resolving stiffness also may be more challenging among some older clients. Your therapy program will maximize opportunities to promote healing so that you can recover function as quickly as possible. In the meantime, it will be important for you to notify us if you are having pain."

EVALUATION TIPS

- Be gentle when touching elderly clients.
- Observe for signs of skin fragility.

Precautions and Concerns

- *Adult norms should not be applied to an elderly population, unless they are age specific.[59]*
- *In cases in which clients have sensory and physical problems, it can be difficult to discern whether their limitation is a result of physical or cognitive causes.[60]*
- *Minimize obstacles in the treatment area that might contribute to the possibility of falling.*
- *Ask about pain, and prioritize treatments to reduce it.*
- *Use extra padding on splint edges.*

The Role of the Therapy Assistant

- *Spend extra time as needed with the client to ensure a successful learning experience in hand therapy.*
- *Explore activities of daily living needs, and provide adaptive devices to maximize function.*
- *Provide extra encouragement as needed if recovery is slow.*
- *Practice and review exercises as determined by the supervising therapist.*
- *Provide splinting based on individual experience and competencies.*
- *Instruct clients in home programs as determined by the supervising therapist.*

CASE Studies

CASE 27-1

E.F. is a 78-year-old, left-hand dominant woman who fell and sustained fractures of her left ring and small finger metacarpals. Her medical history included cancer with left mastectomy and osteoarthritis of both hands. She had significant edema after the injury and was not able to tolerate cast immobilization. She was sent to hand therapy for protective splinting because of the inability to tolerate the cast. E.F. lived alone and worked as a lecturer and writer. She traveled often to give lectures and for book-signing appearances.

E.F. was not able to write or use her left hand for any activities while casted in a forearm-based protective splint. She was also unable to drive. She was able to dress herself and perform one-handed self-care using her non-dominant hand and adapted techniques. Friends helped with her transportation and home chores.

E.F. was highly motivated but experienced significant stiffness throughout all digits of the hand. This was exacerbated by a flare of her osteoarthritis. Fortunately, her edema improved with proximal active range of motion, elevation, and light compressive garments. When she was cleared medically, E.F. performed a home program of gentle active range of motion and blocking exercises for her wrist and all joints of all digits of her left hand. She enjoyed using a hot pack before exercising. Buddy straps were provided for support with exercise and for improved comfort with light self-care tasks. Functional activities with tendon gliding were emphasized. A dorsal drop-out splint was helpful in facilitating pain-free composite flexion motions. When E.F. was cleared medically, a gentle static progressive splint was fabricated for small finger metacarpophalangeal joint flexion. E.F. still had difficulty with handwriting because of the flare-ups of osteoarthritis. A soft wrist wrap was tried, along with a hand-based carpometacarpal joint splint. She found these to be helpful and used them intermittently as needed for symptom relief. Built-up cushions were provided for her pen and her toothbrush. She practiced handwriting for improved pinch strength and range of motion.

E.F. made slow progress. She eventually recovered nearly full range of motion of all digits of the left hand, but at the time of discharge, she still used her wrist wrap and carpometacarpal joint splint as needed for pain relief. She continued to perform her home exercise program. E.F. told the therapist that it had helped her to know initially that although her progress might be slow, she had potential to recover over time. She stated that the encouragement in therapy had been helpful to her and that prioritizing handwriting had been the most important activity for her to work on. At first glance, one might have presumed that ulnar-sided hand range of motion would be most important to work on. Listening to E.F. allowed the therapist to incorporate E.F.'s most important activity of handwriting into the treatment program early.

CASE 27-2

S.P. is a 75-year-old woman who underwent elective surgery for proximal interphalangeal (PIP) joint arthroplasty with radial collateral ligament reconstruction to her left index finger. A history of osteoarthritis had con-

tributed to severe PIP joint ulnar deviation and pain. She attended therapy with her husband. At her first therapy visit, she cried uncontrollably, stating that she and her husband had been fighting about her hand therapy appointments. Her husband was undergoing treatment for cancer and was not feeling well, and she depended on him to drive her to her hand therapy appointments.

S.P. had a medical history of heart disease and diabetes. Her incision was healing slowly, and her physician postponed removal of sutures for this reason. She was frustrated by this and stated repeatedly that she wanted her sutures removed.

S.P. was fitted with a custom-fabricated digit-based volar gutter splint per physician orders, maintaining PIP joint neutral alignment to support the collateral ligament repair. She was instructed to elevate her upper extremity. She was taught to perform proximal active range of motion and active range of motion of the uninvolved digits, as well as index finger PIP joint protected active range of motion from 0 to 20 degrees initially per physician orders. She was taught to stabilize the metacarpophalangeal joint for these exercises. She was instructed not to get her digit wet and to sleep with her splint on at night.

When S.P. returned 2 days later, she was not wearing her splint. She had gotten her digit wet doing the dishes and could not remember the last time she had seen her splint. Her digit was posturing in extreme PIP joint ulnar deviation. Her incision site appeared to be dehiscing somewhat. No redness or other objective signs of inflammation were noted.

The physician was called, and a note describing the findings was faxed to the doctor's office. Another splint was made, and the client's husband was included in all instructions and exercise practice thereafter.

Over the next few weeks, S.P. made slow progress. Her incision site healed, and she wore her splint as instructed most of the time. She and her husband argued regularly in therapy about her exercises and splint use, but they somehow managed to work this out. After 6 weeks, she had excellent PIP joint flexion and extension with 10 degrees of PIP joint ulnar deviation. She was instructed to continue to use her splint at night, and she stated that she would do so. When asked if she was happy with her results, she stated that she was glad to have the improved motion but wished her finger was not deviated.

CASE 27-3

B.C. is a 92-year-old, right-hand dominant man who was volunteering as a driver for persons who needed transportation to their medical appointments. He was assisting a developmentally disabled passenger who became unruly and violent, kicking B.C. repeatedly in the left knee and the left wrist. B.C. lived alone in his house and had been independent in all activities of daily living at the time of the injury. He reported no other medical problems.

B.C. was sent to hand therapy by his family physician with a diagnosis of left wrist pain. He presented with pain 10/10 at rest. Significant edema was noted over the area of the left ulnar head. Forearm rotation and all active range of motion (AROM) of the left wrist was painful. Grip testing was deferred because of pain. Digital AROM was within normal limits in composite flexion and extension.

A circumferential wrist splint was made to immobilize B.C.'s wrist in slight extension, which was his most comfortable position. He was instructed in proximal pain-free AROM, digital AROM within the splint, and elevation of the left upper extremity. He was advised to avoid any use of the left upper extremity that was painful. He also was seen for a trial of ultrasound, which he felt was helpful. After 2 weeks, his pain was resolving, and B.C. began pain-free short-arc AROM for left forearm pronation/supination and for wrist flexion and extension, avoiding radial and ulnar deviation motions, which were painful. Gradually isometric exercises were added, along with increasing arcs of motion for forearm and wrist in pain-free ranges. Two weeks later, small arcs of wrist radial and ulnar deviation were pain-free, so these motions were added but not in extremes of motion because this could have aggravated to his symptoms. Grip strengthening was begun as B.C. was weaned off splint use altogether. After 6 weeks, B.C. reported no pain, and he had resumed full function including return to driving.

SUMMARY

A hand therapist who may be well versed in treatment guidelines for typical client situations can be stymied by unexpected and unique problems presented by older hand therapy clients. We all probably have been frustrated by an elderly client's difficulty with recall or by vague or strange deviations in follow-through.

Despite these frustrations, it is important to reinforce the value and dignity of our geriatric hand therapy clients. Special treatment considerations lead to appropriate and realistic goals, more successful clinical outcomes, more enriching interactions, and an improved sense of competence for therapists and clients. As an added benefit, we also may develop a more accepting attitude toward our own aging process.

Acknowledgment

Thanks to John L. Evarts for thoughtful recommendations and emotional and technical support. This chapter is dedicated to the memory of my father, Herschel A. Cooper, who showed me what graceful aging looks like, and to my mother, Delma P. Cooper, for her ongoing support of my work.

References

1. Franzoi SL, Koehler V: Age and gender differences in body attitudes: a comparison of young and elderly adults, *Int J Aging Hum Dev* 47(1):1-10, 1998.
2. American Association of Retired Persons: *A profile of older Americans*, Washington, 1999, The Association.
3. Manton KG, Blazer DG, Woodbury MA: Suicide in middle age and later life: sex and race specific life table and cohort analyses, *J Gerontol* 42(2):219-227, 1987.
4. Cooper C: Maximizing therapist effectiveness with geriatric hand patients, *J Hand Ther* 6(3):205-208, 1993.
5. Anderson EG: Getting through to elderly patients, *Geriatrics* 46(5):74-76, 1991.
6. Butler RN: Warning signs of elder abuse, *Geriatrics* 54(3):3-4, 1999.
7. Hall GR, Weiler K: Elder abuse, neglect, and mistreatment. In Bradway CW, editor: *Nursing care of geriatric emergencies*, New York, 1996, Springer.
8. O'Connor BP, Rigby H: Perceptions of baby talk, frequency of receiving baby talk, and self-esteem among community and nursing home residents, *Psychol Aging* 11(1):147-154, 1996.
9. Kvitek SDB, Shaver BJ, Blood H et al: Age bias: physical therapists and older patients, *J Gerontol* 41(6):706-709, 1986.
10. Buckwalter JA, Woo SLY, Goldberg VM et al: Current concepts review: soft-tissue aging and musculoskeletal function, *J Bone Joint Surg* 75A(10):1533-1548, 1993.
11. Gerstein AD, Phillips TJ, Rogers GS et al: Wound healing and aging, *Dermatol Clin* 11(4):749-757, 1993.
12. Grove GL: Physiologic changes in older skin, *Clin Geriatr Med* 5(1):115-125, 1989.
13. Malone JL, Rozario N, Gavinski M et al: The epidemiology of skin tears in the institutionalized elderly, *J Am Geriatr Soc* 39(6):591-595, 1991.
14. Fields SD: History-taking in the elderly: obtaining useful information, *Geriatrics* 46(8):26-35, 1991.
15. Fields SD: Special considerations in the physical exam of older patients, *Geriatrics* 46(8):39-44, 1991.
16. Booth FW, Weeden SH, Tseng BS: Effect of aging on human skeletal muscle and motor function, *Med Sci Sports Exerc* 26(5):556-560, 1994.
17. Morris JC, McManus DQ: The neurology of aging: normal versus pathologic change, *Geriatrics* 46(8):47-54, 1991.
18. Kallman DA, Plato CC, Tobin JD: The role of muscle loss in the age-related decline of grip strength: cross-sectional and longitudinal perspectives, *J Gerontol* 45(3):M82-M88, 1990.
19. Gordon T, Pattullo MC: Plasticity of muscle fiber and motor unit types, *Exerc Sport Sci Rev* 21:331-362, 1993.
20. Miles MP, Clarkson PM, Bean M et al: Muscle function at the wrist following 9 d of immobilization and suspension, *Med Sci Sports Exerc* 26(5):615-623, 1994.

21. Haggmark T, Eriksson E, Jansson E: Muscle fiber type changes in human skeletal muscle after injuries and immobilization, *Orthopedics* 9:181-185, 1986.

22. Keen DA, Yue GH, Enoka RM: Training-related enhancement in the control of motor output in elderly humans, *J Appl Physiol* 77(6):2648-2658, 1994.

23. Stevens JC, Cruz LA: Spatial acuity of touch: ubiquitous decline with aging revealed by repeated threshold testing, *Somatosens Mot Res* 13(1):1-10, 1996.

24. Anouti A, Koller WC: Tremor disorders and diagnosis management, *West J Med* 162:510-513, 1995.

25. Findley LJ: Classification of tremors, *J Clin Neurophysiol* 13(2):122-132, 1996.

26. Speechley M, Tinetti M: Falls and injuries in frail and vigorous community elderly persons, *J Am Geriatr Soc* 39(1):46-52, 1991.

27. Rook KS: Encouraging preventive behavior for distant and proximal health threats: effects of vivid versus abstract information, *J Gerontol* 41(4):526-534, 1986.

28. Mulrow CD, Aguilar C, Endicott JE et al: Association between hearing impairment and the quality of life of elderly individuals, *J Am Geriatr Soc* 38(1):45-50, 1990.

29. Keller BK, Morton JL, Thomas VS et al: The effect of visual and hearing impairments on functional status, *J Am Geriatr Soc* 47(11):1319-1325, 1999.

30. Reynolds CF, Jennings R, Hoch CC et al: Daytime sleepiness in the healthy "old old": a comparison with young adults, *J Am Geriatr Soc* 39(10):957-962, 1991.

31. Nesher G, Moore TL, Zuckner J: Rheumatoid arthritis in the elderly, *J Am Geriatr Soc* 39(3):284-294, 1991.

32. Ferrell BA: Pain management in elderly people, *J Am Geriatr Soc* 39(1):64-73, 1991.

33. Kremer JM: Severe rheumatoid arthritis: current options in drug therapy, *Geriatrics* 45(12):43-48, 1990.

34. Dellhag B, Burckhardt CS: Predictors of hand function in patients with rheumatoid arthritis, *Arthritis Care and Res* 8(1):16-20, 1996.

35. Licata AA: Therapies for symptomatic primary osteoporosis, *Geriatrics* 46(11):62-67, 1991.

36. Rikli R, Busch S: Motor performance of women as a function of age and physical activity level, *J Gerontol* 41(5):645-649, 1986.

37. Morey MC, Cowper PA, Feussner JR et al: Two-year trends in physical performance following supervised exercise among community-dwelling older veterans, *J Am Geriatr Soc* 39(6):549-554, 1991.

38. Larson EB: Exercise, functional decline and frailty, *J Am Geriatr Soc* 39(6):635-636, 1991.

39. Champlin L: "Eldercare" goal: integrate health, social needs, *Geriatrics* 46(8):67-70, 1991.

40. Forman WB, Stratton M: Current approaches to chronic pain in older patients, *Geriatrics* 46(7):47-52, 1991.

41. American Geriatrics Society Panel: The management of chronic pain in older persons, *Geriatrics* 53(suppl 3):S8-S24, 1998.

42. Loebel JP, Loebel JS, Dager SR et al: Anticipation of nursing home placement may be a precipitant of suicide among the elderly, *J Am Geriatr Soc* 39:407-408, 1991.

43. Gatz M, Pedersen NL, Harris J: Measurement and characteristics of the mental health scale from the OARS, *J Gerontol* 42(3):332-335, 1987.

44. Moore KA, Babyak MA, Wood CE et al: The association between physical activity and depression in older depressed adults, *J Aging Phys Act* 6:55-61, 1999.

45. Rapp SR, Parisi SA, Wallace CE: Comorbid psychiatric disorders in elderly medical patients: a 1-year prospective study, *J Am Geriatr Soc* 39(2):124-131, 1991.

46. Friedman R, Tappen RM: The effect of planned walking on communication in Alzheimer's disease, *J Am Geriatr Soc* 39(7):650-654, 1991.

47. Hultsch DF, Hammer M, Small BJ: Age differences in cognitive performance in later life: relationships to self-reported health and activity life style, *J Gerontol* 48(1):P1-P11, 1993.

48. Butler RN: Brain preservation, *Geriatrics* 53(11):3-4, 1998.

49. Alexopoulos GS, Mattis S: Diagnosing cognitive dysfunction in the elderly: primary screening tests, *Geriatrics* 46(12):33-44, 1991.

50. Mungas D: In-office mental status testing: a practical guide, *Geriatrics* 46(7):4-66, 1991.

51. Edwards JK: Are there clinical and epidemiological differences between familial and non-familial Alzheimer's disease? *J Am Geriatr Soc* 39(5):477-483, 1991.

52. Goodwin JS: Geriatric ideology: the myth of the myth of senility, *J Am Geriatr Soc* 39(6):627-631, 1991.

53. Jarvik LF, Wiseman EJ: A checklist for managing the dementia patient, *Geriatrics* 46(5):31-40, 1991.

54. Jeste DV, Krull AJ: Behavioral problems associated with dementia: diagnosis and treatment, *Geriatrics* 46(11):28-34, 1991.

55. Falduto LL, Baron A: Age-related effects of practice and task complexity on card sorting, *J Gerontol* 41(5):659-661, 1986.

56. Erber JT: Age-related effects of spatial contiguity and interference on coding, *J Gerontol* 41(5):641-644, 1986.

57. Anderson EG: How not to talk to elderly patients, *Geriatrics* 45:84, 1990.

58. Somerfield MR, Weisman CS, Ury W et al: Physician practices in the diagnosis of dementing disorders, *J Am Geriatr Soc* 39(2):172-175, 1991.

59. Desrosiers J, Hebert R, Bravo G et al: Hand sensibility of healthy older people, *J Am Geriatr Soc* 44(8):974-978, 1996.

60. O'Connor DW, Pollitt PA, Hyde JB et al: The progression of mild idiopathic dementia in a community population, *J Am Geriatr Soc* 39(3):246-251, 1991.

Glossary

A-1 pulley Located at the volar aspect of the metacarpophalangeal joints, it is where the flexor tendons often are constricted in the tunnel below.

abscess Localized collection of pus.

accessory collateral ligament of the proximal interphalangeal joint The PIP joint collateral ligament has two components: the accessory collateral ligament and the proper collateral ligament. The fibers of the accessory collateral ligament insert more volarly on the volar plate. The fibers of the proper collateral ligament insert more volarly and distally on the middle phalanx lateral tubercles.

action tremor An involuntary movement that occurs with intentional use of the extremity and tends to be quiet at rest. Also known as *essential tremor.*

adhesion Attachment of scar tissue to surrounding tissue such as tendon, ligament, fascia, or joint capsule.

adhesive capsulitis Condition characterized by progressive loss of shoulder motion. Also known as "frozen shoulder."

agonists The muscles most directly involved in bringing about a movement. Also known as prime movers.

allodynia Pain from sources that generally do not cause pain; for example, severe burning from a light touch of the involved area.

amyoplasia Absence of development of a muscle during the intrauterine period.

anatomic snuff box The dorsal surface area that lies just distal to the radial styloid process. The tendons bordering it become more prominent when the thumb is extended. Any tenderness elicited on the floor of the snuffbox with palpation suggests a possible fracture of the scaphoid.

angiofibroblastic hyperplasia Pathologic alterations seen in the tissue of clients with the diagnosis of tendonitis. A change in the gross appearance of the tissue is visible.

angiofibroblastic tendinosis Another term for *angiofibroblastic hyperplasia* or for *tendinosis.*

angiogenesis The process of creating new vessels in the tissue of a healing open wound.

ankylosis The stiffening of a joint by disease, injury, or surgery.

annulus fibrosis The multilayered ligamentous exterior of the disk.

antagonists Muscles that assist in joint stabilization, protecting ligaments and cartilaginous surfaces from sustaining potentially destructive forces. The antagonist opposes the agonist. It can slow down or stop the movement.

anterior interosseous syndrome An entrapment neuropathy of the motor branch of the median nerve.

antideformity position Wrist is extended or neutral, metacarpophalangeal joints are flexed, interphalangeal joints are extended, and thumb is abducted with opposition. This position keeps length on the collateral ligaments, which are vulnerable to shortening following injury and swelling. Also known as the *intrinsic-plus position.*

ape hand deformity Classic posture that results from loss of median nerve integrity. It is characterized by loss of thumb opposition and palmar abduction, with the thumb sitting in the same plane as the hand.

aphasia A language disorder resulting from a neurologic impairment that can affect auditory comprehension and oral expression.

arteriole The smallest artery in the body. It often supplies the capillaries and becomes part of the capillary.

arteriole hydrostatic pressure The pressure the blood fluid within the arteriole exerts against the vessel walls.

arthrogryposis multiplex congenita Joint stiffness due to maldevelopment of multiple musculoskeletal tissues (e.g., bones, joints, muscles, ligaments, nerves) involving several areas of the limbs.

arthrokinematics The movement of articular surfaces and movement around a mechanical axis. This is the movement that takes place within the joint.

articular cartilage The hyaline cartilage that lines the ends of articulating bones. Hyaline or articular cartilage has no nerve supply and no blood supply; therefore it depends on joint motion (which bathes it with the rich, nutritious synovial fluid found in the joint capsule) to maintain health.

athetosis Jerky, involuntary, movements of the proximal limb muscles due to cerebral injury during delivery.

authenticity Operating from a core of sincerity and honesty regarding oneself. Being true to oneself and honoring one's own values and unique individuality. Knowing how one's personal attributes can contribute positively to the care of the client.

autonomic instability Sympathetic nervous system irritation.

avulsion injury Forceful pulling away of a piece of bone by the tendon or collateral ligament where it attaches to the bone.

axial skeleton Skeletal components consisting of the skull, rib cage, spine, and pelvis.

axon A process that emerges from the soma of the neuron (at the axon hillock) and that extends to target cells. It transmits action potentials or nerve signals. Typically information travels away from the cell body by way of the axon. Axons can be myelinated or unmyelinated.

axonotmesis A compression lesion to a nerve in which the axons distal to the lesion degenerate. The endoneurial tubes remain, however, so there is typically complete recovery of function.

axoplasmic flow The flow of axoplasm or (cytoplasm) within the axon of the peripheral nerve. The three main flows are fast antegrade flow, slow antegrade flow, and retrograde flow. The role of the axoplasm in nerve homeostasis includes transport of neurotransmitters and transmitter vesicles for use in transmission of impulses at the synapse and carrying recycled transmitter vesicles from the nerve terminal to the soma.

Ballentine's sign The collapse of the distal interphalangeal joints of the thumb and index and long digits when attempting to pinch; it may indicate a neuropathy of the forearm motor branch of the median nerve.

Bankart lesion A lesion consisting of damage to the anterior glenohumeral capsule and glenoid labrum as a result of anterior glenohumeral dislocation.

basal cell carcinoma A malignant epithelial tumor.

base The proximal end of the metacarpal or phalangeal bone.

Bennett's fracture dislocation Intraarticular, unstable, two-fragment fractures of the base of the thumb metacarpal that result in dislocation or subluxation of the carpometacarpal joint of the thumb.

biaxial ellipsoid joint A type of synovial joint that has two axes of motion. An example is the radiocarpal joint, which allows for flexion/extension and radial/ulnar deviation.

bicepital aponeurosis The fibrous tissue that is a continuation of the distal biceps tendon that inserts into the flexor-pronator musculature. It can be palpated medial to the distal biceps tendon with the elbow in resisted flexion and the forearm in supination.

bicondylar Having two condyles.

Bier blocks The arm is exsanguinated with a compression bandage, followed by the inflation of a tourniquet applied proximal to the region involved; and then an intravenous agent (usually a numbing and sympatholytic agent) is injected into the region.

bifocal Referring to fractures consisting of two fracture lines.

blocked exercises Exercises in which proximal support is provided to promote isolated motion at a particular site. Blocked exercises exert more force than nonblocked active range of motion.

body dysmorphic disorder Preoccupation with imagined or innocent variations in appearance.

bony mallet finger injury A fracture of the terminal phalanx of the digit with accompanying terminal extensor tendon injury.

Bouchard's nodes The bony outgrowths at the proximal interphalangeal joints commonly seen in osteoarthritis.

boutonniere deformity Finger posture with proximal interphalangeal joint flexion and distal interphalangeal joint hyperextension. The pathologic condition occurs to the dorsal surface.

bowler's thumb A fibrous enlargement of the nerve from repeated trauma of the thumb against the bowling ball.

bowstringing A tendon that is not supported firmly in place by the pulley system as it crosses a joint and pulls away from the joint as the tendon is being pulled proximally. The tendon strains against the skin, creating the effect of a bowstring.

boxer's fractures Extraarticular fractures of the neck of the metacarpals of the hand; they occur most often at the fourth and fifth metacarpals.

bradykinesia A slowness of voluntary movement and speech.

brawny edema   Firm, thick edema that does not move or become depressed with pressure.

bursa   A fluid-filled sac that decreases friction between structures.

bursitis   Inflammation of the bursa.

calor   A term meaning heat.

camptodactyly   Congenital flexion contracture of a joint in contrast to clinodactyly in which the joint is laterally or medially deviated.

capitellum   The distal lateral articulation of the elbow joint. It articulates with the radial head.

capsular plication   Capsular shortening by suturing or tacking a fold in the articular capsule.

caring moment   The occasion when the therapist and client come together with their unique life histories and enter into the human-to-human transaction in a given focal point in space and time.

caritas   Derived from the Greek word meaning to cherish, appreciate, and give special attention, if not loving attention, to; it connotes something that is very fine, that indeed is precious.

carpal tunnel release   A surgical procedure to decompress the median nerve in the carpal tunnel by cutting the transverse carpal ligament.

carpal tunnel syndrome   Median nerve compression at the carpal tunnel of the wrist.

carpometacarpal boss   An osteoarthritic spur at the base of the second or third carpometacarpal joint. The boss is more evident as a prominent, firm, bony, tender mass when the wrist is flexed.

carpometacarpal interposition arthroplasty   Positioning of a donor tendon or implant in the carpometacarpal joint space usually to stabilize the joint capsule. This is done most often in cases of osteoarthritis at the carpometacarpal joint.

carrying angle of the elbow   The normal valgus presentation of the elbow as the hand deviates away from the body when the upper extremity is observed in anatomic position.

cellulitis   A superficial infection involving the skin and subcutaneous tissue without any localized abscess or pus.

central extensor tendon   Part of the proximal interphalangeal joint dorsal tendon; it attaches to the middle phalanx at the dorsal tubercle.

cerebral palsy   Paralysis of muscles due to brain injury at birth.

cerebral vascular accident   A pathologic condition in which there is a compromise to the cerebral vasculature or blood supply to the brain.

chip bags   Bags containing small pieces of foam of various densities. They are placed inside pressure garments or low-stretch bandages or splints to reduce edema and soften indurated areas.

chondroblasts   Cells that form cartilage; immature chondrocytes.

chondrocytes   Cartilage cells; the functional unit of cartilage.

chronic fatigue syndrome, or chronic fatigue and immune dysfunction syndrome   Fatigue that is unexplained by other diagnoses, persists for more than 6 months, has a definite time of onset, results in decreased activity level but may not be due to ongoing exertion, and is not substantially relieved by rest. At least four minor criteria also must be present.

claw hand deformity   The fourth and fifth digits (in particular) posture into hyperextension at metacarpophalangeal joints and flexion at the interphalangeal joints, which is indicative of an ulnar nerve palsy. This indicates an intrinsic muscle paresis.

clenched fist syndrome   Clients present with tightly curled fingers that are stiff and resist extension. The thumb and index fingers often are spared, enabling the client to maintain a level of function with the involved hand.

clenched fist injury   A wound occurring from a fist to the mouth.

client self-report outcome measures   A questionnaire; a highly structured form of interview designed for the collection of data.

clinodactyly   Congenital medial or lateral deviation of a finger joint in contrast to camptodactyly, in which there is congenital flexion contracture of finger joints.

close packed position   Joint position in which the capsule and ligaments are under the most tension with maximal contact between joint surfaces.

closed chain exercises   Exercises where movement occurs from muscle insertion to origin and the terminal joint is constrained in a fixed position.

cogwheeling   A movement common with clients with Parkinson's disease. It is identified as jerky movements and is considered rigidity superimposed on tremor.

collagen   The most abundant protein in the human body. It is the fundamental component of connective tissue, including fascia, fibrous cartilage, tendon, ligaments, bone, joint capsules, blood vessels, adipose tissue, and dermis.

collateral ligaments   Main restraints to lateral and medial deviation forces. At the proximal interphalangeal joint, they are 2 to 3 mm thick. They are important to the medial-lateral stability of the joint. The two components are the proper collateral ligament and the accessory collateral ligament, which are differentiated by their areas of insertion. The former inserts into bone, the latter into volar plate.

collector lymphatic A three-celled lymphatic vessel having bicuspid-shaped valves every 6 to 8 mm that conduct lymph proximally in the body.

Colles' fracture A complete fracture of the distal radius with dorsal displacement of the distal fragment and radius shortening. It is usually extraarticular, minimally displaced, and stable.

compartment syndrome Compartment refers to closed space for flexor or extensor muscles in the forearm or hand. Syndrome refers to excessive pressure in the compartment that causes vascular compromise of muscles.

complex regional pain syndrome A pain syndrome that can occur after an initiating noxious event or after a nerve injury. The disorder manifests with spontaneous pain that is disproportionate to the initial event, evidence of edema, skin blood flow abnormality, or abnormal sweating. Formerly known as reflex sympathetic dystrophy.

complex tasks Nonrepetitive movements that require input of cognitive processes.

composite motions Combined motions of the wrist, metacarpophalangeal joints, and interphalangeal joints.

compression neuropathy Compression of a peripheral nerve in the limb; it may cause motor or sensory problems.

concentric Muscle contraction resulting in approximation of the origin and insertion.

conditioned responses Cardiovascular, respiratory, gastrointestinal, or immunologic responses that are triggered by heightened perception of environmental stimuli.

condyles The medial and lateral portions of the distal humerus. These regions are proximal to the epicondyles, which are the medial and lateral protrusions of the distal humerus.

congenital clasped thumb Thumb positioned (clasped) into the palm of varied severity and etiologies at birth.

construct validity A comparison between a new measure and an associated measure.

content validity Accurate measurement of a specific domain.

conversion disorder A bodily event such as a seizure or paralysis that is psychological in origin.

cords The pathologic thickening and contracted palmar fascia.

coronoid fossa The volar indentation of the distal humerus that houses the coronoid process of the proximal ulna.

covalent bonds Strong chemical bonds formed by the sharing of a pair of electrons. Mature collagen is stronger than immature collagen because of its covalent bonds.

Cozen's Test The examiner's thumb stabilizes the client's elbow at the lateral epicondyle. With the forearm pronated, the client makes a fist and actively extends the wrist and radially deviates it with the examiner resisting the motion. Severe and sudden pain at the lateral epicondyle area indicates a positive test.

crepitus Grating or popping as the digit flexes and extends.

criterion validity The comparison of a new measure with a gold standard that has been demonstrated as valid for the target population.

cross-bridges In the sarcomere of a muscle cell, the portion of the myosin filaments that pulls the actin filaments toward the center of the sarcomere during muscle contraction.

crush syndrome Compartment syndrome caused by crushing of the arm or leg from heavy building structures in earthquakes and war.

cubital tunnel The groove between the medial epicondyle and the olecranon of the elbow.

cubital tunnel syndrome Compression of the ulnar nerve as it passes through the groove between the medial epicondyle and the olecranon of the ulna.

cutaneous fibrous histiocytoma See *dermatofibroma.*

cyanosis Blue tinge to the skin.

de Quervain's disease Disease evident by pain over the radial styloid process that can radiate proximally or distally. Pain also occurs with resisted thumb extension or abduction, and Finklestein's test frequently is positive. Also known as stenosing tenovaginitis or stenosing tenosynovitis.

degrees of freedom Direction or type of motion at a joint.

dehiscence Wound separation, or the rupture of the sides of an incision.

delta phalanx The extra triangular bone between the proximal and distal phalanx of the thumb found in clinodactyly of the thumb.

demyelinating An inflammatory process that disrupts the myelin sheath that surrounds and insulates the axon of some nerves. The myelin sheath speeds up the signal transmission of the axons and protects the nerve cells.

dendrites Processes that extend from the soma of the neuron and that conduct information toward the cell body. These are the input units of the nerve cell. They are typically tree-shaped processes that receive messages from adjacent neurons.

dermatofibroma An epithelial tumor composed of fibroblastic cells and some scattered histiocytes.

dermofasciectomy Removal of the diseased tissue and the overlying skin.

desensitization The systematic process of applying nonnoxious stimuli to peripheral tissues to reeducate and retrain the nervous system.

diaphragmatic breathing A form of breathing in which air is brought in through the nose with a closed mouth, filling primarily the lower thoracic area. This engages the diaphragm in exhalation and inhalation. The movement of the diaphragm causes thoracic pressure changes in the lower thoracic duct and conducts lymph more proximal within the duct.

diaphysis The central shaft of the bone composed of cortical or dense bone.

diathesis A bodily condition that predisposes someone to a particular disease.

differential digital tendon gliding exercises Exercises used differentially to exercise the flexor muscles. They are a mainstay of conservative management of carpal tunnel syndrome.

digital stenosing tenosynovitis Trigger finger.

directional preference Direction of motion that reduces or centralizes radiating pain of spinal origin.

disease A physiologic or anatomic impairment in the function of a structure or biochemical process.

disease-specific measures Client self-report outcome measures that are intended to be highly responsive for individual diagnoses.

disk herniations Damage to the annular wall of the disk resulting in disk deformity as the nucleus displaces into the lesion.

dissimulation A phenomenon in which clients with somatization disorder become convinced that they have a life-threatening or incapacitating disease or injury.

distal arthrogryposis Limited involvement of the fingers, hand, and wrist and not proximal joints.

distal humerus Distal portion of the humerus that is also the proximal articulation for the elbow joint.

distal interphalangeal extensor lag A finger posture in which the distal interphalangeal joint droops, the client is not able actively to extend the distal interphalangeal joint, but the joint can be corrected passively to neutral.

distal interphalangeal flexion contracture A finger posture in which the distal interphalangeal joint droops and cannot be extended passively to neutral.

distal radioulnar joint The articulation between the distal radius and the distal ulna.

distal transverse arch of the hand The more distal of the two bony transverse arches of the hand. These mobile arches contribute to the normal resting posture (palmar concavity) of the hand and to normal hand function. The distal transverse arch is located at the heads of the digit metacarpals.

dolor A term meaning pain.

dorsal retinacular ganglion The ganglion attached to the first extensor compartment. The client with this ganglion usually has symptoms of de Quervain's tenosynovitis.

dorsal wrist ganglion A ganglion that usually originates from the vicinity of the scapholunate ligament. The most common site for a ganglion cyst is the dorsal radial wrist.

double crush syndrome An irritation to a nerve in more than one place. Minor serial impingements along a nerve have been proposed to have an additive effect that can cause a nerve entrapment lesion distal to the initial lesion site.

dynamic splints Splints that use moving parts such as rubber bands or spring wires to apply a gentle force.

dyscoordinate co-contraction Poor quality of movement that can result from co-contraction of antagonist muscles.

dysesthesias Impairment in sensation.

dyskinesias Distortion of voluntary movements with involuntary muscular activity.

dysphagia Difficulty in swallowing.

eccentric Muscle contraction to stabilize movement resulting in increased distance between the origin and insertion.

ecchymosis Skin discoloration caused by the escape of blood into the tissues from ruptured blood vessels.

ectopic bone formation Pathologic bone growth where it does not belong. It can lead to pain and significant loss of range of motion.

edema A term meaning swelling.

ego self The part of one's self that is focused on the self.

elastic mobilization splints See *dynamic splints*.

Elbow Flexion Test A provocative maneuver designed to reproduce symptoms of ulnar nerve compressin. The elbow is fully flexed for up to 5 minutes; a positive test is symptom reproduction.

Elevated Arm Stress Test Special test used to detect the presence of neurovascular compromise in the thoracic outlet. Abbreviated EAST.

empathy Trying to put oneself in the client's place and identifying with a client's situation in a caring way, without condescension or pitying of the client.

enchondral ossification The process by which the interpositional callus bone (that forms during the second repair stage of bone healing following fracture) gradually is converted to bone tissue by a process of mineralization.

enchondromas The most common primary bone tumors of hand bones; benign cartilaginous lesions. They compose 90% of bone tumors.

endoneurium   The basement membrane that surrounds peripheral nerve fibers. It is closely packed together and serves electrically to insulate axons from each other.

energy conservation   Simplification of a task or activity to minimize the amount of energy used.

epidermal inclusion cyst   Cyst that occurs following injury in which a segment of keratinizing epithelium is forced into subcutaneous tissue, where it produces keratin and becomes a tumor. It occurs most often in men who are between 30 and 40 years of age, with the most common site being the distal phalanx of the left thumb and long finger.

epineurium   The external protective connective tissue covering that surrounds the nerve trunk. It is the outermost covering that functions to surround and cushion nerve fascicles.

epiphyseal distraction (chondrodiastasis)   A method to remodel and align a fracture.

epiphysis   The end of a long bone. This part of the bone is composed primarily of cancellous or spongy bone tissue.

epitendinous suture   Used with pediatric flexor tendon repair to promote easy gliding, reduce gap formation, and for additional strength.

eponychia   An infection that entails the entire eponychium along with one lateral fold. The pus collection usually occurs near the lunula.

equanimity   The quality of being calm and even-tempered, with patience or firmness of mind under stress.

erythema   More redness than usual in the coloration of the skin.

eschar   A thick layer of necrotic collagen over a wound, usually black or dark brown.

essential tremor   The most common movement disorder in which the characteristic tremor occurs with intentional use of the extremity and tends to be quiet at rest. Also known as an *action tremor.*

Essex Lopresti fracture   Fracture of the radial head plus dislocation of the distal radial ulnar joint. It also involves disruption of the interosseous membrane.

extension outrigger splint   A splint created to support the finger in extension that permits a controlled amount of flexion to allow tendon gliding. Slings with elastic attachments support the fingers in extension. An outrigger, or attachment to the sling, is used to direct the angle of pull of the slings.

extensor habitus   Habitual posturing in digital extension. Especially common at the index finger, this posturing can lead to stiffness and functional limitations.

extensor tendon adhesion   The development of restrictive attachments of surrounding scar tissue to the extensor tendon, preventing or limiting gliding of the extensor tendon.

external fixator   A manufactured device for maintaining fracture alignment. It consists of pins, wires, or screws, and it attaches the appropriately aligned and stabilized injured bone to its external low-profile scaffold.

extraarticular   Outside a joint.

extraarticular fractures   Bone fractures that do not involve the joint surfaces.

extracellular matrix   The network of fibrous and fluid material that is excreted by, surrounds, and supports living cells. It is critical to cellular growth and maintenance.

extrinsic extensor tightness   Passive proximal interphalangeal joint/distal interphalangeal joint flexion that is limited when the metacarpophalangeal joint is flexed passively.

extrinsic muscles   Longer muscle-tendon units originating proximal to the hand.

extrinsic tendon tightness   Condition that prevents a normal amount of finger flexion, most notably when the wrist is flexed. The extrinsic tendons are those that originate proximal to the wrist and insert within the hand. Because the extrinsic tendons cross the wrist, when the wrist moves, it will create tightness or slackness in the tendons at the wrist.

exudate   Drainage from a wound that is characterized by a creamy or yellow coloration because of sloughed cells, increased phagocytic activity, and higher protein level.

exudate edema   Edema that is filled with plasma protein molecules.

facet joints   Paired synovial joints of the spine consisting of the articulation between the superior and inferior facets of adjacent vertebrae.

factitious disorders   Disorders that arise out of a psychological need to be sick rather than a conscious effort for material gain. Clients with factitious disorders knowingly cause their own disease but are unaware of the underlying reasons for their behavior.

fasciculations   A muscle twitch, or a small, visible contraction of muscles representing a spontaneous discharge of a number of fibers innervated by a single motor unit.

fasciculus   A bundle of pathway axons within the central nervous system.

fasciectomy   The excision of fascia and palmar aponeurosis.

fasciotomy   The removal of pathologic palmar fascia.

felon   A deep infection of the finger pad involving the tiny compartments of the pulp. Felons are painful.

fibroblasts Cells that respond to mechanical stimulus by producing type I collagen fibers that are found in tendons, ligaments, and joint capsules. They also produce glycosaminoglycans.

fibrolipoma Lipoma with a connective tissue component.

fibromas of the tendon sheath Painless solid tumors that grow slowly over time. Histologically, this tumor has no giant cells.

fibromyalgia A pain syndrome affecting the entire musculoskeletal system. Symptoms include chronic widespread musculoskeletal pain, sleep disturbances, morning stiffness, fatigue, anxiety, and depressive symptoms. The syndrome is often difficult to diagnose.

fibroplasia phase The reparative phase of healing, during which time new tissue is laid down in the wound. The phase begins about day 4 following injury and lasts 2 to 6 weeks. Fibroblasts synthesize scar tissue, with gradual increase of tensile strength. Also known as the *fibroplasia stage*.

fibroplasia stage See *fibroplasia phase*.

fight bite See *clenched-fist injury*.

filariasis Found primarily in the Southern Hemisphere from infected mosquitoes injecting larvae into the bloodstream. The larvae can grown into filarial worms 20 cm long and can destroy lymph nodes and vessels when they die, resulting in severe lymphedema.

flaccidity A form of paralysis in which muscles lack tone. Also known as *hypotonicity*.

flexor tendon adhesions Restrictive attachments of surrounding scar tissue to the flexor tendon, preventing or limiting gliding of the flexor tendon.

fluidotherapy A dry heating device that uses light (sandlike) particles that float around in a heated air environment to warm the extremity, allow motion in the warmth, and help to desensitize sensitive areas.

FOOSH Acronym for a *fall* on *outstretched* *hand*.

force couple Two resultant forces of equal magnitude in opposite directions that produce rotation of a structure.

fracture An impairment of the mechanical integrity of the skeleton that typically leads to functional deficits and pain.

Froment's sign An indicator of an ulnar nerve lesion; one sees flexion of the interphalangeal joint of the thumb as the flexor pollicis longus attempts to compensate for the paralyzed or weak adductor pollicis during lateral pinch.

functional proximal interphalangeal joint stability Joint stability that can be tested actively and passively. If the client demonstrates normal active range of motion (i.e., no subluxation at the proximal interphalangeal joint), there is adequate functional stability of the joint. If, however, there is subluxation with active range of motion, this suggests that major ligament disruption probably has occurred.

functional somatic syndrome A physical illness that is not explained by an organic disease or structural lesion or biochemical change.

fusiform swelling Having tapering at both ends.

Galeazzi's fracture A radial shaft fracture occurring between the middle and distal third of the radius. It also involves a dislocation of the distal radial ulnar joint.

gamekeeper's thumb Acute or chronic ulnar collateral ligament instability of the thumb metacarpophalangeal joint.

ganglion cyst A synovial cyst that arises from the synovial lining of a joint or tendon sheath.

gate theory A hypothesis first proposed by Melzack and Wall in the mid-1960s. It stated that stimulation of the large, myelinated nonnociceptive, A-beta sensory fibers would flood the main pain pathway to higher centers of the brain, effectively gating off pain signals to the cortex and thereby diminishing the perception of pain.

gel sheets Silicone-based sheets of various thicknesses that can be applied to a sensitive area or scar to decrease pressure and touch sensations and to improve appearance and texture of the scar.

generic measures Client self-report outcome measures that are used to compare health conditions and therefore can assist in the analysis of policies and funds distribution.

giant cell tumor The most common solid tumor of the hand. The tumor is grayish-brown with yellow patches. Despite its name, the giant cell tumor does not tend to be located at a tendon sheath and does not contain exclusively giant cells. Also known as *localized nodular tenosynovitis*, *localized pigmented villonodular synovitis*, and *xanthoma*.

ginglymus joint A hinge joint.

glomus body An arteriovenous anastomosis that functions as a thermoregulator and is located in the skin.

glomus tumor Tumor arising from the neuromyoarterial apparatus or the glomus body. It tends to occur subungually (beneath the nail) and in distal finger pads. It causes cold sensitivity, lancing pain, and tenderness. Over time, glomus tumors can lead to erosion of bone.

glycosaminoglycans Monomer proteoglycans produced by fibroblasts and occupying the interstitial space between collagen fibers to provide lubrication and nutrition to the collagen fibers.

gold standard   The best available test to diagnose a condition.

Golgi tendon organ   A spindle-shaped structure at the junction of a muscle and a tendon. The organ senses muscle tension through tendon stretch and inhibits muscular contraction of the agonists and facilitates contraction of the antagonists.

gout   A group of diseases resulting from monosodium urate crystal deposition in the tissues or uric acid in the extracellular fluids.

granulation tissue   The tissue that forms in an open wound and is composed of new collagen and capillary growth, resulting in red coloration. Reepithelialization occurs over granulation tissue in open wounds.

grasp   Involves holding an object between the fingers and palm.

grating   Similar to crepitus and usually at a joint.

grind test   Assessment usually done at the thumb carpometacarpal joint to determine damaged cartilage. The carpometacarpal joint is compressed, and the head of the metacarpal is pressed and gently rotated against the trapezium. Pain and crepitus are positive findings.

ground substance   See *extracellular matrix*.

gunstock deformity   Varus carry angle of the elbow seen in posttraumatic conditions. A loss of the normal carry angle and valgus elbow presentation occur. It is observed as the forearm deviates toward the body while the upper extremity is observed in anatomic position.

Guyon's canal   A superficial passageway between the pisiform and hamate bones of the carpus through which the ulnar nerve and artery pass as they enter the hand.

hard end-feel   Quality of unyielding at passive joint end-range. This is a stiffer joint and less favorable for potential to improve.

head   The distal end of the metacarpal or phalangeal bone.

Heberden's nodes   The bony outgrowths at the distal interphalangeal joints commonly seen in osteoarthritis.

hemangioma   A benign tumor of dilated blood vessels.

hematoma   A confined mass of blood.

hemiarthroplasty   Prosthetic replacement of one joint surface.

hemiparesis   Muscular weakness or partial paralysis restricted to one side of the body.

hemiplegia   Full or partial paralysis of one side of the body.

hemorrhagic   Interruption of the blood supply caused by a break or rupture of a blood vessel in the brain.

Hill-Sachs lesion   A lesion consisting of an osseous defect of the posterolateral portion of the humeral head, caused during traumatic anterior dislocation.

Hoffman-Tinel sign   See *Tinel's sign*.

homeostasis   The condition in which the internal environment of the body remains within certain physiologic limits. Disease is homeostatic imbalance.

homonymous hemianopsia   Loss of visual field in the corresponding right or left half of each eye.

hope   A positive attitude or orientation toward the future.

Horner's sign   Drooping eyelid, constriction of the pupil, redness, and warming of the ipsilateral side of the face often caused from anesthesia to the stellate ganglion.

hydrophilic   Attraction of water molecules, as is the function of plasma proteins in the interstitium.

hyperalgesia   A magnified response to a painful stimulus.

hyperalgia   Increased response to a painful stimulus.

hyperhydrosis   Abnormal sweating often seen along nerve distribution or in an atypical place.

hypermobility   Joint movement that takes place around a physiologic axis but is more than normal.

hyperpathia   Pain that persists after the removal of noxious stimulus; pain that is disproportionately increased by a stimulus, especially a repetitive stimulus.

hypersensitivity   When one experiences pain in response to nonnoxious stimuli.

hypertonicity   A condition in which the muscle is constantly tensed because of increased tone.

hypochondriasis   Excessive concern about minor health disturbances or worry over the possibility of future ill health.

hypomobility   Joint movement that takes place around a physiologic axis but is less than normal.

hypoplasia   Defective development of tissue.

hypotonicity   A form of paralysis in which muscles lack tone. Also known as *flaccidity*.

illness   A client's personal experience of his or her poor health.

imbibition   Primary means of obtaining nutrition for avascular tissues.

immediate active motion   Following a tendon repair, exercises that incorporate an active component of the repaired musculotendinous unit, generally begun within 5 days after repair.

immediate passive motion   Following a tendon repair, exercises that incorporate passive motion in the direction of the tendon repair, generally begun within 5 days after repair.

impingement   Compression of soft tissue structures between bony structures.

indurated   Hardening of tissue such as caused by long-standing congested lymph nodes.

inflammatory phase   See *inflammatory stage*.

inflammatory stage The initial stage of wound healing composed of the immediate vascular and cellular response in an attempt to clear the wound of debris or necrotic tissue. The completion of the inflammatory stage of wound healing facilitates the repair phase of wound healing. Also known as the *inflammatory phase*.

initial lymphatic The smallest of all lymphatic vessels and most superficial in the dermis layer of tissue. It is one cell thick and is lined with overlapping oak leaf–shaped endothelial cells.

innervation density The number of nerve endings in an area.

instability When joint motion occurs around a non-physiologic axis.

intention tremors Rhythmic shaking that occurs in the course of a purposeful movement, such as reaching for an object.

interactional synchrony The way in which two persons behave in pattern and synchrony during a given interaction. Behaviors in the interaction may be nonrandom and patterned after one another in timing and in pattern. For example, when one party leans forward, the other person then leans forward as well.

interosseous muscle tightness Passive proximal interphalangeal joint/distal interphalangeal joint flexion that is limited when the metacarpophalangeal joint is extended or hyperextended passively.

interstitium On a capillary level, the space between the cells.

intervertebral foramen Bony canal that contains the spinal nerve.

intraarticular fractures Bone fractures that involve the joint surfaces.

intracapsular The region within the ligamentous joint capsule.

intraneural scarring Scarring contained within the nerve.

intrathecal/epidural blocks Indwelling or intermittent boluses of local anesthetic and opioid.

intrinsic muscles Small muscles located in the hand.

intrinsic tightness Tightness of the interossei and lumbrical tendons, which originate and insert within the hand. These tendons run volar to the axis of motion at the metacarpophalangeal joint and dorsal to the axis of motion at the interphalangeal joints. Tightness within these tendons limits the position that stretches them, that of metacarpophalangeal joint extension and interphalangeal joint flexion.

intrinsic-plus position Metacarpophalangeal joint flexion with interphalangeal joint extension. Also known as the *safe position*.

ischemia Low-oxygen state; a condition of decreased blood flow to an area. Long-term ischemia may lead to hypoxia and tissue death.

ischemic Insufficient blood supply.

isometric maximum The amount of force that can be maintained by an isometric contraction for 1 second (1 IM).

isotonic contractions Contraction with muscle shortening.

Jeanne's sign An indicator of the presence of adductor pollicis weakness, possibly from an ulnar nerve paralysis.

joint contracture Passive limitation of joint motion.

joint tightness Condition confirmed when the passive range of motion of a joint does not change despite repositioning of proximal or distal joints.

juncturae tendinum Slips of extensor tendon that attach the ring finger extensor tendon to the extensor tendons of the adjacent finger and variably the middle finger tendon to the index finger tendon.

Kanavel's cardinal signs Four signs indicating flexor tenosynovitis: (1) posture with flight digital flexion, (2) uniform volar swelling of the involved digit, (3) tenderness along the tendon sheath, and (4) pain with passive extension of the involved digit.

Keinbock's disease Avascular necrosis of the lunate carpal bone. Manifestations of avascular necrosis include bony sclerosis and osteopenia.

kinesthesia Awareness of the position of body parts in space provided to the central nervous system by proprioceptors, the sensory receptors in muscles, joints, and tendons that monitor length/tension of the musculotendinous complex. Also known as kinesthetic awareness.

Kirner's deformity A specific skeletal deformity characterized by progressive palmar and radial curvature of the distal phalanx of the small finger. The presence of dorsovolar curvature distinguishes Kirner's deformity from clinodactyly of the small finger.

knowing the client Connecting with the client in an intentional and meaningful way; this can take place even within a limited time frame; understanding of the needs of the client and how the client's life as a whole is affect by the client's health condition and treatment.

lability A state of having notable shifts in emotional state, often following a neurologic insult. This frequently presents as uncontrolled crying or laughing.

lag When passive range of motion exceeds active range of motion at a joint.

lateral bands Bands that originate volar to the metacarpophalangeal joint axis. They have intrinsic muscle contributions and join dorsal to the proximal interphalangeal joint axis. They unite to form the terminal extensor tendon.

learned nonuse The phenomenon that commonly occurs when persons who have sustained an injury compensate for their loss by not engaging the affected extremity in activity or rote movements.

Likert scale   A summative scale based on responses to a set of statements; ratings of agreement or disagreement.

limited or selective fasciectomy   Surgical excision of only presently diseased tissue.

lipoma   A common tumor consisting of mature fat cells, characterized by its soft consistency when palpated. Lipomas can occur anywhere that fatty tissue exists, but they occur most commonly in the deep palmar space of the hand.

Lister's tubercle   A bony prominence located at the distal dorsal end of the radius. The extensor pollicis longus tendon passes around the ulnar side of this tubercle.

localized nodular tenosynovitis   See *giant cell tumor.*

localized pigmented villonodular synovitis   See *giant cell tumor.*

locking   During active range of motion, locking of the digit in flexion as the tendon fails to pass through the pulley. The finger usually can be straightened passively.

longitudinal arch of the hand   The longitudinally oriented bony arch of the hand that is composed of a fixed or rigid portion apparent at the carpometacarpal joint of the middle finger.

longitudinal radial ray deficiency   A hand that is radially deviated at the distal forearm in the shape of a golf club. See *radial club hand.*

low transcolumn   The region that involves fractures of the condyles of the distal humerus.

lunula   The white arch visible at the base of some fingernails.

lymph   In the extremities, a clear yellowish fluid filled with water molecules and large molecular substances such as plasma proteins, fat cells, hormones, minerals, ions, bacteria, and tissue waste products.

lymph bundles   Groupings of small lymphatic vessels—that is, the initial lymphatics and collector lymphatics—that generally do not include lymph nodes.

lymph capillary   See *initial lymphatic.*

lymph nodes   Round, oval, or kidney-shaped structures ranging from pin head to olive in size. They are a part of the lymph system with a complex of internal sinuses that are responsible for immunologic functions and filtration of lymph.

lymphangioma   A tumor of lymphatic vessels.

lymphangion   The chamber or space between the valves in the collector lymphatic. As the chamber fills and stretches, the one cell of smooth muscle contracts, and lymph is propelled proximally into the next lymphangion.

lymphangitis   A serious hand infection that progresses rapidly. Although it is much less common than cellulitis, lymphangitis can lead to a generalized infection within just a few hours. Red streaking up the hand and forearm occurs along the lymphatic pathways, and an abscess may form at the elbow or axilla if the problem is left untreated. The causative organism is typically *Streptococcus.*

lymphedema   A permanent loss, destruction, damage, or removal of lymphatic vessels (i.e., lymph nodes) that results in some degree of permanent swelling or potential for swelling. In the United States the term commonly is associated with lymphedema resulting from lymphadenectomy, primary lymph node radiation, or filariasis lymphedema.

lymphotomes   Superficial anatomic lymphatic drainage areas of the body, similar to the concept of dermatomes but not the same areas on tissue.

lymph-venous anastomoses   A joining of small lymphatic and venous vessels.

macrophage   Specific type of cell present in the inflammatory and early fibroplasia phases of wound healing that assists in cleaning the wound of necrotic tissue and debris.

malignant melanoma   Tumor that arises from the melanocytes of the epidermis.

malingering   The intentional presentation of false or misleading health information for personal gain.

mallet finger   A finger posture in which the distal interphalangeal joint droops.

malunion   Growth of the fragments of a fractured bone in a faulty position, forming an imperfect union.

manipulation   Skillful or dextrous treatment or procedure involving use of the hands.

Mankopf's Test   The absence of a rise in heart rate of at least 5% on palpation of a reportedly painful area that suggests symptom magnification.

manual edema mobilization   A method of swelling reduction using light massage and active motion to improve the activity of the intact lymphatic system. The technique was developed by Sandra Artzberger.

manual lymphatic drainage   The manual decongesting of lymph through activating the lymph uptake through massage and low-stretch bandaging programs.

manual lymphatic treatment   A generic term used to describe massage principles for lymphedema that are common to all schools of lymphatic drainage.

maturation phase   Third phase of tissue healing. This phase can last months or years, with changing tissue architecture and improved organization of collagen fibers contributing to increased tensile strength.

mechanoreceptors Specialized nerve endings that transmit information regarding position and motion.

mesoneurium The loose areolar tissue that surrounds peripheral nerve trunks.

metabolites By-products of metabolism; any substance produced by metabolism.

micrographia A change in handwriting evident by uncontrolled small print that is illegible.

Mill's Tennis Elbow Test Originally described as a manipulation maneuver, the technique can be used as a clinical test instead. The client's shoulder is in neutral. The examiner palpates the most tender area at or near the lateral epicondyle and pronates the client's forearm and fully flexes the client's wrist while moving the elbow from flexion to extension. Pain at the lateral epicondyle is a positive finding.

mindfulness The act of paying attention in a particular, intentional way: on purpose, in the present moment, and nonjudgmentally.

minimal detectable change A valid change in score that is not due to chance.

minimally clinically important difference Meaningful change of self-report scores, indicating increased function.

mobilization splints See *dynamic splints*.

mononeuropathy Damage to a single nerve.

Monteggia's fracture A fracture of the proximal third of the ulna in association with anterior dislocation of the radial head.

mucous cyst Cyst ssociated with degenerative arthritis of the small joints of the hand. The distal interphalangeal joint is the most common site of occurrence. Clients are usually between the ages of 50 and 70. Nail longitudinal grooving may be an early clinical sign of a mucous cyst. The cyst is typically 3 to 5 mm and is situated between the dorsal distal interphalangeal joint crease and the eponychium, to one side of the extensor tendon.

multiarticulate Crossing multiple joints.

multiple chemical sensitivies or idiopathic environmental intolerance Having medically unexplained symptoms in response to low-level identifiable environmental exposures.

multiple mononeuropathy Multifocal asymmetric damage to multiple nerves.

multiple sclerosis A chronic and typically progressive demyelinating disease of the central nervous system.

Munchausen syndrome A practice in which clients may cut, bruise, bite, or inject their hands and then give an untruthful history to the medical professionals who care for them.

muscle fiber length equilibrium The length the muscle will maintain when it is unaffected by outside forces.

musculotendinous tightness Tightness confirmed when the passive range of motion of a joint changes with repositioning of adjacent joints that are crossed by that muscle-tendon unit.

myofibroblasts Cells that have a key role in tissue reconstruction after injury. They are highly specialized forms of fibroblasts. They contribute to wound contraction.

neck The area of the metacarpal between the head and the shaft.

negative intracapsular pressure Air pressure inside the joint capsule lower than pressure outside the capsule.

negative ulnar variance A condition in which the ulna is shorter than it should be compared with the radius. This can cause the radius to impinge on the proximal carpal row during forearm rotation and often leads to dorsal and radial wrist pain and an increase in the likelihood of distal radioulnar joint arthrosis developing.

nerve A bundle of pathway axons in the peripheral nervous system.

neural mobility The ability of the neural structures to adjust to changes in the nerve bed length through a combination of gliding and elongation.

neurilemoma Benign nerve tumor. Also known as a *schwannoma*.

neurofibroma Benign nerve tumor.

neurolysis The surgical removal of scar tissue from the nerve.

neuroma A spontaneously firing growth bud from damaged peripheral nerves. Tapping produces a radiating electric shock sensation in the distribution of the nerve.

neuromodulation Altering transmission of nerve impulses.

neuron The basic unit of the nervous system.

neuropathy Pathologic condition of the peripheral nerve.

neuroplasticity The ability of the brain to recover structurally and functionally after injury or disease by nerve cells taking over the function of nerve cells that are no longer functioning.

neuropraxia A local conduction block within a nerve trunk, typically from compression on the nerve.

neurotmesis A complete nerve severance or a nerve injury with such serious internal disorganization that no recovery is expected without surgical intervention.

nociceptive Free nerve endings that are within the mechanoreceptors and that react to painful stimuli.

nociceptors   Specialized nerve endings that transmit pain signals.

nodules   Thickened closed packed collections of cells and the primary pathologic manifestation of Dupuytren's contracture. Also often seen in *rheumatoid arthritis*.

nonunion   Failure of the bone to heal or fuse.

normative data   Client data that has been obtained from groups with specific diagnoses and ability levels.

nucleus pulposus   Pulpy semiliquid center of the disk.

oblique retinacular ligament   Ligament that originates from the flexor sheath, progressing volar to the proximal interphalangeal joint axis and inserting at the terminal extensor tendon dorsally. The oblique retinacular ligament tightens when the proximal interphalangeal joint extends. It provides concomitant proximal interphalangeal joint and distal interphalangeal joint extension and helps prevent hyperextension of the proximal interphalangeal joint.

oblique retinacular ligament tightness   With the proximal interphalangeal joint extended, passive distal interphalangeal joint flexion is limited.

occult dorsal carpal ganglion   Differs from a dorsal wrist ganglion by being small and difficult to palpate. This ganglion may be overlooked in examination. Palpating with the wrist in extreme volar flexion can be helpful. The occult dorsal carpal ganglion is usually disproportionately painful and may be the cause of undiagnosed wrist pain.

O'Donaghue's maneuver   A finding of active range of motion that is greater than passive range of motion, which raises the possibility of symptom magnification.

olecranon   The bony prominence located on the proximal ulna. This is the "point" of the elbow.

olecranon fossa   The channel that houses the olecranon.

oncotic/osmotic pressure   The pressure in the interstitium caused by plasma proteins.

open chain   Movement occurring from muscle origin to insertion with the terminal joint free.

open packed position   Joint position in which the capsule and ligaments are most lax and separation of the joint surfaces is greatest.

osteitis   Inflammation of bone.

osteoarthritis   A gradual loss of articular cartilage caused by degenerative joint disease and chemical factors.

osteoblasts   The functional building blocks of bone. These cells synthesize the organic compounds that mineralize into bone. They are found at the surface of bone tissue.

osteoclasts   Cells responsible for bone dissolution and absorption.

osteocytes   Mature osteoblasts.

osteoid matrix   The noncalcified matrix of young bone; a precursor to bone.

osteokinematics   The movement of the long bone about an axis (*osteo* means bone; *kinematics* is the study of motion).

osteomyelitis   Inflammation of bone and marrow.

osteophytes   Abnormal outgrowths of bone that occur within joints or at other sites where there is degeneration of cartilage. Otherwise known as bone spurs.

osteophytosis   New bone formation occurring as a result of joint erosion.

outrigger   The structure from which the forces of a static progressive or dynamic splint are directed. They can be high profile or low profile.

pallor   Whiter than normal coloration of the skin.

palmar aponeurosis   Normally occurring longitudinal fibrous sheet of the palm.

pannus   Formation of granulation tissue in synovial lining of persons with rheumatoid arthritis.

paresthesia   Abnormal sensation without objective cause, such as numbness, prickling, and tingling.

Parkinson's disease   A progressively debilitating disease that often eventually results in complete loss of independence in activities of daily living. This disease typically is characterized by tremor, rigidity, and bradykinesia.

paronychia   A bacterial infection of the nail fold or the nail plate. Paronychia is the most common hand infection. It may be acute or chronic. The organism in acute paronychia is usually *Staphylococcus aureus*. The organisms in chronic paronychia are usually *Candida albicans* and pyogenic bacteria.

pathway   A chain of communicating neurons in the nervous system. A fasciculus or a tract is a bundle of pathway axons in the central nervous system.

perineural scarring   Scarring between the nerve and the nerve bed.

perineurium   The middle connective tissue covering that surrounds each nerve fascicle. It is a mechanically strong sheath that serves as a diffusion barrier, helping to preserve the specialized microenvironment inside the fascicles.

perionychium   Perionychium is composed of the nail bed and the paronychium. Paronychium is soft tissue around the nail plate.

periosteum   The outer lining or sleeve that envelopes bones. It plays an integral part in bone healing following injury.

peripheral nerve stimulation   Similar to spinal cord simulation but the electrode is positioned in the peripheral nerve instead.

Peyronie's disease Dense fibrous tissue and contracture of the penis.

phagocyte A type of cell that can surround and digest bacteria and other foreign organisms that would be harmful to the body. These cells are essential to the clean-up aspect in the inflammation phase of wound healing.

phagocytosis Removal of dead tissue and foreign bodies.

Phalen's Test A provocative test designed to provoke median or ulnar nerve symptoms in the hand. The wrist is flexed for 60 seconds, and reports of numbness and tingling in the median or ulnar nerve distribution are documented. These symptoms may indicate possible sites of nerve irritation at the wrist. Also known as Wrist Flexion Test.

phasic muscles Muscles that are anaerobic and contract at higher speeds and with greater force than tonic muscles; they fatigue more quickly. They are better suited for short-duration, high-intensity activities.

physis Growth plate at the end of a bone. Injury to the physis can affect growth.

pillar pain Pain experienced on either side of a carpal tunnel incision.

pincer (pinch) grasp Grasping with thumb tip to finger tip.

pinch Grasping between any finger and the thumb.

pitting edema Soft edema that stays depressed after pressure placed on the edematous tissue has been removed. The depressed area is referred to as "pitting."

place and active hold Gentle application of active-assisted and passive range of motion with attempt by client to maintain that position gently after removing the passive assistance.

plane synovial joint Joint with a synovium-lined capsule and relatively flat surfaces.

play skills Involve cognitive input and musculoskeletal activity at different ages.

plexuses Networks of nerves. The human body has four plexuses; the two largest are the brachial plexus and the lumbar plexus.

plyometric exercises Exercises that link strength and speed of movement to produce an explosive-reactive type of muscle response.

plyometrics Exercises in which an eccentric contraction is followed immediately by a concentric contraction, greatly increasing the force generated. If a muscle is stretched, much of the energy required to stretch it is lost as heat, but some of this energy can be stored by the elastic components of the muscle. To express this greater force, the muscle must contract within the shortest time possible. This whole process frequently is called the stretch shortening cycle.

poliomyelitis A disorder caused by a virus that attacks the motor neurons of the anterior horn cells of the spinal cord, resulting in varied symptoms ranging from minor muscle weakness to complete paralysis.

pollicization Surgically converting the index finger (usually) into a thumb.

polyneuropathy Bilateral damage to more than one peripheral nerve. Peripheral polyneuropathy may involve the feet and the hands.

positive ulnar variance A condition in which the ulna is longer than it should be compared with the radius.

postpolio syndrome The late effects of poliomyelitis. Diagnosis is based on a history of poliomyelitis and complaints of a random pattern of increased muscle weakness that does not follow a nerve root or peripheral nerve distribution.

postural tremors Rhythmic shaking that occurs when the muscles are tensed to hold an object or to stay in a given position.

prehension Combination of grasp (or pinch) and release.

premorbid Before injury.

primary healing Following fracture, the use of an internal rigid device that permits direct regrowth of bone across the fracture line allows the fracture to bypass the formation of callus and heal directly with bone tissue. The internal rigid stability offered by a plate and/or screws serves as a substitute external callus, providing the motionless environment required for bone healing.

procollagen Precursor of collagen.

pronator syndrome A condition caused by compression of the median nerve in the proximal forearm, characterized by diffuse pain in the medial forearm.

proper collateral ligament of the proximal interphalangeal joint The PIP joint collateral ligament has two components: the accessory collateral ligament and the proper collateral ligament. The fibers of the accessory collateral ligament insert more volarly on the volar plate. The fibers of the proper collateral ligament insert more volarly and distally on the middle phalanx lateral tubercles.

proprioception The awareness of joint position in space.

proprioceptive neuromuscular facilitation A therapeutic technique that helps initiate a proprioceptive response in entire body or specific muscle groups.

proteoglycans Molecules that are fundamental components of connective tissue. They are composed of sugars linked to polypeptides and are found in the tissues and organs of the body.

proximal interphalangeal flexion contracture A condition in which the proximal interphalangeal joint of the finger is unable to be extended passively or actively.

proximal radioulnar joint The proximal articulation of the radial head and the proximal ulna.

proximal transverse arch The more proximal of the two bony transverse arches of the hand. These arches contribute to the normal resting posture (palmar concavity) of the hand and to normal hand function. The proximal transverse arch is located at the carpus, which has a deep palmar concavity created by the interlocking carpal bones.

pseudarthrosis A false joint that occurs at the site of a nonunion fracture if there is any shearing force present. Abnormal shearing force stimulates undifferentiated mesenchymal cells to produce cartilage at the fracture site.

pseudoboutonniere An injury to the proximal interphalangeal volar plate, usually the result of a proximal interphalangeal joint hyperextension injury. The pathologic condition occurs to the volar surface.

psychogenic tremors A somatization disorder that appears unintentionally and without conscious client awareness of motivation, with shaking of the limbs or body that can appear exaggerated, often improving when the client is distracted.

psychometric properties Attributes of a questionnaire that determine whether it is meaningful and effective for the target population.

pulsatile Having a pulse, as do some vascular tumors.

pump point stimulation A term coined for and unique to MEM (manual edema mobilization), which describes a simultaneous synchronous light massage in two areas of a combination of lymph nodes, lymphatic bundles, and watershed areas.

purulence A viscous, yellowish-white pus that indicates infection.

purulent flexor tenosynovitis Another term for *pyogenic flexor tenosynovitis*.

pyogenic flexor tenosynovitis A term meaning flexor sheath infection.

pyogenic granuloma A lesion that presents as a red mass that bleeds easily. Because it has abundant capillary granulation, it is categorized as a vascular tumor. This lesion is believed to occur after trauma when there also has been an infection.

quadriga effect The effect that occurs when one finger is unable actively to flex that results in the inability of adjacent fingers to flex, especially the distal interphalangeal joints, because of the shared flexor digi-

torum profundus muscle belly. When one flexor digitorum profundus tendon is held out at length by stiffness, adhesions, or splinting, it does not allow the flexor digitorum profundus tendons on either side to be pulled mechanically in a proximal direction by the muscle.

quadriplegia Paralysis of four extremities.

qualitative Information that is subjective and often consists of client narratives. Examples include symptoms, abilities, and participation in daily activities.

quantitative Aspects of evaluation and treatment including those variables that are measured in a standardized fashion and result in numeric data; may be referred to as objective, performance-based, or anatomic. Examples include goniometric measurement, manual muscle testing, and sensory evaluations.

radial club hand So called because it looks like the club of a golfer. Radial club hand is radially deviated like a golfer's club. See *longitudinal radial ray deficiency*.

radial tunnel syndrome A condition caused by compression of the radial nerve in the proximal forearm and characterized by dull aching or burning pain along the lateral forearm.

radiocapitellar joint The lateral articulation of the elbow joint. This is where the head of the radius articulates with the capitellum of the distal humerus.

radiocarpal joint The articulation between the distal radius and the scaphoid and lunate.

reduction Anatomic restoration of bone integrity following bone fracture.

referred pain Pain that is coming from an area other than where it presents.

reflex disturbance Abnormal action of the cell, tissue organ, or organism caused by overstimulation or understimulation.

regional measures Client self-report outcome measures that are designed to demonstrate change at the systems level.

reliability The degree of consistency with which an instrument or rater measures a variable.

remodeling phase The final phase of bone healing following fracture. Repaired bone tissue is replaced and reorganized over months to years to provide the bone with its preinjury strength and structure. Otherwise known as the *maturation phase*.

repair phase The second phase of bone healing following fracture. During this phase, the damaged cells (including the hematoma) are removed and replaced with callus bone.

replant Following amputation, the surgical procedure of reattaching a finger, hand, or arm to the body to reestablish viability and function.

resistance maximal   Maximum resistance that a group of muscles can overcome once (1 RM).

responsiveness   The ability of a test to demonstrate change. It often is referred to as sensitivity to (clinical) change and is established if change in scores accurately represents change in clinical status.

resting tremor   An involuntary movement that tends to abate with functional or intentional hand use but is more present at rest.

revascularization   Surgical procedure to repair severed arteries or veins, restoring blood supply to a limb.

reverse blocking exercises   Exercises that hold the metacarpophalangeal joint in flexion while the interphalangeal joints are extended actively to maximize the extension force to the interphalangeal joints.

rheumatoid arthritis   A systemic disease characterized by synovial inflammation.

rheumatoid nodules   These nodules are made up of granulomatous and fibrous tissue and are seen in 50% of all clients with rheumatoid arthritis. They are often largest at the elbow joint.

rigidity   Stiffness in the limbs or body caused by dysfunction of the basal ganglia and related structures resulting in an increased resistance to the passive movement of a limb.

Roos Test   See *Elevated Arm Stress Test.*

rotator interval   The region between the superior edge of the subscapularis and anterior edge of the supraspinatus tendons.

rubor   A term meaning redness.

rupture of the brachial plexus   Pulling away of nerves due to forceful lateral deviation of the neck as the infant is delivered through a narrow pelvic passage (or as the rider falls from a motor bike).

safe position   Wrist in slight extension, the metacarpophalangeal joints in flexion, and the interphalangeal joints in extension. Also known as the *intrinsic-plus position.*

SAM protocol   Short arc motion protocol; a protocol designed by Evans that allows a small, controlled amount of active motion of the repaired tendon to achieve 3 to 5 mm of tendon gliding.

sarcomas   Cancers arising from muscle, vessels, fat, and fibrous tissue. They are considered rare in the forearm or hand. Sarcomas are categorized by their cell origin, such as fibrosarcoma or synovial sarcoma, and they can metastasize.

scaption   Elevation of the arm in the plane of the scapula.

scapular kinematics   Scapular movement in sequence and proportion to humeral movement.

Schwann cell   A glial cell found only in the peripheral nervous system that provides the myelin that envelops the axon of the nerve.

schwannoma   Benign nerve tumor. Also known as a *neurilemoma.*

secondary healing   The ordered process of bone tissue repair and reorganization orchestrated by a cascade of signaling factors. It involves an intermediate phase in which connective tissue or callus is formed first and then is replaced by bone. Also known as callus healing, indirect healing, or *enchondral ossification.*

second intention   The process of healing an open wound that is not surgically repaired, whereby it closes itself over time.

sensitivity   Few if any clients with the disease have negative test results; a statistical term used to determine validity of diagnostic tests.

serial static splints   Splints that position the tissue for lengthening. They are remolded periodically.

shaft   The diaphysis of the bone.

SHAFT syndrome   The client seeks multiple surgeries in a type of "passive mutilation" performed by well-meaning medical professionals. The acronym stands for sad, hostile, anxious, frustrating, and tenacious.

shoulder-hand syndrome   Pain of the entire upper extremity and shoulder referring into the cervical area.

simple tasks   Compared to complex tasks, refers to repetitive movements (e.g., turning pages).

skier's thumb   Injury to the ulnar collateral ligament of the thumb metacarpophalangeal joint. This is a modern version of gamekeeper's thumb.

sliding filament theory   The cross-bridges on the myosin filament attach to the active site on the actin filament. When all of the cross-bridges in a muscle shorten in a single cycle, the muscle shortens by approximately 1%. Muscles have the capacity to shorten up to 60% of their resting length; therefore the contraction cycle must be repeated multiple times.

Smith's fracture   A complete fracture of the distal radius with palmar displacement of the distal fragment. It is the second most commonly seen distal radius fracture, and it is frequently unstable.

soft end-feel   Quality of a spongy feel at passive joint end-range. This is favorable for potential to improve.

soma   The nerve cell body; the metabolic center of the cell.

somatic blocks   Regional local anesthetic infusion that blocks somatic sensory nerves and causes paralysis. Total paralysis is affected by the amount of anesthetic.

somatization disorders   Persistent or recurrent symptoms with no measurable or objective medical evidence of impairment.

spasticity   An involuntary increase in muscle tone in which abnormal stretch reflexes intensify muscle resistance to passive movements.

specificity All persons who do not have the disease have negative test results; a statistical term used to determine validity of diagnostic tests.

sphygmometer An instrument for measuring grip strength consisting of a soft pressure gauge bulb that the client squeezes.

spinal cord stimulation Procedure during which an electrode is positioned in the epidural space on the spinal cord at the level of the nerve innervating the painful area; electric current is introduced through an implanted battery and helps to suppress pain. Usually a testing period is provided before the permanent implant is inserted.

spinal nerve A peripheral nerve formed from the sensory and motor nerve roots of a spinal segment that join together just as the nerve fibers leave the intervertebral foramen of the spinal column.

spiritual The way in which persons understand their lives in view of their ultimate meaning and value was the definition of spirituality proposed by McLain, Rosenfeld, and Breitbart.

Spurling's Test A special test used to detect the presence of nerve root disease.

squamous cell carcinoma A malignant epithelial tumor.

Starling's equilibrium/balance A balanced movement of fluid out of the arteriole, into the interstitium, and back into the venule or lymphatic vessel functioning on a gradient system from high to low pressure.

static progressive or dynamic Types of splints. See *static progressive splints* and *dynamic splints.*

static progressive splints Splints that apply mobilizing force using nonmoving parts such as monofilament, Velcro, or screws.

static splints Splints used to immobilize tissues, prevent deformity, prevent contracture of soft tissue, and provide substitution for motor function.

steady state respiratory rate When the level of intensity of exercise enables one to sustain equilibrium of the respiratory system that can be maintained over time.

stellate block See *sympathetic blocks.*

Stener's lesion Proximal displacement of the ulnar collateral ligament with interposition of the adductor aponeurosis. This injury requires surgical correction because the interposition prevents healing of the ligament.

subcutaneous ulnar nerve transposition A surgical procedure by which the ulnar nerve is transferred anteriorly and is positioned below the subcutaneous fascia of the anterior forearm, medial to the median nerve.

subepidermal abscesses Infections caused by *Staphylococcus aureus.* They occur on the volar digital pads between flexor creases or in the palm of the hand. If not treated, these infections can become more serious, with involvement of the flexor sheath or deep compartment in the palm.

subluxation A partial dislocation of a joint in which the bones become out of alignment, but the joint itself is still intact. In the situation of a cerebral vascular accident, it is often a term used when the humeral head moves part way out of the shoulder socket.

submuscular ulnar nerve transposition A surgical procedure that involves moving the ulnar nerve and placing it in a well-vascularized muscular bed in the volar forearm. It involves separating the flexor-pronator muscle origin and then reattaching it to its origin on the medial epicondyle.

subungual hematoma Hematoma beneath the nail that causes throbbing and pain.

sudomotor A term meaning sweating.

supraclavicular scalenectomy Surgical removal of the anterior scalene muscle.

supracondylar regions The proximal region of the condyles of the distal humerus.

suture anchor technique A procedure used to attach the distal biceps tendon to the radial tuberosity of the radius following distal biceps tendon ruptures.

swan neck deformity Finger posture with proximal interphalangeal joint hyperextension and distal interphalangeal joint flexion. The metacarpophalangeal joint tends to be flexed.

sweat testing Filter paper is sprayed with ninhydrine reactant 5 and is dried visually to depict sweat patterns compared bilaterally for anhidrosis or hyperhidrosis. Also known as the ninhydrine sweat test.

sympathetic blocks Procedure during which an anesthetic is injected into the volar cervical region and numbs the upper thoracic ganglia. They can be repeated if effective, often with increased analgesia.

sympathetic ganglion Ganglion that supplies most of the autonomic and visceral innervations to the ipsilateral arm.

sympathetically independent pain Symptoms that do not improve with a sympathetic block.

sympathetically maintained pain Pain that is maintained by the sympathetic efferent activity; confirmed when symptoms improve with a sympathetic nerve blockade.

synergistic movements Gross patterns of movement in flexion or extension that occur as a result of interruption in cortical control. All muscles involved are linked neurologically, and when one of these movements occurs, some or all of the other linked muscle groups activate simultaneously.

synovial Pertaining to the lubricating fluid of the joints.

synovial bursa The structure containing synovial fluid surrounding tendons as they cross under pulley systems. The synovial bursa allows smooth gliding of the tendons with less friction, and provides nutrition to the tendon.

synovial tissue Tissue that lines the joints, tendons, and bursae. The tissue produces lubricating fluid.

synovitis Inflammation of the synovial tissue.

systemic lupus erythematosus A systemic auto-immune disease characterized by diverse clinical symptoms caused by inflammation and blood vessel abnormalities.

tendinosis Another term for *angiofibroblastic hyperplasia* or *angiofibroblastic tendinosis*.

tendon gliding A series of exercises that promote flexor tendon glide through full range. The sequence includes fingers straight, metacarpophalangeal joint flexion, hook fist, and flat fist.

tendonitis Tendon injury with classical signs of heat, swelling, and pain. Involved structures are painful with resistance and with passive stretch.

Tennis Elbow Test Another term for *Cozen's Test*.

tenodesis In therapy, mobilization of one or more joints by using the tendinous connections that run past those joints and the relationship between flexors and extensors. Tenodesis is seen with the natural flexion of the fingers that occurs when the wrist is extended, and the natural extension of the fingers that occurs when the wrist is flexed.

tenodesis effect Reciprocal joint movement (flexion or extension of fingers) that occurs at a corresponding distal joint when a proximal joint is extended or flexed respectively (e.g., wrist flexion and finger extension or wrist extension and finger flexion).

tenosynovitis Inflammation of the synovial lining of the tendon sheath.

tensile strength The amount of force required to break a tendon. The tensile strength of a tendon gradually increases following injury and repair.

thermography Equipment that conducts body heat onto elastomesic sheets, causing the sheets to change colors.

thermoplastic splint A splint custom-made usually to increase motion and sometimes to assist motion; when static progressive, the motion is taken to the end-range and held with a static force; when dynamic, the motion is pulled to the end-range using a rubber-band type of force, but the client can release the tension by pulling away.

time-dependent sensitization Repeated stressful episodes make an individual increasingly sensitive to low-level environmental stimuli.

Tinel's sign A temporary tingling or paresthesia experienced with percussion over an injured and/or healing nerve.

tonic muscles The primary dynamic joint stabilizers. Their nutrition comes primarily from delivery of oxygen. They are predominantly type I or slow-twitch muscles and are responsible for sustaining joint arthrokinematics over time.

transcolumn Term used to describe types of distal humeral fractures. It refers to the fracture line crossing both supracondylar regions of the distal humerus.

transpersonal caring relationship The type of relationship that connotes the sharing of authentic self between individuals and within groups in a reflective frame. It conveys a concern for the inner world of another. All parties are changed within the relationship.

transpersonal self Being able to know one's source of strength and meaning and being able and willing to tap into that strength while never assuming the client shares in these values. This approach requires that the therapist be able to sustain healthy personal boundaries and put aside personal concerns in order to care for the client.

transudate edema An edema found in early stages of inflammation or tissue insult when high capillary permeability of vessels has not occurred. It consists mainly of dissolved electrolytes and water molecules.

transverse retinacular ligament Ligament that arises from the lateral band volar surface, envelops the collateral ligaments, and inserts into flexor tendon sheath at the proximal interphalangeal joint, thereby preventing lateral band dorsal displacement.

triangulofibrocartilage ligament A hammocklike structure composed of cartilage and ligaments. It suspends the ulna carpus and acts as a force distributor between the ulnar head and triquetrum and a primary stabilizer for the distal radioulnar joint.

trigger point Palpable taut muscle bands that refer pain when compressed.

triggering Limited digital range of motion caused by dragging of the flexor tendon as it passes through a pulley. The tendon may click or lock during range of motion.

trochlea The medial aspect of the distal humerus. The trochlea articulates with the proximal ulna.

trochoginglymoid joint Joint possessing two degrees of freedom in motion: at the elbow, flexion/extension and supination/pronation.

trophic The characteristics of the skin, including the thickness, moisture, and sheen.

trophic changes Changes in tissue characterized by abnormal hair growth, nail bed changes, cold intolerance, and soft tissue atrophy (most notably at the finger tip pulps).

tropocollagen The basic molecular unit of collagen fibrils composed of three polypeptide chains.

tuft The distal end of the terminal phalanx of the digit.

tumor A term meaning swelling.

two-incision technique This procedure uses an anterior and dorsal incision for biceps tendon repair. A hole is drilled into the tuberosity, and the tendon is pulled through with sutures that are attached to the radial tuberosity with the forearm in neutral.

type III deformity Categorized by Nalebuff, the thumb deformity includes metacarpal adduction, metacarpophalangeal joint hyperextension, and thumb interphalangeal joint flexion. The carpometacarpal joint slides out of its place on the trapezium during pinch activities.

ulnar nerve Nerve arising from the medial cord of the brachial plexus and innervating the majority of the intrinsic muscles of the hand, as well as providing cutaneous sensation to the medial border of the hand and to the fifth and medial half of the fourth digits.

ulnar tunnel syndrome Compression of the ulnar nerve at the wrist within Guyon's canal. Also known as entrapment at Guyon's canal.

ulnocarpal abutment syndrome A syndrome that can develop when the ulna is longer in comparison to the radius and it impinges on the triangulofibrocartilage ligament and ulnar carpus during wrist and forearm motion.

ulnotrochlear joint The medial articulation of the elbow joint where the trochlea articulates with the ulna.

uncinate processes Winglike projections from the superior portion of the cervical vertebra that articulate with the inferior portion of the vertebra above.

uniaxial pivot joint A type of synovial joint that allows 1 degree of motion. An example is the distal radioulnar joint that allows rotatory motion called supination and pronation.

unifocal Referring to fractures consisting of one fracture line.

unstable fractures Fractures that displace spontaneously or with motion.

valgus The presentation of the elbow as the hand deviates away from the body when the upper extremity is observed in anatomic position.

validity The degree to which an instrument measures what it is intended to measure.

varus The presentation of the elbow as the hand deviates toward the body when the upper extremity is observed in anatomic position.

vascular tumor A tumor, usually congenital, that arises when differentiation fails to occur embryonically, resulting in a *hemangioma, lymphangioma,* or congenital arteriovenous fistula.

venule The smallest venous structure; blood passes from the capillaries into the venules and into larger veins.

verruca vulgaris Common wart. They are benign and are caused by the human papillomavirus.

visual analog scale A continuum scale based on responses between two extreme opposites.

visual neglect Clients' inability to perceive entire regions of space contralateral to their brain lesions.

volar plate A fibrocartilaginous structure situated between the collateral ligaments on the volar aspect of the proximal interphalangeal joint.

volar retinacular ganglion The third most common ganglion cyst. This ganglion arises from the A-1 pulley of the flexor tendon sheath of a digit. The volar retinacular ganglion is small, measuring about 3 to 8 mm. It is a tender, firm, palpable mass under the metacarpophalangeal joint flexion crease. It is proximal to the digital nerve.

volar wrist ganglion The second most common ganglion of the hand and wrist. This ganglion can be found at surgery to be much more extensive than originally anticipated. The volar wrist ganglion occurs over the scaphoid tubercle, arising from the scaphotrapezial joint, or over the distal edge of the radius, arising from the radiocarpal joint. Branches of the radial artery may be interwined with the cyst.

Volkmann's angle The digits are held extended with the wrist flexed. Then the wrist is extended with the fingers extended. The angle of wrist flexion so obtained is Volkmann's angle, representing limited wrist extension to less than neutral when the digits are extended.

Volkmann's Passive Muscle Stretch Test See *Volkmann's angle.*

Waddell signs Signs of simulated or exaggerated deficits including extreme reaction to light touch, tenderness that does not conform to established myotomal or segmental patterns, and sensory disturbances that do not conform to established dermatomal or segmental patterns.

Wartenberg's sign An indicator of an ulnar nerve lesion. The fifth digit is postured in abduction, and adduction to the fourth is weak or not possible. Wrist drop deformity is the classic deformity associated with a high radial nerve lesion. When the forearm is pronated, the wrist and digits are unable to extend actively.

watershed areas Drainage areas within the lymphotome that slightly direct the lymph in to a different area. They are not actual structures. An analogy would be the way water flows on either side of a continental divide.

Watson's Test For specifics on this maneuver, which is used to help identify a scapholunate ligament tear or instability, see Terri Skirven's article "Clinical Examination of the Wrist" (*J Hand Ther* 9[2]:96-107, 1996). Also known as the Scaphoid Shift Test.

windblown hand Congenital clasped thumb in association with ulnar deviation of the fingers at the MCP joints.

work of flexion The amount of tension created within the tendon during active flexion. Work of flexion increases with swelling, stiffness, or any internal friction encountered by the tendon because of bulk of repair, tight pulleys, or swelling of the tendons, in addition to the tension normally developed during active flexion.

wrist The multiple articulations that exist between the distal radius, ulna, and eight carpal bones.

xanthoma Another term for *giant cell tumor.*

Index

Page numbers followed by f indicate figures; t,
tables; b, boxes.